The Practice of
Hand Surgery

The Practice of
Hand Surgery

Edited by

D. W. LAMB
MB CHB FRCSE
Senior Lecturer
Department of Orthopaedic Surgery
University of Edinburgh
Consultant Orthopaedic Surgeon
Royal Infirmary, and
Princess Margaret Rose Hospital
Edinburgh

and

K. KUCZYNSKI
MB CHB FRCSE
Senior Lecturer
Department of Anatomy
University of Edinburgh

BLACKWELL SCIENTIFIC PUBLICATIONS
OXFORD LONDON EDINBURGH
BOSTON MELBOURNE

© 1981 by
Blackwell Scientific Publications
Editorial offices:
Osney Mead, Oxford, OX2 0EL
8 John Street, London, WC1N 2ES
9 Forrest Road, Edinburgh, EH1 2QH
52 Beacon Street, Boston
    Massachusetts 02108, USA
214 Berkeley Street, Carlton
    Victoria 3053, Australia

First published 1981

Printed in Great Britain by
Morrison & Gibb Ltd, Edinburgh

DISTRIBUTORS

USA
    Blackwell Mosby Book Distributors
    11830 Westline Industrial Drive
    St Louis, Missouri 63141

Canada
    Blackwell Mosby Book Distributors
    120 Melford Drive, Scarborough
    Ontario, M1B 2X4

Australia
    Blackwell Scientific Book Distributors
    214 Berkeley Street, Carlton
    Victoria 3053

British Library
Cataloguing in Publication Data

The Practice of hand surgery.
    1. Hand – Surgery
    I. Lamb, Douglas W.   II. Kuczynski, Kazimierz
    617′.575   RD559

    ISBN 0-632-00295-6

Contents

INJURIES

Contributors

R. C. B. AITKEN, MD, FRCPE, FRCPSYCH, *Professor of Rehabilitation Studies, University of Edinburgh, Edinburgh, Scotland.*

J. N. BARRON, MS, FRCS, FRCSE, *former Director, Regional Plastic & Maxillo-Facial Centre, Odstock Hospital, Salisbury, England. Past President, British Association of Plastic Surgeons, Past President, British Society for Surgery of the Hand.*

J. A. BOSWICK, Jr., MD, *Professor of Surgery and Chief of Hand Service, University of Colorado, Denver, Colorado, U.S.A.*

A. C. BUCHAN, FRCSE, FDS, RCSE, *formerly Consultant Plastic Surgeon, Bangour General Hospital, Broxburn, West Lothian, Scotland. Past President, British Association of Plastic Surgeons, and Past President, British Society for Surgery of the Hand.*

J. CHALMERS, MD, FRCS, FRCSE, *Consultant Orthopaedic Surgeon, Royal Infirmary, Edinburgh, Scotland.*

T. M. CHALMERS, MB, CHB, FRCPE, *Consultant Rheumatologist, Northern General Hospital, Edinburgh, Scotland.*

J. R. COBBETT, MB, BCHIR, FRCS, *Consultant Plastic Surgeon, Queen Victoria Hospital, East Grinstead, England.*

R. M. CURTIS, MD, *Chief of the Division of Hand Surgery, Union Memorial Hospital, Associate Professor of Plastic and Orthopaedic Surgery, The Johns Hopkins University, Baltimore, Maryland, U.S.A. Past President, American Society for Surgery of the Hand.*

R. A. DICKSON, MA, CHM, FRCS, *Clinical Reader, Nuffield Orthopaedic Centre, Oxford, England.*

J. H. DOBYNS, MD, *Associate Professor of Orthopaedic Surgery, Mayo Medical School, Mayo Clinic, Rochester, Minnesota, U.S.A.*

MARGARET ELLIS, MBAOT, SROT, *District Occupational Therapist, The London Hospital, London, England.*

E. B. FRENCH, MB, BCHIR, FRCP, FRCPE, *formerly Reader, Department of Medicine, University of Edinburgh, Edinburgh, Scotland.*

G. E. FULFORD, MB, BS, FRCS, *Consultant Orthopaedic Surgeon, Princess Margaret Rose Orthopaedic Hospital, Edinburgh, Scotland.*

D. GARLAND, MD, *Chief, Head Trauma Service, Rancho Los Amigos Hospital, Downey, California, U.S.A.*

B. H. HELAL, MCH ORTH, FRCS, FRCSE, *Consultant Orthopaedic Surgeon, The London Hospital, London, England.*

A. W. B. HEYWOOD, MCH ORTH, FRCS, *Orthopaedic Surgeon, Princess Alice Orthopaedic Hospital, Cape Town, South Africa. President Elect, South African Orthopaedic Association.*

J. I. P. JAMES, MS, FRCS, FRCSE, FRACS, *Emeritus Professor of Orthopaedic Surgery, University of Edinburgh, Edinburgh, Scotland. Past President, British Orthopaedic Association, and Past President, British Society for Surgery of the Hand.*

H. E. KLEINERT, MD, *Clinical Professor of Surgery, University of Louisville School of Medicine, Louisville, Kentucky, U.S.A. Past President, American Society for Surgery of the Hand.*

K. KUCZYNSKI, MB, CHB, FRCSE, *Senior Lecturer, Department of Anatomy, University of Edinburgh, Edinburgh, Scotland.*

D. W. LAMB, MB, CHB, FRCSE, *Consultant Orthopaedic Surgeon, Royal Infirmary, Edinburgh, Scotland. Past President, British Society for Surgery of the Hand.*

R. L. LINSCHEID, MD, *Associate Professor of Orthopaedic Surgery, Mayo Medical School, Mayo Clinic, Rochester, Minnesota, U.S.A.*

G. D. LISTER, MD, FRCS, *Professor of Hand Surgery, University of Louisville, Kentucky, U.S.A.*

C. LONG, MD, *Associate Professor of Physical Medicine and Rehabilitation, Co-Director, Department of Physical Medicine and Rehabilitation, Cuyahoga County Hospital, Cleveland, Ohio, U.S.A.*

W. M. McQUILLAN, MB, CHB, FRCSE, *Consultant Orthopaedic Surgeon, Royal Infirmary, Edinburgh, Scotland.*

L. W. MILFORD, MD, *Clinical Professor of Orthopaedics, University of Tennessee, Center for the Health Sciences, Memphis, Tennessee, U.S.A. Past President, American Society for Surgery of the Hand.*

L. H. MILLENDER, MS, *Assistant Chief Hand Service, Robert B. Brigham Hospital, Massachusetts, U.S.A.*

E. A. NALEBUFF, MD, *Associate Professor of Orthopaedic Surgery, Harvard Medical School, Boston, Massachusetts, U.S.A.*

F. V. NICOLLE, MCHIR, FRCS, *Consultant Plastic Surgeon, Hammersmith Hospital, London, England.*

V. L. NICKEL, MD, *Director of Rehabilitation, Sharp Rehabilitation Center, and Professor of Surgery/Orthopaedics and Rehabilitation, University of California, San Diego, California, U.S.A.*

H. MARY PEARCE, DIPCOT, CERTED. *Formerly Head Occupational Therapist, Western General Hospital, Edinburgh, Scotland.*

A. G. POLLEN, MB, BS, FRCS, *Consultant Orthopaedic and Traumatic Surgeon, Bedford General Hospital, Bedford, England.*

A. H. C. RATLIFF, CHM, FRCS, *Consultant Orthopaedic Surgeon, Bristol Royal Infirmary, Bristol, England. President, British Orthopaedic Association.*

J. C. SEMPLE, MB, CHB, FRCSG, FRCSE, *Consultant Hand Surgeon, Western Infirmary, Glasgow, Scotland.*

M. ELIZABETH SHELSWELL, MB, CHB, FRCS, *Consultant Orthopaedic Surgeon, Portsmouth District Hospitals, Portsmouth, England.*

D. C. SIMPSON, MBE, BSC, PHD, FISPO, FRSE, *Emeritus Professor of Orthopaedic Bioengineering, University of Edinburgh, Edinburgh, Scotland.*

R. J. SMITH, MD, *Clinical Professor of Orthopaedic Surgery, Harvard Medical School, Chief of Hand Surgery, Department of Orthopaedic Surgery, Massachusetts General Hospital, Boston, Massachusetts, U.S.A.*

W. A. SOUTER, MB, CHB, FRCSE, *Consultant Orthopaedic Surgeon, Princess Margaret Rose Orthopaedic Hospital, Edinburgh, Scotland.*

A. B. SWANSON, MD, FACS, *Professor of Surgery, Michigan State University, Director of Orthopaedic Training, Grand Rapids, Michigan, U.S.A. Past President, American Society for Surgery of the Hand, Secretary General of the International Federation of Hand Surgeons.*

K. TSUGE, MD, *Professor of Orthopaedic Surgery, Hiroshima University School of Medicine, Hiroshima, Japan.*

R. L. WATERS, MD, *Chairman, Department of Surgery, Rancho Los Amigos Hospital, Downey, California, U.S.A.*

PATRICIA M. WILSON, MCSP, *Senior Physiotherapist, Western General Hospital, Edinburgh.*

T. W. WOLFF, MD, *Clinical Assistant Professor of Orthopaedic Surgery, University of Louisville School of Medicine, Louisville, Kentucky, U.S.A. Former Christine Kleinert Fellow in Hand Surgery.*

RUTH WYNNE-DAVIES, PHD, MB, FRCS, *Reader in Clinical Genetics Research, Department of Orthopaedic Surgery, University of Edinburgh, Edinburgh, Scotland.*

Foreword

That function follows form must be the belief of a hand surgeon. When he corrects the deformities of the skeleton, repairs vessels to nourish the tissue, connects tendons and nerves to give a sensibility and motion to the parts, and restores the covering skin he is practising this belief. To do so he must have some conception of the anatomical relationship of the parts, how they fit together and how they function independently and in co-operation as parts of an organ, the hand. He must know the normal, not only the static anatomy of the lifeless cadaver, but also the dynamic anatomy of the living hand. When manipulating each part to restore it to its normal state, he must visualize it as it should be, not as it was in the dissecting room, but as it will function in the individual.

The complaint that surgeons are lacking in a knowledge of anatomy is a recurrent theme in history. In the 14th century Guy de Chauliac said, 'A surgeon ignorant of anatomy carves the body as a blind man carves wood'. Yet four centuries later, in spite of the influence of Vesalius, the same complaint was heard. Charles Bell, in his effort to unite anatomy and surgery, said: 'I propose to found a system of surgery, founded on anatomy . . . as I everyday see reason to believe that the neglect of surgical anatomy is still a common defect of education.'

Now that interest in surgery of the hand has become world wide and many highly technical procedures have been described, it is fitting that another attempt be made to unite anatomy and surgery. For surgery of the hand requires the utmost skill and, if not based on a thorough knowledge of surgical anatomy, will result in permanent impairment of function of this most important organ.

That this effort should come from Edinburgh and that the study concerns the hand is most appropriate for it follows in the great tradition of the anatomists and surgeons of that city, the birthplace of Charles Bell. His study of comparative anatomy in *The Hand, its Vital Mechanism and Endowment, as Evincing Design,* will always be one of the classics of our speciality.

Professors Lamb and Kuczynski have emphasized the importance of a knowledge of anatomy by combining this material with a discussion of the principles of surgical treatment. Such a contribution requires the combined efforts of a functional anatomist and an experienced surgeon. The principles outlined here should make it possible for young surgeons to provide the care necessary to preserve all possible function in the hand.

Now, over 150 years since Bell decried the neglect of surgical anatomy in the training of surgeons, this work, *The Practice of Hand Surgery,* by its detailed descriptions of the surgical anatomy and the clear delineation of the basic principles of care should put to rest that complaint. At least, it will not be said of hand surgeons, if they use this book as the authors planned it.

Joseph H. Boyes,
MD, FACS, FRCSE, FRACS

Preface

This book originated in response to requests from those attending the instructional course in hand surgery which has taken place annually in Edinburgh over the past twenty years. Following our practice of inviting eminent guest lecturers, we have asked many world authorities to provide us with their unrivalled knowledge and expertise, and we are very grateful to them for their generous and unhesitating co-operation.

The book is primarily intended for surgeons in training, for those staffing casualty and accident departments, and for surgeons in isolated and developing communities who have to deal with trauma of the hand and who would benefit from an account of some of the reconstructive procedures. It is also aimed at the ancillary staff, the nurses, therapists and orthotists, who contribute so much to the quality of recovery from an operation or injury. The importance of team work is stressed throughout and emphasis is placed on a planned combined programme of physiotherapy and occupational therapy in rehabilitation of hand function after injury, disease or operation. No hand surgeon can work in isolation from colleagues in other fields, and chapters on the hand in medicine, the psychology of the deformed hand, medical aspects of rheumatoid disease, and medicolegal assessment are included. The hand cannot be considered in isolation either, and the book therefore contains chapters on the upper limb in stroke, cerebral palsy and spinal cord injury.

A prime object of the book has been to enable the reader to make a diagnosis and an intelligent choice of treatment. As this requires knowledge of normal structure and function and an understanding of their correlation in health and disease, functional anatomy of the hand, its kinesiology and basic evolution, and functional assessment have been considered and introductory basic notes to the chapters on cut tendons, nerves and congenital abnormalities given their place. This should be of particular help to the surgeon in training or preparing for examination. Special emphasis is placed on the practical side of hand surgery, and advice is given not only on methods of treatment but also on their rationale and timing and the technical steps in their application.

It is hoped that experienced surgeons will also find something of interest and benefit in the book. The inclusion of newer developments such as microsurgery of the vessels and nerves, revascularization and replantation, primary repair of flexor tendons and joint replacement should be of value to an experienced surgeon in training his associates and junior staff.

The editing of this book has been a challenge and taken most of our spare time during the past four years. It has been a stimulating experience and we hope will be found to have been worthwhile. We owe a special debt of gratitude to all the registrars with whose training we were concerned over the years, and from whom we have invariably learned much; also to the therapists whose loyal and unremitting work has resulted in much greater success than would otherwise have been achieved. Our special thanks go to Dr Joseph Boyes who very kindly agreed to write a foreword to this book, which we hope may approach, even in small degree, the high standard which he has established for textbooks of hand surgery. We also thank Mr Robert Boome, now returned to his native Cape Town, and Mr Jonathan Redden, at present training in New Zealand, for reading the proofs, Mrs Anne McNeill for many of the line drawings, and Mr M. Devlin for photographic assistance. We should also like to thank our publishers for every co-operation, and in particular Mr Nigel Palmer for his unfailing courtesy and help. Finally, without the forbearance, help and encouragement of our wives, the challenge would never have been accepted and our aims could not have been achieved.

1981

D. W. Lamb
K. Kuczynski

CHAPTER 1

General Anatomy

K. KUCZYNSKI

The upper limb is a mobile system of joints and levers for positioning the hand, a skilful organ capable of complicated tasks of exploration, gripping and manipulation, requiring a great precision, power and accuracy. The versatility of the hand was often regarded in the past as an expression of its primitive, unspecialized character but nowadays is thought to be a highly specialized organ adapted to an infinite variety of tools. Just as there is no 'textbook body' there is no 'textbook hand' either. There are considerable variations associated with many factors, some deviation from the usual arrangement resulting from anomalies of development which, however, do not reach the degree of the congenital deformity.

The hand consists of three parts: the carpus (anatomical wrist*), the hand proper (the dorsum and the palm) supported by the bones of the metacarpus, and five digits, the thumb and four fingers (index, long†, ring and little). The positions which the hand can assume may be considered as:

(1) *Position of rest* (Fig. 1.1), in which there is a moderate degree of dorsiflexion of the wrist with slight ulnar deviation. From index to little finger, there is gradual increase in the flexion of the metacarpophalangeal and interphalangeal joints, while the pulp of the thumb is near the radial aspect of the distal interphalangeal joint of the index.

(2) *Position of function*, which should really be

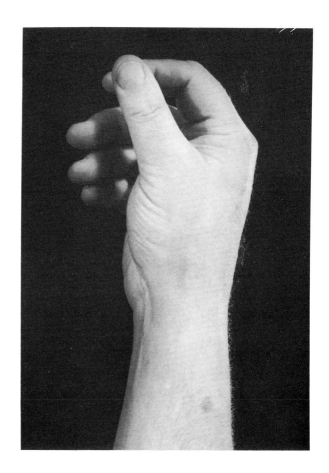

FIG. 1.1. Position of hand at rest. Note the difference from the recommended position of immobilization (Fig. 1.2).

---

* In ordinary speech the distal part of the forearm is called the wrist.
† 'Long' is preferred to 'middle' as the latter can be confused with 'little' during dictation and audiotyping.

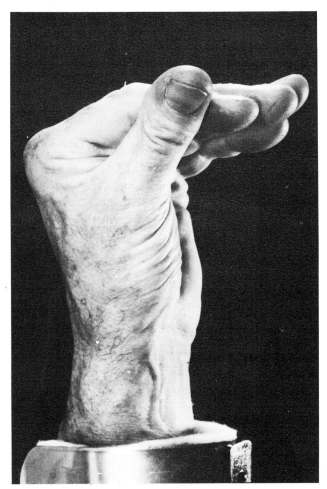

FIG. 1.2. Preferred position of immobilization.

'positions of functions', as there are obviously as many positions as there are varieties of function of the versatile hand.

(3) So-called *functional position of immobilization*, really a position of salvage and compromise, which is employed when the injury is so severe that in spite of treatment we anticipate unavoidable stiffness and therefore select as the future position resulting from this stiffness the one most useful to the individual. It can be compared to the position for arthrodesis.

(4) '*Safer*' *position of immobilization* (Fig. 1.2), which takes into account the fact that, in the metacarpophalangeal joints, the collateral ligaments are slack in extension and stretched in flexion because of the trans-

verse and sagittal cams of the metacarpal heads (see Fig. 1.30), while the collateral ligaments of the proximal interphalangeal joints remain stretched for most of the range of flexion.

From the position of rest the hand can move into an infinite number of optimal positions for any given action.

In general the hand should be regarded as an important *tactile* organ of exploration providing information about ourselves and the surrounding world. It is

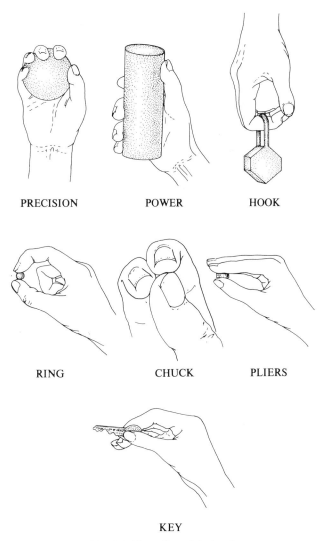

FIG. 1.3. Versatility of the hand.

also a *mobile* organ, its movements being either *non-prehensile* (as when occasionally used for locomotion, in climbing, swimming, or as a weapon, e.g. in karate) or falling into different varieties of the *prehensile movements*. These can be divided into: precision and power grips, hook, ring, chuck, pliers, key or lateral grips (Fig. 1.3). Combinations of these also occur (see p. 64). In most of the prehensile movements a well-opposable and appropriately long thumb in relation to the length of the fingers is of paramount importance.

To carry out its functions in a very finely graduated manner, the hand requires a proper skeletal assembly, motor balance and control, sensory feedback and well-developed higher functional levels of the brain which allow the individual to make a full use of the mechanism of the hand. As a matter of fact each type of tissue makes a special contribution to the functions of the hand.

extension shows proximal increase from the nail and is very marked on the dorsum of the hand. This area has also very considerable transverse mobility to accommodate the displacement due to the movements of the transverse metacarpal arch of the hand (p. 14). The dorsal skin is generously abundant over the back of the interphalangeal joints.

Palmar skin

The palmar skin is thick, unyielding and well fixed to the underlying tissues, particularly in the gripping areas. The keratin layer is thick, compact and laminated (Fig. 1.5). The central area of the palm is usually thickest although there are individual variations, occupation having an important effect.

SKIN

Dorsal skin

In the dorsal skin the keratin layer is thin and forms a loose, flexible covering (Fig. 1.4). The dorsal skin is elastic and mobile. Its mobility during flexion and

Papillary ridges and grooves

The papillary ridges (Fig. 1.6) are thought to have importance in gripping because of their frictional properties, but apparently this seems to be minimal [1]

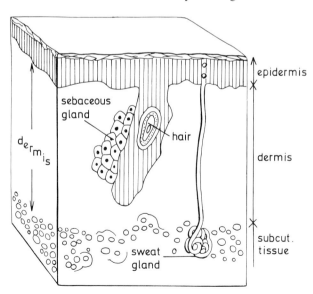

FIG. 1.4. Structure of the dorsal skin.

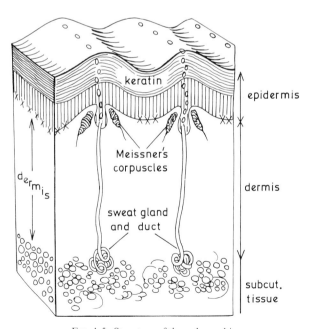

FIG. 1.5. Structure of the palmar skin.

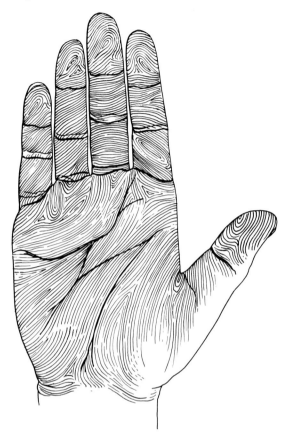

FIG. 1.6. Papillary ridges and grooves.

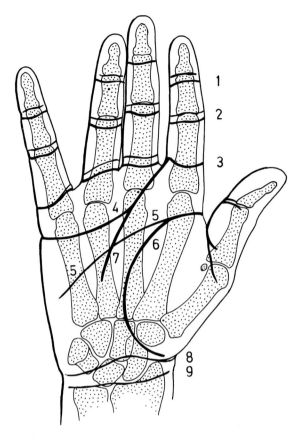

FIG. 1.7. Flexure lines (creases). 1–3, distal, middle and proximal digital creases; 4 and 5, distal and proximal transverse palmar creases; 6 and 7, radial and middle longitudinal palmar creases; and 8 and 9, distal and proximal wrist creases.

except in precision handling. Their importance in sensory feedback is related to the suggestion [2] that they act as mechanisms for transmission of sensory stimuli to the encapsulated and free nerve endings (Fig. 12.7). This mechanism is facilitated by the fact that the keratin of the ridges is softer than anywhere else and that the transmission area of the epidermis is not as well fixed to the dermis as it is opposite the grooves (marked as XXX in Fig. 1.5). The grooves between the papillary ridges contain sweat delivered through openings on the summit of the ridges. This sweat serves to moisten the palmar skin to provide a good gripping surface [3]. It is a well-known fact that in the absence of palmar sweat the hand does not hold well. The palmar sweat glands are not considered to be concerned to a great extent with temperature regulation but react rapidly to emotional stress.

Flexure lines (creases)

At the flexure lines or creases there is no fat in the superficial fascia and the dermis is more directly continuous with the deep fascia (Fig. 1.7 and 1.11). The skin can be folded about these 'skin joints' when movements take place at the articulations of the hand.

Tension (cleavage) lines

Some of the skin lines of the hand are much finer than the flexure creases. These lines, called tension or cleavage lines, are thought to be the result of the manner of arrangement of the collagen network of the dermis

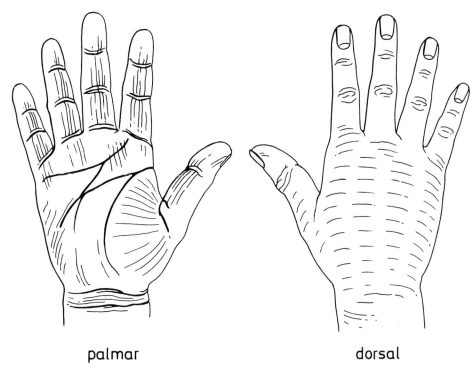

palmar   dorsal

FIG. 1.8. Tension (cleavage) lines. The heavy lines are flexure lines.

showing less extensibility in one direction than in the others. These lines were studied by many workers [4–9], but their significance in the hand is not clear. In other parts of the body their pattern changes with the body build, but in the hand it is variable even in the same type of body build. Generally speaking, they run longitudinally on the palmar aspect and transversely on the dorsal aspect of the hand (Fig. 1.8). On the palmar aspect of the thumb web they converge on the metacarpophalangeal flexure line of the thumb from the radial longitudinal palmar crease. They are absent from the distal pads of the digits and also from their sides. It is possible that the pattern of the tension lines on the gripping pads of the digits and on the web of the thumb is related to the power grip. The gripping pad in front of the phalanx (see Fig. 1.13) is limited anteriorly by the palmar skin with its longitudinal tension lines' pattern. The gripping pad contains an amount of fibrofatty tissue which has a considerable mobility and can be deformed and displaced during power grip (this anatomical arrangement is reflected in the design of the artificial

hand [1]). It seems probable that the displacement of the contents of the gripping pad towards the flexure creases is prevented by fusion of the dermis with the deep fascia at the crease; between the creases the dermal collagen fibres are oriented predominantly longitudinally as the tension lines suggest and, this being the direction of the least extensibility, the contents of the gripping pad are displaced sideways instead of bulging into the flexure creases and interfering with freedom of flexion at the joint. The same concept may be applied to the area of the web of the thumb which is subjected to pressure during power grip. On both sides of the digit the longitudinal tension lines give way to the transverse lines on the dorsum. This junction (Fig. 1.9) is useful in planning incisions particularly as the flexure creases can also be avoided.

Hairs

The palmar aspect is hairless, but hair is present on the dorsum of the hand, growing obliquely, pointing to

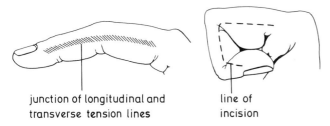

junction of longitudinal and   line of
transverse tension lines   incision

FIG. 1.9. Lateral aspect of a finger.

the ulnar side. The sebaceous glands waterproof the skin by their secretion and assist in its protection against the effects of the elements.

Nails

The nail consists mainly of a semitransparent keratin forming a curved plate surrounded at the sides by folds of skin called nail walls (Fig. 1.10). Nails arise from a modified epidermis called the nail bed. The underlying dermis is highly vascular and is firmly attached to the underlying periosteum of the distal phalanx. The nail bed extends proximally to overlap the attachment of the extensor tendon to the distal phalanx. In the region of the lunula the epidermis is thicker and the underlying dermis looser and less vascular. The lunula marks the

region of the nail bed concerned with formation and growth of the nail. Fingernails grow relatively quickly, the average time for replacement being about 6 months. The nails together with the distal phalanx and a band extending from the base of this phalanx to its ungual tuberosity provide support for the pulp of the digit and thus aid in gripping; they also form part of the tactile mechanism of the digit, as the dermal papillae of the nail bed are well supplied with sensory nerve endings.

SUPERFICIAL FASCIA

Dorsal aspect

On the dorsum the superficial fascia is thin and stretches easily (e.g. oedema, degloving). It is a double layer of scanty superficial fat and a deeper fibrous layer which is separated from the still deeper layers by loose areolar tissue. The superficial fascia enclosing digits and hand like a glove is more intimately adherent to the deeper structures along certain lines: the dorsal aspect of the fifth metacarpal, the dorsum of the first metacarpal and along the sides of the digits (for details see Landsmeer [10]).

Palmar aspect

On the palmar aspect the superficial fascia consists of fatty tissue enmeshed in a network of fibres which are fixed at one end to the skin and at the other to the deep fascia. It forms a sponge-like cushion. The amount and fixation of fatty tissue is variable, depending on the region. At the flexure creases it is absent (Fig. 1.11), over the thenar eminence it is minimal, but it is well

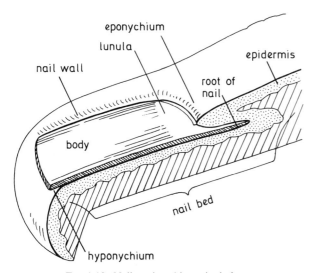

FIG. 1.10. Nail sectioned in sagittal plane.

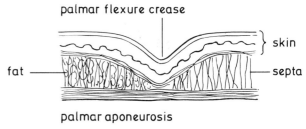

FIG. 1.11. Section of flexure crease.

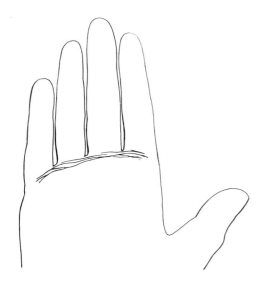

FIG. 1.12. Superficial transverse metacarpal ligament (natatory).

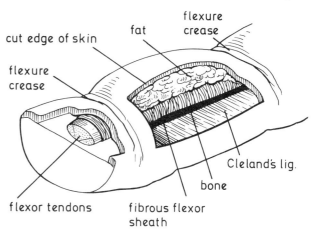

FIG. 1.13. Gripping pad of finger.

developed in gripping areas. The finger web spaces contain pads of fat. Over most of the palmar aponeurosis the fatty tissue is well stabilised in position as it is traversed by the anteroposterior fibres attached at both ends, one to the palmar aponeurosis and the other to the overlying skin (see Fig. 1.11). Fat is more prominent in the medial and distal part of the thenar region, over the metacarpophalangeal joints, in the webs and in the hypothenar area. These gripping pads surround the triangular central area of the palm which is almost free of fat. This arrangement allows the palm to be moulded to the object during power grip. At the level of the finger webs the superficial fascia exhibits transverse fibres which constitute the superficial ligament of the palm lying across the roots of the fingers and the webs between them (Fig. 1.12). In some individuals this ligament may continue for a variable distance in the distal part of the web of the thumb towards its metacarpophalangeal joint. Over the phalanges the palmar superficial fibrofatty tissue is organised into a gripping pad as well. Its walls are: anteriorly the palmar skin, posteriorly the fibrous flexor sheath, the bone and the Cleland's ligaments, while distally and proximally the pad is closed by the digital flexure creases (Fig. 1.13). As already mentioned the contents of this pad have a considerable mobility which can be shown by a normal pinch test; it is absent when the pad is under pressure, e.g. in rheumatoid

affection of the flexor tendon and its sheath. These gripping pads of the digits are very important in prehension as the objects can be imprinted into the pad, particularly during power grip, and securely lodged in their deformable contents which fit round the configuration of the held object. In the distal pulp of a digit the superficial fascia is organized into a compact fat partitioned by firm fibrous septa (Fig. 1.14). The deep fascia is attached to the skin at the distal digital flexure crease closing off the pulp space proximally. The pulp is supported dorsally by the distal phalanx, by the ligaments extending from the base of the phalanx to the ungual tuberosity and by the nail.

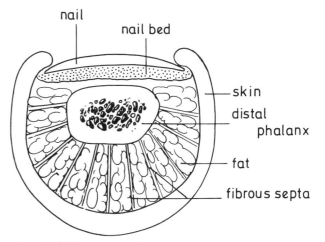

FIG. 1.14. Transverse section through pulp space of distal phalanx. Not all septa are shown as some run in other planes.

DEEP FASCIA

Dorsal aspect

The deep fascia on the dorsum of the hand is usually thought to be arranged in two layers, a superficial layer which covers the extensor tendons and is continuous with the extensor retinaculum, and a deeper layer which covers the interossei. Usually the deep fascia becomes very thin distally and tends to blend with the dorsal superficial fascia. Some authors [10, 11] distinguish the supra-, inter- and infra-tendinous layers of the deep dorsal fascia according to their position in relation to the extensor tendons on the dorsum of the hand (Fig. 1.15). These tendons and the interconnecting bands are embedded in the intertendinous fascia which blends distally with the proximal border of the extensor expansion hood (transverse lamina). In the webs of the fingers this layer often presents a free border marking the point where the dorsal digital vessels enter the superficial fascia (Fig. 1.16). The infratendinous fascia continues distally as far as the capsule of the metacarpophalangeal joint with which it blends and may be attached to the deep aspect of the transverse lamina. The supratendinous layer fuses with the superficial fascia near the distal part of the shafts of the metacarpals. The dorsal fascia covering the interossei may be present as a separate layer or fuse with the infratendinous fascia. Over the dorsum of the first intermetacarpal interval the supra- and infra-tendinous fasciae blend to form an investing layer for the first dorsal interosseus muscle. Over the margin of the thumb web this layer becomes continuous with the anterior interosseous fascia.

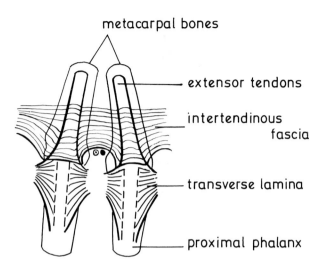

FIG. 1.16. Dorsal fascia at the finger web (modified from Landsmeer).

The deep connective tissue of the hand is also organized in a specific manner for *retention* and *gliding*. The bowstringing of the tendons is prevented in several ways and on the dorsal aspect this function is performed by the *extensor retinaculum*. It is attached laterally to the sharp border between the anterior and lateral surfaces of the distal radius and medially to the medial carpal bones, continuing as an extension round the distal end of the ulna to blend with the deep fascia on the

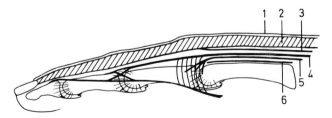

FIG. 1.15. Layers of deep dorsal fascia (modified from Landsmeer). 1, skin; 2, superficial fascia; 3, supratendinous fascia; 4, extensor tendon and intertendinous fascia; 5, infratendinous fascia; 6, interosseous fascia.

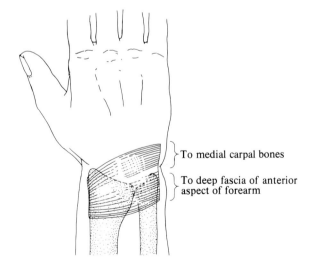

FIG. 1.17. Extensor retinaculum.

palmar aspect of the lower part of the forearm (Fig. 1.17). The septa which extend from retinaculum to the bony points lying deep to it form separate compartments for the tendons.

Palmar aspect

The deep fascia on the palmar aspect of the hand prevents the bowstringing of the tendons in several ways:

(1) The *flexor retinaculum* (transverse carpal ligament) is attached to the bones of the carpus (tubercle of scaphoid, crest of trapezium, pisiform and hook of hamate), so forming a *carpal tunnel* which contains nine long flexor tendons with their synovial sheaths and the median nerve (see Fig. 1.42). An additional attachment to the trapezium forms a tunnel which accommodates the tendon of the flexor carpi radialis and its sheath.

(2) *Palmar aponeurosis* with its ramifications, and

(3) *digital ligaments* are described in chapter 32, p. 472 and Fig. 32.4.

(4) *Fibrous flexor sheaths* (Fig. 1.18) of the fingers are

attached to the sides of the palmar surfaces of the proximal and middle phalanges and to the palmar surface of the distal phalanx. Opposite the metacarpophalangeal joint the sheaths have a rather anular arrangement and are attached to the edges of the volar plates and to the deep transverse ligaments of the palm. At the interphalangeal joints the sheaths are thin and composed of mostly oblique cruciate fibres, while opposite the phalanges they are thick and strong (anular pulleys) and prevent bowstringing of the tendons. These

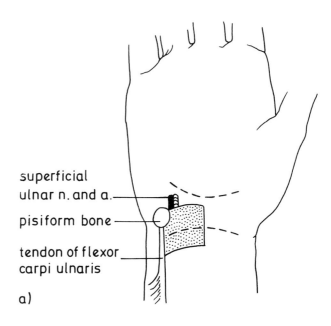

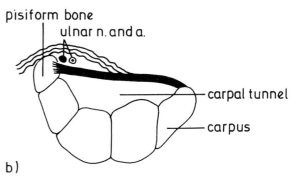

superficial
ulnar n. and a.

pisiform bone

tendon of flexor
carpi ulnaris

a)

pisiform bone
ulnar n. and a.

carpal tunnel

carpus

b)

FIG. 1.19. Guyon's tunnel. (a) anterior view with the extent indicated by stippled area, (b) cross-section.

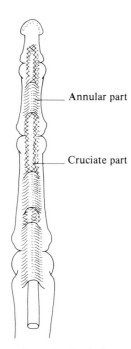

Annular part

Cruciate part

FIG. 1.18. Fibrous flexor sheath of a finger.

osteofibrous tunnels for the flexor tendons are closed distally but open proximally at the level of the metacarpal necks, deep to the palmar aponeurosis.

The thumb has its own fibrous sheath attached to the sides of the proximal phalanx and to the palmar surface of the distal phalanx. There are two anular and one oblique pulleys in the thumb [12]. The most proximal one is at the level of the metacarpophalangeal joint attached mostly to the volar plate of the joint, the second is the important oblique pulley extending from the ulnar side of the base of the proximal phalanx to the radial side of distal part of the shaft of the same phalanx. The third pulley, transverse in its orientation, is near the insertion of the tendon of the flexor pollicis longus.

(5) *Guyons tunnel* is bounded dorsally by the flexor retinaculum, medially by the pisiform bone and the distal part of the tendon of the flexor carpi ulnaris; anteriorly it is roofed by the superficial fibres of the deep fascia extending from the flexor retinaculum in the region of the tendon of the palmaris longus to the pisiform bone and fusing with the deep fascia just proximal to this bone (Fig. 1.19a). On cross-section (Fig. 1.19b) the tunnel is approximately triangular. It overlies the flexor retinaculum only over its proximal parts as its distal edge fuses with the more distal part of the retinaculum. Some of the fibres of the tunnel's roof lie proximally to the retinaculum. The superficial branch of the ulnar nerve leaves the tunnel by passing distally superficial to the fibrous arch of the origin of the hypothenar muscles which is attached to the hook of hamate and the pisiform. The deep branch leaves through the floor of the tunnel passing dorsally into a rather narrow space (deep palmar branch tunnel) between the pisohamate ligament and the above fibrous arch of origin of the hypothenar muscles (site of nerve compression, p. 407).

Gliding

The sliding movements of the tendon are facilitated by the loose connective tissue which forms a paratenon, when more or less straight line movement occurs (Fig. 1.20). Where a tendon slides round a corner or bend the paratenon is replaced by a synovial sheath formed by substitution of the middle areolar layer of paratenon for a space filled with a film of synovial fluid. The

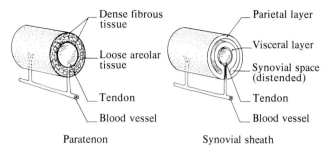

FIG. 1.20. Gliding mechanisms in the hand.

position of the synovial sheaths of the flexor and extensor tendons is described on pp. 25 and 26.

BONES

The *carpus* has a very complicated ligamentous and articular arrangement, only one carpal bone (trapezoid) articulating with a single metacarpal. The carpal groove is maintained by the palmar ligaments which are stronger than the dorsal ones and by the flexor retinaculum. The trapezium and the adjoining part of the scaphoid are turned palmarly carrying the first metacarpal and the thumb in front of the plane of the second and third metacarpal bones. The forward projection on the ulnar side is formed by the pisiform and the hook of the hamate.

The *metacarpus*, with exclusion of the first metacarpal, shows typical small basal facets for the neighbouring metacarpal bases. Again except for the first metacarpal, the dorsum of the shaft widens as it approaches the head. The heads are strong, large, rounded and asymmetrical with distinct tubercles and pits on their sides.

The *phalanges*: all proximal ones have an oval concave facet at the base, while the head is in form of a trochlea with two condyles separated by the intercondylar groove. All the middle phalanges have a double concave facet at the base separated by the intercondylar ridge; the heads are in form of a trochlea. All the distal ones have a double concave facet with the intercondylar ridge at the base while the head consists of a bony expansion forming the ungual tuberosity. The relative length of the phalanges is such that in full flexion the tips of fingers fit together across the plane of the palm. The phalanges of the thumb are like proximal and distal ones of the fingers.

The carpus

The carpal bones can be regarded as arranged around the capitate and are commonly divided into two rows, proximal and distal. More recently a concept of longitudinal chains was introduced: one chain consisting of the radius, lunate and capitate, while the second chain includes the radius, scaphoid and trapezoid with the trapezium [19]. The chains are linked to each other by the articulations and the interosseous ligaments. Not only movement between the elements of each chain is postulated, but also displacement of one chain on the other, e.g. between the scaphoid and lunate. This allows for adjustment of the bones of the carpus in different movements without compromising its stability (compare p. 221). The blood supply reaches the bones of the carpus along the ligaments. Fractures or dislocations which rupture these ligaments may interfere with its blood supply.

The scaphoid (Fig. 1.21a)

The scaphoid has a concave facet for the capitate and a crescentic one for the lunate; it is convex proximally for the radius and distally has a prominent tubercle which projects anteriorly. On the lateral aspect of the tubercle a large slightly convex surface faces the trapezoid and trapezium. Only a narrow strip of bone is non-articular and thus available for the entry of the blood vessels. A fracture in this region may interrupt

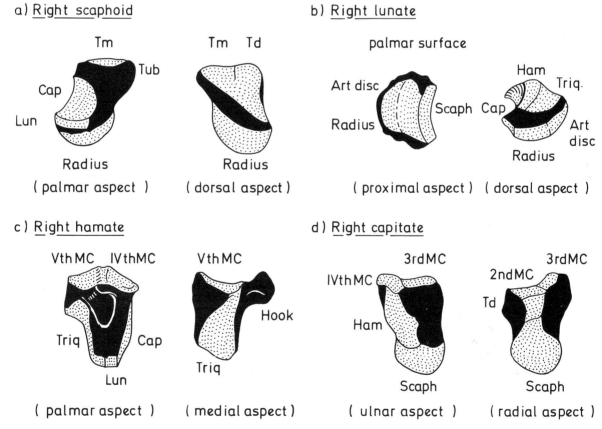

FIG. 1.21. Carpal bones. Tm, trapezium; Cap, capitate; S aph, scaphoid; Lun, lunate; Triq, triquetrum; Ham, hamate; Rad, radius; MC, metacarpal; Tub, tubercle. Articular surfaces are stippled and non-articular are black.

the blood supply to the bone; in a considerable proportion of individuals the blood vessels traverse the bone from the distal part to the proximal and in such cases the proximal fragment may be deprived of the blood supply and undergo an avascular necrosis.

The lunate (Fig. 1.21b)

The lunate has on its ulnar aspect a square facet for the triquetrum and a crescentic one for the scaphoid on its radial side. Distally it is deeply concave for the head of the capitate and convex proximally for the radius. The palmar surface, unlike the other carpal bones, is larger than the dorsal one.

The hamate (Fig. 1.21c)

This bone has a hamulus projecting from its palmar surface. The distal surface articulates with the fourth and fifth metacarpal bones, laterally with the capitate and proximo-medially with the triquetrum. The facets for the metacarpal bases are saddle-shaped, particularly that for the fifth metacarpal.

The capitate (Fig. 1.21d)

The capitate is the central and the largest bone. Its rounded head articulates with the lunate and scaphoid, while the sides articulate with the hamate and trapezoid. The palmar surface is rough for the attachment of the ligaments. The distal surface is set obliquely, the styloid of the third metacarpal fitting into the recessed radial part of this surface. Small facets articulate with the bases of the second and fourth metacarpal bones.

The triquetrum

The triquetrum fits into the angle between the lunate and hamate and thus articulates with both. On the distal part of its palmar surface there is a circular facet for the pisiform. The ulnar aspect is rough for the attachment of the ulnar collateral ligament of the wrist while its proximal part is smooth for articulation with the distal surface of the triangular disc in adduction.

The pisiform

This articulates with the preceding bone. The flexor carpi ulnaris tendon surrounds the bone and is continued distally as pisohamate and pisometacarpal ligaments.

The trapezoid

The trapezoid is a small, irregular bone which fits between the second metacarpal base, the capitate, scaphoid and trapezium.

The trapezium

The trapezium is described on p. 41.

The metacarpals

The first metacarpal is described on p. 41.

The remaining four metacarpal bones have many

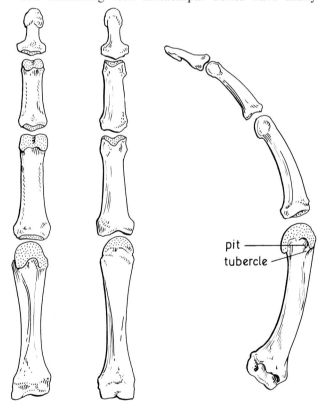

palmar ,   dorsal ,   lateral view of digital ray

Fig. 1.22. Bones of the digital ray.

features in common (Fig. 1.22). (1) The *head* projects palmarly from the plane of the shaft, and its articular surface extends further proximally on the palmar than on the dorsal aspect to allow for considerable flexion at the joint. The dorsal tubercles on the sides of the head and the hollow areas just palmar and distal to them give attachment to the collateral ligaments of the metacarpophalangeal joints. The transverse diameter of the heads is greater palmarly and thus influences the tension of the collateral ligaments in different positions of the joint (see Fig. 1.30, p. 18). The heads of the four medial metacarpal bones show considerable differences, particularly in the degree and nature of their asymmetry. The head of the index metacarpal is deviated in relation to the shaft towards the ulnar side, while those of the fourth and fifth metacarpals deviate towards the radial side. This fits well with the prehensile pattern. The presence in the head of a shoulder on one side together with the contralateral slope of the head (Fig. 1.23) is another expression of this asymmetry (see ulnar shoulder and radial slope in the second and third metacarpal heads, and radial shoulder and ulnar slope in the fifth metacarpal head). The tubercles and the pits on the metacarpal heads are also asymmetrical resulting in different degrees of obliquity of the collateral ligaments and thus determining the direction and range of the rotation at the metacarpophalangeal joints during opposition. All these features should be taken into account when inserting artificial joints. (2) The *shafts* are curved, being longitudinally concave towards the palm (Figs. 1.22 and 1.24a). The sides of the shafts provide area for attachment of the interosseous muscles, while the medial part of the anterior surface of the fifth and the lateral of the first are occupied by the opponens

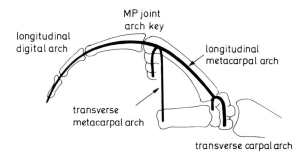

a) Arches of the hand

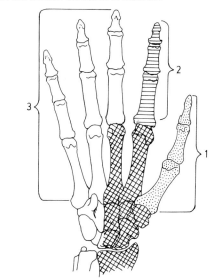

b) Fixed and mobile elements of the hand

FIG. 1.24. Assembly of the skeletal elements.

muscles. The palmar aspect of the third metacarpal is taken by the transverse head of the adductor pollicis. Nutrient foramina are on the radial aspect of the palmar surface of the shaft in the third, fourth and fifth metacarpals and on the ulnar aspect of the first and second metacarpals. (3) The *bases* articulate with the distal row of the carpus and with each other. There are considerable differences between the bases, the two medial ones, particularly the fifth showing flattened saddle-like facets which allow some degree of mobility of these metacarpals on the carpus (see mobile metacarpal arch, p. 14).

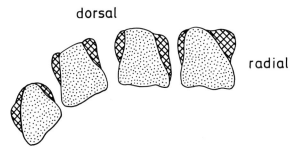

dorsal

radial

FIG. 1.23. End-on view of the metacarpal heads of right hand.

The phalanges

The phalanges of the thumb are described on page 41.

The *proximal phalanx* (Fig. 1.22) is slightly concave palmarly along its whole length (see arches, Fig. 1.24a). It is also slightly concave across the palmar aspect, but it is markedly convex from side to side across the dorsal surface. The longitudinal edges of the palmar aspect are raised for the attachment of the fibrous flexor sheath and the 'check ligaments' associated bilaterally with the edges of the palmar plate of the proximal interphalangeal joint (Fig. 1.33) [27]. The head presents a bilateral slope from the dorsal aspect towards the sides. These slopes accommodate the lateral bands of the extensor tendons. The side of the head shows a pit for the attachment of the collateral ligament. The heads exhibit differences in the deviation, tilt and torsion in relation to the main longitudinal axis of the shaft and differ also in the degree of extent and roundness of their condyles. These asymmetrical differences allow other movements in the joint beside those of flexion and extension [24]. These small additional movements are of some importance in adjustment of the phalanges during prehension.

The bases of the *middle phalanx* (Fig. 1.22) exhibit dorsolateral and dorsomedial slopes for the lateral tendons during movements at the joint. On each side of the attachment of the palmar plate of the proximal interphalangeal joint there is a small palmar tubercle which gives attachment to the fibres of the lateral part of the capsule, to the 'check ligaments' and to a part of the cruciate fibres of the fibrous flexor sheath; these structures are usually found permanently shortened in flexion contracture of the joint. The margins of the palmar surface of the shaft are raised for the insertion of the tendon of the flexor digitorum superficialis and for the fibres of the flexor sheath. The distal part of these margins is flat as there are no 'check ligaments' in the distal joint.

The base of the *distal phalanx* is relatively large, with a raised dorsal margin for the attachment of the extensor tendon and a pitted area palmarly for the tendon of the flexor digitorum profundus. The thin shaft tapers to an expanded racket-like ungual tuberosity.

Blood supply of the phalanges: nutrient foramina for the shafts, usually two in number, lie on each side of the palmar aspect nearer the distal end and point towards the finger-tips.

Ossification in the hand

The cartilaginous skeleton of the hand appears about the seventh week of the intrauterine life (see Fig. 24.2). The rudiments of the ossa centralia are usually present and may remain separate. The general pattern of ossification (see Fig. 24.3) is as follows. The primary centres for the distal phalanges appear first near the distal end of the phalanx, then the centre for the proximal phalanx and lastly that for the middle one. The distal phalanx of the thumb is the first to show the centre in its shaft, i.e. it is the earliest ossification centre in the hand. The trapezium is at first smaller than the trapezoid. The sesamoid bones are cartilaginous in the child and begin to ossify about the thirteenth year of life. Variations include: the radial os centrale which may fail to fuse with the scaphoid; the hook of hamate may remain separate; the secondary ossification centre of the first metacarpal may be in the head of the bone; the styloid process of the third metacarpal may be separate; the distal phalanges may occasionally be bifurcate; the thumb may have three phalanges.

Assembly of the skeletal elements

The following arches of the hand (Fig. 1.24a) can be recognized.

(1) Transverse carpal arch, fixed and rigid.

(2) Transverse metacarpal arch: second and third metacarpals fixed, first, fourth and fifth mobile.

(3) Longitudinal metacarpal arch represented by the fixed concavity of the metacarpal shaft.

(4) Longitudinal metacarpophalangeal and digital arch, mobile and continuous with the longitudinal metacarpal arch. The principal *fixed axis of the hand* is continuous with the radius through the fixed carpal arch and consists of the second and third metacarpal bones, which are positioned and fixed for function by synergistic action of the radial extensor and flexor muscles of the carpus. Around this principal axis the mobile elements can be moved into many positions. These mobile elements (Fig. 1.24b) are:

(1) The first metacarpal with the bones and joints of the thumb, which possesses the greatest mobility.

(2) The index finger which has considerable independence from the other fingers.

(3) The fourth and fifth metacarpal bones together with the long, ring and little fingers.

Line of impact

A fall on the outstretched hand or striking a blow causes an impact which is usually taken by the third metacarpal bone, from which it is usually transmitted to the capitate and scaphoid bones, the force passing up from there along the radius.

JOINTS OF THE HAND

Radioulnar joint

The distal radioulnar joint is included here because of its close proximity and frequent communication with the radiocarpal joint through a disc perforation [13]. The head of the ulna articulates with the ulnar notch of the radius and with the proximal surface of the articular disc, which is a thick, firm, fibrocartilaginous plate, attached to the distal margin of the notch of the radius and to the base of the ulnar styloid. A lax capsule is represented by weak transverse fibres which unite the front and back of the radius and ulna. The synovial lining envelops the distal end of the ulna; it can be visualized as a triangular double-layered tent or sail with

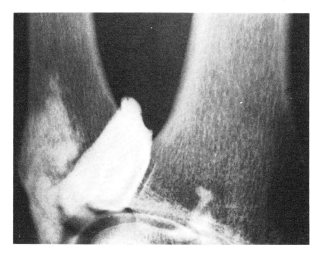

FIG. 1.26. Radiograph of distal radioulnar joint following injection with an opaque medium.

its apex proximal (sacciform recess) and its distal margin bent around the ulna (Figs. 1.25 and 1.26). No communication is found between the joint and the extensor tendon sheath to the little finger. In young people the disc is intact, presenting healthy articular cartilage which at its periphery merges imperceptibly with the synovial lining. In older people the perforation of the disc is quite common, accompanied by degenerative changes in the disc and related articular surfaces. Nerve supply of the joint is derived from the anterior and posterior interosseous nerves.

Radiocarpal joint

In the radiocarpal joint the convex surface, composed of the scaphoid, lunate and triquetrum, articulates with the concave ellipsoid surface of the radius and the disc (Fig. 1.27). In the usual position only scaphoid and part of the lunate articulate with the radius, the remainder of the lunate is opposite the disc and the triquetrum is in contact with the capsule. In adduction the latter bone lies opposite the disc. The capsule is attached near the articular surfaces and surrounds the joint. The ligaments are much stronger on the palmar aspect and the capsule is weakest posteriorly. The *palmar radiocarpal ligament* extends from the radius obliquely and medially to the proximal carpal row and to the capitate; it imparts considerable stability to the wrist. The weaker dorsal

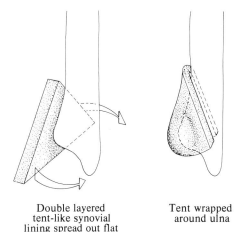

Double layered
tent-like synovial
lining spread out flat

Tent wrapped
around ulna

FIG. 1.25. Distal radioulnar joint.

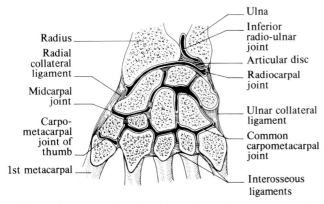

FIG. 1.27. Section through radiocarpal, carpal, carpometacarpal and intermetacarpal joints.

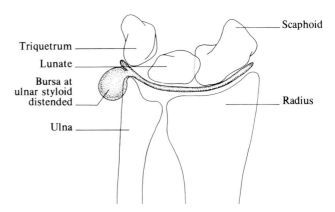

FIG. 1.28. Tracing of arthrogram of the radiocarpal joint.

radiocarpal ligament unites the posterior edge of the lower end of the radius to the first carpal row and particularly to triquetrum. The *radial collateral ligament* extends from the radial styloid to the scaphoid and the weaker one, the *ulnar collateral ligament*, from the ulnar styloid to the triquetrum. There has been recent detailed description of the ligaments of the wrist [14]. *Synovial membrane*: the joint cavity does not extend between the carpal bones because of the presence of the interosseous ligaments which are flush with the carpal articular surface. The synovium lines the palmar and dorsal aspects of the capsule and also the collateral ligaments on their inner aspects. The cavity extends a little further distally along the ulnar collateral ligament than along the radial one. A well developed bursa is present at the ulnar styloid, as noted previously [13]. It communicates by a channel with the radiocarpal joint (Fig. 1.28). It is related on the medial side to the ulnar collateral ligament at its attachment to the ulnar styloid, it is protected dorsally by the tendon and sheath of the extensor carpi ulnaris and it faces the flexor carpi ulnaris as it approaches the pisiform; at its radial end it is related to the tendon and sheath of the extensor to the little finger. The bursa probably facilitates the play of the tendons in this region. Extension of the pathological (e.g. rheumatoid) processes through this channel is a possibility. In this joint the synovial folds and fringes are well developed and numerous, particularly at the dorsal and palmar articular margins. They lie on the underlying fibrous bundles of the dorsal and palmar ligaments and are associated with the blood vessels

destined for the carpal bones. All main nerves of the region give branches to the joint [15, 16].

The intercarpal joints

The midcarpal joint is between the proximal and distal carpal rows. Most of the joints between the individual bones are gliding although the capitate rotates as well. The individual bones of each row are united by interosseous, palmar and dorsal intercarpal ligaments. The *pisotriquetral joint* has a separate synovial cavity, which is relatively large. The capsule is thin and strong, reinforced by strong pisohamate (to the hook of hamate) and pisometacarpal (to the base of the fifth metacarpal) ligaments. *Midcarpal joint*. In the lateral part (Fig. 1.27) a shallow concave saucer of trapezium and trapezoid faces the rounded distal surface of the scaphoid; in the larger medial part of the joint the capitate and hamate occupy a deep concavity formed by the triquetrum, lunate and medial aspect of the scaphoid. If the transverse line of the medial part of the joint is extended laterally it cuts across the waist of the scaphoid. Palmar and dorsal intercarpal ligaments between the two rows of the carpal bones are concentrated mostly on the capitate. The *intercarpal joint cavity* is extensive and complex. Offshoots of the midcarpal cavity extend between the three proximal and between the four distal carpal bones. Occasionally in deficiencies of the interosseous ligaments a communication may exist between the midcarpal and radiocarpal or carpometacarpal joints. The synovial folds and fringes are present but not as well developed as in the radiocarpal joint. Very little synovium is present on the palmar aspect of the lateral, gliding part of the midcarpal joint. The nerve supply to these joints is derived from the main nerves of the region.

Movements at the radiocarpal and intercarpal joints are complex [17–19]. Most sources agree that these joints constitute one functional unit, that the scaphoid and lunate most of the time move synchronously and that the scaphoid link (including the scapholunate ligament) provides stability resulting in the co-ordinated movements of the proximal and distal carpal rows. The first metacarpal, trapezium and scaphoid may be considered as a 'jointed strut' concerned with movements of the thumb (p. 221) and is the commonest site of post-traumatic arthritis in the wrist. According to Fisk [17], in dorsiflexion the first two-thirds of movement occurs in the radiocarpal joint and the last third in the mid-carpal joint, thus a fall on the outstretched hand results in the impact being taken in the midcarpal region across the waist of the scaphoid. In palmar flexion the first half of movement takes place in the midcarpal joint. Adduction occurs almost entirely at the radiocarpal joint, while in abduction the midcarpal joint and particularly movement of the head of the capitate in the cup of the scaphoid and lunate are important. In both movements the axis is anteroposterior through the centre of the capitate. The range of movements at the wrist is subject to individual variation but on average is as follows: dorsiflexion (extension) – 70°, palmar flexion – 75°, adduction (ulnar deviation) – 40° and abduction (radial deviation) – 20°. Combination of all the above movements is known as circumduction.

Carpometacarpal joint

The common carpometacarpal joint (Fig. 1.27) is formed by the distal carpal row and the bases of the four medial metacarpal bones. It is surrounded by a fibrous capsule and may have an interosseous ligament between the capitate and hamate proximally and the bases of the third or fourth metacarpals or both. The cavity of the joint extends proximally between the four distal carpal bones and distally into the three intermetacarpal joints; these extensions are quite small compared with the other carpal joints. The base of the second metacarpal fits well into a recess formed by the trapezium, trapezoid and capitate; in this area there is only a little synovium. The only part which shows an extensive synovial surface is between the bases of the third and fourth metacarpals corresponding to the interosseous ligament. When a fresh amputation specimen is injected with an opaque medium hardly any space can be found in the lateral part in contrast to the ulnar part as the joints between the bases of the fourth and fifth meta-carpal bones and to some extent between the bases of the third and fourth metacarpals have a slight slack in the capsule. This difference is probably related to the tight fit of the fixed axis of the hand (second and third metacarpals) while the ulnar part of the joint has a more extensive lining to accommodate the anteroposterior movements of the fourth and fifth metacarpals when the transverse metacarpal arch (p. 14) is actively formed; some degree of opposition is possible in the joint between the fifth metacarpal base and the hamate which is of flattened saddle variety [20].

Generally speaking, there is only a small amount of synovium between the individual bones of one carpal row and also between the two carpal rows, while the lining of the dorsal and palmar walls, especially of the radio-carpal but also of the midcarpal, and to some extent of the ulnar part of the carpometacarpal joint, is extensive.

Digital joints

The digital joints exhibit the independence of the inter-phalangeal from the metacarpophalangeal joints. The latter are linked together to form one system (Fig. 1.29), while the interphalangeal joints are set separate in their fingers. However the proximal and distal interphalangeal joints of the same finger are linked functionally by the oblique retinacular ligament (p. 30). In a majority of individuals the proximal interphalangeal joint cannot be hyperextended while the distal one can (see p. 22). The differences in setting of the digital joints, their asymmetry, particularly of the metacarpophalangeal joints, the additional movements possible in the interphalangeal joints, all contribute to the direction which a finger assumes if flexed separately, namely towards the scaphoid.

Metacarpophalangeal joints of the fingers

The metacarpophalangeal joints of the fingers are of the ball-and-socket variety; the concave surface of the base

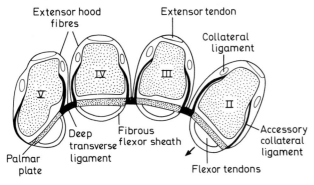

FIG. 1.29. End-on view of metacarpal heads and related structures.

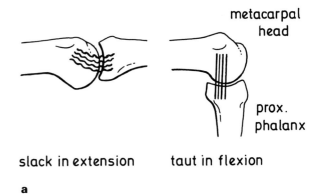

a

of the proximal phalanx receives the rounded meta-carpal head covered by the articular cartilage distally and anteriorly. The phalangeal articular surface extends on to the palmar ligament which is attached very strongly to the base of the phalanx and is covered by cartilage where it faces the head of the metacarpal. The *capsule* is strengthened on each side by a collateral ligament which is attached to the tubercle and impression of the head of the metacarpal (see Fig. 1.22) and to the side of the base of the proximal phalanx. The course of the ligament and configuration of the head of the meta-carpal is such that, owing to the presence of the sagital and transverse cams, the collateral ligaments are slack in extension and taut in flexion (Fig. 1.30). The fibres of the capsule palmar to the collateral ligament have a fan-shaped disposition, are attached to the edge of the palmar plate and are known as accessory collateral ligaments. The palmar plates are attached only loosely to the necks of the metacarpals but are continuous at the sides with the three deep transverse ligaments of the palm (Fig. 1.29) which unite the palmar plates of the medial four metacarpophalangeal joints and thus indirectly the heads of the four medial metacarpal bones. Many other mobile structures are attached to the palmar plates: tendon and muscle fibres of the interossei, extensor expansion hood fibres and those of the palmar aponeurosis. The asymmetry of the metacarpal heads (p. 13), the degree of strength of the ligaments, their course and attachments [21–23] result in greater ulnar than radial deviation in the index and the long fingers, while the ring finger is equal in that respect and the metacarpophalangeal joint of the little finger shows radial deviation. Direction in which axial rotation takes

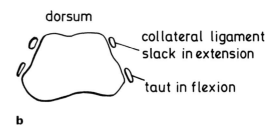

b

FIG. 1.30. (a) Effect of the sagittal cam of the metacarpal head on the collateral ligaments. (b) Spreading effect of the transverse cam of the metacarpal head on the collateral ligaments.

place depends on the oblique course of the collateral ligaments [24].

Synovial membrane. The dorsal pouch extends 1 cm in the index, but less in the other fingers, proximally in the median line from the joint interval. The palmar pouch extends in the median line for about 1.25 cm proximally in the index finger, less in the remainder of the fingers. The proximal edge of the palmar plate is continuous with an area of softer and pliable tissue which is attached to the neck of the metacarpal and which is lined with the synovium on the surface facing the joint cavity. On each side of the palmar plate there are extensions of the palmar pouch which reach further than the plate both proximally and anteriorly. On each side of the meta-carpal head there is a curved strip of bone covered by synovium between the attachment of the capsule and the articular margin. This strip is much wider on the ulnar side. *Nerve supply* of the joints of index and long fingers is derived from the median and radial nerves,

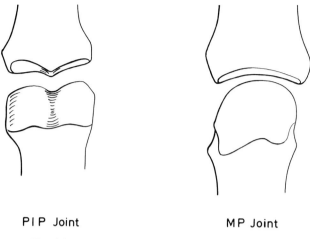

PIP Joint   MP Joint

FIG. 1.31. Anterior view of the fit of articular surfaces.

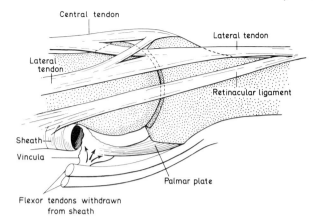

FIG. 1.32. Lateral and palmar relations of proximal interphalangeal joint.

while those of the remaining two fingers have branches from the ulnar nerve.

Movements. In addition to flexion and extension (90°) the joints allow hyperextension, particularly passive, some rotation, abduction and adduction and circumduction. These joints are important in prehensile movements of the hand. Owing to the manner of attachment of the collateral ligaments and the profile of the metacarpal head (Fig. 1.30) it is clear that if the ligaments should, through disease, become permanently shortened when the joint is in extended position, flexion of the joint is impossible and the power grip against the palm is lost and against the thumb is very much less efficient.

Proximal interphalangeal joints

The proximal interphalangeal joints are of bicondylar variety (Fig. 1.31) and only a little movement is possible other than flexion and extension. These small additional movements result from slight deviation, torsion and asymmetrical curvatures of the surfaces and provide adaptive displacements when gripping irregular objects and when making a fist or using a power grip [24]. The *capsule* on the dorsum is replaced by the extensor expansion which overlies the synovial membrane (Fig. 1.32). On the palmar aspect the capsule consists of the palmar plate which is continuous proximally with a pliable, much softer and bulkier band of connective tissue extending to the neck of the proximal phalanx.

At the sides of the plate there are tougher fibres which are continuous with the most dorsal parts of the cruciate bundles of the fibrous flexor sheath (see Fig. 1.18, p. 9); some of them are deeper parts of the attachments of the sides of the palmar plate to the neck of the proximal phalanx and are known also as 'check ligaments' (Fig. 1.33). On the medial and lateral aspects the capsule can be divided into three areas: the band of the collateral ligament (area 2), a triangular area above it (area 1) and a triangular fan-shaped area below it (area 3) (Fig. 1.34). Some of the dorsal fibres of area 3 are attached to the lower part of the lateral tubercle while some of them continue towards the small

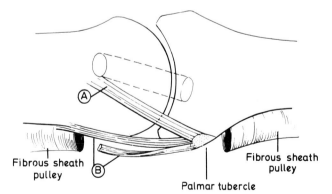

FIG. 1.33. Check ligaments: A, fibres of lower part of collateral aspect of the capsule attached to palmar tubercle; B, fibres of cruciate part of fibrous sheath.

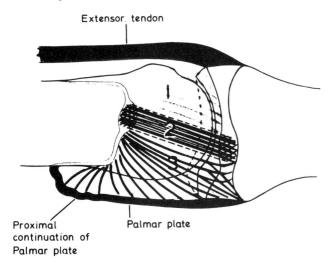

Extensor tendon

Proximal
continuation of
Palmar plate

Palmar plate

FIG. 1.34. Parts of capsule of the proximal interphalangeal joint:
1, upper area; 2, collateral ligament; 3, lower area.

tubercle on the palmar aspect of the base of the middle
phalanx where they meet the most dorsal fibres of the
flexor sheath ('check ligament') as they cross the joint.

Laterally, the oblique retinacular ligament lies anterior
to the lateral tendon. In addition there are the digital
cutaneous ligaments (p. 472) which extend from the
periosteum to the skin and contain the neurovascular
bundles. Anterior to the palmar plate there is flexor
tendon sheath with its contents. The vinculum breve of
the superficialis tendon and the vinculum longum of the
profundus tendon are continuous with the connective
tissue proximal to the palmar plate. The collateral
ligaments are slightly slackened when the joint is in full
extension, become taut after the first 10–15° of flexion
and remain taut throughout the rest of the range of
movement except for a few degrees in the final range
of flexion [25]. Thus when immobilization of the joint
is unavoidable, the 'safer position' is in almost full
extension, as further flexion does not result in increased
tightness of the collateral ligament but puts at risk of
contracture more palmarly situated structures. *Synovial
membrane*: the general arrangement of the dorsal and
palmar pouches is similar to that of the metacarpophalangeal joints except that they do not extend so far
proximally (8 mm on average). Range of *movement* is

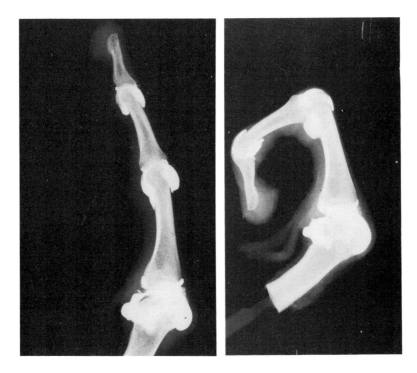

FIG. 1.35. Arthrogram of the digital joints of a finger injected with an opaque medium.

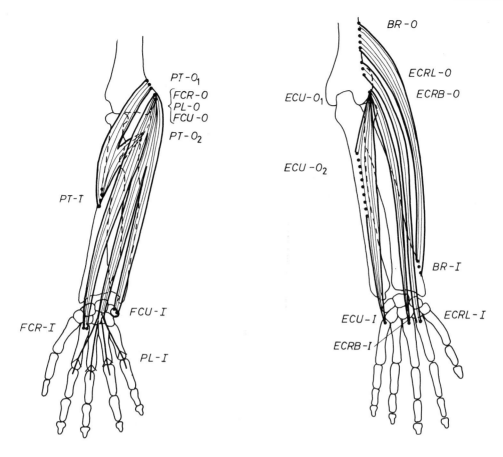

Fɪɢ. 1.36. Superficial muscles of the forearm.

Pronator teres (*PT*)

PT-O₁ Humeral attachment: lowest part of medial supracondylar ridge, medial epicondyle.

PT-O₂ Ulnar attachment: coronoid process.

PT-I Middle of lateral surface of radius.

Flexor carpi radialis (*FCR*)

FCR-O Common flexor origin on the medial epicondyle.

FCR-I Base of second metacarpal.

Palmaris longus (absent in 10%) (*PL*)

PL-O Medial epicondyle.

PL-I Flexor retinaculum and palmar aponeurosis (see later).

Flexor carpi ulnaris (*FCU*)

FCU-O Medial epicondyle, medial border of olecranon and upper part of posterior border of ulna.

FCU-I Pisiform bone.

Brachioradialis (*BR*)

BR-O Upper thirds of lateral supracondylar ridge.

BR-I Lateral side of lower end of radius.

Extensor carpi radialis longus (*ECRL*)

ECRL-O Distal third of lateral supracondylar ridge.

ECRL-I Base of second metacarpal.

Extensor carpi radialis brevis (*ECRB*)

ECRB-O Lateral epicondyle of humerus (common extensor origin).

ECRB-I Base of third metacarpal.

Extensor carpi ulnaris (*ECU*)

ECU-O₁ Lateral epicondyle.

ECU-O₂ Middle part of posterior border of ulna.

ECU-I Base of fifth metacarpal.

100° on average. Usually no hyperextension is possible but some individuals may exhibit some even with active 'swan neck' position shown.

Distal interphalangeal joints

The distal interphalangeal joints are also of bicondylar type. Their anteroposterior extent is smaller than that of the proximal joint. The palmar extension of the articular surface on the head of the middle phalanx is also relatively smaller than that on the corresponding part of the proximal phalanx. These joints have similar ligaments to those of the proximal joint but attachment of the palmar plate to the neck of the middle phalanx is of such nature that some degree of hyperextension, particularly passive, is possible. No definite 'check ligaments' are demonstrable in this joint [26]. The joint is related dorsally and palmarly to the massive terminal portions of the extensor and profundus tendons. The average length of the dorsal and palmar pouches is 5 mm. The range of movement varies from 60–90°.

Figure 1.35 shows the radiographic appearance of the synovial cavities of the digital joints in a fresh amputation specimen of a finger in which they were injected with an opaque medium. It is equally distributed between the dorsal and palmar pouches in all three joints in extension, but in flexion the dorsal pouches in the interphalangeal joints are squeezed almost flat while those of the metacarpophalangeal joints are maintained or even slightly increased. This is probably due to the fact that the fibres of the proximal edge of the extensor expansion are drawn off the dorsal pouch of the metacarpophalangeal joint during flexion allowing the pouch to expand dorsally on each side of the extensor tendon. The distension of this dorsal synovial pouch may be important in considering the effects of the increased intra-articular pressure in pathological (e.g. rheumatoid) processes [23].

MUSCLES CONCERNED WITH MOVEMENTS OF THE HAND

Muscles acting on the thumb are described on pp. 46–49.

The flexor carpi radialis, palmaris longus, flexor carpi ulnaris and extensor carpi radialis longus and brevis

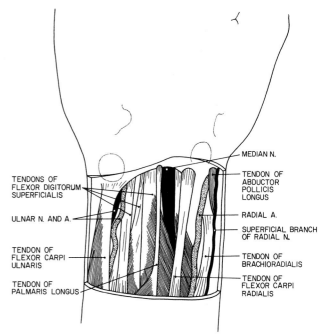

FIG. 1.37. Anterior aspect of the wrist. From Passmore, R. and Robson, J. S. (1976) *A Companion to Medical Studies*, Volume 1. Blackwell Scientific Publications: Oxford.

act only at the wrist (see Fig. 1.36). Tendons at the wrist are shown in Fig. 1.37.

Muscles acting on the fingers and on the wrist secondarily are two long flexors of the fingers and three extensors: digitorum, indicis and digiti minimi.

Flexor digitorum superficialis

This arises from the medial epicondyle of the humerus, ulnar collateral ligament, medial border of the coronoid process and upper two-thirds of the anterior border of the radius. Four tendons arise from the muscle about half way down the forearm: two for the long and ring fingers lie superficial to those for the index and little fingers. This position of the tendons is maintained as far as the palmar part of the carpal tunnel where the tendons diverge to reach the entry into the fibrous flexor sheath in company with the tendon of the profundus. About the level of the metacarpophalangeal joint each tendon of the superficialis splits into two, each half passing posteriorly to the tendon of the profundus to be inserted into the margins of the palmar

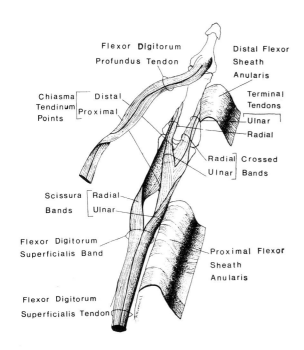

FIG. 1.38. Components of the flexor digitorum superficialis tendon.

surface of the middle phalanx, some of the fibres decussating posteriorly to the profundus tendon (Fig. 1.38). The tendons of the superficialis are also attached by vincula brevia and longa which take part in conducting small blood vessels to the tendons (see Fig. 11.1). Vinculum breve is a small triangular band in the interval between the terminal part of the tendon and the front of the proximal interphalangeal joint and distal part of the proximal phalanx. Vincula longa are variable slender bands extending from the tendon to the proximal part of the proximal phalanx. In the little finger the superficialis tendon is absent in about 20 per cent of hands and in the remainder it is less developed in proportion to the finger length than its counterpart in the radial three fingers [33]. It may be replaced by a slip from the ulna, flexor retinaculum or palmar fascia.

Nerve supply is from the median nerve in the forearm (C7, C8; T1).

Actions. As it crosses elbow, wrist, metacarpophalangeal and proximal interphalangeal joints, it may assist in flexion of all of them but its main action is on the last-named. It is difficult to be sure that it is working as the profundus can produce all actions of the superficialis. However, EMG studies [34] suggest that it is used when an additional effort is required as in a strong hook grip (e.g. when carrying a heavy suitcase). It can also be considered as an important check on hyperextension stress in the proximal interphalangeal joint [33].

Flexor digitorum profundus

This arises from the upper two-thirds of the anterior and medial surfaces of the ulna and from the adjoining half of the interosseous membrane. Half way down the forearm the most radial part of the muscle forms a separate tendon for the index finger giving it some degree of independence. The remainder of the muscle forms the tendons to the rest of the fingers near the flexor retinaculum. In the carpal tunnel they lie posterior to those of the superficialis. Each tendon of the profundus enters the fibrous flexor sheath behind that of the superficialis, which it perforates opposite the proximal phalanx. Vincula brevia are attached to the capsule of the distal interphalangeal joint and longa to the tendons of the superficialis and their vincula brevia (see Fig. 11.1, p. 154). The terminal part of the tendon is inserted into the base of the distal phalanx.

Nerve supply. The medial half of the muscle (to the ring and little fingers) is supplied by branches of the ulnar nerve (C8 and T1), while that for the index and long fingers is supplied by branches of the anterior interosseous nerve (C7, C8; T1). Occasionally either of the above nerves may supply the whole muscle.

Actions. It helps to flex all the joints it crosses but its primary action is to bend the distal interphalangeal joints.

Extensor digitorum

The extensor digitorum arises from the anterior surface of the lateral humeral epicondyle, from the fascia covering the muscle and from the intermuscular septa. The muscle ends in four tendons proximal to the wrist, which pass deep to the extensor retinaculum. On the dorsum of the hand the tendons are interconnected by very variable oblique bands. The tendon to the index is frequently free of that to the long finger while those to the ring and little fingers are usually closely attached as far distally as the metacarpophalangeal joint. The tendons may be reduced in number but more commonly they may be doubled or trebled. The long extensor tendon at the level of the metacarpophalangeal joints divides into three bands. Its direct continuation proceeds along the dorsum of the proximal phalanx, while the transverse (shroud) fibres embedded in the proximal edge of the hood of the extensor expansion (see later), encircle the metacarpal head to fuse with the deep transverse ligament of the palm. This attachment of the long extensor limits its proximal retraction. The main portion of the tendon gives a slip, variable and very often absent, to the dorsal part of the capsule of the metacarpophalangeal joint and then continues towards the proximal interphalangeal joint. Before reaching it, the tendon divides into three terminal bands. A central one is attached to the base of the middle phalanx. Two lateral bands, which at first lie in the grooves over the lateral part of the dorsum of the proximal interphalangeal joint, converge to be attached to the base of the distal phalanx. All these elements of the extrinsic tendinous component are bound together by oblique and transverse fibres embedded in the flat triangular extensor expansion with its hood, and proximal and distal wings (Figs 1.39 and 1.40).

Actions (see also p. 30). The muscle primarily extends the metacarpophalangeal joints. In hyperextended position of these joints it has a tendency to abduct the fingers from the line of the long finger. It assists also in extension of the interphalangeal joints (see later). As it crosses the wrist and elbow joints it can extend the former, but flexion effect on the latter is negligible.

Extensor digiti minimi

This arises from the anterior surface of the lateral humeral condyle and from its own fascia. Its tendon traverses a special compartment of the extensor retinaculum, splits into two – the lateral half joining the tendon of the extensor digitorum to the little finger – all three bands inserting into the extensor expansion on the dorsum of the proximal phalanx.

Actions are similar to those of the extensor digitorum.

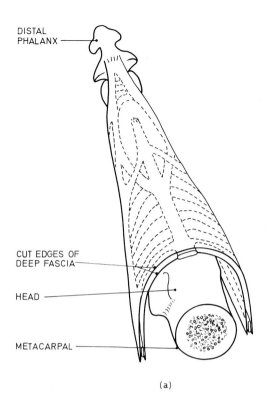

(a)

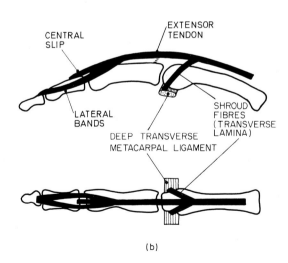

(b)

Fig. 1.39. (a) Extensor expansion, (b) extensor extrinsic component.

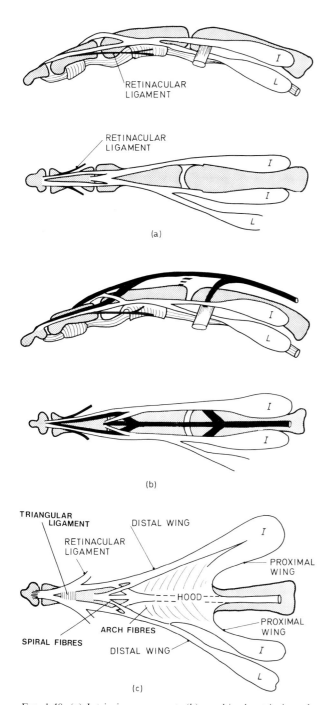

FIG. 1.40. (a) Intrinsic component, (b) combined extrinsic and intrinsic components, (c) the extensor expansion spread out flat. L, lumbrical; I, interosseous muscle.

Extensor indicis

The extensor indicis arises deep in the forearm from the lower part of the ulna and adjoining interosseous membrane. Its tendon passes through the extensor retinaculum in company of extensor digitorum. In the hand the tendon lies on the ulnar side of the index tendon of the extensor digitorum and is inserted into its expansion.

Actions are similar to those of the extensor digitorum, except that it can produce independent extension of the index.

Nerve supply of the above three muscles is derived from the posterior interosseous (deep radial) nerve (C7, C8).

Synovial sheaths in the wrist and the hand

In front of the wrist there are usually three synovial sheaths: (1) for the tendon of the flexor carpi radialis, (2) of the flexor pollicis longus (radial bursa), and (3) common flexor sheath (ulnar bursa) for the eight tendons of the long flexor of the fingers, which are invaginated into the bursa from the radial side (Fig. 1.41). In the carpal tunnel the invaginated tendons form three potential pockets of the ulnar bursa: one in front of the tendons, the second between the two layers

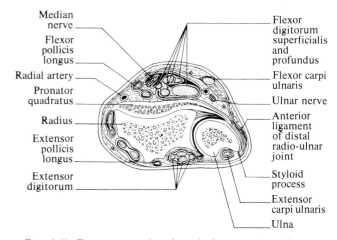

FIG. 1.41. Transverse section through forearm above flexor retinaculum showing the relation of the synovial sheaths to the tendons.

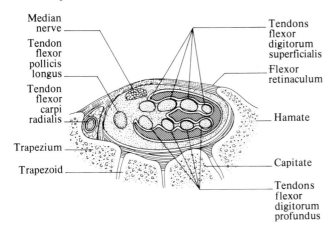

FIG. 1.42. Transverse section through the distal row of carpal bones showing the flexor retinaculum and arrangement of the synovial sheaths of the flexor tendons.

and the third between the profundus tendons and the floor of the carpal tunnel (Fig. 1.42). Mesotenons of the ulnar bursa tendons are on the radial side. All three synovial sheaths on the front of the wrist begin approximately 2 to 3 cm proximal to the flexor retinaculum (Fig. 1.43). The first two end at the insertion of the tendons while the common flexor sheath terminates about the

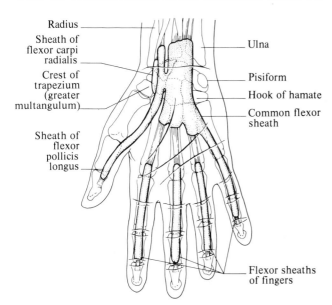

FIG. 1.43. Tendon sheaths at the palmar surface of the right hand shown in relation to skeleton and surface markings.

middle of the palm, except for the little finger in which its digital sheath in about 70 per cent of individuals is continuous with the common sheath. The digital synovial sheaths line the osteofascial canals on the front of the fingers. They terminate distally at the insertion of the profundus tendon and extend proximally in the three radial fingers to the metacarpal necks. The remnants of the mesotenons are represented by the vincula. The flexor pollicis longus sheath may communicate at the level of the wrist with the common flexor sheath in about 80 per cent of individuals and the index profundus tendon may possess a separate palmar sheath.

On the *dorsum* the synovial sheaths begin just proximal to the extensor retinaculum. Those of the tendons attached to the metacarpus extend distally to their insertions, while the others reach half way down the hand (Figs 1.44 and 1.45). Six sheaths are present on the dorsum of the wrist which surround the following tendons: (1) abductor pollicis longus and extensor pollicis brevis, (2) extensor carpi radialis longus and brevis, (3) extensor pollicis longus, (4) extensor digitorum and extensor indicis, (5) extensor digiti minimi, and (6) extensor carpi ulnaris.

The intrinsic muscles of the fingers are hypothenar muscles, interossei and lumbricals.

Hypothenar muscles

Abductor digiti minimi

The abductor digiti minimi (Fig. 1.46) arises from the tendon of the flexor carpi ulnaris, from the pisiform and its ligaments and also from a fibrous arch spanning from the pisiform to the hook of hamate and serving as a common origin of the abductor and the short flexor of the little finger. It is inserted into the medial side of the base of the proximal phalanx of the little finger and its extensor expansion.

Actions. It abducts the little finger and assists in flexion of the metacarpophalangeal joint and by its insertion into the expansion helps in extension of the interphalangeal joints. It is quite a strong muscle. Its origin has to be stabilized by the flexor carpi ulnaris for the muscle to have a full effect; if it is paralysed the contraction of the flexor carpi ulnaris may cause abduction of the little finger.

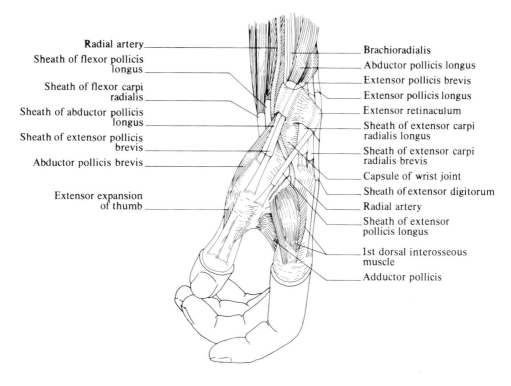

Radial artery — Brachioradialis
Sheath of flexor pollicis longus — Abductor pollicis longus
Sheath of flexor carpi radialis — Extensor pollicis brevis
— Extensor pollicis longus
Sheath of abductor pollicis longus — Extensor retinaculum
Sheath of extensor pollicis brevis — Sheath of extensor carpi radialis longus
Abductor pollicis brevis — Sheath of extensor carpi radialis brevis
— Capsule of wrist joint
— Sheath of extensor digitorum
Extensor expansion of thumb — Radial artery
— Sheath of extensor pollicis longus
— 1st dorsal interosseous muscle
— Adductor pollicis

FIG. 1.44. Dissection of the lateral side of left wrist and hand showing synovial sheaths of tendons.

Opponens digiti minimi

The opponens digiti minimi (Fig. 1.46) arises from the hook of hamate and the flexor retinaculum. It is inserted into the distal two-thirds of the medial half of the palmar aspect of the fifth metacarpal. It is often split into two layers by the deep branches of the ulnar artery and nerve.

Actions. It deepens the hollow of the palm by pulling the metacarpal anteriorly and rotating it laterally. It also takes part in movement of opposition of the little finger and the thumb.

Flexor digiti minimi brevis

This variable muscle may be fused with its neighbours or be absent in 20–30 per cent of people. When present it arises from the flexor retinaculum, hook of hamate and the fibrous arch which unites it to the origin of the

abductor. It is inserted into the medial side of the base of the proximal phalanx of the little finger.

Actions. It flexes the little finger ray at the carpometacarpal and metacarpophalangeal joints.

Nerve supply of the above three muscles is from the deep branch of the ulnar nerve (T1).

Palmaris brevis

This is a small subcutaneous muscle which arises from the medial border of the palmar aponeurosis and is inserted into the skin of the medial border of the hand, thus protecting the ulnar nerve and vessels. It is supplied by the superficial branch of the ulnar nerve. It deepens the hollow of the hand assisting in the palmar grip; its contraction causes wrinkling of the skin at its insertion.

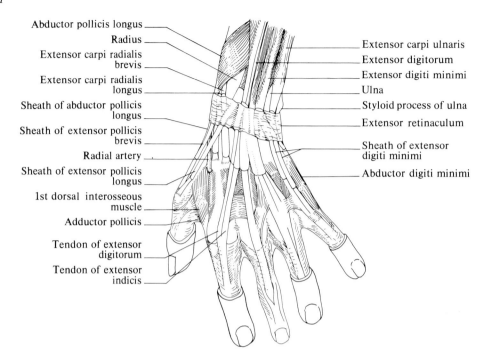

Abductor pollicis longus

Radius

Extensor carpi radialis brevis

Extensor carpi radialis longus

Sheath of abductor pollicis longus

Sheath of extensor pollicis brevis

Radial artery

Sheath of extensor pollicis longus

1st dorsal interosseous muscle

Adductor pollicis

Tendon of extensor digitorum

Tendon of extensor indicis

Extensor carpi ulnaris

Extensor digitorum

Extensor digiti minimi

Ulna

Styloid process of ulna

Extensor retinaculum

Sheath of extensor digiti minimi

Abductor digiti minimi

FIG. 1.45. Dissection of back of forearm, wrist and hand showing synovial sheaths of tendons.

Lumbricals

The two lateral ones arise from the lateral side of the profundus tendons to the index and long fingers; the medial two arise by two heads from the adjacent sides of the profundus tendons to the long, ring and little fingers (Fig. 1.47). Variations in origin or insertion of lumbricals are common [35]. The second arises from two tendons in 20–30 per cent of people, their number may be increased or, rarely, reduced to three, with the third usually being absent. These small cylindrical muscles join the lateral edge of the extensor expansion (Fig. 1.40). A lumbrical may split into two going to two fingers.

Nerve supply. The two lateral ones are usually supplied by the median nerve (T1), the medial two by the ulnar nerve (T1). The number of those supplied by the median may be reduced to none or increased to three.

Actions. The line of pull of each lumbrical lies palmar to the axis of the metacarpophalangeal joint and dorsal to the axes of the interphalangeal joints. The lumbricals therefore extend the latter joints and with the fingers extended at the interphalangeal joints they flex the metacarpophalangeal joints. Acting from their insertion they slacken the tension in the tendons of origin. They also serve as an adjustable, contractile link between the flexor and extensor systems of the fingers where their muscle spindles [36] can function as an important proprioceptive feed back mechanism.

Interossei (Fig. 1.47)

There are three *palmar* muscles. (The classical first palmar interosseus is considered to be a small negligible slip belonging either to the oblique head of the adductor pollicis or to the deep head of the flexor pollicis brevis). They arise from the metacarpals of the fingers on which they act: the first one from the ulnar side and adjoining palmar aspect of the second metacarpal, the two remaining from the radial aspect and adjoining palmar surface of the fourth and fifth metacarpal shafts respectively. They are inserted into the extensor expansion (see below). The four *dorsal* interossei are twice the size of the

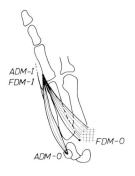

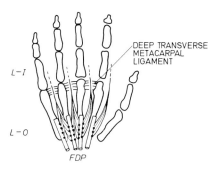

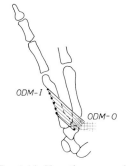

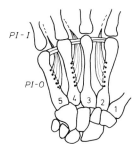

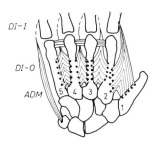

FIG. 1.46. Hypothenar muscles.

FIG. 1.47. Intrinsic muscles of the fingers.

Abductor digiti minimi (*ADM*)

ADM-O Pisiform bone.
ADM-I Base of proximal phalanx.

Flexor digiti minimi brevis (*FDM*)

FDM-O Flexor retinaculum and hook of hamate.
FDM-I Base of proximal phalanx of little finger.

Opponens digiti minimi (*ODM*)

ODM-O Flexor retinaculum, hook of hamate.
ODM-I Medial aspect of fifth metacarpal.

Lumbrical muscles (*L*) **of the right hand**

L-O Tendons of flexor digitorum profundus (*FDP*).
L-I Distal wings of extensor expansion.

Palmar interossei muscles (*PI*)

PI-O Palmar aspect of second, fourth and fifth metacarpal shafts.
PI-P Almost all fibres inserted into the distal wings of the extensor expansion (like lumbricals).

Dorsal interossei muscles (*DI*)

DI-O Adjacent sides of two metacarpal bones. Abductor digiti minimi (ADM) completes the series.
DI-I Considerable variation as distal attachment is divided in variable amounts between: base of proximal phalanx, proximal and distal wings of extensor expansion.

palmar ones and arise from the adjacent metacarpals: the first from the first and second metacarpal shafts by two heads [37] which form an interval transmitting the radial artery into the palm. The dorsal interossei show a considerable variation in the degree in which they divide the fibres of their insertion between the base of the proximal phalanx and the extensor expansion [37–

42]. The third dorsal usually inserts only into the expansion.

Nerve supply. All are supplied by twigs (T1) from the deep branch of the ulnar nerve. In 10 per cent the first dorsal is supplied by the median nerve.

Actions. The dorsal muscles abduct the fingers away from an imaginary line drawn along the longitudinal axis of the long finger. The first dorsal can rotate the index finger at the metacarpophalangeal joint. The palmar interossei adduct the fingers towards the line of the long finger. Although interossei are posterior to the deep transverse ligament of the palm, they lie anterior to the axis of flexion at the metacarpophalangeal joint and so flex this joint. By their insertion into the extensor expansion they extend the interphalangeal joints.

The extrinsic and intrinsic components of the dorsal apparatus are applied through the complicated mechanism of the *extensor expansion* (Figs. 1.39 and 1.40). This lies in a shallow connective tissue bed, gliding immediately beneath the skin and closely related to the bones and joints of the fingers, and is therefore vulnerable. It can be visualized as a plexiform arrangement of bands and flat thin membranes sandwiched between two thin layers of connective tissue in which it can slide not only longitudinally but also transversely, changing the position of one band in relation to the others and also to the axes of the joints over which they act. Before the function of the dorsal apparatus is discussed, the retinacular ligament should be considered. It is composed of two parts: (1) a *transverse* layer, a broad, thin ligament which passes across the dorsum and sides of the proximal interphalangeal joint, superficial to the extensor apparatus, and which reaches on each side the fibrous flexor sheath on the palmar surface of the proximal phalanx; (2) the *link* or *oblique retinacular ligament* (Fig. 1.40) passes underneath the transverse part and is a strong fibrous band extending from the palmar aspect of the fibrous flexor sheath and the adjoining bone; it passes obliquely on the palmar side of the axis of the proximal interphalangeal joint towards the dorsum of the finger, joining the lateral band of the dorsal expansion, dorsal to the distal interphalangeal joint axis. The mechanical effect of this ligament can be seen when passively flexing the distal interphalangeal joint; this causes the ligament to become taut and forces

the proximal interphalangeal joint into flexion simultaneously and automatically (see Fig. 1.48a and observe on your own finger). If now the proximal interphalangeal joint is passively extended, the distal interphalangeal joint is brought into extension as well. With this link it might be thought unnecessary to have muscles for active extension of the distal interphalangeal joint, since this would be automatically accomplished by the extensor muscles of the proximal interphalangeal joint. However, passive extension of the distal joint is only partial and some active force is necessary to complete it.

When measured along the dorsum, the finger is about 2.5 cm longer in flexion than in extension. This is because of the palmar projection of the heads of the metacarpals and phalanges. Obviously this feature augments the effect of the retinacular ligament during flexion, but diminishes it when the flexed finger is extended. Complete extension at the distal interphalangeal joints is due to the tension in the terminal parts of the lateral bands and follows the contraction of the muscles attached to

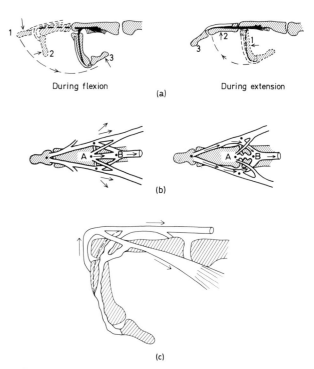

During flexion   During extension

(a)

(b)

(c)

FIG. 1.48. Mechanism of extension of interphalangeal joints.

the distal wings of the extensor expansion. This contraction relaxes the central band so that force (A-B, Fig. 1.48b) of the long extensor is transferred to the lateral bands to act on the distal interphalangeal joint and complete its full extension. This resembles a servo-mechanism, since the force from the long extensor has its point of application changed from the proximal to the distal interphalangeal joint by the contraction of the muscles attached to the distal wings of the extensor expansion.

When extending the fully flexed finger, contraction of the long extensor extends the metacarpophalangeal joint; it is also involved in the extension of the inter-phalangeal joints by a more complex mechanism. In the fully flexed position of the proximal interphalangeal joint the distal wings and lateral bands of the extensor expansion lie on the sides of the head of the proximal phalanx (Fig. 1.48c). In these circumstances the pull of the extensor muscles is applied to the central slip and extends the middle phalanx at the proximal inter-phalangeal joint, and not to the lateral bands which in the flexed proximal interphalangeal joint are relaxed as they lie along the short cut, i.e. in the line of the shortest distance to the base of the distal phalanx. Any further pull on the lateral bands in this position shifts them more towards the palm and make them less able to extend the distal joint. Thus the pull on the central fibres extends only the proximal interphalangeal joint, but as a result of this extension the retinacular ligament partially extends the distal joint. After extension of the proximal interphalangeal joint, the lateral bands have moved dorsally and the distal wing muscles now pull on them to cause the active final extension of the distal joint.

In summary, the normal phalangeal movements are co-ordinated by the retinacular ligament, while the metacarpophalangeal joint moves independently, being extended by extensor digitorum, extensor digiti minimi and extensor indicis and flexed by the long flexors and intrinsic muscles.

INNERVATION OF THE HAND

Functional microanatomy of the peripheral nerve trunks and the nerve endings are described on p. 181. The nerve supply of the thumb is given on p. 51.

The nerve supply of the hand is obtained through the brachial plexus from the lower four cervical and first thoracic nerves.

Sensory innervation

The pattern of distribution of the median, ulnar and radial cutaneous branches in the hand is shown in Fig. 1.49. Important variations are shown in Fig. 1.50. The afferent impulses from the skin, joints and muscles are of great importance for sensory feedback, and for protection against injury. The sensory function of the hand can be classified as: (1) informative of position, shape, weight, etc. of objects, (2) 'grip sight' for fine sensory appreciation and tactile discrimination both in precision and power grip, (3) protective.

The dorsal branches of the radial nerve do not extend beyond the middle phalanx, while the dorsal branches from the palmar digital nerves supply the dorsum more distally, the digital nerves to the thumb and to the little finger being usually an exception. Area of sensory loss following section of the radial nerve is usually quite small.

The skin of the palmar aspect of the ring finger may show variation in the extent of supply by ulnar and median nerves.

Dermatomes

The central area of the skin of the hand, both palmar and dorsal, approximately along the axis of the long finger ray, is supplied by C7, the area on the radial side by C6 and on the ulnar side by C8 dermatome.

Cutaneous branches from the ulnar nerve

The dorsal cutaneous branch

The dorsal cutaneous branch winds dorsally deep to the tendon of the flexor carpi ulnaris to supply the ulnar side of the dorsum of the hand and of the medial one and a half fingers as far as the middle phalanges.

The palmar cutaneous branch

The palmar cutaneous branch is given off just proximal

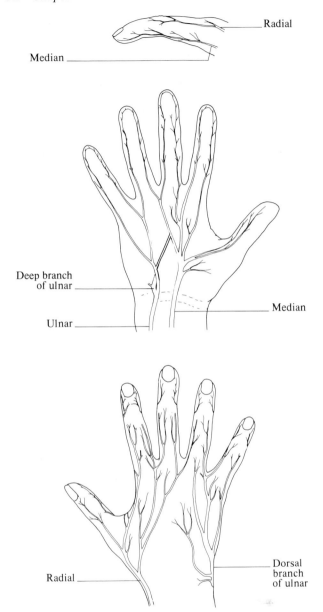

FIG. 1.49. Distribution of cutaneous nerves.

to the wrist and supplies the ulnar side of the wrist and hand.

Two palmar digital branches

Two palmar digital branches of the superficial division

of the ulnar nerve supply the skin of the medial one and a half fingers on their palmar aspect as well as part of the dorsal surface including the nail bed.

Cutaneous branches from the median nerve

The palmar cutaneous branch is given off 5 cm above the wrist, pierces the deep fascia and descends superficial to the flexor retinaculum. It supplies a small area of the skin and fascia of the palm and adjoining thenar eminence.

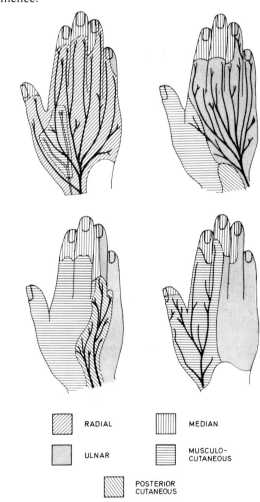

FIG. 1.50. Variation in the pattern of the cutaneous nerves to dorsum of the hand. From Grant, J. C. B. (1962) *An Atlas of Anatomy*. London, Baillière.

The palmar digital branches

The palmar digital branches arise near the distal border of the flexor retinaculum. Usually there are: one *proper digital nerve* to the radial side of the index and three *common digital nerves* which more distally divide into proper digital nerves to both sides of the thumb (p. 51), to the adjacent sides of the index and long fingers and to the radial side of the ring finger. The dorsal branches of these nerves supply the distal halves of the fingers.

Motor innervation

The *muscular* branches to the intrinsic muscles of the hand are derived from the ventral ramus of the first thoracic nerve with a variable contribution from that of the eighth cervical.

Like cutaneous nerves the muscular branches conduct many afferent proprioceptive fibres from the joints, tendons and muscles and also contain postganglionic sympathetic fibres.

Nerve supply to the muscles of the hand is shared between the ulnar and median nerves; many variations of the average pattern described below and innervation solely by ulnar or by median nerve have been reported ('all median' and 'all ulnar' hand).

Ulnar nerve

Ulnar nerve (C8, T1) often receives a contribution from C7 either through the lateral cord or through the lateral root of the median nerve. It follows the course of the axillary and brachial arteries as far down as the middle of the upper arm, where it deviates from the artery by piercing the medial intermuscular septum. In a considerable number of people [43] the nerve passes through an arcade and between the internal brachial ligament of Struthers and the medial intermuscular septum, see also p. 402. The nerve reaches the posterior aspect of the medial humeral epicondyle; it passes into the cubital tunnel between the two heads of the flexor carpi ulnaris, lying on the medial collateral ligament of the elbow joint beneath a fascial band which bridges the distal part of the gap between the two heads (p. 402). In the forearm it is deep to the flexor carpi ulnaris and lies on the flexor digitorum profundus, pierces the deep fascia just proxi-

mal to the flexor retinaculum, passes superficial to it, enclosed in Guyon's tunnel (see Fig. 1.19), and enters the hand between the pisiform medially and the hook of the hamate laterally [44]. In the hand it divides into its two terminal branches, superficial and deep. The *superficial branch* leaves the distal end of Guyon's tunnel superficial to the fibrous arch of the common origin of the abductor and flexor of digiti minimi [44], supplies palmaris brevis and divides into two palmar digital nerves already described. The *deep branch* leaves the tunnel through the interval in its floor between the fibrous arch of the common origin of the abductor and flexor [44] (which are both supplied by it) and the pisohamate ligament (deep palmar branch tunnel), frequently splits the opponens digiti minimi into two laminae (supplying both of them) and passes laterally between the proximal parts of the metacarpal bones and long flexor tendons to run with the deep palmar arch between the two heads of the adductor pollicis and ends in the first dorsal interosseous. It supplies all interossei and the two medial lumbricals. It has a considerable sensory component [45]. Occasionally a branch is given off from the deep division of the ulnar nerve distal to the pisohamate ligament, which carries contribution to the digital branch of the superficial division of the nerve destined for the little finger [46]. This rare variation may be clinically relevant.

Median nerve

The median nerve (C5, 6, 7, 8, T1) is formed by the union of two roots, one from the medial and one from the lateral cords of the brachial plexus. It descends through the arm in company with the brachial artery, enters the forearm between the two heads of the pronator teres and then under the fibrous arch of origin of flexor digitorum superficialis (it may be compressed at both sites); it continues along the midline of the forearm closely attached to the deep surface of the flexor digitorum superficialis. Shortly after entering the forearm it gives off the *anterior interosseous nerve* either from the posterior or radial aspects, which passes in relation to a connective tissue arch arising from the deep head of the pronator teres [47]. Anastomoses between the ulnar and median nerves in the forearm (Martin–Grüber), present in 10–15 per cent of people, often arise from the anterior interosseous nerve. At the wrist the median nerve lies deep to the palmaris longus tendon, between the tendons of the flexor digitorum superficialis and of the flexor carpi radialis. After giving its palmar branch (already described), it enters the carpal tunnel where it lies near the deep surface of the flexor retinaculum (see Figs. 1.41 and 1.42). At the point of emergence from the carpal tunnel (Fig. 1.51) it gives off a muscular branch which follows a *recurrent* course to supply the muscles of the thenar eminence (p. 48). Variations in the region of the carpal tunnel [48] include: accessory branches in the carpal tunnel, high division of the median nerve, accessory branches proximal to the tunnel and variations in the course of the recurrent branch, which may be given off distal to the tunnel, in the tunnel, or may pierce the flexor retinaculum.

The digital branches of the median nerve have been described. They usually supply the two lateral lumbricals.

The radial nerve (C5, 6, 7, 8, and T1)

Contributions from the C5 and T1 are small and inconstant. The nerve divides just above the elbow into its two terminal branches: superficial and deep.

The *superficial branch* takes part in supply of the dorsum of the wrist, hand and the lateral three (or two) and a half fingers.

The *deep branch* (posterior interosseous nerve) winds round the neck of the radius between the superficial and deep layers of the supinator muscle and supplies the extensor digitorum, extensor carpi ulnaris, extensor digiti minimi, abductor pollicis longus, extensor pollicis brevis and longus, extensor indicis and extensor carpi radialis brevis. The long carpal extensor is supplied by a branch from the main trunk of the radial nerve.

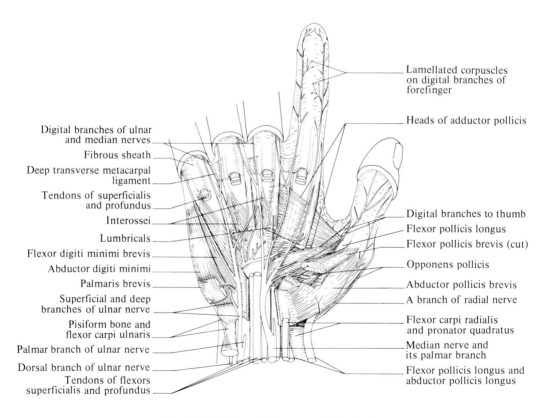

FIG. 1.51. Median and ulnar nerves in the hand.

Autonomic innervation

There are no parasympathetic fibres in the upper limb. The efferent fibres of the sympathetic system are distributed to the blood vessels, sweat glands and to the arrectores pili muscles. The preganglionic fibres are derived from the lateral horn of the upper thoracic spinal cord, and they synapse in the first thoracic and inferior cervical sympathetic ganglia, and probably in the middle cervical ganglion. From these ganglia the postganglionic fibres, transmitted mostly in the lower trunk of the brachial plexus, accompany the peripheral nerves and are distributed in their field of supply. The vessels of the upper limb have, however, a double source of sympathetic fibres as some of the postganglionic fibres are distributed directly, often by the ansa subclavia, to the subclavian artery to form a periarterial sympathetic plexus on the wall of the artery. These fibres do not extend far distally and continuation of this plexus on the arteries of the limb is provided by contributions from adjacent peripheral nerves.

BLOOD SUPPLY AND DRAINAGE OF THE HAND

The details of the blood supply of the thumb are given on p. 49.

The supply is very good, excellent anastomoses being present (Fig. 1.52). There are four transverse anastomoses which unite the radial and ulnar arteries: superficial and deep palmar arches and dorsal and palmar carpal arches (the last one is usually small). There are also longitudinal links with the anterior and posterior interosseous arteries via carpal arches. Communications exist between the arteries of the palm and dorsum through the proximal and distal perforating branches in each of the three medial intermetacarpal spaces. At the distal end of a digit, its two palmar arteries join to form an arch which gives off numerous fine branches to the pulp and the nail-bed. Palmar digital arteries are the main supply of the digit; they anastomose with small dorsal arteries.

Blood supply of the hand is derived chiefly from the distal parts of the radial and ulnar artery but also to a small degree from the interosseous arteries.

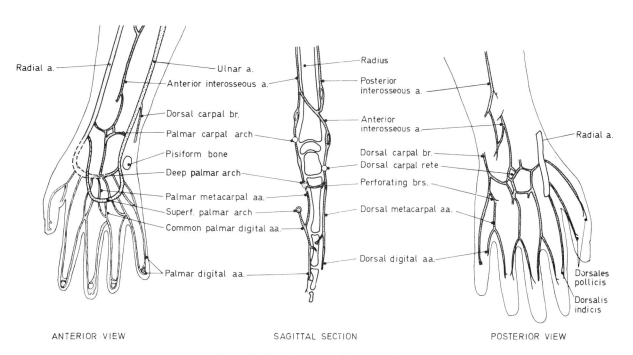

ANTERIOR VIEW   SAGITTAL SECTION   POSTERIOR VIEW

Fig. 1.52. Named arteries of the upper limb.

Radial artery

The *radial artery* (Fig. 1.52) runs down the forearm to the lateral aspect of the wrist, where it curves round to the back of the hand before passing anteriorly between the two heads of the first dorsal interosseous muscle through the first intermetacarpal space. Entering the palm between the two heads of the adductor pollicis it ends by anastomosing with the deep branch of the ulnar artery to form the deep palmar arch. In the anatomical snuff-box it lies superficial to the radial collateral ligament, scaphoid and trapezium. It may pass occasionally superficial to the extensor tendons. Its palmar branches are: palmar carpal, a variable superficial palmar which may take part in formation of the superficial palmar arch, and branches to the thumb (p. 49). The dorsal branches are two to the thumb and one to the radial side of the index (p. 50) and the dorsal carpal branch given off at the side of the distal part of the carpus to the dorsal carpal rete.

Ulnar artery

The *ulnar artery* (Fig. 1.52) accompanied by two venae comitantes lies to the radial side of the ulnar nerve above the wrist; it enters Guyon's canal superficially to the flexor retinaculum and ends at the radial side of the pisiform by dividing into its deep palmar branch and the superficial palmar arch. It gives palmar and dorsal carpal branches which join the respective carpal arches. The anterior and posterior interosseous arteries, derived from the ulnar, complete the blood supply of the hand by their contribution to the hand anastomoses (Fig. 1.52). The anterior interosseous artery gives off a long, slender, usually small calibre median artery, which however may be quite large and end as the digital arteries or by joining the superficial palmar arch. The *deep palmar branch* leaves Guyon's tunnel through its floor in company of the deep branch of the ulnar nerve, between the pisohamate ligament and the fibrous arch of origin of the abductor and short flexor of the little finger.

Superficial palmar arch

The *superficial palmar arch* is the main branch of the ulnar artery in the hand. Accompanied by two veins it lies immediately dorsal to the palmaris brevis and to the palmar aponeurosis, in front of the branches of the median nerve and the long flexor tendons. The arch is often incomplete (Fig. 1.53) and its radial component is variable. The main branches of the arch are: the palmar digital artery to the medial side of the little finger and three common palmar digital arteries which divide into proper digital branches for the adjacent sides of the four fingers. At first the arteries are anterior to the digital nerves, but near the webs are on a slightly dorsal plane to them; on the sides of the fingers they lie behind the corresponding digital nerves and in this position they give off dorsal branches which anastomose with the dorsal digital arteries. At the level of the metacarpal heads each common palmar digital artery is joined by a palmar metacarpal artery from the deep palmar arch and by a distal perforating branch from the dorsal metacarpal artery.

Deep palmar arch

The *deep palmar arch* is the radial artery continued into the palm, where it anastomoses with the deep branch of the ulnar artery. It lies deep to the long flexor tendons and their synovial sheaths at the level just distal to the metacarpal bases. It gives branches to the thumb, radialis indicis and also to three palmar metacarpal arteries which pass distally to join the common palmar digital arteries. Three small proximal perforating branches join the dorsal metacarpal arteries and small recurrent branches run to the palmar carpal arch. In this way the radial and ulnar arteries, palmar carpal arch, palmar digital arteries and dorsal metacarpal branches of the dorsal carpal arch are all interconnected.

Dorsal carpal arch

The *dorsal carpal arch* lies at the back of the wrist at the level of the midcarpal joint. It is formed by the dorsal carpal branches of the radial and ulnar arteries and the terminal branches of the anterior and posterior interosseous arteries (Fig. 1.52). It gives off a dorsal digital artery to the ulnar border of the little finger and three dorsal metacarpal arteries which receive proximal and distal perforating branches from the palm. Each dorsal metacarpal artery divides at the webs between the

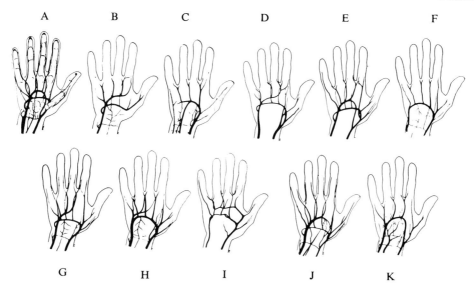

FIG. 1.53. The commoner variation of the arterial supply to the hand. After Strickland, B. and Urquhart, W., Digital Arteriography. *British Journal of Radiology*, **36**, 465, 1963. (A) Usual normal pattern. (B) Absent radial artery. (C) Ulnar artery absent or small. (D) Absent radialis indicis and princeps pollicis replaced by branch from superficial arch or superficial palmar artery. (E) As in (D) replaced by first dorsal digital artery. (F) Absent superficial arch. (G) Superficial arch incomplete as superficial palmar artery ends in thenar muscles. (H) Ulnar artery ends in deep arch with small superficial branch. Main supply to fingers from deep arch. (I) Superficial arch formed by branches from the radialis indicis, ulnar artery ending in deep arch. (J) Superficial arch larger than deep. The arch may be completed by the superficial palmar artery, the radialis indicis or the princeps pollicis, or the median artery. (K) Absent deep arch replaced by branches from the superficial arch, the anterior carpal arch or the perforating branches from the dorsal metacarpal arteries. From *The Hand*, **4**, 8, 1972.

fingers into two dorsal digital arteries for the adjacent sides of the four fingers; these arteries do not extend far beyond the proximal interphalangeal joints.

The *palmar carpal arch* lies deep to the flexor tendons, in front of the lower end of the radius and the proximal carpus. It is formed by the union of the palmar carpal branches of the radial and ulnar arteries. It is joined by twigs of the anterior interosseous artery and recurrent branches from the deep palmar arch.

Veins of the hand

The veins of the hand can be divided into superficial ones which lie outside the deep fascia and the deep veins found inside it. The *deep veins* are in pairs and accompany the arteries; they possess valves and lie on each side of the artery communicating across it by numerous anastomoses. The *superficial veins* (Fig. 1.54) are inconspicuous in the palm as most of the venous drainage of the hand occurs through the dorsal route. Paired palmar digital veins, which communicate with each other across the surface of the digit drain a fine plexus in the superficial layers. Most of the drainage is directed towards the dorsal digital veins and particularly through the intercapitular veins (Fig. 1.54b). The dorsal digital veins, one on each side, anastomosing freely with each other and with the palmar veins, join at about the level of the metacarpal heads to form the dorsal metacarpal veins. Their pattern is extremely variable as they form the dorsal venous network (Fig. 1.54b) on the back of the hand. The cephalic vein issues from the radial end of this network and the basilic vein arises from the ulnar end. Thus most of the venous return from the palm goes to the dorsum, particularly through the intercapitular veins between the heads of the metacarpal bones and around the margins of the hand.

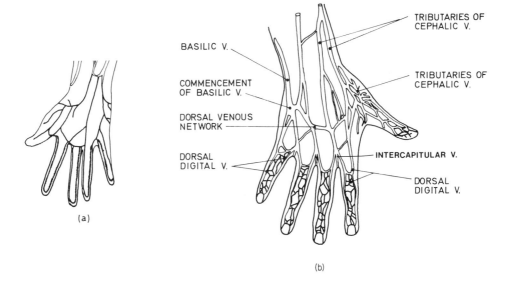

FIG. 1.54. (a) Superficial veins on flexor aspect of right hand. (b) Superficial veins on dorsum of hand and digits.

Lymph drainage of the hand

The collecting system is arranged in superficial or sub-cutaneous and deep layers, which remain practically separate until the main trunks of the superficial set pierce the deep fascia in the upper arm. The palmar surface of the digits and the palm itself (Fig. 1.55) have a rich plexus of *superficial lymphatics*. Most of these drain into the vessels of the dorsum around the sides of the digits, margins of the palm and through the interdigital clefts. In their further course they accompany the main superficial veins. The *deep lymphatics* follow main neurovascular bundles, but are less numerous than the superficial ones. Most of the lymph from the upper limb passes into the lateral group of the axillary nodes.

Mechanism of fluid return

The main bulk of the centripetal flow of the fluid passes from the dorsal aspect of the hand through the venous and lymphatic channels of the limb. Compression of these channels by the active contractions of the muscles within the fascial compartments creates a pumping action which maintains this backflow, its direction being determined by the valves in the vessels. In the upper limb this mechanism is particularly active in the axilla and hand. In the hand, the veins can be emptied by repeated clenching of the fist; the venous blood and lymph are squeezed into the dorsal region of the hand where they can accumulate since the connective tissue is loose and mobile on the back of the hand. Interference with normal movement of the shoulder and hand therefore causes swelling. As there is just enough skin on the hand, any accumulation of fluid on the dorsum makes the skin tighter, thus impairing the range of flexion, making the pump mechanism of the hand less efficient, and so creating a vicious circle. It is important to realise that immobilization of the shoulder and the hand has its inherent risks and if possible in injury or disease one or both of these regions should be kept mobile.

THUMB

The importance of the thumb lies in its being capable to oppose not only to the pulps of the other digits but also to be brought into functional contact with the other surfaces of the fingers and with a part of the palm. It is of great importance in many varieties of pre-hension and manipulation enhancing very considerably

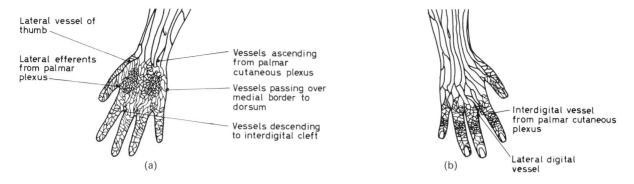

FIG. 1.55. Superficial lymph vessels of (a) anterior and, (b) posterior surface.

their accuracy and precision. The thumb possesses a great mobility but at the same time can be securely stabilized in an optimal position for any given action. It is of advantage to consider the bony and articular chain of the thumb as one functional unit not only with regard to range of movement in any particular joint but also with regard to the arrangement of the connective and muscular tissues. Absence of the thumb is often considered to constitute almost a 50 per cent disability as far as the whole hand is concerned. Even if the thumb is present but affected by a severe contracture of the first web the hand is disabled to a very great extent.

The first metacarpal is tethered to the second by skin and fasciae covering the walls of the first intermetacarpal interval and surrounding the first metacarpal, which cannot move away from the second metacarpal further than the intermetacarpal structures allow (normally the angle between the first and second metacarpals in full abduction is about 40°). The muscles which connect the first metacarpal to its partners have the same effect. Here it is important to remember that the muscle is not composed only of muscle fibres but also contains a considerable amount of connective tissue which may undergo contracture.

The skin of the first web presents tension lines which on the dorsal aspect are arranged in a criss-cross network, while on the palmar aspect the tension lines converge from the radial longitudinal palmar crease ('skin joint') onto the metacarpophalangeal flexion crease of the thumb. These converging lines run at approximately right angles to the flexion creases and are thought to represent the direction in which the local skin is

least extensible. This may be related to the direction in which the contents of the web are displaced during power grip in order to avoid their encroachment towards the flexion creases which would diminish freedom of flexion at the joints. The skin of the palmar aspect of the first web is not fixed to the underlying structures like that of the hypothenar region.

The fasciae of the first web

The superficial fascia encases the first intermetacarpal interval deep to the skin and is adherent to the dorsum of the first metacarpal. In the distal and ulnar part of the thenar region the fatty content of this layer is increased, forming together with the metacarpophalangeal, fingerweb and hypothenar fatty pads a gripping system surrounding the central area of the palm. In some individuals there may be a continuation of the superficial transverse ligament of the palm (see Fig. 1.12) for a variable distance into the margin of the first web. In other cases a band of fibres may be seen extending into the radial part of the first web margin from the region of the metacarpophalangeal flexion crease of the thumb. On the dorsum the superficial fascia consists of a double layer of superficial fat and deeper fibrous layer which is connected to the deeper fascia by loose areolar tissue.

On the dorsum of the first web the two layers of the deep fascia present over the rest of the metacarpal bones, namely supratendinous and infratendinous layers, fuse together deep to the superficial fascia of the web.

Distally they fuse with the epimysium situated in the interval between the adductor pollicis and the first dorsal interosseous and then continue into the deep palmar fascia of the thenar eminence. This thenar fascia in its turn is continuous with the radial edge of the palmar aponeurosis. On the dorsum of the first metacarpal the deep fascia splits to enclose the extensor tendons, the deep layer being attached to the bone. Oblique septum, extending from the radial margin of the palmar aponeurosis to the third metacarpal, is found in most cases to be rather frail and insignificant. In some hands there is a contribution from the deep transverse layer of the palmar aponeurosis extending for a variable distance into the thenar fascia (Fig. 32.1). In some cases the longitudinal slip of the superficial layer of the palmar aponeurosis extends into the thenar fascia from the tendon of the palmaris longus (Fig. 32.1). In both instances these extensions fade away inside the thenar fascia without any attachment to the deeper structures. There are no special fascial or aponeurotic sheets inside the first intermetacarpal interval except for the epimysia covering the muscles; these epimysia may be considerably thickened in pathological conditions like the rest of the connective tissue of the muscle. In broad, well-muscled hands there may be a considerable area of the deep surface of the palmar aponeurosis, just distal to the flexor retinaculum, which gives rise to the strong aponeurotic fibres of origin of flexor pollicis brevis.

Other fasciae of the thumb

The arrangement of fasciae in the rest of the thumb presents some differences from those of the fingers. The gripping fat pads are situated over the palmar aspect of the proximal phalanx and over the proximal third of the distal phalanx. These pads are not as thick as in the fingers and in the distal phalanx the pad has an oval shape and is situated transversely just distal to the interphalangeal flexion crease. The oblique tension lines extend at the side of the distal phalanx towards the nail walls. In this position they overlie the interosseous ligament extending from the lateral tubercle of the base of the distal phalanx to the lateral aspect of the ungual tuberosity (Fig. 1.56). This tough band can be considered as a continuation of the digital ligaments

(corresponding to Cleland's and Grayson's ligaments in the fingers, p. 472) present along the proximal phalanx, both bands providing mechanical support for the palmar pads of the thumb. The palmar aspect of the pulp of the thumb in its distal two thirds is similar in structure to the terminal pads of the fingers but is more extensive. Numerous septa fix the skin of the pad to the underlying structures and thus a very great number of the sensory endings are placed favourably for reception of the tactile stimuli. The ulnar half of the terminal pulp of the thumb is more frequently used as it meets the radial halves of the terminal pads of the fingers during opposition.

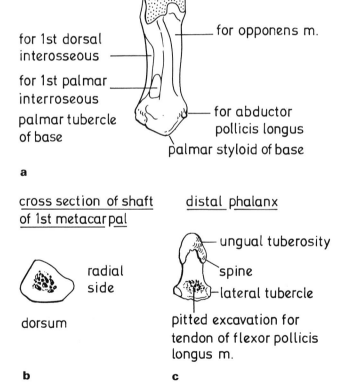

Fig. 1.56. Bones of right thumb. (a) Palmar aspect of the first metacarpal. (b) Cross-section of the shaft of the first metacarpal. (c) Palmar aspect of the distal phalanx.

The deep fascia of the palmar aspect of the thumb is organized for the retention of the tendon of the flexor pollicis longus. The fibrous sheath for this tendon commences at the level of the base of the proximal phalanx and extends over the base of the distal phalanx. It is strong and anular with many oblique fibres opposite the shaft of the proximal phalanx (p. 10) but weaker and more cruciform opposite the joint. The synovial sheath of this tendon is very much longer than the fibrous one as it extends from the distal phalanx as far proximally as the lower forearm.

The bones of the thumb

Trapezium

The trapezium presents four articular surfaces for: (1) first metacarpal, (2) second metacarpal, (3) trapezoid and (4) scaphoid. The last three are slightly concave uniform planes, while the first one is of a typical saddle-shaped variety (Fig. 1.57). On the anteromedial surface of the bone a deep groove for the tendon of the flexor carpi radialis is flanked by two prominent lips to which the flexor retinaculum is attached. The radial lip is called the crest of trapezium and its enlarged distal end is the tubercle of trapezium. The posterior surface of the bone shows two dorsal tubercles, radial (more prominent) and ulnar. Between the two the surface of the bone gives attachment to the lateral ligament of the wrist and supports the radial artery.

First metacarpal

The first metacarpal is shorter than the others and its shaft is broader and flatter. It is also more mobile than the others and is separated from them by a wide first intermetacarpal interval. Its dorsal surface faces in a more lateral direction than the others. The *base* shows a prominent palmar tubercle just distal to a projecting lip of the palmar styloid process (Fig. 1.56). At the opposite side of the base a less prominent dorsal styloid is felt. Between the two, on the radial aspect of the base the tendon of the abductor pollicis longus muscle is attached. The *shaft* is almost as broad as the base and its dorsal surface is only very slightly rounded. The cross-section of the shaft is triangular. The palmar aspect

of the shaft presents a blunt margin which divides the surface into two strips: a larger radial one to which the opponens muscle is attached, and a medial one for one of the heads of the first dorsal interosseous muscle. The *head* of the first metacarpal is wide and has the usual markings for attachment of the collateral ligaments. The palmar surface of the head is not as extensive as that in the other metacarpal bones.

Phalanges

The phalanges of the thumb are similar to the proximal and distal phalanges of the fingers but are shorter and broader. The distal tuberosity of the distal phalanx of the thumb provides support for the broad nail; the phalanx is particularly thick and rough on the palmar surface for the attachment of the fibrofatty terminal pad of the thumb. The distal phalanx has a blunt, wide and projecting dorsal margin at the base for the attachment of the extensor apparatus, while the proximal third of

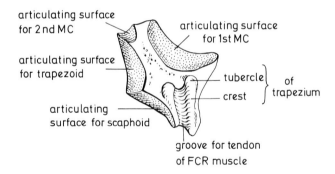

palmar view (anteromedial)

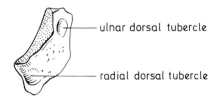

dorsal view

FIG. 1.57. Right trapezium.

the palmar surface consists of a pitted and rough excavation for the attachment of the tendon of the flexor pollicis longus.

The joints of the thumb

The three joints of the thumb (carpometacarpal – CMC, metacarpophalangeal – MP and interphalangeal – IP) can be regarded as one functional unit, as there is a considerable variation in the contribution which each joint makes to the total movement in different subjects. Although the three joints which the trapezium makes with the second metacarpal, trapezoid and scaphoid do not usually contribute to a great extent to the final range of the thumb movements, their consideration may be important in pathological conditions in which the stresses are transmitted through the trapezium more proximally.

Carpometacarpal joint of the thumb

The detailed description of this joint has been given elsewhere [28, 29] and can be summarized as follows. The joint is usually considered to be of a saddle variety in which the two saddles fit recriprocally (Fig. 1.58b). However, the movement in this joint would be easier to visualize if the metacarpal saddle was applied by its underside to the upper surface of the trapezial saddle pommel to pommel and cantle to cantle (Figs. 1.58c and 1.59).

The two sellar surfaces of the joint show many matching features, but also some differences which may be important in the mechanism of the thumb movements.

The groove of the metacarpal surface, which corresponds to the ridge of the trapezial surface, is longer but has the same general direction as the ridge. However, the radius of curvature in the plane of the ridge is smaller in the metacarpal than in the trapezium. The greater length of the metacarpal groove is due to extension of the articular cartilage on to the anterolateral and posteromedial aspects of the metacarpal base. In abduction the most convex part of the trapezial ridge is withdrawn from the most concave part of the metacarpal groove and the flatter anterolateral surfaces of both saddles are free to slide on each other (Fig. 1.59c). In the adducted position the deepest part of the metacarpal concavity fits over the most convex part of the trapezial

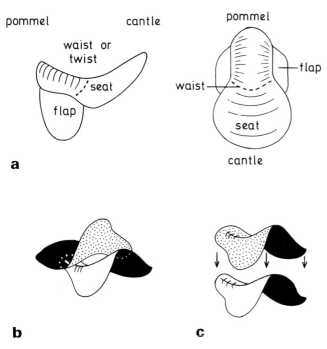

FIG. 1.58. Carpometacarpal joint. (a) Parts of the saddle, (b) and (c) fit of the trapezial and metacarpal saddles.

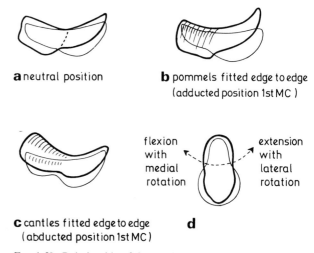

FIG. 1.59. Relationship of the saddles in movements at the joint.

ridge (Fig. 1.59b), the range of movement between the two surfaces becoming limited; thus the position of adduction is the most stable.

The capsule of the joint has considerable slack and the articular surfaces can be distracted by as much as 3 mm when the muscles and tendons are removed. The dissection of the ligaments of the joint in the fresh amputation specimen shows that most of them are disposed obliquely (for details see Fig. 1.60). It would appear that coaptation of the articular surfaces in this joint depends to a great extent on the presence of muscles and tendons. Their removal in fresh amputation specimens allows for distension of the joint with an opaque medium (Fig. 1.61) which is difficult otherwise. There is a definite slackness of the synovial lining on coaptation; it can be stretched on distraction of surfaces and produces a roll-like collar when the distracting force is removed. This excess of the lining can be seen in formalin-fixed specimens as definite folds and fringes which during life are probably neither permanent nor constant in position.

Abduction and adduction occur along the line of the

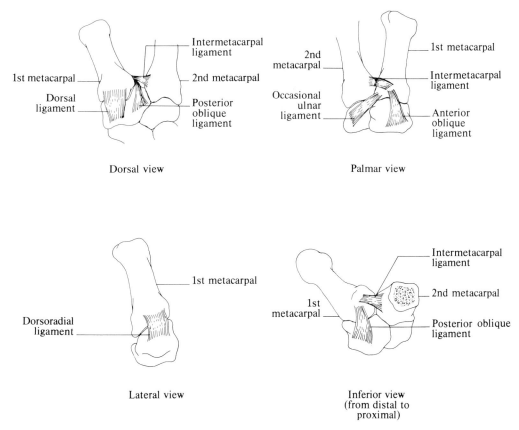

FIG. 1.60. Ligaments of carpometacarpal joint of thumb.
Dorsal ligament extends from the dorsal radial tubercle of the trapezium to the dorsal styloid and adjacent margin of the first metacarpal. *Dorsoradial ligament* is continuous with the previous one (they may be considered one ligament). It is attached to the radial margins of the base of the first metacarpal and of the trapezium. *Anterior oblique ligament* extends from the palmar tubercle of the trapezium to the palmar tubercle of the first metacarpal. *Posterior oblique ligament* is attached to the ulnar dorsal tubercle of the trapezium and to the palmar tubercle of the first metacarpal. The *intermetacarpal ligament* extends from the lateral aspect of the base of the second metacarpal to the palmar tubercle of the first metacarpal.
Inconstant *ulnar ligament* extends from the distal margin of the flexor retinaculum to the palmar tubercle of the base of the first metacarpal.

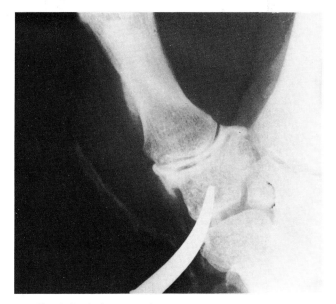

FIG. 1.61. Arthrogram of carpometacarpal joint of thumb.

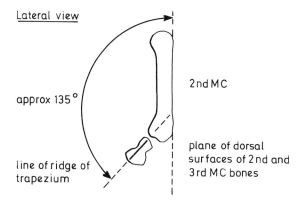

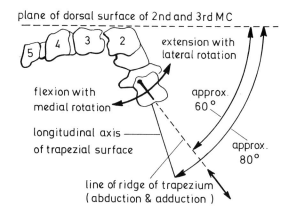

FIG. 1.62. Angles of orientation of the trapezium to the fixed axis of the hand.

ridge of the trapezial surface and as this ridge is concave from one end to the other, the base of the metacarpal moves in the opposite direction to its head (for example in abduction the base moves towards the second metacarpal while the head moves away from it). The axis of these movements changes along the line of the ridge of the trapezial surface as it is curved anteromedially, but the approximate plane in which they occur is about 60° anterolateral to the plane of the dorsal surfaces of the second and third metacarpal bones (Fig. 1.62).

The first metacarpal moves in a curved path parallel to the groove of the trapezial surface and thus flexion is of necessity accompanied by medial rotation and extension by lateral rotation (Fig. 1.62). The movements of flexion and extension are limited by the capsule and ligaments of the joint at the extremes of their range with the result that no point on the base of the first metacarpal can traverse the whole length of the trapezial groove. Further rotation is added by riding up of the first metacarpal on the trapezium, a movement which is allowed by the loose capsule. These two mechanisms (travel in the trapezial groove and riding up of the surfaces) are combined during movements of the thumb but it is not clear whether they can occur simultaneously at any point in the trapezial groove or whether the

second mechanism occurs only at the two ends of the trapezial groove.

Metacarpophalangeal joint of the thumb

This joint is formed by a slightly concave surface of the base of the proximal phalanx and the articular surface of the head of the first metacarpal which is very much less rounded and less extensive, particularly on its palmar aspect, than the heads of other metacarpal bones (Fig. 1.63). This joint also differs from the other MP joints by the presence of the two constant sesamoids (radial and ulnar) in the palmar plate which articulate with the head of the first metacarpal. The collateral ligaments are under the cover of the dorsal expansion

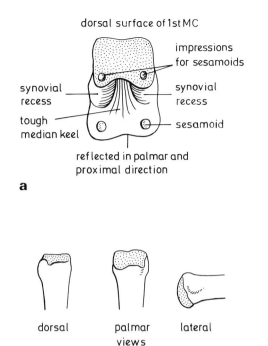

dorsal surface of 1st MC

impressions for sesamoids

synovial recess

synovial recess

tough median keel

sesamoid

reflected in palmar and proximal direction

a

dorsal

palmar views

lateral

b

FIG. 1.63. (a) Metacarpophalangeal joint of the thumb, (b) Articular surface of the head of the first metacarpal.

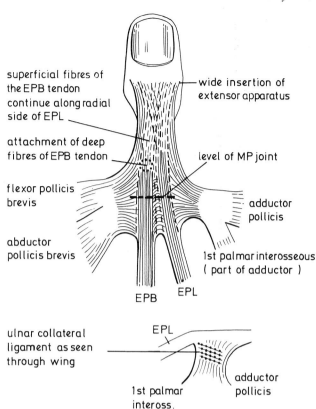

superficial fibres of the EPB tendon continue along radial side of EPL

wide insertion of extensor apparatus

attachment of deep fibres of EPB tendon

level of MP joint

flexor pollicis brevis

adductor pollicis

abductor pollicis brevis

1st palmar interosseous (part of adductor)

EPB

EPL

ulnar collateral ligament as seen through wing

EPL

1st palmar inteross.

adductor pollicis

FIG. 1.64. Extensor expansion of the thumb.

of the thumb and as the ulnar wing of the expansion is narrower than the radial (Fig. 1.64) it provides less protection for the ulnar collateral ligament which, if ruptured or detached by injury, may slip over the outer surface of the expansion, preventing reduction and repair. The fan-shaped fibres of the collateral aspect of the capsule just proximal to the bands of the collateral ligaments are attached to the margins of the palmar plate and are strongly fixed to the sesamoids, joined here by the part of the insertion of the short muscles of the thumb. The tendon of the flexor pollicis longus lies between the sesamoids on its way to the proximal entrance to the flexor fibrous sheath. As in other MP joints the palmar plate is strongly attached to the proximal phalanx but only loosely to the neck of the first metacarpal.

The synovial arrangement of this joint reflects considerable variation in its structure. The dorsal pouch is on average about 5 mm long and the palmar pouch is not much longer. There is hardly any bone at the side of the head of the metacarpal which is covered by the synovial membrane except on the ulnar aspect where a small synovial recess is present. There is also a small recess extending distally over the dorsum of the base of the proximal phalanx.

The variations in structure go hand in hand with great individual differences in mobility of the joint. In some people the joint is almost immobile while in others it approaches the mobility of a ball-and-socket joint. On average, flexion and extension are about 50–60° while hyperextension may be about 5–10° although some people exhibit here almost a 'double joint'. Abduction and adduction which may vary from 0–20° are usually associated with rotation which may reach 20° and may contribute considerably to the movement of opposition.

Interphalangeal joint of the thumb

This is a massive hinge in which wide and strong attachments of the extensor and flexor tendons to the distal phalanx surround the joint interval from one collateral ligament to the other. The palmar plate may contain sesamoids in many people and the joint itself shows considerable variation in structure. The dorsal synovial pouch may measure 10 mm with a fringe hanging down into the joint; in other cases the pouch may be 5 mm or even less. The palmar synovial pouch shows the same degree of variation, in some cases having an additional palmar recess extending distally for 2 or 3 mm.

The movements in this joint are essentially flexion and extension which may reach 90° (average about 80°). Hyperextension on average is about 10° but may reach more in people who use the thumb habitually for exerting pressure, e.g. glaziers, potters, sculptors.

The muscles of the thumb

The terminology of the thumb muscles more than anywhere else reflects only very partially and imperfectly their function and the contribution which they make to the coordination and balance evident in almost every movement of this very mobile digit. The muscles of the thumb can be compared to the stays attached to a mobile articulated mast. They are in a state of balance from which movements are carried out by contraction of some and relaxation of others. This complexity is well reflected in an extensive representation of the thumb in the brain.

The long muscles and their tendons, which cross more than one joint of the thumb, have multiple actions and because most of the short muscles of the thumb have multiple insertions (e.g. into the lateral tubercle of the base of the proximal phalanx, into the sesamoid of the palmar plate, into the dorsal expansion of the thumb – all from one muscle) they can also act on many joints, the resulting action depending upon which set of the antagonists is contracting or relaxing, e.g. abductor pollicis brevis can flex and rotate medially the first metacarpal in the CMC joint, can flex and rotate at the MP joint and can extend at the IP joint; it can also abduct at CMC and MP joints. Owing to the configuration of the articular surfaces in the CMC joint all flexors at this joint are also medial rotators and all extensors rotate laterally. As the long extensor approaches the thumb from the medial side it can adduct it particularly in later stages of its action. The short

extensor approaches the first metacarpal from the radial side and thus can abduct it in the CMC joint. The role of the long abductor is complex and not clear owing to a very considerable variation in the manner of insertion of its tendon (into the trapezium, into extensor tendons, into the thenar muscles and the flexor retinaculum). It does not act as a stay-wire supporting a mast, but it seems that it stabilizes the lateral aspect of the CMC region. It is also a strong abductor of the wrist. As it is attached to the base of the first metacarpal quite near the joint interval, strictly speaking it cannot be considered as an abductor at the CMC joint because by pulling the base of the metacarpal laterally in the concavity of the trapezium it would move the head of the first metacarpal towards the second metacarpal. On the other hand it may pull the first metacarpal bodily as far as the loose capsule allows. It could be made a true abductor of the first metacarpal in the CMC joint if its insertion were moved more distally along the shaft of the metacarpal. Some abduction is also possible when the tendon gives a slip to the abductor pollicis brevis.

Long muscles of the thumb

Flexor pollicis longus

Flexor pollicis longus is attached deeply in the forearm to the radius and the interosseous membrane. It may have an occasional slip arising from the medial part of the coronoid process of the ulna. The muscle fibres extend along the radial side of its tendon to the level of the carpus. It may communicate with the other digital flexors. The tendon of the flexor pollicis longus enters the carpal tunnel deep to the tendon of the flexor carpi radialis and spirals round the latter near its insertion. This results in the superficial fibres of the flexor pollicis tendon having an appearance of going round both sides of the more deeply placed tendon fibres and becoming more posterior to them distally; these originally superficial tendon fibres are inserted dorsal to the deeper fibres which more distally in their course become superficial and exhibit a longitudinal palmar groove near the insertion. The tendon of the flexor pollicis longus runs between the two sesamoids of the metacarpophalangeal joint of the thumb and enters the fibrous flexor sheath at the base of the proximal phalanx. The synovial sheath of this tendon extends proximally into the lower forearm (Fig. 1.43). It communicates with the sheath of the fingers with the frequency given from 50 to 85 per cent. The tendon has a well developed vinculum breve. The tendon is inserted into the deep excavation on the palmar aspect of the base of the distal phalanx (Fig. 1.56). The nerve supply of this muscle is derived from the anterior interosseous nerve (C8, T1). It is the only flexor of the interphalangeal joint of the thumb. It positions the distal phalanx of the thumb in varying degrees of flexion and thus controls the type of the pinch (e.g. pincers or pliers-like). It assists also in flexion of the remaining joints of the thumb and also of the wrist.

Abductor pollicis longus

Abductor pollicis longus is attached deeply in the forearm to the dorsal aspects of the radius, ulna and intervening interosseous membrane. It becomes superficial in the distal forearm and together with the tendon of the extensor pollicis brevis crosses the tendons of the carpal radial extensors of the wrist; it occupies the most lateral compartment deep to the extensor retinaculum in a common synovial sheath with the tendon of the short extensor of the thumb. It crosses the radial artery superficially and becomes attached (sometimes by several slips) to the principal point of its insertion, the lateral side of the base of the first metacarpal. Its other attachments and its action have been already discussed. It is an important muscle in positioning and stabilizing the thumb both in power and precision grips. Its nerve supply is derived from the seventh and eighth cervical nerves through a branch from the posterior interosseous nerve.

Extensor pollicis brevis

Extensor pollicis brevis arises from the radius and the interosseous membrane, crosses the wrist in the same compartment with the abductor pollicis longus tendon and is inserted into the dorsal aspect of the base of the proximal phalanx where it helps to replace the dorsal capsule of the metacarpophalangeal joint of the thumb. The superficial fibres of the tendon continue distally along the radial side of the tendon of the long extensor in the extensor expansion (Fig. 1:64) often reaching the base of the distal phalanx. The muscle is occasionally absent (in 5 per cent of people); it may often have multiple tendons. It may be fused with the abductor pollicis longus. Its nerve supply is derived from the seventh and eighth cervical nerves through a branch from the posterior interosseous nerve. It extends and abducts the carpometacarpal joint, extends the metacarpophalangeal and may extend the interphalangeal joint of the thumb. It also assists in flexion and abduction of the wrist.

Extensor pollicis longus

Extensor pollicis longus arises from the dorsal surfaces of the ulna and the interosseous membrane. It lies in a special compartment of the extensor retinaculum on the ulnar side of the dorsal tubercle of the radius, where it changes its direction to oblique, crosses superficially the tendons of the radial extensors of the wrist, replaces part of the dorsal capsule of the metacarpophalangeal joint and continues in the dorsal expansion of the thumb (Fig. 1.64) to be inserted widely into the dorsal aspect of the base of the distal phalanx. It derives its nerve supply from the seventh and eighth cervical nerves through a branch of the posterior interosseous nerve. It extends all joints of the thumb and rotates the first metacarpal laterally at the same time. Owing to its oblique course and side-to-side displacement of about 10 mm. it can also adduct the thumb in the late stages of its action. It assists also in extension and abduction of the wrist and in supination.

Short muscles of the thumb

First palmar interosseous muscle

First palmar interosseous muscle is a small slip which extends from the ulnar aspect of the base of the first metacarpal to the base of the proximal phalanx and the extensor expansion of the thumb. It becomes continuous with the tendon of the adductor pollicis and is regarded by many as a part of the latter. Its nerve supply comes from the first thoracic nerve through a branch from the deep part of the ulnar nerve. It assists the adductor pollicis in its actions (see below).

First dorsal interosseous muscle

First dorsal interosseous muscle. Its deep part is confined to the second digital ray, while the superficial part arises from the shafts of the first and second metacarpal bones (Fig. 1.47). Its nerve supply (T1) is from the deep branch of the ulnar nerve. It assists in adduction of the thumb.

Abductor pollicis brevis

Abductor pollicis brevis is the most superficial muscle of

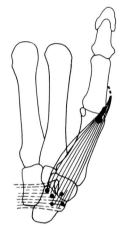

abductor pollicis brevis

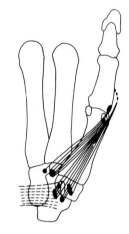

flexor pollicis brevis

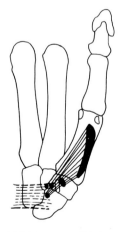

opponens pollicis

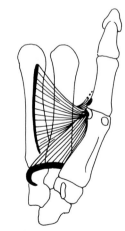

adductor pollicis

Fig. 1.65. Short muscles of the thumb (see text).

the thenar group. It arises from the flexor retinaculum, scaphoid, trapezium and by a frequent slip from the tendon of the abductor pollicis longus and also from palmaris longus. It is inserted into the lateral tubercle of the radial side of the base of the proximal phalanx, into the radial sesamoid of the metacarpophalangeal joint and into the extensor expansion of the thumb (Figs 1.64 and 1.65). It may have a double muscle belly. The recurrent branch of the median nerve supplies it with fibres derived from the first thoracic nerve. It abducts the thumb both in the carpometacarpal and metacarpophalangeal joints; when the thumb is fully abducted the angle between the first metacarpal and the proximal phalanx may reach 30°. It assists also in flexion and medial rotation of the carpometacarpal and meta-carpophalangeal joints. Through its wide insertion into the extensor expansion of the thumb it assists in extension of the interphalangeal joint of the thumb.

Opponens pollicis

Opponens pollicis lies deep to the abductor pollicis brevis, being overlapped by its proximal and radial part. It arises from the flexor retinaculum and trapezium (Fig. 1.65) and is attached to the radial half of the shaft of the first metacarpal, some fibres reaching the palmar aspect of the metacarpophalangeal joint. The nerve supply comes from the first thoracic nerve through the recurrent branch of the median. It is most active during abduction and medial rotation of the first metacarpal in the carpo-metacarpal joint. It assists the flexor pollicis brevis when opposing the ulnar fingers and it may also assist the adductor pollicis in the final stages of opposition to the radial fingers.

Flexor pollicis brevis

Flexor pollicis brevis may be partly fused with the opponens or may have three heads. Usually there are two (Fig. 1.65): (1) superficial head, arising from the flexor retinaculum, trapezium and the sheath of the flexor carpi radialis and occasionally from the deep aspect of the palmar aponeurosis, and (2) deep head which arises from the capitate and trapezoid where it is continuous with the origin of the oblique head of the adductor pollicis. The two heads unite and are inserted into the lateral tubercle of the radial side of the base of the proximal phalanx, into the radial sesamoid of the meta-carpophalangeal joint and into the extensor expansion of the thumb (Fig. 1.64). The nerve supply is from the first thoracic nerve; it may reach the muscle through the recurrent branch of the median, through the deep branch of the ulnar nerve or through both. The muscle flexes and rotates medially the first metacarpal at the carpometacarpal joint, assists in flexion, medial rotation and abduction at the metacarpophalangeal joint and through the extensor expansion assists in extension of the interphalangeal joint.

Adductor pollicis

Adductor pollicis arises by two heads (Fig. 1.65): (1) oblique head from the sheath of the flexor carpi radialis, bases of second, third and fourth metacarpal bones, from the trapezoid and capitate bones; and (2) transverse head from the shaft of the third metacarpal. It is inserted into the tubercle on the ulnar side of the base of the proximal phalanx, into the ulnar sesamoid of the metacarpophalangeal joint and into the extensor expansion of the thumb (Fig. 1.64). The nerve supply is from the eighth cervical and first thoracic nerves through the deep branch of the ulnar nerve. The muscle adducts the thumb into the plane of the palm; it is important in strong pinch acting together with another strong muscle, i.e. flexor pollicis longus in the late stages of opposition. Owing to the insertion into the extensor expansion it assists in extension at the interphalangeal joint of the thumb; it can also assist in adduction and lateral rotation at the metacarpophalangeal joint.

The complexity of arrangement of the muscles of the thumb is particularly well illustrated by the important movement of *opposition*. In this movement the thumb as a whole is abducted at first, then flexed and medially rotated; finally adduction brings the terminal part of the thumb into contact with the distal pulp of a finger. All joints and most of the muscles of the thumb are involved in this composite movement, some of the muscles contracting to act as stabilizers, some as the prime movers, while the reciprocally innervated antagonists either relax to exert an important control of fine adjustment by graded paying-out or contract to prevent that part of the action of the prime movers which is not wanted at the moment. It is thus important to think of any muscle of the thumb as a member of a functional group associated at any given time with other muscles for a specific purpose and not as an individual separate unit.

Blood supply of the thumb

There is a considerable variability of the arteries of the thumb [30]. Most of the thenar muscles are supplied by the superficial palmar branch of the radial artery; this branch may continue its course to complete the superficial palmar arch or it may end in the substance of the muscles.

The proper digital arteries of the thumb are well developed only on the palmar aspect; the dorsal arteries are very small except in rare cases; they are usually distributed only as far as the tissues related to the proximal phalanx. Before the radial artery reaches the tendon of the extensor pollicis longus it usually gives a small dorsal digital artery to the radial border of the thumb and just before it disappears between the two heads of the first dorsal interosseous muscle, gives a dorsal branch to the ulnar side of the thumb (Fig. 1.66a).

The ulnar and radial palmar digital arteries run along the corresponding margins of the thumb and anastomose with each other transversely deep to the tendon sheath of the flexor pollicis longus about the midpoint of the shaft of the proximal phalanx. They also anastomose to form an arch across the distal phalanx; this arch provides a fine network of the vessels which enter the distal pulp of the thumb and the bed of the nail. The palmar digital arteries also send dorsal branches to the more distal part of the thumb.

The palmar digital arteries may be derived from: (1) princeps pollicis artery, which is the most common source of their origin, (2) superficial palmar arch and (3) dorsal metacarpal artery of the thumb.

Princeps pollicis artery (Fig. 1.66c) (also called the first palmar metacarpal) is one of the terminal branches of the radial artery as it passes through the adductor pollicis muscle. It runs distally along the ulnar aspect of the palmar surface of the shaft of the first meta-carpal, often under cover of the first palmar interosseous muscle, to the interval between the adductor and flexor pollicis brevis. It gives two circumflex perforating branches which run dorsally around the radial and ulnar

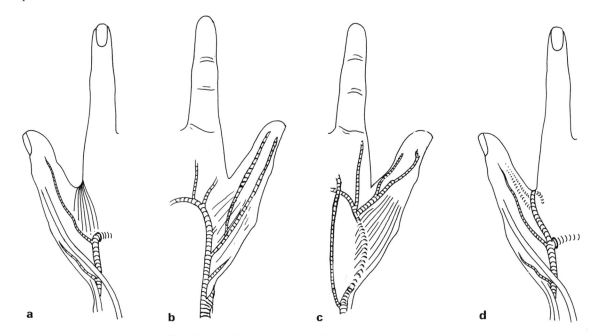

FIG. 1.66. Variations in blood supply to the thumb. (For explanation see text.)

sides of the neck of the first metacarpal to anastomose with the dorsal digital arteries. Princeps pollicis artery divides into its two terminal branches, namely palmar digital arteries, under cover of the tendon of the flexor pollicis longus; these branches become superficial on each side of the tendon, the radial branch passing behind the tendon to take up its position dorsal to the radial digital nerve. The size of the princeps pollicis artery varies considerably; sometimes it is very small and may be replaced to a great extent by an unusually well developed dorsal metacarpal artery of the thumb (see below).

In about 30 per cent of people the palmar digital arteries of the thumb arise from a branch or branches of the *superficial palmar arch*, the princeps pollicis being quite small (Fig. 1.66b).

In about 20 per cent of people the *dorsal metacarpal artery* of the thumb (Fig. 1.66d) arises from the radial artery before the latter passes between the heads of the first dorsal interosseous muscle and runs along the dorsal surface of the muscle to pass anteriorly around the distal margin of the adductor pollicis to join the palmar arteries. This artery may be the principal source of the

blood supply to the thumb and is vulnerable in wounds or procedures involving the dorsum of the first web [31].

Venous drainage of the thumb

The dorsal superficial veins are larger than those on the palmar aspect; they lie along the margins of the back of the thumb and are connected by irregular venous arches. There is usually a well developed perforating vein on the dorsum of the proximal part of the first web and there are several perforating palmar veins just proximal to the base of the thenar eminence. The deep veins accompany the arteries. They are relatively small and in some people may take the form of a fine venous network running along the neurovascular plane of the digit.

Lymph drainage of the thumb

The cutaneous plexus is well developed on the palmar aspect and is very fine and dense; some of its efferents join the vessels on the lateral aspect of the forearm. A few superficial efferents pass from the palmar aspect of the base of the thenar directly into the lymphatics accompanying the median vein of the forearm, however most of the superficial lymphatics join the vessels on the dorsum of the hand which then pass from the back to the front of the limb around the lateral border of the forearm. The deep lymph vessels accompany the deeper blood vessels.

Nerve supply of the thumb

Cutaneous branches to the thumb

The cutaneous branches to the thumb as in the rest of the body contain also sympathetic efferent fibres and the digital nerves carry also sensory fibres to the joints, ligaments and bones. The proximal part of the skin of the ball of the thumb is supplied by twigs from the lateral cutaneous nerve of the forearm and the palmar branch of the median nerve. The palmar digital nerves of the thumb supply the distal part of the thenar eminence and the rest of the palmar surface of the thumb. Each of these nerves terminates by dividing into two branches, one to the pulp and the other to the bed of the nail. The two dorsal digital nerves of the thumb, ulnar and radial, supply the skin of the back of the thumb; they are derived from the terminal part of the superficial branch of the radial nerve, subject to frequent variations in the supply to the dorsum of the hand (see p. 32). The terminal part of the dorsum of the thumb may be supplied by small twigs which come from the palmar digital nerves, but the extent is variable. The branches of the radial nerve may reach the root of the nail and in some people may even innervate the pulp of the thumb to such an extent that, in spite of a complete division of the palmar digital branches of the thumb, there is enough sensation provided by the radial nerve to allow the thumb a satisfactory grip function.

Nerve supply to the muscles of the thumb

The nerve supply to the muscles of the thumb has been given with the description of the muscles. The variation in this supply includes the median nerve supplying the first dorsal interosseous muscle, double nerve supply (median and ulnar) to the thenar muscles, commonest of these being the innervation of the flexor pollicis brevis already mentioned. The extent of contribution which the eighth cervical nerve makes to the nerve supply of the muscles of the thumb is also variable.

SURFACE ANATOMY OF THE HAND

The *head of the ulna* stands out prominently in pronation; on its posteromedial aspect the *styloid process* can be felt. The *anterior border of the lower end of the radius* is felt as a distinct transverse ridge on the front of the forearm about 2 to 3 cm proximal to the base of the thenar eminence. The *styloid process of radius* may be felt projecting down from the lateral aspect of the distal end of the radius and its tip is 1 cm distal to the tip of the ulnar styloid. The *dorsal radial tubercle* (of Lister) can be felt on the back of the distal end of the radius in line with the second intermetacarpal space. The four points of the main attachments of the flexor retinaculum can be identified on the palmar aspect of the carpus: the *tubercle of the scaphoid* can be felt at the proximal border of the thenar eminence and the *crest of the trapezium* immediately distal to it; the *pisiform* is a prominence felt at the base of the hypothenar eminence and the *hook of the hamate* lies 2 to 3 cm distal and lateral to the pisiform, in line with the ulnar border of the ring finger. The whole of the radial border and most of the dorsal aspect of the second metacarpal can be readily palpated. The dorsal surfaces of the third, fourth and fifth metacarpal bones are covered by the extensor tendons, but the *styloid process of the third metacarpal* can be felt about 3 cm distal to the level of the dorsal tubercle of the radius. When a fist is made the proximal row of knuckles is made by the metacarpal heads and the more distal ones by the heads of the phalanges.

Tendons near the palmar aspect of the *wrist* (Fig. 1.37) can be easily palpated. From the radial to the ulnar side they are: tendon of the flexor carpi radialis, which crosses the distal palmar wrist crease at the junction of its lateral third and its medial two thirds, where it passes in front of the scaphoid tubercle; then the tendon of the palmaris longus (absent in 10 per cent), of the flexor digitorum superficialis and of the flexor carpi ulnaris. The surface markings of the palmar synovial sheaths are shown in Fig. 1.43, p. 26. The tendons and their sheaths on the dorsal and lateral aspects are shown in Figs. 1.44 and 1.45. The *anatomical snuff-box* is a hollow at the lateral aspect of the wrist between the styloid process of the radius and the base of the first metacarpal. It is bounded anteriorly by the tendons of the abductor pollicis longus and of the extensor pollicis brevis while the posterior boundary is made by the tendon of the extensor pollicis longus. In the depth, on the floor of the snuff-box are the scaphoid and trapezium with the lateral collateral ligament of the wrist, crossed here superficially by the radial artery; its pulsation can be felt on applying light pressure. The roof of the snuff-box is crossed under the skin by the branches of the superficial division of the radial nerve, which can be rolled on the surface of the tendons.

The *palmar skin creases* are shown in Fig. 1.7. At the wrist the *proximal palmar skin crease* overlies the radiocarpal joint while *the distal crease* is over the proximal border of the flexor retinaculum marking at both ends the position of pisiform and scaphoid bones. The *proximal transverse crease of the palm* extends from the junction of the head and shaft of the second metacarpal bone to cross obliquely the distal third of the third metacarpal shaft, middle of the fourth and proximal third of the fifth metacarpal shafts. The *distal transverse crease of the palm* lies across the junctions of the heads and shafts of the fourth and fifth metacarpal bones, then crosses obliquely the head of the third metacarpal ending at the cleft between the index and long fingers. The *radial longitudinal palm crease* extends from the junction of the head and shaft of the second metacarpal to the ulnar margin of the proximal part of the third metacarpal and from there it curves as far as the trapezio-scaphoid joint. The *basal digital creases* lie approximately at the junction of the proximal one third and distal two thirds of the proximal phalanx. Of the two *middle digital creases*, the distal one usually overlies the proximal interphalangeal joint, while the *distal digital crease* lies proximal to the distal joint. In some cases an additional more distal crease overlies this joint. In hands engaged in heavy manual work, the digital creases are more proximal than in those with longer, softer and more supple fingers, where the distal lines of the digital creases represent accurately the lines of the joints.

Pulsation of the *radial artery* can be felt between the tendons of the flexor carpi radialis and of the abductor pollicis longus. The *ulnar artery* in Guyon's tunnel is not easily felt pulsating. The *superficial palmar arch* runs obliquely distally and laterally from between the pisiform and the hook of the hamate to reach the midpoint between the base of the long finger and the distal palmar wrist crease (its further course is variable). Thus it reaches as far distally as the lower border of the extended thumb. The *deep palmar arch* is about 1.5 cm proximal to the superficial arch. It can be mapped out by feeling on the dorsum of the hand the proximal end of the first intermetacarpal space and transferring this point to the palm; a line across the palm from this point to the hook of the hamate, slightly convex distally represents the deep arch. The trunk of the *median nerve* is found at the midpoint of the distal wrist crease; it cannot be palpated as it is deep to the fasciae and the tendon of the palmaris longus. Deep to the nerve at this point is the lunate bone which may compress the nerve if it is dislocated into the carpal tunnel. The trunk of the *ulnar nerve* with the ulnar artery to its radial side is found near the radial aspect of the pisiform; division into the superficial and deep branches occurs near the hook of the hamate. The *recurrent branch of the median nerve* emerges at the area which is 3 to 3.5 cm directly distal to the point on the distal wrist crease at the junction of its lateral third with the medial two thirds, where it crosses the tubercle of scaphoid. The *bifurcation of the common palmar digital nerves* occurs just distal to the level of the superficial palmar arch, while the corresponding arteries bifurcate near the webs of the fingers at the level of the bases of the proximal phalanges. In the fingers the *neurovascular bundles* lie against the fibrous flexor sheath, palmar to the line joining the ends of the palmar digital creases, from dorsal to palmar being vein, artery and nerve, the last being nearest to the midline of the digit. On the palmar aspect, the level of the *metacarpophalangeal joints* is 2 cm proximal to the edge of the webs of the fingers; on the dorsum they are 1 cm distal to the knuckles, while the *proximal interphalangeal joints* are 0.5 cm and the *distal joints* 0.25 cm from their knuckles.

Fig. 1.67. Progress in ossification of the bones of the hand. (a) newborn, (b) at $1\frac{1}{2}$ years, (c) at $2\frac{1}{2}$ years (note the epiphyses of the digital rays), (d) at $4\frac{1}{2}$ years, (e) at $9\frac{1}{2}$ years, (f) at 13 years.

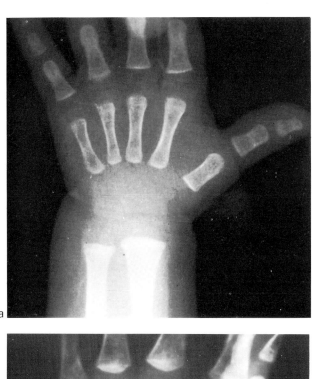

a

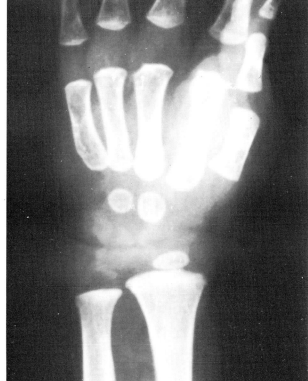

b

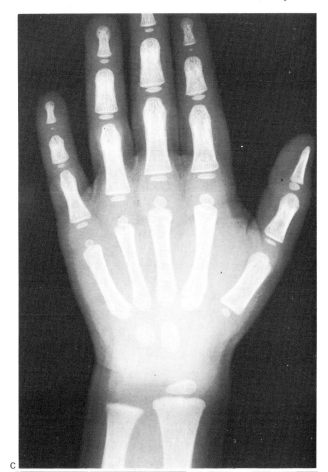

c

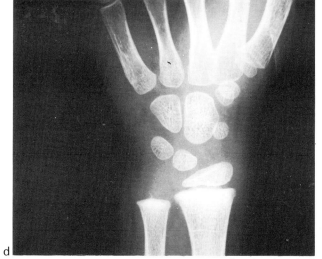

d

[*continued overleaf*

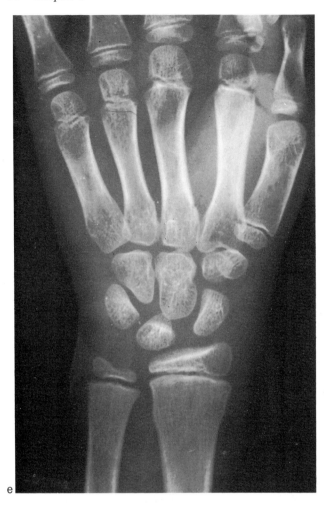

e

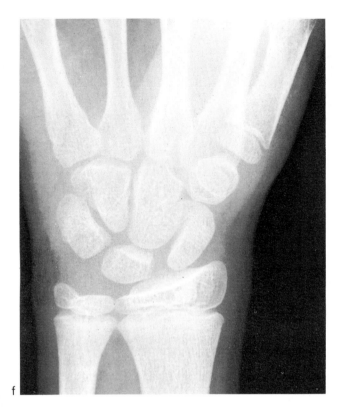

f

FIG. 1.67 (*continued*).

RADIOGRAPHIC ANATOMY OF THE HAND

The hand and the wrist are easily accessible to X-ray examination with the radiographs being sharp and clear. Not only the usual information is obtained about injury and disease, but also ossification data (Fig. 1.67) can be employed to study the skeletal age and progression towards maturity [49]. The digital bones are well ossified at birth, and the subsequent ossification of the carpus occurs usually in an orderly fashion making this region the most suitable for assessment of the age of the developing skeleton.

There are many special views employed for radio-graphic examination of the hand [50, 51]. The following are the standard views:

The hand. Posteroanterior view (Fig. 1.68) with the hand pronated, i.e. palm towards the film; *lateral view* (Fig. 1.69) with the hand at 90° to the film; *oblique view* (Fig. 1.70), i.e. posteroanterior view with the pronated hand at 45° to the film.

The fingers. Posteroanterior view (Fig. 1.71a) and *lateral view* of separate fingers (taken to avoid overlapping) (Fig. 1.71b). *Special views* of the metacarpal heads [52] are used to show the rheumatoid changes (Fig. 1.72a & b), with the back of the fingers against the film, the

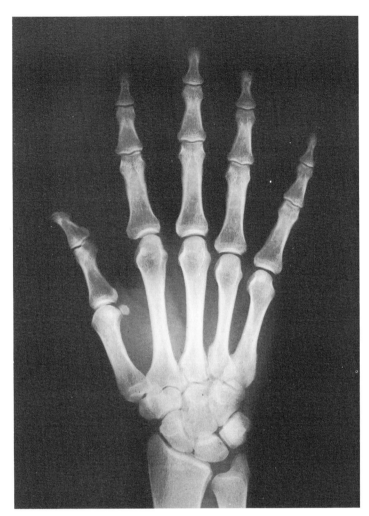

FIG. 1.68. Posteroanterior view of the hand.

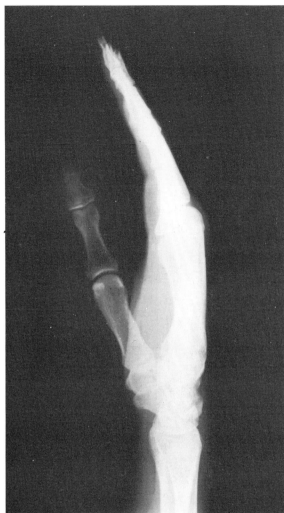

FIG. 1.69. Lateral view of the hand.

metacarpophalangeal joints at 70° of flexion, the thumb fully extended and the central X-ray beam along the longitudinal axis of the metacarpals and directed from a point 15° to the ulnar side of the hand.

The thumb. Lateral view (Fig. 1.73a) with the hand in pronation and the palm raised on a non-opaque pad to bring the lateral surface of the thumb in contact with the film; *posteroanterior view* (Fig. 1.73b) with the hand in the lateral position (as in Fig. 1.69) and the thumb supported in abduction (p. 44) on a non-opaque pad.

The carpometacarpal joint of the thumb is not easily accessible to the radiographic examination, particularly when a view along the ridge of the trapezial saddle (p. 44) is required. The author is developing a rigid perspex box into which the upper limb including the hand and elbow can be firmly tied; the box can be rotated 360° and tilted either away or towards the X-ray tube (Fig. 1.74a & b). This method can also be used for detailed analysis of the carpal bones and joints. It ensures a fixed position of the hand during radiography and one which can be repeated accurately.

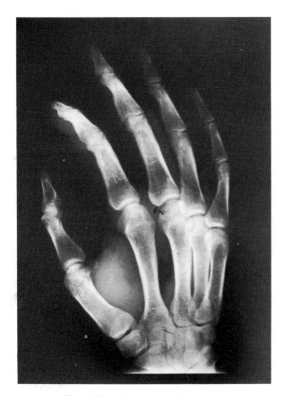

FIG. 1.70. Oblique view of the hand.

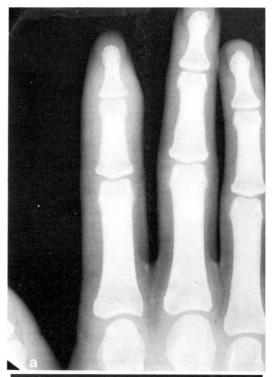

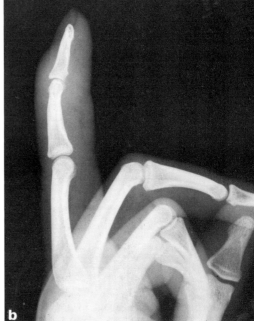

The wrist. Posteroanterior view (Fig. 1.75a) with the hand pronated, i.e. palm towards the film; *lateral view* (Fig. 1.75b) with the hand at 90° to the film; *posteroanterior oblique view* (Fig. 1.75c) with the wrist midway between the posteroanterior and true lateral views, the ulnar side to the film and *antero-posterior oblique view* (Fig. 1.75d) with the hand and wrist rotated back from the previous position by 90°. For visualization of the *carpal tunnel* an *axial view* (Fig. 1.76) is used with the palm on the film and the wrist dorsiflexed to about 45° with some degree of ulnar deviation.

FIG. 1.71. Views of the fingers; (a) posteroanterior, (b) lateral.

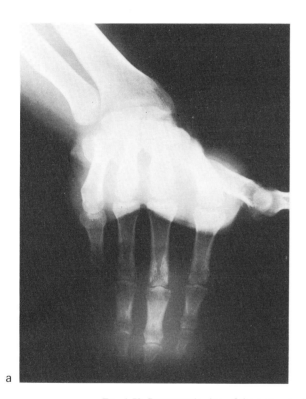
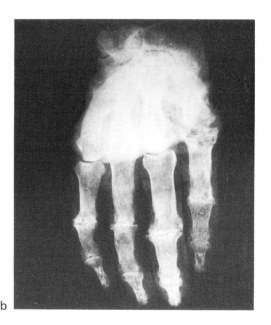

FIG. 1.72. Brewerton's view of the metacarpal heads. (a) normal, (b) rheumatoid hand.

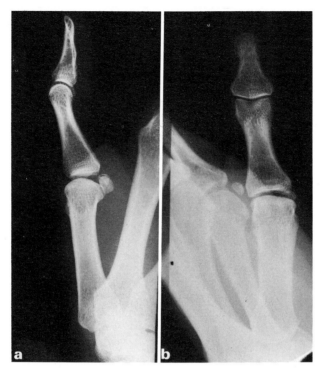

FIG. 1.73. (a) Lateral view of the thumb, (b) posteroanterior view of the thumb.

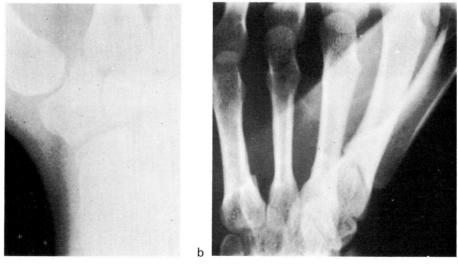

FIG. 1.74. Special views of the carpometacarpal joint of the thumb (KK); (a) across the ridge, (b) along the ridge of the trapezial saddle (p. 44).

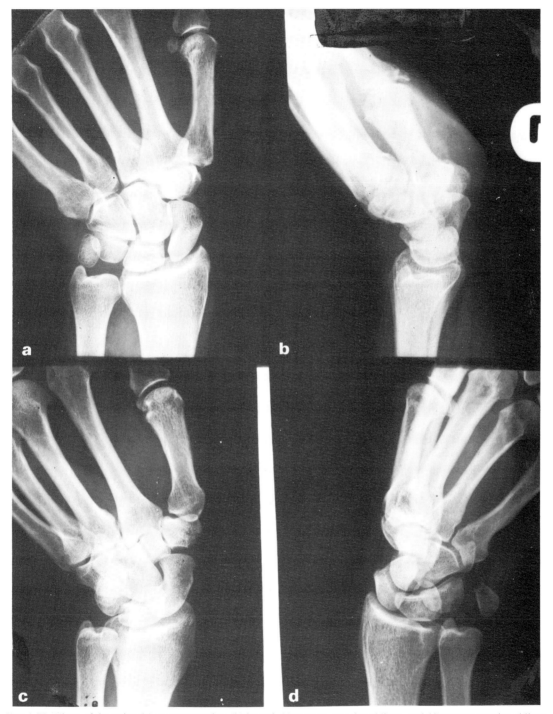

FIG. 1.75. Views of the wrist; (a) posteroanterior, (b) lateral, (c) postero-anterior oblique, and (d) anteroposterior oblique.

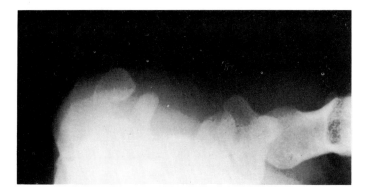

Fig. 1.76 Axial view of the carpal tunnel.

REFERENCES

[1] SIMPSON, D. C. Gripping surfaces for artificial hands. *The Hand*, 1971, **12**.

[2] CAUNA, N. Nature and functions of the papillary ridges of the digital skin. *Anatomical Record*, 1954, **119**, 449.

[3] CAUNA, N. The mode of termination of the sensory nerves and its significance. *Journal of Comparative Neurology*, 1959, **113**, 169.

[4] LE GROS CLARKE, W. E. *The Tissues of the Body*. Oxford, Clarendon Press, 1971.

[5] DUPUYTREN, G. *Traité théoretique et pratique des Blessures per Armes de Guerre*. Paris, 1834.

[6] LANGER, A. K. Sitzungberchte der Kaiserlichen, *Akadamie der Wissenschaften in Wien*, 1861, **44**, 1946.

[7] JONES, W. F. Tension lines, cleavage lines and hair tracts in man. *Journal of Anatomy*, 1941, **75**, 248.

[8] COX, H. T. The cleavage lines of the skin. *British Journal of Surgery*, 1941, **29**, 234.

[9] GIBSON, T. Physical properties of skin. *Journal of Anatomy*, 1969, **105**, 183.

[10] LANDSMEER, J. M. F. Anatomical and functional investigations on the articulations of the human fingers. *Acta anatomica*, 1955, Suppl. 24.

[11] ANSON, B. J. *An Atlas of Human Anatomy*. Saunders, Philadelphia, 1950.

[12] DOYLE, J. R. AND BLYTHE, W. F. Anatomy of the flexor tendon sheath and pulleys of the thumb. *Journal of Hand Surgery*, 1977, **2**, 149.

[13] KESSLER, I. AND SILBERMAN, Z. An experimental study of the radiocarpal joint by arthrography. *Surgery, Gynecology and Obstetrics*, 1961, **112**, 33.

[14] TALEISNIK, J. The ligaments of the wrist joint. *Journal of Hand Surgery*, 1976, **1**, 110.

[15] WILHELM, A. Zur innervation der gelenke der obern extremität. *Zeitschrift für Anatomie und Entwirklungsgeschichte*, 1958, **120**, 331.

[16] BUCK-GRAMCKO, D. Denervation of the wrist joint. *Journal of Hand Surgery*, 1977, **2**, 54.

[17] FISK, G. R. Carpal instability and the fractured scaphoid. *Annals of the Royal College of Surgeons of England*, 1970, **46**, 63.

[18] LINSCHEID, R. L., DOBYNS, H. J., BEABOUT, J. W. AND BRYAN, R. S. Traumatic instability of the wrist. *Journal of Bone and Joint Surgery*, 1972, **54A**, 1612.

[19] LANDSMEER, J. M. F. *Atlas of Anatomy of the Hand*. Churchill Livingstone, Edinburgh, 1976.

[20] PETRIE, P. W. R. AND LAMB, D. W. Fracture-subluxation of base of fifth metacarpal. *The Hand*, 1974, **6**, 82.

[21] LANDSMEER, J. M. F. Anatomical and functional investigations on the articulations of the human fingers. *Acta anatomica*, 1955, Suppl. 24.

[22] HAXTIAN, R. W. AND TUBIANA, R. (1967) Ulnar deviation of the fingers. *Journal of Bone and Joint Surgery*, 1967, **49A**, 299.

[23] KUCZYNSKI, K. The synovial structures of the normal and rheumatoid joints. *The Hand*, 1971, **3**, 41.

[24] KUCZYNSKI, K. Less known aspects of the proximal interphalangeal joints of the human hand. *The Hand*, 1975, **7**, 31.

[25] KUCZYNSKI, K. The proximal interphalangeal joint. Anatomy and causes of stiffness in the fingers. *Journal of Bone and Joint Surgery*, 1968, **50B**, 656.

[26] LANDSMEER, J. M. F. The proximal interphalangeal joint. *The Hand*, 1975, **7**, 30.

[27] WATSON, H. K., LIGHT, T. R. AND JOHNSON, T. R. Checkrein resection for flexion contracture of the middle joint. *Journal of Hand Surgery*, 1979, **4**, 67.

[28] KUCZYNSKI, K. Carpometacarpal joint of the human thumb. *Journal of Anatomy*, 1974, **118**, 119.

[29] KUCZYNSKI, K. The thumb and the saddle. *The Hand*, 1975, **7**, 120.

[30] MURAKAMI, T., TAKAYA, K. AND OUTI, H. The origin,

course and distribution of arteries to the thumb. *Okajimas folia anatomica Japonica*, 1969, **46,** 123.

[31] MUTZ, S. B. Thumb web contracture. *The Hand*, 1972, **4,** 236.

[32] FETROW, K. O. Practical and important variations in sensory supply of the hand. *The Hand*, 1970, **2,** 178.

[33] SHREWSBURY, M. M. AND KUCZYNSKI, K. Flexor digitorum superficialis tendon in the fingers of the human hand. *The Hand*, 1974, **6,** 121.

[34] LONG, C. Intrinsic-extrinsic muscle control of the fingers. Electromyographic studies. *Journal of Bone and Joint Surgery*, 1968, **50A,** 973.

[35] MEHTA, H. J. AND GARDNER, W. U. A study of lumbrical muscles in the human hand. *American Journal of Anatomy*, 1961, **109,** 227.

[36] RABISHONG, P. The proprioceptic innervation of the lumbrical muscles of the human hand. *Revue de chirurgie orthopedique*, 1962, **48,** 234.

[37] KUCZYNSKI, K. The variations in the insertion of the first dorsal interosseous muscle and their significance in the rheumatoid arthritis. *The Hand*, 1972, **4,** 37.

[38] EYLER, D. L. AND MARKEE, J. E. The anatomy and function of the intrinsic musculature of the fingers. *Journal of Bone and Joint Surgery*, 1954.

[39] LANDSMEER, J. M. F. Anatomical and functional investigations on the articulations of the human fingers. *Acta Anatomica*, 1955, Suppl. 24.

[40] LE DOUBLE, A. F. *Traité des variations du système musculaire de l'homme*. Paris, Schleicher Frères, 1897.

[41] SALSBURY, C. R. The interosseous muscles of the hand. *Journal of Anatomy*, 1937, **71,** 395.

[42] STACK, H. G. A study of muscle function in the fingers. *Annals of the Royal College of Surgeons of England*, 1963, **33,** 307.

[43] SPINNER, M. AND KAPLAN, E. B. The relationship of the ulnar nerve to the medial intermuscular septum in the arm and its clinical significance. *The Hand*, 1976, **8,** 239.

[44] MCFARLANE, R. M., MAYER, J. R. AND HUGILL, J. V. Further observations on the anatomy of the ulnar nerve at the wrist. *The Hand*, 1976, **8,** 115.

[45] DYKES, R. W. AND TERZIS, J. K. Functional anatomy of the deep motor branch of the ulnar nerve. *Clinical Orthopaedics*, 1977, **128,** 167.

[46] DENMAN, E. E. An unusual branch of the ulnar nerve in the hand. *The Hand*, 1977, **9,** 92.

[47] MAEDA, K., MIURA, T., KOMADA, T. AND CHIBA, A. Anterior interosseous nerve paralysis. *The Hand*, 1977, **9,** 165.

[48] LANZ, U. Anatomical variations of the median nerve in the carpal tunnel. *The Journal of Hand Surgery*, 1977, **2,** 44.

[49] GREULICH, W. W. AND PYLE, S. I. *Radiographic Atlas of Skeletal Development of the Hand and Wrist*, 2nd ed. Stanford, 1959.

[50] CLARK, K. C. *Positioning in Radiography*, 9th ed. London, Heinemann Medical, 1973.

[51] MESCHAN, I. *An Atlas of Normal Radiographic Anatomy*, 2nd ed. Philadelphia, 1959.

[52] BREWERTON, D. A. A tangential radiographic projection for demonstrating involvement of metacarpal heads in rheumatoid arthritis. *British Journal of Radiology*, 1967, **40,** 233.

CHAPTER 2

Muscle and Tendon Kinesiology

C. LONG

The intricacies of hand kinesiology have fascinated many scientific observers over the centuries. In the recent historical past, Duchenne contributed some astute reasoning to the knowledge of hand behaviour [1]. Many of his conclusions concerning kinesiology of the hand are being verified today. Bunnell and Kaplan in this century have extrapolated clinical and laboratory findings into workable hypotheses [2, 3]. Most recently, the addition of electromyographic methods in the mid 1940s has allowed direct examination of muscular activity in the normal or pathologic moving hand. Methods of using and interpreting electromyographic examinations have been published [4, 5]. This chapter will delineate the roles adopted by various muscles and tendons in controlling the hand and wrist. This summary is a synthesis of laboratory electromyographic findings and other observations.

THEORY OF MOVEMENT PATTERNS IN THE UNLOADED HAND

There are four basic patterns of muscle synergy to move fingers and these can be applied to any motion of any finger. They obtain while the finger is in motion, or while it is held at the defined terminal position of the motion. The synergistic muscles generally operate synchronously rather than sequentially.

Opening motions

These include activities of the hand in which the fingers are moving toward, or are held at, the position of extension of metacarpophalangeal and interphalangeal joints. The active muscles are the extensor digitorum and lumbricals.

There is an absolute synchrony of extensor digitorum and lumbricals, which operate together at all times when the finger is undergoing an opening motion. The explanation is related to viscoelastic contributions in hand kinesiology. The resting position of the fingers is flexed (p. 1); the major contributors to this flexed position are the long finger flexors, especially the flexor digitorum profundus. In an attempt to extend the finger (open the hand), contraction of the extensor digitorum loads the finger with two forces, the flexor one resulting from passive flexor digitorum profundus viscoelasticity and the extensor one resulting from the extensor digitorum voluntary contraction. Landsmeer has developed a mathematical theory of metacarpophalangeal–interphalangeal joint control [6]. The theory dictates that the direction of metacarpophalangeal–interphalangeal motion, with forces applied on both the extensor and flexor side of the finger, is *predetermined by the anatomy of the bones and extensor aponeurosis. The finger under these conditions of loading will move toward metacarpophalangeal extension/interphalangeal flexion (Fig. 2.1).*

Under conditions of attempted opening, with contraction only of the extensor digitorum, the finger will therefore 'claw' because of the simultaneous volar loading by the viscoelasticity of the flexor digitorum profundus. *For opening motion to be completed it is essential that the lumbricals contract.* The lumbricalis applies forces at its origin on the flexor digitorum

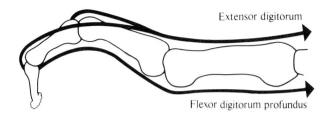

Extensor digitorum

Flexor digitorum profundus

FIG. 2.1. Claw position is a result of loading the extrinsic tendons. From Long and Brown [5].

profundus that cancel the viscoelastic forces of the profundus on the volar finger. The removal of these flexion forces within the profundus by contraction of the lumbricalis enable the extensor digitorum to operate unencumbered as an extensor of the interphalangeal joints as well as the metacarpophalangeal joint. The major function of the lumbricals in opening motions is the removal of flexor digitorum profundus viscoelastic flexion forces from the finger, but it also assists interphalangeal extension.

Closing motions

These are the activities of the hand in which the fingers are moving toward, or are held at, the position of full flexion of the metacarpophalangeal and interphalangeal joints. The active muscles are the flexor digitorum profundus and the extensor digitorum.

The most striking find here is the absolute absence of lumbrical participation. Unloaded closing motions of the finger are accomplished by the extrinsics alone. The profundus is always predominant, unless the subject willingly prevents distal interphalangeal flexion, thereby intensifying superficialis contributions. In closing motions, the superficialis probably contributes significant viscoelastic flexion forces, which are reduced as the wrist is used in a more flexed posture. With the wrist flexed, increasing superficialis voluntary activity is noted as it substitutes a voluntary force for its reduced viscoelasticity in the finger flexion equation.

The absence of lumbrical contribution [7] in the closing motion is one of the major concepts of 'the new kinesiology' in the hand. Because of the recurrent

finding in numerous normal hands, the absence of lumbrical participation in this motion must be taken as fact. Details of the total equation of finger control have been published [8]. The behaviour of the lumbricals in all aspects depends on its origin which dictates its ability to relieve the viscoelastic pull of the profundus at the metacarpophalangeal joint. Because of this, contraction of the lumbrical cancels out its own tendency to flex the metacarpophalangeal joint; the muscle subtracts from the flexion force of the flexor profundus (by pulling distally) exactly what it adds to metacarpophalangeal flexion (by pulling proximally). *Whenever the interphalangeal joints are flexing or held flexed the lumbrical is inactive.*

The extensor digitorum consistently acts as a brake against too rapid flexion of the metacarpophalangeal joints during full finger flexion. It also counteracts volar subluxation of the first phalanx at the metacarpophalangeal joint due to forces generated by the flexor digitorum profundus [9].

Landsmeer's theory [6] suggests that the finger will claw when loaded by extensor digitorum and flexor digitorum profundus as in the closing motion. Obviously, these same two muscles can produce closing; the exact explanation for this ability is still obscure. Forces must flex the metacarpophalangeal joint (moving it away from its natural direction of rotation into extension). The present explanation invokes viscoelastic forces in the bi-articular interossei, as the metacarpophalangeal joint flexes in closing the hands. As the finger is flexed by the profundus, the interossei are stretched, thereby adding flexion force at the metacarpophalangeal joint. The flexion forces cannot derive from the lumbrical.

Clawing motion

These include activities in which the fingers are moving toward, or are held at, the position of metacarpophalangeal extension/interphalangeal flexion. The active muscles are the extensor digitorum and flexor digitorum profundus, the same as in closing the hand.

The clawing motion is the most 'pure' example of Landsmeer's theory. If the hand intends to reach the clawed position, its best choice of muscles is the two extrinsics (flexor and extensor). These produce rotation towards the theoretical 'end positions' of metacarpophalangeal extension/interphalangeal flexion (the claw position), as in Figure 2.1. The rationale obtains, regardless of the starting position of the finger.

Reciprocal motions

These are activities in which the fingers are moving toward, or are held at, the position of metacarpophalangeal flexion/interphalangeal extension. The active muscles are the interossei and the lumbricals (for any single finger these are designated the 'intrinsic triad').

The reciprocal position exemplifies the major forces necessary to drive the finger away from the end positions imposed by finger and tendon anatomy. *Since the finger tends to rotate under extrinsic power into interphalangeal flexion/metacarpophalangeal extension, a major function of the intrinsics is to rotate the finger away from these positions.* In reaching the terminal position of metacarpophalangeal flexion/interphalangeal extension, both metacarpophalangeal flexion and interphalangeal extension forces are required. Interphalangeal extension is provided by the lumbricals and those interossei inserting into the extensor mechanism (all the palmer interossei and dorsal II, III and IV to greater or lesser extent). Metacarpophalangeal flexion in reciprocal motion is the function of all the interossei.

The thumb in unresisted motion

A particularly elegant review of thumb motions and subsequent electromyographic studies was performed by Ebskov [4]. A device measured six degrees of translational and rotational freedom in thumb motion during the simultaneous recording of multichannel electromyograms from the muscles driving the thumb. Figure 2.2 summarizes the findings. The diagrammed actions relate to motions of the whole thumb ray, not to the individual motions of metacarpophalangeal and interphalangeal joints.

Two muscles behave somewhat differently than might be expected on the basis of their anatomical capabilities: the flexor pollicis longus does *not* participate in motions of the unloaded thumb metacarpal; the first dorsal interosseus is *not* active in moving the unloaded thumb metacarpal. Ebskov's dissertation can be consulted for further analyses of muscular action and dynamic bone and joint measurements under all conditions of thumb motion. It also includes a thorough history of the

nomenclature of thumb motions, and the purported anatomy of the thumb as related by different observers.

THEORY OF MOVEMENT PATTERNS IN THE LOADED HAND

The technique for studying the resisted hand [10, 11] in the laboratory varied from that reported in the freely moving hand. The details of this method have been published [12–14].

Resisted hand motions require careful classification, such as that derived partially from Napier's [15] and Landsmeer's descriptions of power grip and precision handling [16]. *Power grip* is the grasping of an object by the fingers and thumb acting firmly against the palm. *Precision handling* is the manipulation of an object by fingers and thumb to produce a new position of the object.

Power grip is further divided into [13] *squeeze grip* (including simple squeeze, hammer squeeze and screwdriver squeeze with rotation), *hook grip, disc grip* and *spherical grip*. Precision handling includes *precision rotation* and *precision translation*; each precision handling activity can be performed in a tip-to-tip, pad-to-pad or pad-to-side mode.

Muscles acting during resisted motion

In general, the *extrinsic muscles* produce few surprises in either power grip or precision handling. The extrinsic muscles [12] across the hand increase their activity in proportion to the external load (in proportion to the strength of power grip, or the resistance or speed in precision handling). The only significant exception is the abductor pollicis longus, which is considerably less active than other extrinsics in most forms of power grip; apparently the abductor stands-by during these motions to reduce its tendency to pull the first metacarpal out of the palm.

By contrast, the *intrinsic muscles* vary in their participation in power grip and precision handling, and actually determine the character of the hand's behaviour. In *power grip*, the intrinsics add to the strength of extrinsic grasp, as well as producing adjustments of finger position. In *precision handling* the intrinsics mainly guide the course of finger motion during manipulation of the object.

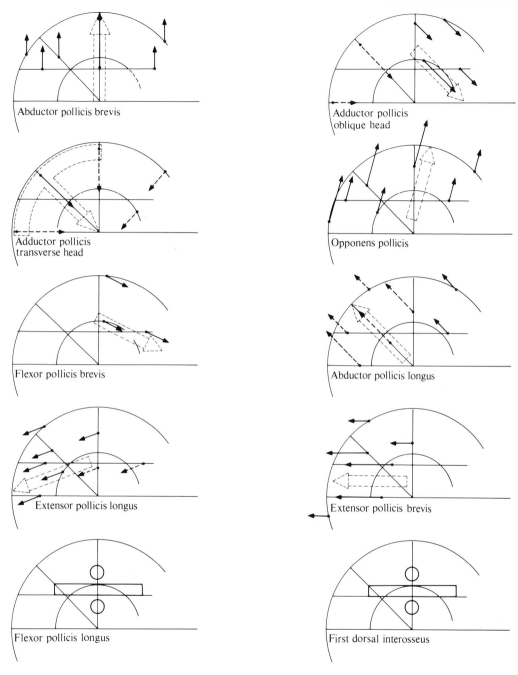

FIG. 2.2. Spectrum of activity of thumb muscles, from Ebskov [4]. Small arrows indicate directions of muscle influence on the thumb. The large arrows suggest the probable prime function of the muscle in relation to the unloaded thumb.

In all types of *power grip*, the interossei carry the major burden of the load. They mainly provide flexion power at the metacarpophalangeal joint, but also rotate the finger (via the first phalanx) to adjust to the shape of external objects and thereby allow most efficient application of extrinsic power. Additionally, in some motions, an interosseus acting primarily as a metacarpophalangeal flexor inadvertently creates a tendency toward rotation of the finger; the paired interosseus of that finger then acts to prevent the unwanted rotation. With the occasional exception of the fourth, the lumbricals do not participate in power grip at all.

Precision handling is another matter. Here the lumbricals join the thenar muscles to provide the necessary equipment for the fingers and thumb to manipulate objects. In *precision rotation* the interossei provide rotation of the manipulated object by abducting or adducting the finger. The lumbricals apparently contribute to counter-clockwise rotation (right hand) by metacarpophalangeal abduction in the index and middle fingers. The thenar triad of abductor brevis, opponens and flexor brevis assist in counter-clockwise rotation of objects (right hand).

Precision translation moves an object directly towards or away from the palm. Translation away from the palm heavily involves the intrinsic triad, as would be expected in this *reciprocal motion*. The motion towards the palm shows some activity of the first lumbrical which is yet unexplained.

Muscle actions at the wrist

Hand position in space is determined by the shoulder and elbow, and the wrist provides a graduated device for hand positioning. This versatile joint allows the adoption of special positions for special functions, as in writing (extension) or holding a beer can (flexion). It further provides a very fine, continual, and automatic adjustment of the balance of viscoelastic forces in the extrinsic muscles operating the fingers. Wrist position in part determines that share of finger flexion or extension power derived from voluntary contraction versus the share derived from viscoelastic forces. For instance, wrist flexion imposes a requirement for voluntary digital flexion while permitting a large level of passive (viscoelastic) extension. These shifts in balance, particularly

in relation to increased viscoelastic contribution, have been termed 'tenodesis effect' because of the resemblance to tenodesis surgery.

Seven muscles affect wrist position as a primary function: flexor carpi radialis and ulnaris, palmaris longus, extensors carpi radialis longus, brevis and ulnaris, plus the abductor pollicis longus. Each moves the wrist in the expected anatomic direction, close to that attributed to Braus in the diagram reproduced by Steindler in his classic book on kinesiology [17].

Individual wrist muscles do not act alone but in concert with finger operators and with each other. Electromyography shows a clear pattern of synergy between some of the wrist muscles and those moving the fingers [11, 18, 19]. In general, closing motions of the hand are accompanied by activity of the wrist extensors which provide a force to counteract the tendency of the finger flexors to flex the wrist. The most active wrist extensor in this synergy is the extensor carpi radialis brevis, and next the extensor carpi ulnaris. The extensor carpi radialis longus is relatively inactive in this synergy. The relationship of extensor carpi radialis brevis to flexor digitorum profundus activity is very clear and can easily be verified by palpation of one's own wrist. As the hand is closed into a fist, the activity of the extensor carpi radialis brevis increases to a maximum. This activity stops as soon as the fist begins to open (flexor digitorum profundus activity ceases). The surgical implications of this fact are clear; the extensor carpi radialis brevis is a natural synergist of the flexor digitorum profundus, relaxing when the flexor digitorum profundus relaxes. The extensor carpi radialis brevis therefore makes a logical choice as an in-phase muscle transfer when finger flexion is needed [11, 20], other factors being equal.

During opening motions of the hand both the flexor carpi radialis and extensor carpi ulnaris are active. The flexor carpi radialis, centrally located, is a direct synergist to the finger extensors. The extensor carpi ulnaris, although seemingly paradoxical in its action, may be providing ulnar deviation forces important to keep the hand in the midline, as well as providing a simple support function to free the extensor digitorum for its essential role in opening the hand. These demonstrable synergies again point to a natural surgical conclusion; other factors being equal, the in-phase choices for transferred muscles to open the hand are the flexor carpi radialis and the extensor carpi ulnaris.

REFERENCES

[1] DUCHENNE, G. B. A. *Physiology of Motion, 1885*. Translated by E. B. Kaplan. Philadelphia, W. B. Saunders, 1959.

[2] BUNNELL, S. *Surgery of Hand*, 2nd Ed. Philadelphia, J. B. Lippincott, 1949.

[3] KAPLAN, E. B. *Functional and Surgical Anatomy of Hand*. Philadelphia, J. B. Lippincott, 1953.

[4] EBSKOV, B. *De Motibus Motoribusque Pollicis Humani*, Copenhagen, 1970.

[5] LONG, C. AND BROWN, M. E. Electromyographic kinesiology of the hand: muscles moving the long finger. *Journal of Bone and Joint Surgery*, 1964, **46A,** 1683.

[6] LANDSMEER, J. M. F. AND LONG, C. The mechanism of finger control, based on electromyograms and location analysis. *Acta Anatomics*, 1965, **60,** 330.

[7] BACKHOUSE, K. M. AND CATTON, W. T. Experimental study of functions of lumbrical muscles in human hand. *Journal of Anatomy*, 1954, **88,** 133.

[8] THOMAS, D. H., LONG, C. AND LANDSMEER, J. M. F. Biomechanical considerations of lumbricalis behavior in the human finger. *Journal of Biomechanics*, 1968, **1,** 107.

[9] SMITH, E. M., JUVINALL, R. C., BENDER, L. F. AND PEARSON, J. R. Role of the finger flexors in rheumatoid deformities of the metacarpophalangeal joints. *Arthritis and Rheumatism*, 1964, **7,** 467.

[10] LONG, C. II, CONRAD, P. W., HALL, E. A. AND FURLER, S. L. Intrinsic-extrinsic muscle control of the hand in power grip and precision handling, an electromyographic study. *Journal of Bone and Joint Surgery*, 1970, **52A,** 853.

[11] LONG, C. II. *Normal and Abnormal Motor Control in the Upper Extremities*. Final Report, Social and Rehabilitation Services, Grant No. RD-2377-M, December 1, 1966 to April 30, 1970, Cleveland, Ohio, 1970.

[12] CONRAD, P. W., JR. *Electromyography of the Extrinsic Muscles of the Hand in Power Grip*. M.S. Thesis, Physical Therapy Curriculum, Case Western Reserve University, Cleveland, Ohio, 1969.

[13] HALL, E. A. AND LONG, C. Intrinsic hand muscles in power grip: an electromyographic study. *Electromyography*, 1968, **8,** 397.

[14] MEIBUHR, S. L. (FURLER, S. M.). *Electromyography of Intrinsic Muscles of the Hand During Precision Handling*. M.S. Thesis, Physical Therapy Curriculum, Case Western Reserve University, Cleveland, Ohio, 1969.

[15] NAPIER, J. R. The prehensile movements of the human hand. *Journal of Bone and Joint Surgery*, 1956, **38B,** 902.

[16] LANDSMEER, J. M. F. Power grip and precision handling. *Annals of the Rheumatic Diseases*, 1962, **21,** 164.

[17] STEINDLER, A. *Kinesiology of the Human Body Under Normal and Pathological Conditions*. Springfield, Charles C. Thomas, 1955.

[18] MCFARLAND, G. B., KRUSEN, U. L. AND WEATHERSBY, H. T. Kinesiology of selected muscles acting on the wrist: electromyographic study. *Archives of Physical Medicine and Rehabilitation*, 1962, **43,** 165.

[19] RADONJIC, D. AND LONG, C. II. Kinesiology of the wrist. *American Journal of Physical Medicine*, 1971, **50,** 57.

[20] LIFFERT, R. D. AND MEISTER, M. Patterns of neuromuscular activity following tendon transfer in the upper limb: a preliminary study. *Journal of Hand Surgery*, 1976, **1,** 181.

CHAPTER 3

Evolution of Basic Features of the Human Hand, its Kinaesthetics and Control

D. C. SIMPSON

The hand of man is so capable of intricate tasks that it is often thought of as being unique; an example of specialization given to man, as Sir Charles Bell said, because of his intellect. Even superficial study of the hands of man's nearer relatives amongst the primates does not support this view, and it might be more accurate to say nowadays that it is the unconscious component of man's brain which has made an ordinary hand into one of the most competent pieces of biological structure.

Although man now lives in a very different environment from his evolutionary past, it was that which influenced his development; the hand of modern man still has most of its original features and though they have lost their original importance, they have determined the design of man's artefacts. It is, therefore, important as well as rewarding to look at the past, although much must be conjecture.

General remarks

During evolution many small anatomical changes occur and these mutations due to cosmic radiation, viral infections, chemical action or some other injury, may cause a marginal difference in the struggle to live long enough to reproduce. Those individuals whose characteristics are slightly changed to provide a better 'fit' to the existing or new environment will be more likely to succeed. Consequently not only will there be a tendency for a surviving population to improve its relationship to the environment during times of steady environmental conditions, but there will also be a tendency for a group to emerge as a specially successful one following an environmental change if a previously inconsequential anatomical change had occurred: a pre-adaptation. Anatomical changes which lead to a greater short-term advantage are usually along the line of increasingly specialized characteristics. Man has specialized in versatility, and of all evolutionary specializations this is the only one which could have prevented him reaching the evolutionary dead-end, trapped by his own specialization, the fate of so many species. Man has moved through the stage when he was at risk and can now 'evolve' in an extracorporeal fashion through his machines and his intellect to meet any threat to his existence.

Any evolutionary changes are slight and progress linearly on previous anatomical structure and evolution. Lateral moves onto alternative paths of development are rarely possible. The moves are almost invariably towards increased specialization because the bias in the selection is towards improvement in efficiency as well as in function in any system over a period. In practice, evolution parallels industrial design processes towards a natural goal of population increase or dominance.

Man is inevitably a living record of his evolutionary experience and displays this in his characteristics. One of the most influential experiences of his ancestors must have been the arboreal one. In this environment the critical functions are the ability to grasp quickly, with hands and feet, to position the hands and feet accurately in space, and to be able to appreciate relative positions of objects in space, and more particularly of moving objects in a 'moving' space. There was an obvious necessity to have a secure grasp.

Hand-arm positioning system

It is not possible to consider the kinaesthetics of the hand alone; the hand and arm, with their attached muscles, are so intimately linked together in their function with the central nervous system which is involved in their control that it is more logical to discuss a 'hand–arm' system than a limb. Viewed in this way it is easier to see the advantages given by that system, and why its function has properties which might be unexpected.

The role of the hand is, or was, to take part in locomotion, to acquire, to defend, to hold or to release, to assist in feeding, to groom and, more generally, to act not only towards the owner but to act outwards towards the exterior environment, while the role of the rest of the limb has been to position and orientate the hand. This requires six degrees of freedom: three spatial (near, far; up, down; left, right) and three rotational about these three orthogonal axes X, Y, Z (Fig. 3.1a).

The wider the field of influence of the hands the greater the success achieved, and so it is worth looking at the arm as if it had been designed as a hand positioning mechanism to meet that need. The movements of the upper arm relative to the trunk are obtained by muscles attached in a distributed way to the trunk, while what is effectively a single smoothly operating socket joint, allowing a very wide range of angle movement, is obtained by the auxiliary movement of scapula and clavicle.

This doubles the range of movement of the gleno-humeral joint and works with it. Scapula and clavicle also act as the direct and essential skeletal link in the proprioceptive chain between the humerus and the rest of the skeleton. The wide range of movement at the shoulder has had such an advantage that the less secure joint which resulted did not apparently prove to be a disadvantage of importance.

At the elbow, where the modified hinge allows the arm to fold on itself, the skeletal structure branches in two components, the radius and the ulna, which provide a forearm rotational mechanism in which muscular forces achieve axial rotation of carpus and hand. The non-axial rotating articulation of ulna to humerus and of radius to carpus with the rotation of the heads of both radius and ulna gives the necessary stability to allow smooth orientation of the hand and provides almost the only conceivable type of axial rotational mechanism which could be provided in a single section of a biological structure made up of linked cylinders. The eight carpal bones function as a universal joint which transmits this rotation to the hand with its division into five rays, a primordial feature which has persisted since the five ray pectoral fin of the coelacanth.

As a positioning mechanism, the arm appears effective, and when we consider the possible ways in which the limb might have evolved, it can be seen that its structure of two hinged cylinders with a specialized joint at each

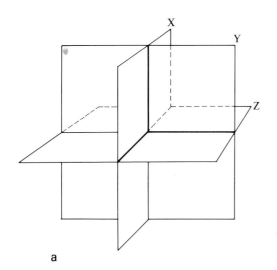

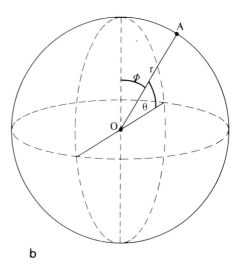

a   b

FIG. 3.1. Orientation of the hand-arm system. (a) X, Y, Z system. (b) Spherical polar system ($OA = r$).

end is not only effective, but is possibly the most appropriate arrangement to work with the central nervous system. Hand movements occur relative to the body, and relative to objects in the space surrounding the body, and the body itself moves in this space. For this to be possible, the central nervous system which controls the movement must hold a concept of spatial relationships at the unconscious level.

There is no way of knowing what this concept is but, of the principal concepts of space used by mathematicians, the most likely candidate is the spherical polar system where the length of a radius vector and its angles of rotation about the origin in two planes at right angles to each other (e.g. elevation and azimuth) are the three coordinates (r, θ and ϕ) (Fig. 3.1b).

Both spherical polar coordinates and eye spatial function are 'egocentric' and both lend themselves directly to controlling and positioning a jointed mechanical system; the human upper limb contains all the features which are required in a sophisticated manipulator operating on these lines. If the arm is viewed in this light and in terms of spherical polar coordinates, then, if the origin is taken to be the shoulder, the elbow can be seen clearly as a simple device to make the arm a 'hand–shoulder distance-varying mechanism' of the folded strut type. The two coordinate angles of the spherical polar system, θ and ϕ, now apply, not to the upper arm, but to an imaginary line linking the hand to the shoulder, whose length is altered by wrist, elbow and shoulder; that is, the 'true arm' is a 'line of sight' from shoulder to wrist. The upper and lower parts of the arm are not themselves involved because the control of position refers to the wrist–shoulder relationship.

If such a system does represent the organization of the arm, it provides an explanation of why, for example, the elbow is a hinge while the shoulder is a socket joint and the wrist is of the universal type; if the folding strut has a length reducing function only, its action must be to bring the wrist and shoulder together and with any other type of joint at the elbow this would not necessarily occur. The simple function of the elbow in reducing the length of the radius vector gives that joint a minor role in the planning of movement by the central nervous system; the important position is that of the hand, whereas the position of the elbow is normally of little consequence. Similarly, it is often remarked that with the elbow extended the hand can be rotated through about

360° but, when the elbow is flexed, this is reduced to 180°. If, however, the wrist, while rotating is kept at one point in space and the elbow is moved in a circular path round an imaginary axis joining wrist to shoulder, the full potential rotation of the hand is restored, because humeral rotation not only gives added rotation of the hand but, with shoulder movement, it can rotate the position of the fold of the strut (the elbow) out of the way of obstacles without affecting the processing of hand control information. The socket joint allows movement of the upper arm in the angular dimensions, and rotation, whereas the wrist allows only angular movement; the hand takes its rotation from the forearm.

If the arm indeed does act to position the hand in terms of distance, elevation and azimuth (r, θ, ϕ), it would mean that the 'mechanical' component, the upper limb, would be working on the same, or at worst a very similar, basis of spatial relationship to the eye, and the most that might be required would be to transfer the origin of the polar system from one point to another. The advantage that this would have for rapid eye–hand coordination would be enormous and certainly the performance in practice is excellent; a consistent neural concept of space would explain why the present skeletal structure of the arm provides the advantage necessary for the persistence of that form.

The hand

The human hand differs from most anthropoid apes by having greater thumb:finger length ratio. This is because the fingers are proportionally shorter, which is an advantage. Because of their orthograde bipedal locomotion, man and the gorilla can have fingers which are relatively short because they do not have to grasp the large branches necessary to hold their adult weight.

The shorter finger gave an easier thumb to finger-tip apposition, in turn giving greater manipulative ability, and, therefore, a greater versatility. Although even the most superficial study of the anthropoids who retain the long fingers will show they have no mean ability in manipulation and exploratory skills, the shorter fingers of man have made the grasping of smaller objects simpler. The important factor is that this was an improvement on the former situation and resulted in a definite step away from anatomical specialization.

Specialization was, of course, occurring, but it was in holding tools and, although the handles had to be made to fit the characteristics of his hand and thus generally meant a cylindrical or branch-like shape, the design of the tool itself allowed him to change his characteristics and 'evolve' at will.

Many features of the hand survive almost unchanged from the earlier environment and have had a profound influence on current hand use. The necessity for a firm grasp of hanging branches meant that differentiation of the thumb from the fingers to oppose all the fingers was critically important and gave survival advantage. This has become of immense importance in holding and in manipulating irregularly shaped objects. The last results partly from the axial rotational mobility of the digits at the metacarpophalangeal joints which increases from the radial to the ulnar side. This was important because the ring and little fingers had a following or adaptive role in support; the index and long, as befitting the principal apposing parts to the thumb, were the most stable (p. 14), while the other two allowed a measure of rotation to allow the hand to adapt to hold an object, their position in turn being safeguarded when hanging on a vertical creeper or branch by the firmness of the other two. The transverse metacarpal arch (p. 14) has a primary function among anthropoid apes in allowing maximum hand surface in contact with the object cradled between the thenar and hypothenar eminences, or thenar and fingers. With the shorter fingers, the arch gives easy finger to thumb apposition, and has been of particular importance in the new environment. A cylinder forced between thumb and index finger also acts to close the hand quickly by reacting on the web, driving the grasp closed, a useful mechanism when trying to catch branches but this web also gives a surprising symmetry which makes for versatility in tool holding.

The principle of increasing the maximal surface area in contact with different shapes became much more important when the finger length reduced, but the need for a secure grasp shown by all primates also produced, at the next level, the 'passive' gripping mechanism of an adaptable finger pulp (p. 7). The ridged volar skin, normally slightly damp with sweat and therefore with a high coefficient of friction has limited properties of stretch. It covers a closed volume and so, when depression of the skin of the finger pads by an object reduces that volume, the increase in pressure stiffens the pad into a form which is moulded to the object. For the small forces involved this gives an astonishingly secure grip, and it is surprising that it is only recently that this concept has been employed in man-made gripping tools.

Role of the nervous system

The mechanical aspects of hand anatomy provide for a prehension apparatus which is of great adaptability at the level of hand and finger and therefore of potentially great versatility. The role of the hand in a brachiating or semi-brachiating creature is so important that its structure has had, of necessity, to be intricate, but the real complexity lies with the controlling system in the central nervous system which must receive all the information necessary for its operation with the minimal dependence on visual information. The eyes must estimate the position in space of a branch with respect to the observer and to estimate its suitability, but the arm must position the hand correctly and the hand, in grasping, has to investigate and report the dimensions of the branch, its rigidity and texture or the frictional forces without the further involvement of the eyes, because the safety of the individual depends on this. It is, therefore, not surprising that the finger pads are areas with a very high tactile discrimination (p. 180). A reminder of its original importance is seen today in the reluctance of many individuals to allow tactile information from the fingers to adapt out; the fingers are kept in motion exploring or 'fidgeting'. Similarly, the fingers had to be very good at detecting slip, a characteristic which has survived and is so established that there appears to be a fixed relationship between strength of grip used and the force at which slip would just occur.

The hand had an additional role in gathering information. Quality and texture of objects could be tested by small movements of the evenly ridged and sensitive finger tip but detecting the shape of objects is simply an extension of gauging branch size. The basic grasping principle of hand shape adaptation to give the maximum area of the hand in contact with an object has the result that the hand envelops and so takes the shape of the part of the object it holds. The proprioceptive information of the finger configuration is extremely accurate; the same hazardous arboreal progression which required accuracy would have eliminated mutations which would have degraded the accuracy. The position of the fingers holding an object therefore indicates to the central nervous system the shape of the object and further exploration of that object improves the quality and completeness of that information by the collection of a number of configurations which build up a spatial description which becomes progressively more and more complete.

An arboreal environment requires a very developed sense of position of the limbs and of three dimensional space but, because of the rapidly changing situation, it also means that visual information tends to dominate the proprioceptive sources and takes a higher ranking when there is a clash between them; normally there is no clash and the kinaesthetic information from different channels reinforce each other.

In a system of jointed rods such as the skeleton, in order to have internal information about the position of the most distal part, there must be no breaks in the chain and there must be information about every joint angle to allow the computation of a picture of the structure. A break in the chain or a gap in the information somewhere along the line to the hand would make the estimation of hand position impossible but, because of the vital importance of proprioceptive information, there are many sources giving similar information, each supporting the other. Of those concerned with joint angle, the joint receptors almost certainly give the most accurate information, supported by corresponding information from tendon, and particularly from skin.

This system of relying on more than one channel ensures that the organism is protected against failure of any channel and this is particularly marked in the hand. If damage occurs in one channel, the body is said to adapt; the mechanism of adaptation may be no more complex, however, than the dropping of the priority of the affected source and the upgrading of another, with a possible diminution of the accuracy of the resultant position determination.

It is the 'extension' of man's proprioception outside the body to objects held in the hand, however, which is his most remarkable and unique characteristic.

Proprioceptive information received by the central nervous system must be processed before it can be used in limb control and, although the concept of extensive computation and processing of data in the brain may be somewhat difficult to accept, there is no doubt that this does occur and without any involvement of the conscious mind. In man there is an additional property of being able to extend his proprioception, e.g. by a stick held in the hand. This extra computational ability appears to be the particularly human one which gives him a disproportionate advantage over other animals. Proprioception as a monitoring mechanism in body movements appears to give greatest attention to the most distal part and the ability to extend out into a tool allows this tool to be used as if it were within the biological envelope. It is impossible to overestimate the importance of this.

The hand of man, because of a change in his evolutionary path, has become the most versatile of all; its obvious principal characteristics are the ability to adapt at finger and hand level to the shape of objects, to hold and manipulate but not to let slip, and to gather information about objects with which it is in contact. Its real characteristic is that it enables man to hold tools and therefore become an ultra-adaptable animal; it allows him to control the machines and instruments which he can design and construct. The increased ability to 'do', which comes from his machines, and his extended intellectual capacity, which comes via his use of tools, from books, machine storage and computer manipulation of knowledge, have allowed him to evolve in the last few thousand years from primitive tool user and recorder of his ideas into the most powerful creature in the world. It would seem to come very largely from his capacity to extend his proprioception out from his grasp into the tool he holds. His conscious intellect enables him to plan his strategy but most of the hand function that is now necessary for survival in today's environment could be carried out with only one finger pad and an apposing finger, the common grasp of the chimpanzee.

CHAPTER 4

The Hand in Medicine

E. B. FRENCH

The hand, directed by the mind, is largely responsible for the dominant position of man in the animal kingdom. It is such a highly developed structure that its area of representation on the cerebral cortex is disproportionately large. The palmist has been tempted to read more from the hand than is justified, yet experience enables us to make a surprisingly accurate assessment of people from the appearances of the face and hands. The firm determined grip or the soft flabby handshake often reflects the personality. The manicured or the careworn hand, the tobacco stains, the bitten nails, the nervous tremor, the rings and the tattoo each tell their story. The use of gesture in speech, though variable from one culture to another, is universal, and the deaf and dumb can communicate through the hands alone. Even more remarkable is the one-handed language of the blind, deaf and dumb. During the clinical interview, hand gestures can be most informative. Thus the headache which is shown by the flat of the hand pressed over the vertex usually indicates a psychogenic symptom, of something weighing on the mind. The pain of peptic ulcer is commonly indicated by the finger tips in the epigastrium, whereas the flat of the hand rubbed to and fro is more likely to imply a functional dyspepsia. An epigastric pain due to the agony of gallstones is recalled by the hand or the fist pressed firmly over the area. The gestures made by patients suffering from the lightning pains of tabes dorsalis or the retrosternal pain of angina pectoris are even more informative than words.

The rewards of examination are proportional to the care taken. A methodical approach is essential and noting every variation leads to the appreciation of less obvious, but not necessarily less important, phenomena which are often missed by a cursory examination. It is both an instructive and a chastening experience to record independently with three or four colleagues all imperfections in a patient's hand. Total agreement rarely if ever occurs. The diagnostic features on examination of the hand range from minor details like tobacco stains to signs of major potential significance such as clubbing of the fingers. Some diagnoses can be made beyond all reasonable doubt from inspection of the hand alone. For example, liver failure with cirrhosis is present if clubbing of the fingers is accompanied by melanin pigmentation, palmar erythema, leuconychia, spider telangiectases and flapping tremor. Some would add Dupuytren's contracture to the list, but this disorder is so common with advancing years in healthy Caucasians and so rare in some other races that the recorded association may be an example of looking for something in special circumstances. At least one book has been devoted to the subject [1], but this single chapter gives account of some hand abnormalities during a description of a routine examination and adds a few examples to show that something of value can be learned with regard to all specialties.

Abnormal movements

Abnormal movements of the hand are often noticed while the history is being taken. These include hyperkinesia, fine or coarse tremors, choreiform or athetoid movements and tetany.

Hyperkinesia refers to the agitated movements, the twisting and twining of a handkerchief or the overhasty efforts to undo buttons which characterize thyrotoxicosis or nervousness. It contrasts with the immobile puffy hands of myxoedema.

Fine rapid tremor at a rate of about 10 per second, which is an exaggeration of physiological tremor, often indicates nervousness, but it is also seen in thyrotoxicosis and acute hypoglycaemia. In each case it is an adrenaline effect and it can be abolished by a β-adrenergic blocker [2].

The most characteristic *coarse tremor* is that of Parkinson's disease. Rhythmic movements of about 5 per second affect the thumbs, fingers and hands. The tremor worsens with excitement and usually stops for a short time after making a movement. It may be due to other disorders affecting the basal ganglia. A coarse rapid tremor made worse by movement is a feature of chronic alcoholism and is a warning of impending delirium tremens. Benign familial tremor can be distinguished from it only by its duration and familial occurrence, while the facies does not show other signs of alcoholism. Sudden, darting, irregular movements of the outstreched hands and fingers is not only characteristic of the flapping tremor of liver failure already mentioned, but occurs also in chronic respiratory and renal failure. It can be of such a severity as to cause objects to be flung out of the hand.

Choreiform and athetoid movements result from lesions of the basal ganglia. They are seen predominantly in Sydenham's and Huntingdon's chorea, in hepatolenticular degeneration and as a sequel to kernicterus or occasionally vascular lesions or injury.

The spasm of tetany is recognized by the characteristic main d'accoucheur, with the fingers extended at the interphalangeal but flexed at the metacarpophalangeal joints. It is often accompanied by pain in the forearms and paraesthesiae in the fingers. The commonest cause is alkalosis due to hyperventilation, which may be an indication for psychiatric assessment. Any other cause of alkalosis or a reduction in the serum ionized calcium may also lead to tetany.

In addition an *intention tremor* may be noted while the patient is undressing and this calls for formal neurological tests to distinguish between sensory and cerebellar ataxia.

Posture

The posture of the hand may be characteristic as exemplified by the flexed hand and arm of hemiplegia or the way in which both hands are flexed with a lack of natural spontaneity of movement in Parkinson's disease. Unilateral or bilateral wrist drop suggests radial nerve palsy and lead palsy respectively. Ulnar nerve paralysis results in 'la main en griffe', with the little finger curled and the ring finger partly so, like a talon. It may be confused with Dupuytren's contracture, but readily distinguished from it by absence of hard, nodular thickening of the palmar fascia and by the sensory impairment over the ulnar third of the hand and weakness of most of the small muscles.

General observations may lead to useful information about occupation of the patient, shape and size of the hand, colour, temperature and sweating.

Occupation

Of particular diagnostic value sometimes are the typical blue marks caused by coal dust in a miner who has not divulged his occupation. The lesions may draw attention to pneumoconiosis as an explanation for dyspnoea or for diffuse opacities in a radiograph of the chest. It is worth bearing in mind also that a recent tattooing may have been the source of type B viral hepatitis. In each case the blue colour of the tattoo is due to black particles (coal dust and Indian ink), changed in appearance by the scatter of light as it passes through and is reflected back from the skin. In the atrophic skin in rheumatoid disease, with prolonged steroid therapy or in old age, the tissues may be so thin that the red colour of the blood shows clearly.

Manual work of various kinds produces characteristic callosities at specific sites, while sawyers are apt to lose fingers. Conversely, a knowledge of the occupation may help to identify unusual lesions such as pilonidal sinuses in the finger webs of barbers due to the implantation of hairs, erysipeloid of butchers or anthrax following the handling of imported bonemeal.

Shape and size

Examples of unusual shapes include those associated with Marfan's and Turner's syndromes and pseudohypoparathyroidism. The long thin fingers of *Marfan's syndrome* should strongly suggest the diagnosis of dissecting aneurysm of the aorta in a young man with sudden retrosternal pain. Short fourth and fifth metacarpals would be evidence in favour of *Turner's syndrome* in a woman complaining of amenorrhoea. Brachydactyly, in conjunction with a round face and short stature adds supportive evidence of *pseudohypoparathyroidism*.

Enlargement of the hands can provide confirmation of *acromegaly* which has been suspected from the facies.

Colour

Pallor of the nails and palmar creases gives a useful clinical estimate of anaemia. If the hand is cyanosed and warm it can be deduced, in a temperate climate, that arterial oxygen saturation is reduced. An exception to this is polycythaemia rubra vera in which the density of the colour leads readily to a cyanosed appearance which may be eliminated only by the patient breathing 100 per cent oxygen in association with maximal vasodilation [3]. Vitiligo commonly affects the hands and may be associated with pernicious anaemia and other auto-immune disorders.

Pallor or darkening of the skin due to a decrease or an increase in melanin content from generalized causes is apt to be most evident in the hands and face. White hands with a smooth, soft skin are seen in conjunction with similar changes in the face in hypopituitarism. Included among the causes of unusual darkening are Addison's disease, Nelson's syndrome, MSH secreting bronchial carcinoma, haemochromatosis and chronic poisoning by silver or arsenic. In the case of arsenic, characteristic spiky hyperkeratoses also develop on the palms. While the usual statement that the palmar creases are apt to be pigmented from these systemic causes is true, it must be borne in mind that brown palmar creases, and buccal pigmentation too, are sometimes seen in healthy people with dark hair and brown eyes [4].

Temperature

In a temperate climate the temperature of the patient's hand is a good guide to the mean blood flow through it. In most patients with heart failure the hands tend to be cold due to vasoconstriction in response to a low cardiac output. If they are warm with heart failure the sign is of particular value in drawing attention to occult thyrotoxicosis or some other cause of high output failure. It is of interest and value that the clinician's hand, in spite of its variations in temperature, can usually detect even a modest fever from the feel of the trunk or brow of the patient.

Sweating

Thermal sweating has little effect on the palms [5]. During acute hypoglycaemia the hands, including the palms, take part in generalized sweating. Hot, moist palms often indicate thyrotoxicosis and contrast usefully with cold clammy hands due to nervousness.

COMPONENTS OF THE HAND

These general observations can be followed fruitfully by careful consideration of the individual components of the hand, each of which may singly or in combination be affected by a variety of local and systemic disorders. An indication of this variety is given by reference to a few examples of disorders affecting different structures.

Skin

The smooth hairless hands of a boy should change to the lined and hairy hand of the adult male unless hypogonadism is present. In the elderly, atrophy leads to wrinkling and frequently to senile purpura characterized by large flat purple areas due to bleeding from rupture of unsupported vessels [6]. This is largely confined to the backs of the hands and forearms and is accompanied by white stellate scars following subepidermal tears and brown patches due to iron deposits. These senile changes, when found with transparent skin are similar to those produced by adrenocorticosteroids and both reflect the degree of osteoporosis present [7].

Superimposed on any age changes there may be lesions indicating specific skin disorders or dermatological manifestations of systemic disease. *Scabies* is an example of the former in which a suspected diagnosis is greatly supported by the distribution of lesions between the fingers and on the volar aspect of the wrists. It is often possible to extract the mite from the blind end of one of the thin sinuous lines which indicate a burrow. An example of the latter is the raised, slowly spreading, ringed eruption of *granuloma annulare* on the backs of the hands; its occurrence should lead to a check for diabetes mellitus. The backs of the hands are also sites of election for dermatitis artefacta, self-inflicted lesions which are an appeal for help and an indication for psychiatric attention.

Nails

A transverse groove (Beau's line) at a similar level on each of the nails dates a systemic disturbance and occasionally discloses a recent illness which has not been mentioned. Koilonychia accompanying anaemia indicates chronic iron deficiency. Splinter haemorrhages in the nails have for long been quoted as a feature of infective endocarditis. The fact that one or two such haemorrhages are often present in healthy subjects has erroneously led to the discredit of this sign. If infective endocarditis is under consideration, then the observation of splinter haemorrhages beneath several of the nails is strong supportive evidence.

Subcutaneous tissue

Of interest rather than of importance are the firm painless nodules which occur in rheumatoid disease. Clinically similar but more sinister and less persistent nodules are a feature of acute rheumatic fever, especially over the dorsum of the hands; they are indicative of significant involvement of the heart.

Tendons

Lesions of particular interest are the xanthomatous deposits which are apt to occur in Types II and III hyperlipidaemia. They are seen more readily by examination of the clenched fist, when the nodular thickenings become prominent. Affected subjects are liable to peripheral vascular disease, myocardial infarction and other ill effects of atherosclerosis.

Muscles

Wasting is common in rheumatoid disease or in cachexia. Otherwise wasting of muscles is secondary to lower motor neurone damage or, rarely, to muscle diseases. Generalized wasting of the muscles of both hands with fasciculation is common in motor neurone disease. Lesions affecting the first thoracic root or ulnar nerve affect most of the muscles of the hand. Selective wasting of the thenar muscles occurs with a median nerve lesion, the commonest cause of which is compression in the carpal tunnel. It should be borne in mind that the carpal tunnel syndrome, though usually of unknown cause, may be due to a systemic disorder, such as myxoedema or rheumatoid arthritis.

Bones

Clinical evidence of involvement of the bones of the hand by systemic disease is comparatively rare though the causes are many, including tuberculosis, syphilis, sarcoidosis, tuberous sclerosis or sickle cell disease. A characteristic and at times very useful diagnostic sign is pseudo-clubbing of the fingers in hyperparathyroidism. It is due to absorption of the terminal phalangeal bones so that the unsupported nails become curved and the soft tissues redundant and therefore bulbous. The condition may be mistaken for clubbing, but the distinction is clear if the shortening of the terminal phalanges and the preservation of the angles between the nails and the nail beds are observed.

Nerves

With symmetrical polyneuritis distal sensory impairment of glove and stocking distribution characteristically affects both hands and feet. With subacute combined degeneration of the spinal cord, the hands alone may be affected [8]. Several other neurological lesions affecting the hands have already been described.

Blood vessels

It need hardly be mentioned that the radial pulse is a source of information about the heart rate, rhythm and stroke volume. A hard artery is usually due to medial sclerosis and occlusive arterial disease in the hand is comparatively rare. The transient occlusion of Raynaud's phenomenon is due to vasospasm induced abnormally readily by cooling. It is commonly idiopathic, but when it develops in a teenage female it can be the first feature in the development of systemic lupus erythematosus. In this disease there may also be tiny red lesions in the skin over the nail bases due to arteriolar occlusions.

Joints

The joints of the hands are frequently involved in rheumatoid disease, osteoarthrosis, psoriatic arthritis and gout. The differential diagnosis depends largely upon the history and the distribution and symmetry of the joints involved. For example, rheumatoid disease and psoriatic arthritis may be very similar, except that the terminal interphalangeal joint is much more commonly involved in psoriasis. This joint is also most commonly involved in generalized osteoarthrosis, giving rise to Heberden's nodes.

CONCLUSION

The conditions already mentioned have a bearing on two dozen specialties in medicine and surgery. Even the forensic expert, in league with the police, may be able to identify a body or a crime from the fingerprints. Indeed it was this fact that led Dr. Ruxton to attempt to conceal the identity of his victims by removing, among other things, their terminal phalanges [9].

While attention could be drawn to many other aspects, this chapter demonstrates sufficiently the diagnostic value of a careful examination of the hand, which can truly be a 'mirror of disease'.

REFERENCES

[1] BERRY, T. J. *The Hand as a Mirror of Systemic Disease*. Philadelphia, F. A. Davis, 1963.

[2] MARSDEN, D. C., FOLEY, T. H., OWEN, D. A. L. AND MCALLISTER, R. G. Peripheral β-adrenergic receptors concerned with tremor. *Clinical Science*, 1967, **33**, 53.

[3] CORRAL, R. J. M. Personal communication.

[4] Personal observation.

[5] KUNO, Y. *The Physiology of Human Perspiration*. London, Churchill, 1934.

[6] SHUSTER, S. AND SCARBOROUGH, H. Senile purpura. *Quarterly Journal of Medicine*, 1961, **30**, 33.

[7] MCCONKEY, B., BLIGH, A. S., FRASER, G. M. AND WHITLEY, H. Transparent skin and osteoporosis, *Lancet*, 1963, **i**, 693.

[8] MAWDSLEY, C. Personal communication.

[9] GLAISTER, J. AND BRASH, J. C. *Medico-Legal Aspects of the Ruxton Case*. Edinburgh, Livingstone, 1937.

CHAPTER 5

Clinical Examination

R. J. SMITH

This chapter is not meant to be a comprehensive analysis of the examination of all injuries, deformities and abnormalities of the hand. Details of the examination and the findings to be anticipated after specific injuries, with rheumatoid disease, in the congenitally deformed hand and with various neurological abnormalities are covered in the sections dealing with these conditions. Rather, a general approach and description of a plan of examination is outlined. Certainly, this plan may be varied depending upon the surgeon, the patient and the condition to be evaluated. However, if a meaningful history and physical examination are to be performed which do not overlook important details and yet are not unnecessarily tedious and exhausting, a basic routine should be employed.

The value of radiography, laboratory and electrical studies in diagnosing disorders of the hand cannot be overestimated. Yet, it is the clinical examination which serves as the basis for all treatment. It is at the initial examination that the hand surgeon's responsibilities begin, and the accuracy of his findings greatly influences the results of subsequent treatment. Because of the enormous complexity of anatomical structures which contribute to the versatility and power of the hand, the surgeon must follow an orderly plan of investigation if he is to perform a comprehensive and meaningful clinical examination. Only then can he be confident that he has gathered all the information necessary to analyze structural disorders and to formulate an intelligent plan of surgical reconstruction.

HISTORY

Most patients give a notoriously poor history of their injury or illness. With the slightest encouragement they tirelessly relate countless irrelevant details. Their memory of significant events is often vague, distorted or totally inaccurate. To some, pain is either absent or intolerable. If a meaningful history of an illness is to be obtained the patient's jargon must be translated into relatively precise and accurate data. The 'first joint of the third finger' to one patient is the 'last joint of the fourth finger' to another. Therefore, fingers must be identified by name rather than number. The 'tip joint, middle joint and knuckle joint' are less ambiguous than the 'first, second and third joint'. Symptoms can be quantitated by various means. 'Terrible pain' can be better evaluated if the patient is asked whether it is of such severity as to interfere with the ability to sleep, to work, or to engage in athletics. The blood loss after an injury may be estimated by inquiring with what material the hand was bandaged and whether the bandage was soaked through and had to be changed. Even such subjective symptoms as those relating to the appearance of the hand might be better judged if the patient is asked whether he is self-conscious when with strangers, whether gloves are worn to hide the hand or whether the hand is kept constantly in the pocket. If the hand is 'terribly stiff in the morning' the patient may be asked whether he is able to dress, or prepare breakfast, or drive to work. As there is hardly a symptom or complaint which cannot be related to some everyday nonscientific yardstick, it is the surgeon's obligation to make these comparisons with all relevant portions of the history.

The following plan has proved helpful in obtaining a complete initial history:

(1) History of illness or injury
   (a) When?
   (b) Where?
   (c) How?
   (d) What progress?
(2) Present condition
   (a) Pain
   (b) Stiffness or swelling
   (c) Weakness
   (d) General function
(3) Chief complaint
(4) General information
   (a) Dominant hand
   (b) Occupation
   (c) Hobbies
(5) General medical history
   (a) Previous injuries
   (b) Past illnesses
   (c) Immunization
   (d) Present medication
   (e) Allergies
   (f) Contributory family history

History of illness or injury

When? Determine as accurately as possible when the illness or injury occurred. If the patient is unsure or vague, the memory can usually be jogged by relating dates in the medical history to other important events. Frequently, medical milestones can be pinpointed by holidays or vacations.

Where? 'Did it occur at work?' is most important for medicolegal purposes. Did the accident occur in the street, in the hospital or in the farmyard? This information is essential to determine the nature and severity of contamination.

How? With machine accidents much can be learned about the nature of the injury by determining the function of the machine. Was it hot or cold, did it repeat,

is it the type of machine which tears, crushes, pulls or cuts, how long did the hand remain in the machine before it was extricated? The cleanliness of the machine or object which inflicted the wound should be determined. Was it coated with chemicals, grease or plastic? Could a portion of the machine have broken and become lodged in the wound?

What is the progress? The immediate effects of injury, the initial treatment and the progress of the abnormality must be carefully noted. Original radiographic reports, photographs, electrical and laboratory studies should be obtained. What medical treatment was given and with what effect? Was the patient originally treated in a hospital and if so, was surgery performed and what was the postoperative care? What were the results of this treatment, and in what way has the condition improved or worsened since the abnormality was first noted? Although much valuable information can be obtained from the records of previous surgeons, emergency rooms and hospitals, the patient's evaluation of progress should be sought and recorded.

Present condition

Careful inquiry must be made into the state and function of the hand at the time of examination. The following questions are often helpful.

Pain. The patient should be asked when the pain is most severe, precisely where it is located and what is its type. Is it burning, shooting or throbbing? What makes it better and worse? Is medication required, and if so, how much, what kind and when? Is it relieved by steroids or tranquilizers?

Stiffness and swelling. When is it worse? When is it better? Where is it located? Does it improve with medication?

Weakness. What is the patient unable to do? What can be done with difficulty?

General function. Is the patient working? If so, what is the regular job? Can the patient engage in athletics, take care of the house, or dress?

Chief complaint

With all patients other than those who recently sustained an acute injury, the reason for seeking treatment must be established clearly. This is particularly true with long-standing deformities or disabilities. The surgeon must not attempt to guess what bothers the patient the most. If a young lady with cerebral palsy has decreased sensibility and poor motor control, she may be more eager to have her wrist brought out of palmar flexion for better appearance than to have surgery to improve hand function. A patient with severe rheumatoid deformities of the hand may be bothered more by the locking of the fingers in flexion and extension than with the ulnar drift. Following malunion of an intra-articular fracture of the proximal interphalangeal joint of the index finger, one patient may be most concerned with pain, another may object to its appearance and a third may complain of stiffness which is incompatible with his work. Whether the treatment should be arthrodesis, arthroplasty or amputation may depend upon these complaints. Often a most important part of the history is the ability of the surgeon to determine what the patient expects from treatment. Although treatment may not be dictated by the patient's wishes, the surgeon must be cognizant of them as they may serve as a guide to care.

General information

Much general information about the patient may be as important in selecting a plan of treatment as the anatomical abnormalities within the hand itself. These data should be obtained preoperatively if appropriate care is to be planned.

Which is the *dominant hand*? If ambidextrous, which hand is used for writing and which for heavy grip?

What are the patient's *occupation* and *hobbies*? Is there 'light work' at the place of employment? Is the patient totally without income when disabled? Does a mother have help at home? Are there any infants?

General medical history

This is of course essential. The surgeon must carefully determine if there have been any previous injuries to the upper limbs. Medical and surgical history must include questions about diabetes, gout and arthritis. Has previous *immunization* been received, particularly against tetanus? Is any *medication* taken for medical or psychiatric disorders? Is there a *contributory family history* of illness, *allergy* or congenital deformity?

Once a comprehensive history is obtained, the surgeon should be able to arrive at a provisional diagnosis. The physical examination should further refine that diagnosis and allow a treatment plan to be determined.

PHYSICAL EXAMINATION

Patients are frequently somewhat apprehensive during a physical examination. If injury is recent there is often fear of pain when the bandages are removed and when injured parts are manipulated. If the abnormality is long-standing, the patient knows that pain may be exacerbated by stretching stiff joints, manipulating painful scars or the inevitable repeated poking with steel pins to determine sensory patterns. The fear of pain is greatly magnified in the mind of a child. Therefore, the examination of the hand must be performed gently, methodically and in plain view of the inquisitive eyes of the patient. There should be no attempt to hide the hand in order to improve the objectivity of the examination as this will only add to the patient's apprehension. Except for the most trivial injuries, the entire limb should be examined from the shoulder distally. The surgeon and the patient should be seated opposite each other across an examining table. If the patient has just suffered an acute injury he may prefer to lie comfortably on an examining table. A small child may prefer the security of sitting on the mother's lap. An infant is much more patient and tolerant of the examination if held in the mother's arms.

Examination should proceed from the uninjured to the injured parts. A recent severe wound should not be probed in an emergency ward. The risk of contamination and the pain caused by such an examination are not justified by the surgeon's curiosity. The wound should only be examined in a sterile setting and under appropriate anaesthesia. Even less extensive wounds should be examined only on a sterile field with the surgeon appropriately masked and gloved.

A most valuable, rapid and accurate means of record-

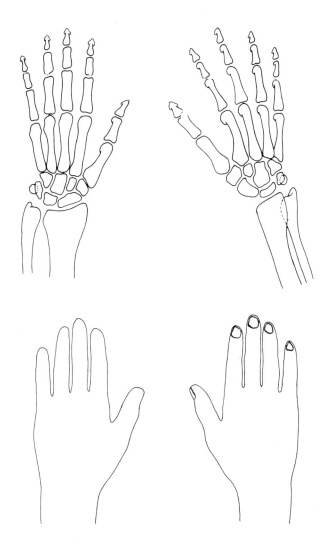

FIG. 5.1. A diagram sheet which enables areas of injury, deformity and sensory impairment to be noted accurately and rapidly at the time of the examination.

ing the findings of an examination of the hand is the use of a sketch. The hand should be drawn as it is seen with landmarks of digital and palmar creases noted, and with all wounds, scars, deformities and abnormalities appropriately shown (Fig. 5.1).

'Eyeball' measurements are notoriously inaccurate and should be avoided. A few simple and inexpensive measuring devices suffice for most clinical examinations of the hand. These include a goniometer and ruler, tape measure, two point caliper (or paper clip), blunted pin, dynamometer and pinch meter (Fig. 5.2). A goniometer is essential for accurate determination of joint motion. A 'range of motion form' further simplifies recording these findings (Fig. 5.3). The length of scars should be measured, sensory abnormalities should be mapped and areas of increased sensitivity and tenderness precisely determined and identified. Strength should not be recorded as 'good' or 'fair' but rather should be measured with dynamometers which objectively determine power (p. 88 and see Fig. 5.11a).

Infants and children should be observed carefully while the history is being obtained to determine the attitude of the hands, and how they handle toys and dolls. Much of the examination can be in the form of a game. A child can be asked to see how rapidly paper clips can be picked up, paper torn, objects placed on his fingertip drawn or identified rather than being subjected to the tedium of repeated flexion and extension of the fingers. The face must never be covered during the examination as the worst will be suspected.

A useful and systematic method of examination of the hand may consist of the following:

Inspection

Posture. The position of the fingers, thumb and wrist are noted with the hand at rest. With the wrist in mild dorsiflexion, the fingers normally lie adjacent and parallel to each other and fingertips form a gentle curve with gradually increasing flexion to the ulnar side of the hand. If this curve is broken, a tendon laceration or rupture may be suspected. If the nails are not parallel, the rotational deformity may signify a spiral fracture of the metacarpal or phalanx. Normally, the thumb lies perpendicular to the index fingertip and there is mild flexion of its metacarpophalangeal and interphalangeal joints. With median nerve palsy, the thumb is supinated and adducted.

The forearm is then pronated and the wrist allowed to fall into palmar flexion. If the extensor tendons are intact, the fingers and thumb gently extend at the metacarpophalangeal joints.

Atrophy. Normal convexity at the thenar and hypothenar eminences, when the injured hand is compared with the

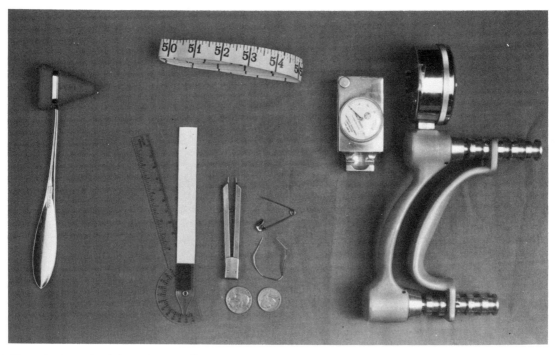

FIG. 5.2. These simple 'tools of the trade' are sufficient for most clinical examinations of the hand. A goniometer accurately measures range of motion. The coins, paper clip, dulled safety pin and blunted calipers are used for sensibility testing. Pinch and squeeze dynamometers determine objectively hand strength. The tape ruler measures the circumference of arm and forearm in order to evaluate atrophy or hypertrophy. The percussion hammer is used for neurological tests.

uninjured one, suggests intact median and ulnar nerves. The thenar muscles frequently have dual innervation. The examiner should, therefore, be particularly alert to shallowness in the region of the abductor pollicis brevis at the most radial side of the thenar eminence. Concavity in this region suggests abnormal median nerve function as the abductor brevis usually is supplied by the median nerve alone (Fig. 5.4). At the dorsum of the hand, the borders of the metacarpal shafts are usually not well visualized as they are surrounded by the bulk of the inter-osseous muscles. The hypothenar muscles clothe the ulnar side of the fifth metacarpal. Atrophy of these muscles may suggest either a muscular disease, injury to the ulnar nerve, or injury of the C8/T1 nerve roots. Atrophy of the forearm or arm may suggest nerve or muscle injury or disuse. Circumference of the two limbs should be measured and compared. As a rule, the circumference of the arms is measured 8 cm proximal to the epicondyles and the forearms measured 6 cm distal to the

epicondyles. Usually, the dominant limb circumference is about 1 cm greater than that of the assistive limb.

Swelling. Absence of digital creases may indicate swelling of the adjacent joint or soft tissues. All fingers gently taper to their tips. A lack of symmetry suggests tumour or inflammation in this area. The palmar skin is firmly held by the palmar fascia beneath it. If the mid-palmar concavity is lost, infection or inflammation should be suspected. At the dorsum of the hand the skin is looser and thinner. With diffuse swelling, there is often loss of venous filling and a puffiness which is bounded by the deep fascial attachments to the first and fifth metacarpal shafts. Uneven swelling may suggest inflammation of the tendon sheaths, a local pocket of fluid or perhaps syno-vitis within the wrist itself. Wrist synovitis is most likely to be poorly defined and the extensor tendons can usually be identified gliding above or beside it. With extensor tenosynovitis (particularly in rheumatoid disease) there

HAND EXAMINATION CHART

MASSACHUSETTS GENERAL HOSPITAL

Patient's Name:
Unit Number:
Chart Number:

Date:
Symptomatic Hand:
Major Hand:

		Active Motion							
		MP		PIP		DIP		Lacks MPL (cms)	
		R	L	R	L	R	L	R	L
Thumb	Extension								
	Flexion								
Index	Extension								
	Flexion								
Middle	Extension								
	Flexion								
Ring	Extension								
	Flexion								
Little	Extension								
	Flexion								

		Right	Left				Right	Left
Wrist	D.F.				Forearm	Pronation		
	P.F.							
	R.D.					Supination		
	U.D.							
Thumb	ABD				Elbow	Extension		
	ADD							
	PRO					Flexion		
	SUP							
Pinch (kg/lbs)					Circumference (in cms.)	Biceps		
Grip (kg/lbs)						Forearm		

Note: With Joint Measurements:

0° = STRAIGHT LINE (FULL EXTENSION). Other figures refer to angles from full extension. Thus, 30/70 = lacks 30° of extension and flexes to 70°. 40/40 = ankylosed in 40° of flexion.

FIG. 5.3. A hand examination chart is used for initial examinations and for follow-up purposes. Normal is always compared with abnormal. Boxes which are left empty are assumed to indicate a normal range of motion. If only passive motion is measured, this is indicated at the top of the examination chart.

is often a dumbbell shaped swelling from which the extensor tendons emerge distally (see Fig. 25.1a). The extensor tenosynovium is compressed in the region of the wrist joint by the extensor retinaculum.

Skin changes. The texture and moisture of the skin should

be noted. Smooth, shiny and dry skin may result from nerve injury. Increased redness, sweating and warmth are suggestive of infection or sympathetic dystrophy. If there are areas in the hands of a working person which are not ingrained with dirt or grease, these portions are probably not used because of pain, stiffness or weak-

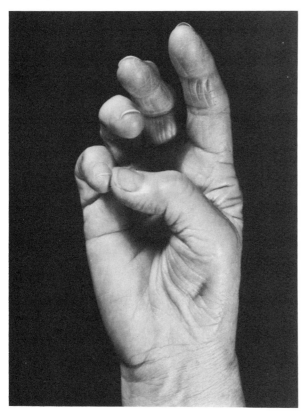

FIG. 5.4. This woman complained of numbness of the radial three digits and awkwardness of the use of her thumb. Atrophy of the abductor pollicis brevis is seen by the shallowness to the radial side of the thenar eminence.

ness. The colour of the skin may be a valuable sign in cases of arterial insufficiency, vasospasm or Raynaud's phenomenon.

Deformity. Shortening, amputation, deviation or rotation of the wrist or of the digits should be sketched and measured. In all cases, the two hands should be compared. In order to be accurate, measurements should be made from an identifiable reference point. The length of a finger may be measured from its proximal flexion crease; angulation of the digit should be measured in relation to an unaffected proximal bone; rotational deformities of the digit may be measured by the angle the nail makes with that of the adjacent finger. If the hand appears flat, or the finger is clawed, or the wrist deformed

as with the 'silver fork' appearance following a Colles' fracture, this appearance should be noted and sketched.

Palpation

Masses. The surgeon should gently palpate areas of swelling. Interstitial oedema which is recent and reversible often pits on pressure. Chronic oedema with intracellular fluid changes is more likely to feel brawny and indurated. If swelling is in the subcutaneous tissues, the skin above it may feel relatively soft and supple. An isolated firm swelling at the base of the finger which does not move with flexion or extension may well be a ganglion of the digital pulley. A nodule which moves proximally and distally with finger motion may be caused by inflammation of the tendon sheath. A digital nerve tumour or vascular malformation may move from side to side but may be fixed longitudinally. The nature of a mass often can be diagnosed by determining whether it is warm, pulsatile, firm or fluctuant, whether it is multilocular, changes in size with elevation or dependency of the limb and whether there is crepitation with flexion and extension of the finger.

Instability. Joint stability may be tested by holding the more proximal bone and moving the more distal bone gently but firmly in an anterior, posterior, medial and lateral direction (see Chapter 14). Angulatory stability should be tested in both extension and flexion. With joint lesions, crepitation may be elicited by gently grinding the more distal bone against the more proximal one. This is performed by compressing the two bones together and gently rotating the more distal one on the more proximal.

Vascular patency. Vascular patency at the wrist may be tested by means of the Allen test. The examiner compresses the radial and ulnar arteries just proximal to the wrist. As firm pressure is applied to these vessels the fingers are alternately flexed and extended four or five times. With the fingers fully extended, the palm is blanched. The radial artery is then released. Pink colour should return to the hand within four or five seconds. If there is a delay, the radial artery may not be patent. The same procedure is then performed with the release of the ulnar artery. The vascular patency of the finger can be similarly tested by compressing its radial and ulnar digital arteries and rapidly flexing and extending the fingers several times. Again the arteries are alternately released and the colour of the finger noted.

Passive motion

Each joint tested should be measured in all its natural planes of motion. Forearm pronation and supination are measured with the elbows firmly fixed to the patient's side. The wrist is rotated into pronation, then supination, and the angle of the dorsum of the hand with a vertical plane is measured. The forearm is considered in neutral position when the dorsal plane of the hand is vertical.

Wrist dorsiflexion is measured by placing one limb of the goniometer on the palm of the hand and the other at the volar aspect of the forearm (Fig. 5.5a). Palmar flexion is measured by placing the goniometer at the dorsum of the hand and forearm (Fig. 5.5b). When the dorsum of the hand and forearm are colinear, the angle is considered to be at zero degrees. Radial and ulnar deviation of the wrist is measured by placing one arm of the goniometer over the third metacarpal and the other parallel to the radius (Fig. 5.5c). Thumb abduction is the angle between the first and second metacarpals when the thumb is brought fully away from the palm. Adduction of the thumb is the angle between the first and second metacarpals with attempts to bring the thumb close to the palm. Neutral or zero rotation of the thumb is the position at which the thumb nail is perpendicular to the

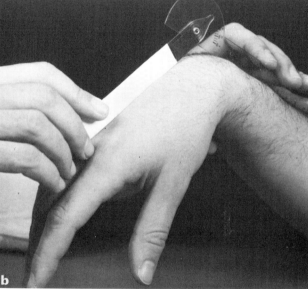

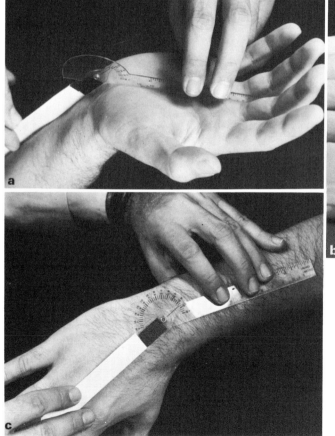

FIG. 5.5. Measurement of passive motion.

(a) Wrist dorsiflexion is measured by applying one limb of the goniometer at the volar aspect of the forearm and the other in the palm.

(b) Wrist palmar flexion is measured by applying one limb of the goniometer at the dorsum of the forearm and the other at the dorsum of the third metacarpal.

(c) Radial and ulnar deviations of the hand are measured by the angle of the third metacarpal and the shaft of the radius.

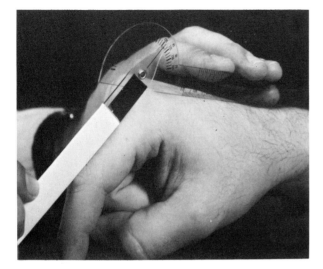

FIG. 5.6. Motion at the metacarpophalangeal and interphalangeal joints is measured by the angle between the dorsum of the bones which form the joints.

plane of the palm. Pronation ('medial rotation') of the thumb is measured by the angle between the plane of the thumb nail and the palmar perpendicular.

When the metacarpophalangeal and interphalangeal joints are completely straight, they are considered to be at zero degrees. Flexion and extension of the metacarpophalangeal and interphalangeal joints are measured by the angle at the tested joint with the goniometer resting on the dorsum of the finger (Fig. 5.6). Range of motion of the two sides (normal and abnormal) should be compared.

Active motion

In determining muscle-tendon function, the examiner resists motion at the insertion of the structure to be tested while the other hand palpates the muscle or tendon just proximal to the joint (Fig. 5.7a, b, c). For example, in testing the abductor pollicis brevis, the examiner will apply resistance to the radial side of the proximal phalanx of the thumb with one hand while palpating the abductor brevis with the other. The patient is asked to abduct strongly against the resistance and the tone of the tested muscle can be palpated (Fig. 5.7c). In testing the flexor digitorum profundus of the index finger, resistance is applied to the distal phalanx of the finger with one

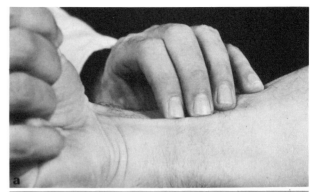
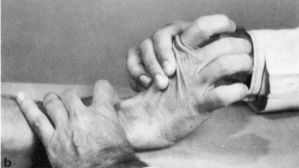
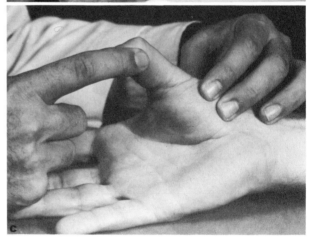

FIG. 5.7. In order to test the power of a muscle-tendon unit, the examiner resists motion at the insertion of the tested structure while palpating the muscle or tendon just proximal to the joint with the other hand.

(a) Flexor carpi radialis, and (b) extensor carpi radialis brevis are being tested.

(c) Testing the power of the abductor pollicis brevis. With resistance applied to the radial side of the proximal phalanx, the patient is abducting the thumb strongly. The abductor brevis is palpated.

hand while stabilizing the middle phalanx with the other. The tendon can be palpated by the hand which stabilizes the middle phalanx. Flexor digitorum superficialis is tested by passively extending all the fingers which are adjacent to the one which is to be examined. By this manoeuvre, the profundus is pulled distally and proximal interphalangeal joint flexion can be produced only by the flexor digitorum superficialis (Fig. 5.8).

As a rough guide to finger flexion, the distance by which the fingertips fail to reach the mid-palmar crease may be used to determine cumulative finger motion.

Thenar muscles supplied by the median nerve are probably best tested by having the patient place the dorsum of the hand upon the table and asking him to point the thumb tip to the ceiling. This motion is accomplished almost exclusively by the abductor pollicis brevis and the radial head of the flexor pollicis brevis. These muscles can be palpated as described above. This is a better test of median nerve function than opposition of the thumb, which is a complex motion partly achieved by ulnar innervated muscles.

Function of the adductor pollicis may be tested by asking the patient to hold a paper or card between the thumb and index finger as it is being pulled away. With weakness of the adductor, the thumb flexes acutely at the interphalangeal joint as the flexor pollicis longus substitutes for loss of the adductor of the thumb in an attempt to maintain strong pinch (Froment's sign) (Fig. 5.9). The two sides should be compared.

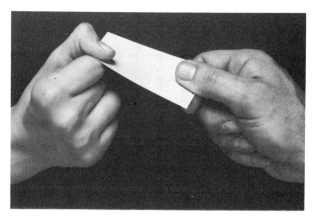

FIG. 5.9. Weak adductor pollicis is shown by the 'Froment sign'. With an attempt to forcefully pinch against resistance, the interphalangeal joint of the thumb flexes acutely.

In testing for interosseus muscle function abduction and adduction of the fingers should be performed on a flat plane with the fingers in complete extension (Fig. 5.10). The muscle bellies should be palpated adjacent to the metacarpal shafts while resistance is applied against the tested finger. If the fingers are not stabilized in

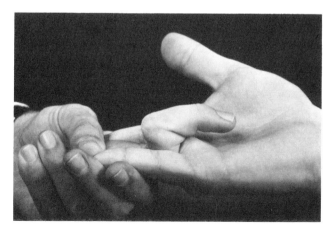

FIG. 5.8. Flexor digitorum superficialis is tested by passively extending the adjacent fingers to relax profundus to the tested digit.

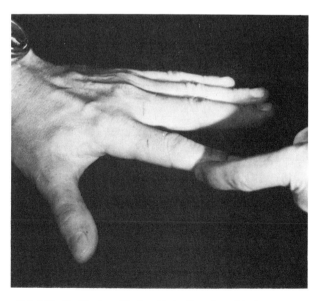

FIG. 5.10. Positioning of the hand to test function of the interosseus muscle.

extension. they converge with flexion and diverge with extension often giving the mistaken impression of the presence of weak interosseus muscle function. The extensor digiti quinti proprius is an excellent abductor of the little finger, even with total absence of the hypothenar muscles and its function must not be interpreted as intrinsic muscle return.

Strength of the muscles of the hand should be tested by means of a dynamometer and pinch meter in order to obtain a valid and reproducible quantitative evaluation of muscle strength. The handles of most dynamometers can be adjusted and should be placed so that the patient can readily grasp and squeeze them. The patient is seated comfortably with the forearm resting on the examining table and then asked to squeeze the dynamometer as hard as possible, first with one hand, and then the other. The test is repeated three times and the average grip strength of each hand is noted (Fig. 5.11a). Pinch strength can be valuable in determining the progress of ulnar nerve recovery and in evaluating intrinsic muscle weakness. Accurate and reproducible measurements of pinch strength depend largely upon the manner in which it is tested. Three main types of pinch are tested in most cases: (1) thumb pulp against radial side of index tip (pulp-to-side pinch); (2) thumb pulp against index and middle finger pulp (three point chuck pinch); and (3) thumb tip against index tip (tip-to-tip pinch). Of the three, we have found pulp-to-side pinch most valuable as a functional guide and a test for intrinsic muscle power. As with the grip test, the two sides are compared and three readings are taken and averaged (Fig. 5.11b).

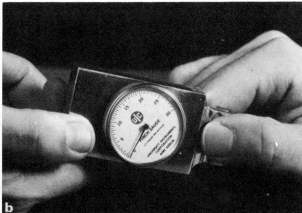

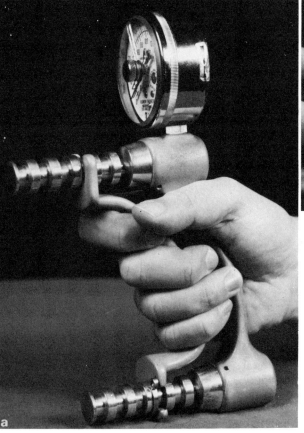

FIG. 5.11. Testing the strength of muscles.

(a) The handles of the dynamometer are adjusted to permit the patient to grip as powerfully as possible. The forearm and the dynamometer rest on the table, the elbow is in mild flexion. Power of both hands is compared.

(b) While the examiner (left) supports the pinch gauge the patient pinches as strongly as possible. Here pulp-to-side pinch is being tested.

Sensory examination

There are various modalities of sensibility. All must be carefully evaluated in cases of central nervous system disease such as cerebral palsy. A patient with spastic hemiplegia may have excellent pinprick and light touch sensibility but lack proprioception, two point discrimination and stereognosis. In judging peripheral nerve injury, however, sharp/dull sensibility and fine discrimination tests may be sufficient to make the diagnosis and to judge recovery. The examination should first be performed in the uninvolved areas of the hand. The patient should not be asked to close the eyes or turn away while being tested. When the questionably involved areas of the hand are being tested, the examiner's assistive hand may be used as a shield so that the patient does not inadvertently receive visual clues.

A useful preliminary test is to ask the patient to differentiate between the milled edge of one coin and the smooth edge of another (Fig. 5.12). The examination then continues by asking the patient to discriminate the *sharp* from the *dull* end of the pin. Avoid using hypodermic needles for the test as they are painful and cause unpleasant puncture wounds. A blunted safety pin is usually ideal. The pin tip should touch the skin and not be inserted into it. The patient is requested to make a response each time even if unsure as to what end of the pin is being used. Eight out of ten correct responses indicates good pinprick discrimination. If sharp/dull discrimination is not possible, the conclusion is that the tested sensory nerve is abnormal.

Two point discrimination may be tested by the use of dulled calipers or a paper clip. Again, the normal areas of the hand are tested first, with the calipers spread about 10 mm. One should be certain that the area to be tested rests comfortably on the table or other flat surface and the patient is instructed not to move the finger during the examination. Both points of the caliper are applied to the skin simultaneously and are best oriented longitudinally. The pressure applied should be sufficient to slightly indent the skin without blanching it (Fig. 5.13). A random pattern of two point and one point pressure is applied and the patient encouraged to 'guess two or one' with each testing even if he is uncertain. The narrowest caliper width at which eight out of ten correct responses are obtained is considered the two point discrimination. 'Normal' two point discrimination varies according to the finger being tested, the side of the hand being tested, and the amount of callus or thickening of the skin which may reflect the patient's hobbies or occu-

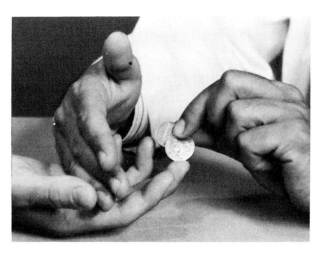

FIG. 5.12. An effective and rapid method of preliminary sensibility examination is the coin test. The patient is asked to differentiate the roughened edge of one coin from the smooth edge of another. This test is particularly useful for children who fear any sharp objects and prefer this game to pinprick testing.

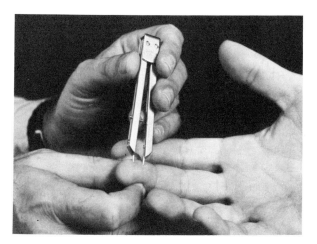

FIG. 5.13. Two-point discrimination may be performed with a paper clip or with the dulled points of a caliper. The points are applied simultaneously, longitudinally and with just sufficient pressure to indent the skin gently. The patient is asked whether he is being touched with two points or one point. The tested finger should be supported to prevent the fingertip from flexing into the caliper points.

pation. The involved and uninvolved hand should, therefore, be compared.

In order to test *proprioception* of the finger, the proximal phalanx is stabilized by the examiner who then gently grasps the involved fingertip by its sides, flexes and extends it several times and finally maintains the finger in a flexed or extended position. The patient is then requested to imitate this position with the uninvolved hand. If the finger is held by its pulp, deep pressure sensibility may offer the patient a clue as to the position of the finger even with total loss of proprioception. Each finger is tested several times, and it is important that the patient not be permitted to receive visual clues while the test is being performed.

An excellent and rapid functional test of skin sensibility is the *pick-up test*. Several small objects such as pins, small screws and nuts, coins or marbles are placed on a table top and the patient is asked to pick them up rapidly and place them in a small saucer or cup. The test is performed first with the uninvolved hand, then the injured hand. The patient is timed during a visual performance of this test, and then blindfolded and the test repeated. Often subtle sensory changes in the median nerve distribution can be detected by this test by an astonishing delay in pick-up time of the involved hand as compared to the normal hand when blindfolded. Substitution patterns with the use of ulnar innervated fingers will also signal median nerve involvement.

Percussion over the site of nerve injury usually causes paraesthesia in the sensory distribution of the nerve. This sign is due to a relative lack of nerve myelinization and is *not* the sign of nerve regeneration. *Tinel's sign* was originally described as a test of nerve regeneration. With a positive Tinel's sign paraesthesia in the sensory distribution of a nerve occurs when the nerve is percussed *distal* to the site of repair.

If a sensory nerve has been divided, the skin it supplies becomes smooth and red and often lacks perspiration. One of the signs of recovery after nerve injury is the return of perspiration through reinnervation of the sweat glands by the recovering sympathetic nerves.

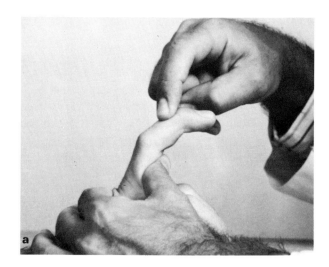

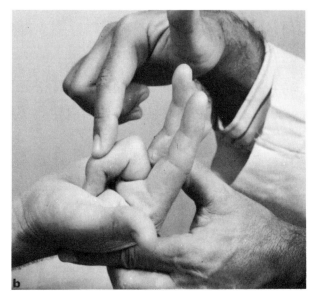

FIG. 5.14. This patient has limited flexion at the proximal interphalangeal joint of the middle finger. There is less proximal interphalangeal flexion when the metacarpophalangeal joint is extended (a) than when it is flexed (b). Proximal interphalangeal joint stiffness is therefore due to tightness of the intrinsic muscles which are further tightened with metacarpophalangeal extension.

Contractures

Contractures may result from intra-articular joint ab-

normality, capsular contraction, fibrosis of muscles, tendon adhesions, fascial thickening or skin scar. Most frequently, several of these factors are responsible for contractures in the hand. If contracture or stiffness is intra-articular due to bone abnormality, the radiographs usually show an articular deformity. In addition, a firm resistance is felt in attempting to correct the deformity passively. The position of the more proximal or distal joints does not influence the deformity.

If joint deformity is due to capsular contracture, attempts to correct the contracture passively produce a firm, rubbery resistance. The deformity is not influenced by the position of the more proximal or distal joints. Radiographs are frequently normal.

If muscle contracture has caused a joint deformity, the contracture may often be lessened by passively positioning a more proximal joint so that the contracted muscle is relaxed. Thus, with Volkmann's contracture of the flexor digitorum profundus, acute flexion of the interphalangeal joint may be lessened by flexing the wrist. When the wrist is brought into dorsiflexion, the fingers become more tightly flexed. This is known as the *tenodesis effect*. Muscle spasm such as seen in stroke or cerebral palsy causes a similar tenodesis effect. Peripheral nerve block often relaxes the spasm and allows the joint to move more freely. With tightening of the intrinsic muscles of the hand, extension contracture of the proximal interphalangeal joint is relaxed by flexion of the metacarpophalangeal joint, since the tendons of the interossei lie volar to the axis of metacarpophalangeal joint motion and dorsal to the axis of proximal interphalangeal motion. If the metacarpophalangeal joint is held in full extension, proximal interphalangeal flexion will be diminished (Fig. 5.14a, b).

With contractures due to tendon incarceration, as with a locked trigger finger, passive mobility is often possible when the metacarpophalangeal joint is flexed. Active motion is usually considerably less than passive motion. Similarly, in tendon adhesions, the contracture may be released by appropriately positioning the hand or finger to relax the offending tendon.

With fascial contracture, as with Dupuytren's contracture, the fascial band is usually palpable. Appropriate positioning of the finger may relax the contracture although joint relaxation and the tenodesis effect is not found if the fascia has intimately involved the volar capsule of the joint.

Contractures due to skin scars are usually visible and are sometimes relaxed by flexing the more proximal joints of the affected portion of the hand.

Tenderness

Defining an area of tenderness is often critical in diagnosing accurately the site of infection, tumour or nerve injury. The hand must always be placed at rest and the examination should proceed from the uninvolved to the involved region. Gentle palpation is the rule. The examiner must be certain that he is not causing pain by moving more proximal or more distal joints in palpating for an area of tenderness. For example, in examining a patient with a suspected flexor tenosynovitis of the middle finger the surgeon must map the precise area of tenderness. The palm is palpated beginning first over the fifth metacarpal head and then gradually progressing radially. The skin is gently depressed by the examiner's finger and the patient is asked whether there is much pain. When the skin over the third metacarpal head is depressed, the patient will note increased tenderness. In palpating the finger itself, it is stabilized by being gently held with one hand dorso-laterally while the examiner's other hand palpates distally over the volar side of the finger. If the finger is not stabilized by this means even the gentlest palpation will force it into extension and the examiner will have difficulty in differentiating the volar tenderness of tenosynovitis from pain that could result from joint infection, cellulitis or a subcutaneous abscess, all of which would be exacerbated by finger extension.

EXAMINATION OF THE HAND UNDER SPECIAL CIRCUMSTANCES

When a patient is admitted to an accident ward with severe injuries to the hand, the wisdom of performing a detailed examination of all structures may be questioned. Much of the history can often be obtained from a fellow worker or family member. Appropriate radiographs are obtained of all serious hand injuries. However, the physical examination of the hand should not be overly traumatic or tedious. The surgeon should inspect the attitude and active motion of the digits and note the circulation of tissues distal to the site of injury. Pin-prick perception at the finger tips may provide sufficient information of nerve injury to serve as an excellent guide to the initial treatment without the necessity of probing the wound. The preoperative examination should be sufficient to alert the surgeon and anaesthetist as to the general duration and magnitude of the imminent operation and the possible need for extensive flaps or grafts which may influence the preoperative preparation of the patient.

Frequently, an injury to the hand is associated with more severe injuries elsewhere. The physical examination of the hand even in the unconscious patient can be most informative. Fractures and tendon injuries often can be diagnosed by the posture of the hand and the position of the digits with wrist palmar flexion and dorsiflexion. Deep tendon reflexes can give considerable information regarding the integrity both of the peripheral nerves and of the muscle–tendon units. Sensory nerve injuries may be diagnosed by carefully examining for deficient areas of perspiration. Crepitation or false motion at the site of a deformity indicates areas of fracture which may then be confirmed by appropriate radiographs. Of course life-saving procedures must take priority in the treatment of seriously injured patients, but fractures can be splinted, wounds can be cleansed and damaged structures can be repaired despite serious injuries elsewhere.

The examination of the hand postoperatively is as important as any phase of the postoperative care. Much can be learned without removing dressings, casts or splints. The fingertips must not be encased in dressings which preclude their examination. The colour of each finger is noted. Capillary refill time should be checked: normally, gentle pressure upon a fingertip causes it to blanch, while pink colour should return within two or three seconds. If colour return is delayed more than six or seven seconds, there may be vascular embarrassment due either to constrictive dressings, oedema or haematoma. The cause must be promptly diagnosed and released. Sensibility of the fingertips should be noted. Hypoaesthesia in one area of the hand may be due to the effects of a peripheral nerve block following supra-clavicular or axillary anaesthesia, it may represent neura-praxia or axonotmesis following the prolonged use of a tourniquet, it may indicate nerve injury due to surgery, the positioning of the hand or constrictive dressings. Accurate recording of the location and progression of hypoaesthesia is essential for both its diagnosis and treatment.

The surgeon should be trained to check the limb proximal to the dressings for signs of infection following surgery. Lymphangitis or lymphadenitis should be noted promptly by the telltale red streaks up the arm or painful nodes about the elbow or axilla. The presence of an odour in a dressing several days postoperatively is frequently an ominous sign indicating discharge of haematoma or infection. The alert surgeon judiciously sniffs the dressing as a routine part of his postoperative examination.

PHOTOGRAPHS

Photographs of the hand should be an integral part of the patient's record. Aside from the immense value of photographs in teaching, they serve an important role in evaluating the patient's progress. In developing a large library of clinical photographs, the following system may prove valuable:

(1) A relatively inexpensive camera and lighting system should always be available in the clinics and in the operating rooms. The same camera model and lighting system should be used for all photography.

(2) The use of colour transparencies is considered best for clinical photography. Colour slides can be used for conferences and for teaching. They can be printed into colour photographs or transposed into black and white prints with little loss of fidelity. Medium speed (ASA 64) film has proven satisfactory both for lack of graininess and adequate contrast.

(3) The same background should always be used. A dark blue towel is an excellent backdrop as it is pleasing when shown in colour and provides good contrast when converting colour slides into black and white photographs. In photographing patients with dark skin, the use of a light green towel as a background is more suitable.

(4) All photographs are taken with a camera so directed that the fingers are pointing up; thus, the shadows on all photographs are similar.

(5) The hand should not rest on a table or background when the photographs are taken. The hand should be several inches above the background so that the fingers and wrist are unsupported. Photographs are taken showing maximum active motion in both the anteroposterior and lateral planes.

(6) In taking operative photographs additional time should be taken to clean and clear the field. All sponges, extraneous clamps and forceps are removed, the skin is

cleansed with a moist sponge and a clean blue or green background (sterile towel or sheet) is placed behind the hand to be photographed.

(7) A notebook is kept with the camera case to record the names of all patients photographed. As soon as the slides are returned from the laboratory, they are labelled and filed. It is best to file photographic slides under the patient's name rather than by clinical diagnosis. A cross-index with clinical diagnosis is valuable.

To keep the slides and photographs clean and intact they are never loaned; duplicates are produced on a slide copier when needed by others. All originals of slides are kept at home or in a locked cabinet at the hospital. The patient is not told that we have photographs of his operation, to prevent him from requesting them for lawyers, friends or photo albums. A junior house officer or junior assistant who is assigned to take photographs and label them is free to make duplicates of any film he wishes. This increases his interest in photography and assures a more complete collection of photographs for both the surgeon and his assistant.

FURTHER READING

[1] BASMAJIAN, J. V. *Muscles Alive, Their Functions Revealed by Electromyography*. Baltimore, Williams & Wilkins, 1974.

[2] FLATT, A. E. *The Care of Congenital Hand Anomalies*, St. Louis, C. V. Mosby, 1977.

[3] KENNEY, W. E. The importance of sensori-perceptual gnosis in the examination, the understanding and the management of cerebral palsy. *Clinical Orthopaedics*, 1966, **46**, 45.

[4] LANDSMEER, J. M. F. Power grip and precision handling. *Annals of Rheumatic Diseases*, 1962, **21**, 154.

[5] LISTER, G. *The Hand: diagnosis and indications*. Edinburgh, Churchill Livingstone, 1977.

[6] MOBERG, E. Evaluation of sensibility in the hand. *Surgical Clinics in North America*, 1960, **40**, 357.

[7] NAPIER, J. R. The prehensile movements of the human hand. *Journal of Bone and Joint Surgery*, 1956, **38B**, 902.

[8] SEDDON, H. *Surgical Disorders of the Peripheral Nerves*. Baltimore, Williams & Wilkins, 1975.

[9] SMITH, R. J. AND LEFFERT, R. D. Open Wounds. In: J. Edward Flynn, *Hand Surgery*, 2nd Ed. Baltimore, Williams & Wilkins, 1975.

[10] TACHDJIAN, M. O. AND MINEAR, W. L. Sensory disturbances in the hands of children with cerebral palsy. *Journal of Bone and Joint Surgery*, 1958, **40A**, 85.

CHAPTER 6

Functional Assessment

F. V. NICOLLE and R. A. DICKSON

As the prehensile unit of the upper limb the hand is one of the most important organs in the body, but because of its complexity its overall function is extremely difficult to assess in a meaningful, accurate and objective fashion. The summation of several variables is necessary to provide a comprehensive functional assessment. These variables are sensory function, muscle power, tendon function, joint function, and dynamic function, both subjective and objective.

Sensory function

Sensory perception in the human hand has developed to a very highly specialized degree. We are capable of recognizing objects by feel alone. This sensory power is known as tactilegnosis [1]. This freely developed sensory power is produced by four sources of different sensory nerve impulses in the hand–skin, joint, tendon, and muscle spindles. Nerve impulses transmitted from the skin will clearly be of prime importance in our fine appreciation of touch and recognition of small objects whereas the characteristics of an object such as its weight, movement and size will be mainly transmitted by nerve impulses from joints, tendon organs and muscle spindles. There are by tradition four types of nerve receptor: the tactile receptor of Meissner, Pacinian receptors for pressure, end bulbs of Kraus for perception of coolness, and organs of Ruffini for perception of warmth. However, these may not be so specific and there exist in the skin numerous unencapsulated nerve endings which

also transmit the sensations of touch, temperature and pain (p. 181).

The assessment of sensory function is important in determining the extent of nerve injuries and in the monitoring of subsequent recovery. Seddon [2] classified nerve injuries according to the extent of damage:

(1) neuropraxia, a mild disturbance of brief duration,

(2) axonotmesis, in which the endoneurial tubes remain intact but the axon undergoes degeneration,

(3) neurotmesis, complete severance of the nerve.

Frequently, however, it is difficult to diagnose precisely the type of nerve injury because the lesions may be of a mixture of types. Furthermore there is no immediate clinical means of distinguishing between a neurotmesis and axonotmesis, both initially showing complete loss of sensory function. It is important to remember that loss of sensation in part of the hand can frequently be a greater handicap to the patient than loss of mobility since the latter can be more easily compensated for by an additional contribution from an adjacent joint or digit. Furthermore disturbance of sensation is often associated with pain which adds further to the degree of disability.

Tests for sensation

It is important when testing for sensation and muscle power that the part to be investigated is warm and that the interest, cooperation and concentration of the subject should be obtained. Different stimuli should not follow each other too quickly. This is important because when conduction is delayed the response may then refer to the previous stimulus. The area of altered sensation should be mapped out with a continuous line for light touch and a dotted line for pin prick [3]. It is convenient to record these areas on a stencilled stamp of the dorsal and volar surface of the hand.

Two point discrimination is the most valuable test at present available in determining the quality of sensory nerve recovery [1], and the method of demonstrating this is described on p. 89.

The *pick-up test* is also of great value and described on p. 90. Familiarization markedly affects this test which is at the most subjective only.

McQuillan's *vibration test* [4], although in the experimental stage, may prove to be a useful semi-objective method of determining sensory function. Vibratory stimuli of increasing amplitude are applied to the pulps of the fingers and the thresholds of perception documented serially.

Muscle function

Voluntary muscles may act as prime movers, antagonists, fixators or synergists. There are many methods of assessing muscle power but the most consistent and reliable is that recommended by the Medical Research Council Nerve Injuries Committee [3]. This is as follows: 0–no contraction, 1–flicker or trace of contraction, 2–active movement with gravity eliminated, 3–active movement against gravity, 4–active movement against gravity and resistance, 5–normal power. Methods of assessing muscle function in the hand are shown in Chapter 5, pp. 86–88.

The power of each individual muscle under suspicion must be tested, graded and recorded. This form of testing may also yield additional information. In hysterical states muscles may function synergistically although showing no prime mover action. When a muscle is recovering function following re-innervation it may show evidence of fixator activity before it demonstrates prime mover action. This information should be documented on the MRC grading record. It is important that the examiner should not only look for but feel the contraction of these hand muscles, almost all of which are freely accessible for this purpose. It is recommended that the MRC method be adhered to as this technique

eliminates trick movements. By serial examinations it is possible to determine the progression of recovery following injury.

Electrophysiology (see also p. 181)

Damage to the main nerves of the upper limb frequently impairs hand function. It is often useful to assess the type of nerve damage, its progression, and response to treatment by electrophysiological methods. More subtle changes can frequently be detected in this manner than by serial motor and sensory testing. Furthermore, the anatomical level of nerve damage can be accurately localized, and this may be extremely important as hand function can be impaired by nerve entrapment as proximal as the cervical spine and as distal as the carpal tunnel, with very similar clinical manifestations. These techniques may be invaluable in deciphering conflicting signs due to anomalous nerve distribution. However, they must be used and interpreted with skill and some reservation. The two techniques most commonly used and most simple to interpret are nerve conduction studies and electromyography.

Nerve conduction studies

The principle of this technique is to stimulate by electrode a peripheral nerve at a point on its course, and to record an action potential at another point in the distribution of the nerve. Information about both motor and sensory function can thereby be obtained. In order to examine motor nerve function a nerve can be stimulated at a point along its course and the action potential recorded by another electrode inserted into a muscle supplied by that nerve, e.g. the median nerve and the abductor pollicis brevis muscle. There are many electrophysiological variables that can be measured, but the two most commonly recorded are the amplitude of response and delay between stimulus and response. Accurate calibration and recording is essential, and comparison should be made with the normal side or the laboratory control if the condition is bilateral. In a case of right carpal tunnel syndrome after stimulation of the median nerve above the wrists on both sides, the normal side may show a short delay between stimulus and response and an action potential of normal magnitude.

The affected side may show a prolonged latency between stimulus and response and a low amplitude response indicative of nerve compression at a point between stimulus and response. In general this distal motor latency is a more meaningful measure than amplitude and can accurately localize the site of the lesion, which may be the wrist, elbow, brachial plexus or cervical spine according to the nature of the disease.

Similarly, sensory activity can be determined in a retrograde fashion by stimulating the sensory nerve endings in the pulp of the fingers and picking up action potentials at a proximal point on the course of the nerve. Sensory and motor function can, therefore, be monitored by this electrophysiological technique.

Electromyography

Needle electrode recording of the activity of a muscle may provide useful information about its behaviour and, combined with nerve conduction studies, may indicate muscle or nerve lesion as the incriminating condition. A quiet low level of activity indicates normal resting muscle whereas fasciculation may indicate nerve degeneration. Maximum voluntary effort evokes a normal amplitude potential in a normal muscle but no such response occurs if the nerve supply is inadequate. Of more importance than one solitary recording are serial recordings timed appropriately. For example, electromyography performed early after damage will yield nothing of value as nerve degeneration will not yet have occurred. As in nerve conduction studies, timing, skill, calibration and interpretation are most important if the technique is to be meaningful. These electrophysiological techniques are sophisticated methods of investigation and the advice of the clinical neurophysiologist should be sought.

Inter-relation between tendon and joint

The purpose of tendons is to secure a firm attachment to bone and thus facilitate the movements of joints by muscles. In this respect tendon and joint function are intimately related. After a laceration of the volar aspect of a digit it is simple to decide the integrity of the long flexor tendons by testing their function according to the MRC principles. Indeed this is mandatory after such an injury. Such testing is, however, frequently neglected in relation to other forms of reconstructive surgery. One of the conditions governing a satisfactory tendon transfer is that the tendon transferred should be that of an adequately functioning muscle. A prerequisite for a successful prosthetic joint replacement is an intact tendon mechanism. These points are most important but not always appreciated. If there is any clinical suspicion of flexor tenosynovitis then these tendons must be cleared and seen to function satisfactorily prior to joint replacement [5]. Similarly, metacarpophalangeal joint surgery should not be performed in the presence of a painful unstable wrist or when there is a question of the integrity of the dorsal extensor tendon mechanism. These problems should be resolved first by thinking and working in a proximal to distal direction in the planning of surgical intervention. The intricate interdependence of function at several levels demands this form of critical assessment if optimal results are to be consistently obtained.

Joint function

The prime function of a joint is that it should move through a useful range, and measurement of range of joint motion is an important objective assessment parameter in hand function. Where appropriate, therefore, joint mobility should be preserved, but there are sites in the hand where mobility is less important than stability, which is vital [6]. It is a critical determination of hand function that the difference between active and passive ranges of motion be appreciated. Prior to tendon repair it is essential that the joints served by that tendon mechanism are capable of a useful range of passive motion. If not then even a perfect tendon repair will not restore good joint function. Of much greater significance is the active range of motion, which is the arc of motion that the patient creates: this reflects much more meaningful function. If an excellent passive range of joint motion exists prior to tendon surgery but only limited active movement is achieved postoperatively then there is a very poor functional result. This is also of considerable importance in relation to prosthetic joint replacement. Analysis of the active range of motion following arthroplasty for arthritic conditions has clearly shown that, while the osteoarthritic individual makes the best use actively of his passive range of motion, the rheumatoid arthritic uses actively only a fraction of the previous passive arc [7]. Clearly the results of prosthetic replacement based solely upon available passive range must be interpreted with extreme caution if accepted at all. Attention to relevant objective measures is surely the only way that meaningful data can be collected and used to the advantage of both patient and surgeon.

Dynamic function

The commonly used methods of assessment are shown in Table 6.1. Assessing the dynamic state of the hand by subjective methods is liable to great variability in what constitutes a patient's important functions. However a suitable record of the patient's views, the performance of his everyday tasks, his predominantly important functions and any special disabilities is recommended [8]. Ideally, individuals should be scrutinized at work and in the performance of essential everyday tasks at home. By this means we can learn precisely what the functional disabilities are and can design a suitable treatment programme. This has already been shown to be of value in the functional assessment of the results of total hip replacement [9]. Methods of grading pain have been suggested [8], but it seems unlikely that grading of such a subjective impression can be of any real quantitative value. Some authorities believe that the best cosmetic hand is also the best functional hand. This may well be the case, but lack of evidence precludes cosmesis as more than a superficial standard for assessment purposes. It

is important in using these subjective assessment methods that the help of the professionally trained occupational therapist be obtained.

The *clinical appraisal* of the hand has been described fully on pp. 80–90. It is emphasized that photography is a most useful method of documenting appearance. Additional advantages of routinely photographing each hand before and after treatment are for medicolegal purposes and to build up a comprehensive teaching slide collection. The dynamic state of the hand can be more effectively documented by cine-photography.

Measurement of the grip and pinch strengths of the hand are important methods of quantitative assessment [1], and are described on p. 88.

When the hand loses the function of effective pinch, as it may do in rheumatoid disease, it loses 80 per cent of its value [10]. If only one digit is affected by trauma or disease, grip strength may not be altered either before or after corrective surgery; measurement of individual digital forces is therefore all the more important [11]. The thumb, index and middle fingers have been described as the dynamic tripod of prehension [12]. *Pinch strength* is therefore a most useful measurement of the function of the hand, particularly when surgery is performed on the thumb. Table 6.2 shows the pinch forces of the index, middle, ring and little fingers against the thumb before and three months after fusion of the metacarpophalangeal joint of the thumb for Barron stage III rheumatoid disease [13]. A 50 per cent improvement in pinch strength has been achieved.

The measurement of the *density of the individual bones* of the hand may be a very accurate method of determining how much the hand is used. There is circumstantial evidence to suggest that the incriminating factor in bone loss in the hands of patients with rheumatoid disease is progressive loss of hand function. Local disuse osteopenia occurs after fracture and occurs unilaterally

TABLE 6.1 Methods of assessment.

Subjective	Objective
Patient's views	Clinical appraisal
Everyday tasks	Photography
Important functions	Cine-photography
Pain grades	Radiography
Cosmetic appearance	Range of motion
	Active
	Passive
Occupational therapy assessment	Grip strength
	Pinch strength
	Bone density

TABLE 6.2 Digital pinch forces before and three months after thumb metacarpophalangeal joint fusion.

Digit	Index kgf	Middle kgf	Ring kgf	Little kgf
Preoperative	4·0	4·5	3·7	2·9
Postoperative	6·1	6·0	5·7	4·1

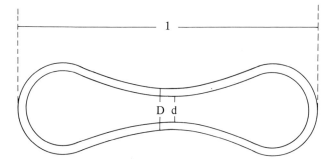

FIG. 6.1. Measurement of bone density. D, total bone width; d, medullary width; 1, length of bone. D. and d are measured at the mid-shaft.

$$\text{Area index} = \frac{D^2 - d^2}{DL}$$

TABLE 6.3 Changes in bone density and pinch force before and after metacarpophalangeal joint synovectomy.

	Bone (%)	Force (%)
Mean annual loss preoperatively	25·6	37·1
Mean annual gain postoperatively	13·6	21·7

in long-standing hemiplegia [14]. Metabolic studies of patients with paralytic acute anterior poliomyelitis have shown generalized osteopenia [15]. Gravity has been shown to have an effect on the length and shape of bones [16], and there is a reduction in bone density when exposed to a reduced barometric pressure [17]. That such a mechanism of bone loss can occur in the hand has been shown in a study of manual versus non-manual workers [18], where calcification of bone near a joint depended very much on occupational stress applied to the bone over an appreciable period. The progression of osteoporosis of the proximal phalanx has been correlated in rheumatoid disease with loss of grip power of the hand [19]. This relationship between osteoporosis and hand function has been extended to the individual digital level and the individual hand bones have been shown to lose up to 50 per cent of their bone in one year's progress of rheumatoid disease

[20, 21]. A positive relationship has been shown in the normal hand between the strength of the digit and its bone density; the stronger the digit the greater its density [22]. It has also been shown that surgical intervention in rheumatoid disease can lead to a considerable improvement in both function and density [23]. Certain drugs, by improving the state of rheumatoid disease in the hand, have also been shown to improve the density of the individual bones [24]. It is therefore suggested that measurement of bone density may be a useful parameter for the assessment of hand function. On a standard anteroposterior radiograph, certain corticomedullary ratios can be measured with sensitive Vernier calipers. Figure 6.1 shows the measurement of area index and dimensionless ratio, variables known to correlate well with ash weight. In general, area index is the most useful but dimensionless ratio may be of value when comparing the density of bones of markedly different sizes. Table 6.3 shows the changes in area index and pinch force in fifteen digits which underwent metacarpophalangeal joint synovectomy. During the preoperative year there was a significant reduction in bone density and pinch force and after surgery a significant increase, although it can be observed that they never reverted to their initial magnitudes.

REFERENCES

[1] MOBERG, E. Evaluation of sensibility in the hand. *Surgical Clinics of North America*, 1960, **40,** 357.

[2] SEDDON, H. J. *Peripheral Nerve Injuries.* Medical Research Council Special Report Series No. 282. London, HMSO, 1954.

[3] MEDICAL RESEARCH COUNCIL. *Aids to the Investigation of Peripheral Nerve Injuries.* London, HMSO, 1943.

[4] NEILSON, J. M. M., BOARDMAN, A. K., McQUILLAN, W. M., SMITH, D. N., HAY, R. L. AND ANTHONY, J. K. F.

Measurement of vibro-tactile threshold in peripheral nerve injury. *Lancet*, 1969, **ii,** 669.

[5] TUBIANA, R. Personal communication, 1973.

[6] NICOLLE, F. V. Recent advances in the management of joint disease in the rheumatoid hand. *Hand*, 1973, **5,** 91–95.

[7] KETTELKAMP, D. B., LEAVERTON, P. E. and MISOL, S. Gait characteristics of the rheumatoid knee. *Archives of Surgery*, 1972, **104,** 30.

[8] SAVAGE, O. Measurement in rheumatoid arthritis. *Proceedings of the Royal Society of Medicine*, Supplement, 1966, **59,** 85.

[9] HOWARTH, R., BENTLEY, G. AND NICHOLS, P. J. R. Functional end-results after total hip replacement for degenerative arthritis of the hip. *Orthopaedics*, 1975, **8,** 51.

[10] ARDEN, G. P., HARRISON, S. H. AND ANSELL, B. M. Surgical treatment in rheumatoid arthritis. *British Medical Journal*, 1970, **IV,** 604.

[11] DICKSON, R. A., PETRIE, A., NICOLLE, F. V. AND CALNAN, J. S. A device for measuring the face of the digits of the hand. *Biomedical Engineering*, 1972, **7,** 270–273.

[12] CAPENER, N. The hand in surgery. *Journal of Bone and Joint Surgery*, 1956, **38B,** 128.

[13] BARRON, J. N. Assessment of suitability for surgery in general timing of operation. *Annals of Rheumatic Diseases*, Supplement, 1969, **28,** 74.

[14] HODKINSON, H. M. AND BRAIN, A. T. Unilateral osteoporosis in longstanding hemiplegia in the elderly, *Journal of the American Geriatric Society*, 1967, **15,** 59.

[15] WHEDON, G. D. AND SHORR, E. Metabolic Studies in Paralytic Acute Anterior Poliomyelitis. Alterations in Calcium and Phosphorus Metabolism. 1957.

[16] TULLOH, N. M. Relation between carcass composition and live weight of sheep. *Nature*, 1963, **197,** 809.

[17] HUNT, R. A. AND SCHRAER, H. Skeletal response of rats exposed to reduced barometric pressure. *American Journal of Physiology*, 1965, **208,** 1217.

[18] KEANE, B. E., SPEIGLER, G. AND DAVIS, R. Quantitative evaluation of bone mineral by a radiographic method. *British Journal of Radiology*, 1959, **32,** 162.

[19] VIRTAMA, P., HELELA, T. AND KALLIOMAKI, J. L. Osteoporosis in rheumatoid arthritis; a follow-up study. *Acta Rheumatologica Scandinavica*, 1965, **14,** 276.

[20] DICKSON, R. A. AND NICOLLE, F. V. The assessment of hand function. Part I—Measurement of individual digits. *The Hand*, 1972, **4,** 207.

[21] DICKSON, R. A., PAICE, F. AND CALNAN, J. S. The quantitative colour television image analyser. A new method of measuring bone density. *Journal of Bone and Joint Surgery*, 1973, **55B,** 359.

[22] DICKSON, R. A., PAICE, F. AND NICOLLE, F. V. The assessment of hand function. Part II—Forces and bone density, a relationship in the hand. *The Hand*, 1973, **5,** 15.

[23] DICKSON, R. A. AND NICOLLE, F. V. The assessment of hand function. Part III—The final analysis. *The Hand*, 1976, **8,** 110.

[24] SCHORN, D. Personal communication, 1977.

CHAPTER 7

Basic Surgical Techniques

L. W. MILFORD

Preoperative care

A final examination of the patient, prior to hospital admission may reveal changes in the pathological condition or healing process which could influence the surgeon. Also, the patient has an opportunity to ask the surgeon any pressing questions. Advice is given again as to what to expect in terms of length of hospital stay, the type of anaesthetic and the surgical procedure that is anticipated. The patient and family are also advised of the approximate time of the operation in order to allay unnecessary anxiety.

The patient awaiting surgery should be isolated in a comfortable anteroom or induction room. Should a local anaesthetic be used, it is extremely important that there is no careless conversation that would increase the patient's anxiety. Remarks such as 'Are we still out of such and such?' or 'Has such and such been repaired?' should not be spoken in front of the patient who is awake. If an unusually long delay occurs in the operative schedule, the relatives must be advised accordingly.

Outpatient surgery

At times it is of benefit, by reducing time and cost, for the surgery to be undertaken on an outpatient basis. There should be an established routine, for the patient to be prepared and await surgery in an appropriate room, and to have someone accompany him home afterwards. This routine is well established in many hospitals. It reduces complications following surgery, and difficulties, such as

the patient becoming faint or weak, bleeding occurring through a dressing, or nausea experienced or anxiety magnified, can be handled by a friend or family member; otherwise a return to the emergency room may be necessary.

The operating theatre

It is erroneous to think that, since the operative field is small, the operating room should be likewise. The fact is that, since the patient is operated on in an outstretched position of both arms, one extended for intravenous use and the other for the surgical procedure, a larger operating room will be required than one that accommodates, for example, an abdominal surgery procedure.

The operative field (Fig. 7.1)

Stability of the operative field is essential for efficient surgery. The patient is placed supine on a regular operating table, and an operating hand table is placed to support the patient's arm in the appropriate position. This hand table must have a supporting leg so that there is no springboard effect to the operating area, permitting the surgeon to stabilize his hands by pressing his elbows on the table surface. The surgeon should sit routinely on the same side, preferably the axillary side, in order to present the same anatomical orientation for each procedure. The table should be adjusted to the surgeon's elbow level so that he is sitting firmly, with the knees level with the hips and the feet flat on the floor. The

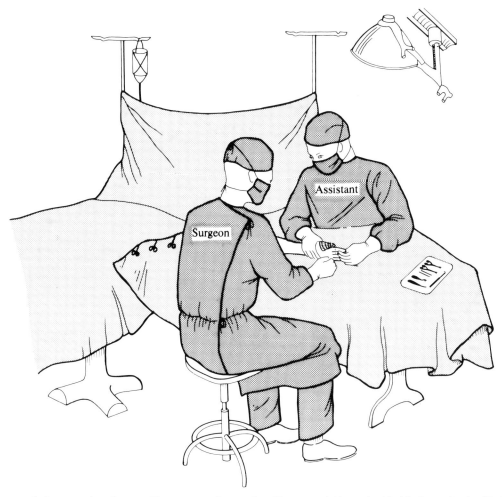

Fig. 7.1. Layout of the operating theatre. The surgeon sits comfortably on a rigid stool with his knees level with his hips. His elbows press on the table surface to stabilize the hands. The assistant should be a few inches higher for a better view, holding the patient's hand firmly. The basic instruments should be accessible with minimal effort and the patient's hand and the anaesthetist should be screened by a drape to prevent contamination. After Crenshaw, A. H., ed. *Campbell's Operative Orthopaedics*, 5th Ed. St. Louis, Mosby, 1971.

assistant must sit a few inches higher to give a clear view of the operative field. Stabilizing 'hand holders', such as a lead template, are excellent for certain procedures such as excision of small tumours in the palm and Dupuytren's contracture. Other procedures, such as tendon grafts and tendon transfers, that require mobility of the field, do not lend themselves to the fixed position of a hand-holding apparatus. An assistant willing to become catatonic to hold the patient's hand so that the surgeon can see best is much more efficient.

The surgeon's stool should have some surface other than hard metal; either wood or a pad of rubber is less fatiguing. It should not be too large for comfort, since bending forward on its edge may cause pressure on the surgeon's sciatic nerve, and it must be stable enough not to waver with weight-shifting. A constant balancing

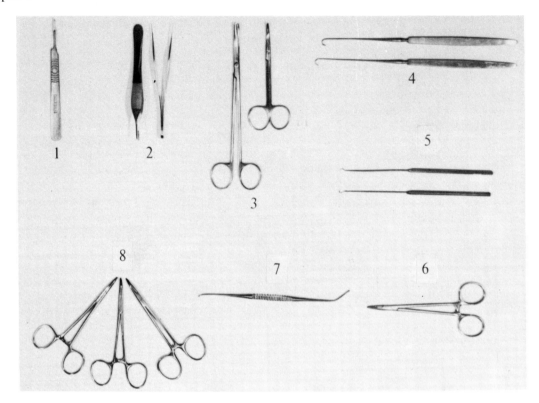

FIG. 7.2. Instruments used in hand surgery.
Basic hand tray: (1) Scalpel with size 15 blade, (2) toothed and non-toothed Adson dissecting forceps, (3) long and shorthandled dissecting scissors, (4) nerve hooks, (5) skin hooks, (6) needle holder, (7) Watson Cheyne dissecting probe, (8) mosquito artery forceps.

effort on the part of the surgeon causes early muscle fatigue. Should the operating table be too low, the surgeon must bend forward, tiring his back; should it be too high, he is unable to see without standing or stretching.

The ideal operating table has an extending shelf that holds certain basic instruments: scissors, knife, forceps and three or four haemostats, with one or two additional instruments such as a probe and a couple of skin retractors (Fig. 7.2). These can be reached by the surgeon with minimal effort and do not require additional handling by the nurse, thus eliminating two steps: the request for the instrument and the transfer of it by the nurse. On a separate large table there are other instruments that *might* be needed. This should be sufficiently close to the nurse so that she can readily hand the surgeon any additional instruments needed.

Draping

A tourniquet is placed well above the elbow over the arm padded with cotton rolls. This tourniquet should contain no large unyielding buckle but preferably a Velcro-like smooth covering. It should be tested routinely for leakage by inflating momentarily prior to surgery. A sterile pad is placed over the operating hand table. Since the operative field should always extend from above the patient's elbow to the fingertips, a standard draping can be used in all procedures which leaves the hand unencumbered for moving. Therefore, the preparatory solution is used over the entire hand and as far as an area above the elbow taking care not to permit its flow under the tourniquet. Betadine is a useful solution but may provide a slightly sticky surface. Tincture of iodine, half strength, followed by a solution of alcohol, is also satisfactory and has been used for many years. Occasionally alcohol alone can be used on infants' hands and hands of old people that have been adequately prepared before surgery with soap and water. Any solution containing mercury should not be used because of the occasional severe allergic reaction.

These solutions should be applied with a sponge by an assistant with gloved hands. A sponge on long forceps is less efficient and will not cover the surface as smoothly. After appropriate skin preparation draping is carried out to provide an operative field from just above the elbow distally, and the anaesthesiologist is shielded with an adequate screen. The draping should be routine for all hand operations. A soft-coloured draping material is more satisfactory than a white one, which causes harsh reflections.

Lighting is placed so as to provide maximum viewing by the seated surgeon. Sterile operating light handles are helpful because they can be adjusted during the operation if necessary.

It is the assistant's duty to anticipate the needs of the surgeon after routine draping has been carried out. Skin incisions may be outlined with a commercially available sterile skin pencil. Only after skin preparation, incision-marking and lighting adjustments is the tourniquet inflated. The arm is first exsanguinated with a Martin bandage wrap or by elevating the extremity for a minimum of 2 minutes. This provides partial exsanguination but not a completely dry field. Some surgeons feel this is an advantage since veins and arteries can be seen more clearly when divided and clamped properly.

Instrumentation and haemostasis

Hand surgical instruments have smaller working terminal parts than those generally used in orthopaedics or general surgery. However, this does not mean that the hand-holding end should be reduced to the point of being inconvenient for the surgeon to grasp and control the instrument. As stated previously the four basic instruments used in hand surgery are the knife, dissecting scissors, forceps and haemostat (Fig. 7.2). Most surgeons prefer a No. 15 curved blade with occasional use of a No. 11 blade Bard-Parker. For large incisions on the forearm and for cutting skin flaps, a No. 10 blade is useful. Frequent changes of blade should be anticipated to provide a continual efficient working-edge and two

knife handles should be available at all times. The scissors are those that have been used traditionally in ophthalmology, and have a double curved surface with a slightly blunted tip. The pickup forceps, again are those used frequently by ophthalmologists, 1·5 mm in size, or smaller for small nerve and vascular work. Jewellers' pointed forceps have been popularized recently for nerve and vascular work and are used for holding the needle of a 10/0 nylon suture. The haemostats are generally the so-called 'mosquito' size with curved ends. This permits more accurate grasping of the bleeding vessel without crushing surrounding tissue. Another very useful tool is the dissecting probe. This curved pointed probe is excellent for passing and pushing tendons through pulleys and exploring under bone surfaces for fusions and adhesions. Double-hooked retractors are generally preferable to the single-hooked retractors except when handling skin flaps. These double hooks are excellent in most incisions on the palm and finger surfaces. Needle holders with smooth jaws to avoid cutting the suture material are preferred, as it is much more efficient to tie sutures with a needle holder than with the surgeon's unassisted hand. The bone instruments may consist of short Ochner clamps which act as miniature Lane bone-holding forceps. Towel clips are set aside for this purpose only to save other instruments. The use of electric cautery makes the operative field much less bloody and can be used with efficiency if great care is taken not to overheat surrounding nerve tissue.

Incisions (Fig. 7.3)

Skin incisions may be made anywhere on the palmar or dorsal surface of the hand, as long as certain principles are observed. In general, they should parallel the major creases of the hand as closely as possible and not cross these creases at or near a right angle. This avoids tension lines being created along the healed scar causing hypertrophy. This does not imply that the deeper incisions for dissection should be in the same direction. Most of the underlying dissections parallel the tendons or neurovascular bundles. Any incision should be sufficiently extensive to avoid excessive traction on the skin edges in attempting to expose underlying structures. Most incisions are curved since most skin creases of the hand

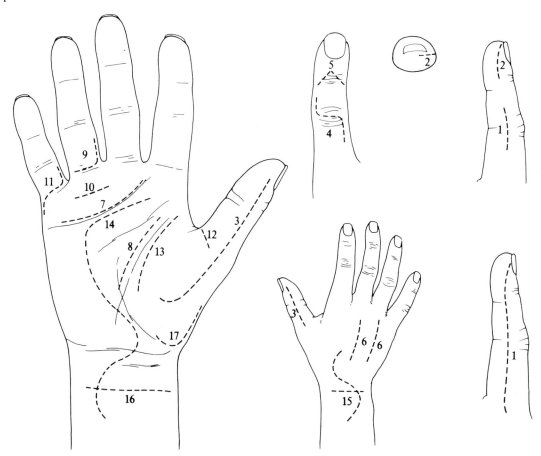

FIG. 7.3. Correct skin incisions in hand; (1) midlateral incision in finger; (2) incision for draining pulp infection; (3) midlateral incision in thumb; (4) incision to expose central slip of extensor tendon; (5) inverted V-incision for arthrodesis of distal interphalangeal joint; (6) incision to expose metacarpal shaft; (7) incision to expose palmar fascia distally; (8) incision to expose structures in middle of palm; (9) L-incision in base of finger; (10) short transverse incision to expose flexor tendon sheath; (11) S-incision in base of finger; (12) incision to expose proximal end of flexor tendon sheath of thumb; (13) incision to expose structures in thenar eminence; (14) extensive palmar and wrist incision; (15) incisions in dorsum of wrist; (16) transverse incision in volar surface of wrist; (17) incision in base of thumb. After Bunnell, S. *Journal Bone and Joint Surgery*, **14**, 27, 1932; and Bruner, J. M. *British Journal Plastic Surgery*, **4**, 48, 1951.

are also curved, and must be more critically placed than on any other part of the body, with the exception of the face. This is done most accurately by drawing the proposed incision with a skin pencil prior to the inflation of the tourniquet. The incision is carried directly through the underlying subcutaneous fat to the fascial layer, after which the opening is converted to an oval shape or an ellipse to permit better exposure of the underlying structure. The skin on the palmar aspect is less mobile than on the dorsum and requires a longer incision to expose the same underlying area. Curved or S-shaped incisions may be slow to heal in the older patients and in rheumatoid disease. Incisions should be made so that extension is possible later, should the occasion demand.

Care should be taken that multiple incisions are not too close together, since this would tend to impair the blood supply of the skin between the incisions. Only experience helps to determine this interval.

Scars do not stretch but hypertrophy as the result of intermittent tension and, therefore, must not cross flexion creases.

Finger incisions

There are two basic skin incisions, the mid-lateral, more accurately defined as dorsal lateral, and the volar zig-zag incision (Fig. 7.4). The latter has been utilized more recently.

The posterior lateral incision crosses none of the flexor creases of the finger and is placed dorsal to the flexor creases at their most dorsal margin (Fig. 7.3–1 and 3). It extends from the point of the junction of the matrix of the nail into the lateral pulp then proximally to a point posterior to the distal flexor crease and to the middle flexor crease, then extending on to the lateral aspect of the metacarpophalangeal joint (Fig. 7.5). After incising through the skin, it is deepened through the underlying fat. There is very little underlying fat at the lateral aspect of the proximal interphalangeal joint, making it easy to enter the joint accidentally. The incision continues through the fatty area until an interval is reached deep to the neurovascular bundle and superficial to the bone or joint, and then is carried forward to enter the flexor

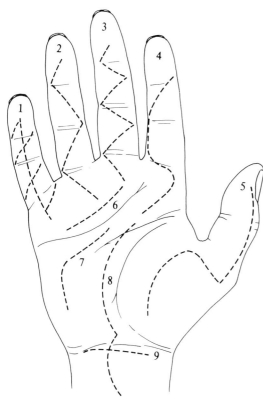

FIG. 7.4. Additional correct skin incisions in hand. (1) Z-plasty incision often used in Dupuytren's contracture (McGregor); (2) and (3) Zigzag incisions for Dupuytren's contracture or exposure of flexor tendon sheath; (4) volar flap incision; (5) incision to expose structures in volar side of the thumb and thenar area; (6) incision in distal palm for trigger finger or other affections of proximal tendon sheath; (7) incision to form flap over hypothenar area; (8) incision to expose structures in middle of palm; it may be extended proximally into wrist; (9) short transverse incision in volar surface of wrist. After Crenshaw, A. H., ed. *Campbell's Operative Orthopaedics*, 5th Ed. St. Louis, Mosby, 1971.

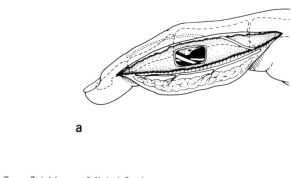

a

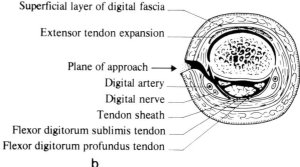

b

FIG. 7.5. (a) Midlateral approach to expose flexor tendon sheath. On radial sides of index and middle fingers and on ulnar side of little finger is dorsal branch of digital nerve that should be preserved if possible. Volar flap containing neurovascular bundle has been developed and reflected. Window has been cut in sheath to show relations of flexor tendons. (b) Cross-section of finger to show midlateral approach. After Crenshaw, A. H., ed. *Campbell's Operative Orthopaedics*, 5th Ed. St. Louis, Mosby, 1971.

tendon sheath if required, taking the neurovascular bundles forward within the flap (Fig. 7.5). On the radial aspect of the index finger, care should be taken to avoid the dorsal branch of the digital nerve as this supplies the radial aspect of the index fingertip. It is possible to obtain exposure to the flexor tendon sheath throughout the digit and also to the neurovascular bundle, not only of the side of the incision, but of the opposite side as well. The finger is opened as an envelope; the dorsal margin of the skin may be dissected by slightly undermining it, permitting a more even closure.

The second basic incision is the zig-zag incision (Bruner) which extends from the distal to the proximal portion of the finger (Fig. 7.4–2 and 3). It crosses skin creases but not at a right angle. The advantage of this incision is that it permits a direct anterior exposure to the flexor tendon sheath and both neurovascular bundles. This is offset by the danger that both neurovascular bundles might be damaged by an inaccurate exposure or a remaining neurovascular bundle severed resulting in necrosis of the skin flap. This incision is used electively to expose flexor tendons and nerves within the finger and can be easily extended into the palm; however, in fingers that have flexion contractures, the incisions do not permit extension of the finger without placing undue tension on the incision itself. To overcome this, Z-plasties (Fig. 7.4–1) or skin grafts are better employed.

Thumb incisions

A lateral incision similar to that of the finger, especially on the radial side of the thumb (Fig. 7.3–3) makes most underlying structures accessible. This may be extended proximally to the mid-portion of the thumb metacarpal and then angled across the thenar eminence (Fig. 7.4–5). Care should be taken to avoid severing the dorsal branch and the superficial radial nerve that frequently supplies a portion of the radial pulp of the thumb. Fat is scanty over the lateral aspect of the metacarpophalangeal joint and distal joint of the thumb, and because of this the joint can be easily entered and the volar plate dissected from its mooring by mistake. This incision is utilized for tendon grafts and exposing other deep-lying structures. The flap created has minimal fat and usually has sufficient healing power not to concern the surgeon when using this flap over the thenar area.

A transverse incision in the skin crease of the meta-carpophalangeal joint of the thumb (Fig. 7.3–12) is useful in releasing a trigger thumb; however, both digital nerves at this level lie surprisingly anterior and must be carefully avoided.

Palmar incisions

Elective palmar incisions parallel the flexor creases (Figs. 7.3 and 7.4); to extend into the digital area, variations must be carried out so as not to cross a skin crease at a right angle. This is done by adjusting the incision to cross the skin creases at a 45° angle and extending it on up into the digits as far as necessary, either laterally or utilizing the volar zig-zag incision. It is desirable to dissect palmar skin margins away from the fascia and create an ellipse revealing the underlying fascia in the separate plane. The palmar fascia may then be excised or incised knowing that there is no structure of critical importance superficial to this except the recurrent motor branch of the median nerve. The bones are generally exposed from the dorsal aspect of the hand. It should be remembered that the pre-tendinous fascia over the metacarpal heads does not extend completely over the palm and there is some herniation of fat normally on each side of the metacarpal heads. This, therefore, is not the safety barrier that it is in mid-palm. Incisions in the proximal palm should parallel the thenar crease, and the exact topography of the recurrent motor branch of the median nerve must be remembered. This can be located by extending an imaginary line from the mid-portion of the thumb web to the pisiform bone, and transecting this with the line extending proximally from the radial side of the middle finger. (See also surface anatomy, p. 52.) At the transection point, the median nerve can usually be found just distal to the flexor retinaculum.

Incisions extending from the palm to the wrist should not cross the wrist flexor creases at a right angle but should be diverted to the ulnar side to avoid the palmar branch of the median nerve between the flexor carpi radialis and palmaris longus tendons.

Wound closure

It is usually possible to carry out a primary closure of any incised tidy wounds, thus lessening the chances of infection or excessive scarring which would destroy the gliding mechanisms underneath. Wounds that are severely contaminated or crushed, such as high velocity missile wounds, human bites or crushing machine-inflicted wounds, should not be closed primarily. When in doubt, the wound, after careful excision under general anaesthesia, should be left open temporarily. It is inspected after 24 or 48 hours and any necrotic tissue excised. Closure may then be carried out within the first 3–5 days, usually by skin graft, although secondary suture may be possible if tension is not too great. The wound should preferably not be left open to granulate by scar.

Wounds may have to be reopened should there be haematoma, excessive swelling and tension or infection. Any patient with severe pain following wound closure or who has discharge, odour or fever, should have the wound inspected.

Underlying tissue such as joint cartilage, exposed fractures or tendons, will not often survive without adequate cover. It is, therefore, necessary to provide coverage for these as soon as, in the judgement of the surgeon, it is safe to do so.

Basic skin techniques (see also Chapter 9)

Only experience determines what constitutes too much tension. Skin stretched to the point of becoming white is under too much tension and will cause delayed healing and further necrosis of skin edges. This aspect must always be considered at the time of wound closure and the surgeon must be well versed in the techniques of skin grafting. Little harm is done by waiting 3–5 days, should the wound not be deemed safe to close. However, after 5 days, collagen is produced rapidly causing late secondary wound contractures.

Free skin grafts

Free skin grafts are necessary when there is an area defect within the dermis. This defect should be closed by free grafts without attempting Z-plastys or local rotational flaps in the recently damaged hand. Split thickness grafts may be used for temporary coverage, a more definite coverage being undertaken at a later date. Split grafts often contract up to 50 per cent of the total area, which may not be acceptable in some instances. Free grafts are destroyed by haematoma, inadequate im-

mobilization and infection, so that wound care must provide the bed required for a successful take. Full thickness grafts are seldom used on hands, especially with potential contamination. Fingertips may, however, support a full thickness graft, particularly in children. A thick split graft is desirable over the wearing surfaces of the palm. 'Pinch' grafts should never be used. The donor site for free grafts should be carefully selected. The upper inner arm for small grafts is the most acceptable. For techniques of grafting of skin and use of flaps see Chapter 9.

Basic bone techniques

The maintenance of reduction of manipulated fractures should be carried out by simple splinting or by K-wire internal fixation, which are placed by either open reduction or percutaneous pinning. Treatment of fractures by traction is rarely if ever indicated. Internal fixation enables the dressings to be removed and reapplied without jeopardizing the alignment of the reduced fracture. Sites of osteotomy and arthrodesis are, likewise, best maintained by internal fixation.

The insertion of Kirschner wires does not require excessive equipment; a drill that will hold four different sizes of Kirschner wires (0·035–0·054 of an inch) is mandatory. A battery-operated drill, is extremely useful. The Kirschner wire should be sharpened at both ends. A cutter should be available to nip the wires at the desired level close to the bony cortex. Other instruments, such as a Kocher clamp, used towel clip, or Lewin clamp are useful to maintain bone reduction. Dental chisels, small rasps, bone cutters and rongeurs are also used routinely. Very thin osteotomes with sharp cutting surfaces are much easier to use than a chisel. In a compound fracture or in open reduction it is easier to insert the wire retrograde from the fracture until the Kirschner wire is projecting out beyond the cortex and one point is left within the fracture. After reduction of the fracture or site of arthrodesis, the wire is redirected in reverse for fixation. Kirschner wires should be cut off beneath the skin or left out a few millimetres through the skin and covered with the sterile dressing. Tenting the skin up with a cut Kirschner wire will invariably enable it to migrate painfully through the skin. Skin infection following use of a Kirschner wire is not common unless there is motion between the wire and skin. To avoid rotation it is best to have Kirschner wires placed parallel for fixation as wires placed criss-cross tend to hold the ends apart. Kirschner wires can be removed under a local anaesthetic.

Basic tendon techniques (see also Chapter 11)

It is necessary to suture cut tendons and to maintain the anastomosis while healing is taking place. Regardless of the type of suture employed or the material used,

anastomosis cannot be maintained without additional splinting to ensure relaxation of the muscle. Intermittent passive or even active finger joint movement during this phase of healing is permitted by some in an attempt to reduce adherence of the tendon to its surrounding sheath and other tissues. Complete agreement has not been reached as to whether or not this is beneficial. During repair of the tendon, it must not be crushed by instruments unless plans are made to excise this crushed part eventually. Tendon end excision will cause shortening and undesired tension on the musculotendinous unit. At any point where tendons are touched with a sharp

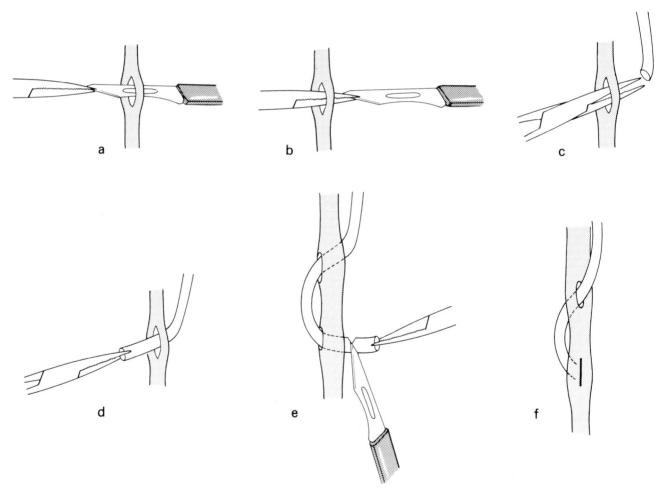

FIG. 7.6. Steps in technique of end-to-side anastomosis. Note in (f) that end of tendon has been buried. Sutures will be appropriately placed to fasten tendons together. After Crenshaw, A. H., ed. *Campbell's Operative Orthopaedics*, 5th Ed. St. Louis, Mosby, 1971.

instrument, there is the likelihood of adhesion formation.

Many techniques have been used to repair tendons. Problems may arise from the breakage of suture material, the loosening of knots or the suture cutting out or being too reactive. At present, monofilament wire suture and synthetic fibres are most acceptable. Wire is more difficult to handle but retains its knot better than the synthetic fibres.

There are four basic instances in which tendon sutures may be employed: end-to-end anastomosis, end-to-side anastomosis, tendon sutured to multiple tendons and attachment of tendon to bone.

End-to-end suture

End-to-end suture may be necessary in the cut tendon or in the attachment of a tendon graft. The Bunnell criss-cross stitch has been used with success but extensive exposure may be needed for this suture technique. The method of Kessler provides a good grasping suture and needs a smaller area of exposure (see Fig. 11.4, p. 157). There are many variations of these; in any case, a needle applied with an atraumatic eyeless end is highly desirable and care should be taken to tie an exact square knot.

End-to-side anastomosis (Fig. 7.6)

This technique is usually needed when one motor unit must activate several distal tendon segments (see Fig. 35.15, p. 510). Great care should be taken to avoid greater tension on one tendon than on the others. Individual through-and-through mattress sutures are used to hold the transfer to each tendon. Tension is always a critical factor and should be carefully considered at the time of suture.

Attachment of tendon to bone

This is best done by abrading the bone, drilling a hole

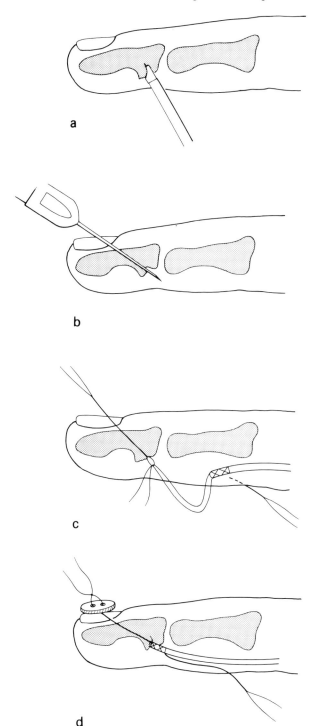

FIG. 7.7. One method of attaching a tendon to bone. (a) Small area of cortex is being raised with osteotome. (b) Hole is being drilled through bone with Kirschner wire in Bunnell drill. (c) Bunnell crisscross stitch has been placed in end of tendon, and wire suture is being drawn through hole in bone. (d) End of tendon has been drawn against bone, and suture is being tied over button. After Crenshaw, A. H., ed. *Campbell's Operative Orthopaedics*, 5th Ed. St. Louis, Mosby, 1971.

through it and using a Bunnell pullout suture, which is very useful at this site (Fig. 7.7). The pullout should be easy to remove; otherwise it may tend to distract the bone and tendon anastomosis.

Multiple tendon lacerations

Multiple tendon lacerations at the palm or wrist level are best sutured with a single separate stitch. These sutures may be either the Kessler stitch or a single double-right angle suture.

Fishmouth suture

The Pulvertaft method (Fig. 11.16) of applying a smaller tendon diameter to a larger one is useful, but it may be more difficult to obtain smooth ends than with the other types of sutures.

Extensor tendons (see also Chapter 11)

Extensor tendons divided about the metacarpophalangeal joint may be sutured with a simple roll stitch using No. 34 monofilament wire. This suture is passed through the skin and rolls around the proximal and distal tendon segments and out of the skin from the opposite border (Fig. 7.8). This enables the tendon stitch to be withdrawn

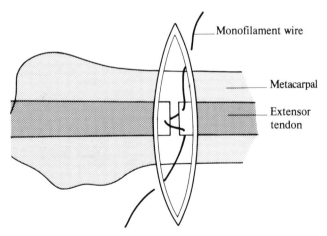

Monofilament wire

Metacarpal

Extensor tendon

FIG. 7.8. Roll stitch is useful in repairing an extensor tendon that has been divided near a metacarpophalangeal joint. After tendon has healed, the suture is removed by pulling on one of its ends. After Crenshaw, A. H., ed. *Campbell's Operative Orthopaedics*, 5th Ed. St. Louis, Mosby, 1971.

at a later date and maintains good apposition when the hand and wrist is splinted. It should be maintained for a minimum of 4 weeks.

ANAESTHESIA

J. CAMPBELL SEMPLE

The hand lends itself well to a number of techniques in anaesthesia. Local anaesthesia can be used as well as regional blocks or general anaesthesia. The selection of these will depend upon the desire of the surgeon, the temperament of the patient and the availability of the anaesthetist. General anaesthesia is probably the quickest method of obtaining consistent and complete anaesthesia but may require admission to hospital. A local anaesthetic is immediately available and may be managed by the surgeon, but it is generally not feasible in large surgical procedures requiring lengthy operating time.

Local anaesthesia

Almost all hand surgery can be carried out under local anaesthesia [1], although for reasons of tradition and convenience most elective surgery in Britain is carried out under general anaesthesia. Some hand surgery is better performed under local anaesthesia; for example, following tendon repair under general anaesthetic, the patient may produce considerable tightness or tremors when recovering from the anaesthetic, whereas a long-acting proximal nerve block will allow a steady, controlled return of sensation and function with no danger of suture line rupture from uncontrolled movement of the finger or hand.

Various local anaesthetic agents are available but fall into two main groups, short-acting lignocaine, lasting for approximately 1 hour, and bupivicaine which lasts for 8–10 hours, although it takes rather longer to produce its initial effect. These agents are simple, easy to use, and quite safe as long as the toxic dose of 200 mg lignocaine is not exceeded. An excess may produce cardiac irregularities or cerebral irritation manifested as minor epileptic seizures, although probably the most common effect of lignocaine overdosage is that the patient becomes nervous and agitated.

To get the best use out of local anaesthesia it is often combined with additional drugs:

(1) *Adrenalin* (Epinephrine) in a dilution of 1 in 10 000 can be added to produce vasoconstriction, and thereby delay the diffusion and resorption of the anaesthetic and prolong its effect. However, this advantage is more than outweighed by the very serious danger of digital necrosis following such an injection, and it is recommended that *no lignocaine/adrenalin mixtures be used in hand surgery.*

(2) *Hyalase.* To obtain rapid action of a local anaesthetic, the addition of 1 or 2 ml of hyalase will speed the diffusion of the injected material in the tissues.

(3) In most surgical situations, anxiety is allayed by an additional premedication, such as injection of *valium* and *pethidine* (Demerol).

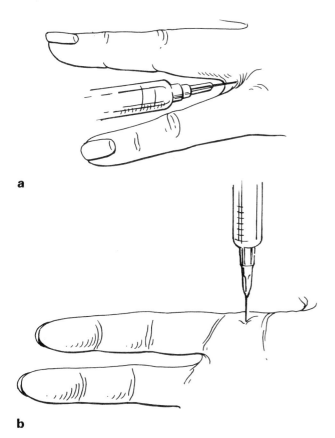

a

b

Fig. 7.9. Injection sites in (a) digital block, and (b) radial digital block to index finger.

Lignocaine and bupivicaine, properly used, should provide complete anaesthesia for the duration of surgery. If the patient is uncomfortable or is aware of pain during the operation, it is due to the inexpert use of these agents. Time spent in learning the following techniques is well spent in terms of the future comfort and efficiency of both emergency and elective hand surgery. It must be stressed that these agents take time to act; lignocaine takes about 10 minutes to act fully, particularly when being used as a nerve block [2], and bupivicaine takes 20–30 minutes before achieving its full effect. There is no excuse for putting the local anaesthetic in and proceeding immediately with the operation. If, after an appropriate interval, the patient is still feeling pain, a carefully repeated injection of local anaesthesia will be necessary.

Local infiltration

This is only of value in the emergency room and only in certain sites, usually where the tissues are fairly slack, such as the dorsum of the hand and forearm. It is not advised on the front of the hand or in the fingers, as the injected solution produces far too much tension and swelling of the tissues, thus making good surgery almost impossible. Lignocaine 0·5 per cent is sufficient to produce anaesthesia by this method, and the spread of the anaesthetic solution may be aided by the addition of hyalase.

Digital block (Fig. 7.9)

The digital block is probably the most commonly used anaesthetic technique in the emergency room, and properly carried out will produce excellent anaesthesia of the finger for approximately 1 hour. An injection of about 2 ml of 1 per cent solution of lignocaine on either side of the finger, in the interdigital web at the base of the finger, reaches the region of the digital nerve. A final 2 ml should be injected across the dorsum of the finger to block the branches of the nerve which supplies the dorsum of the finger. It is inadvisable to inject at the base of the finger itself, as it is possible to produce considerable tension in the finger which can embarrass the circulation. On no account should anaesthetic solutions containing adrenalin be used in a digital block, as there is a really significant danger of producing arterial spasm and necrosis of the digit.

Median nerve block (Fig. 7.10)

The median nerve can be very effectively blocked just proximal to the wrist creases. It is not advisable to try to block it in the carpal tunnel itself, as injecting solution through the tough and fibrous flexor retinaculum is difficult particularly as the nerve breaks up into its branches at this point. However, just proximal to the wrist creases, the nerve lies just under the skin between palmaris longus and flexor carpi radialis tendons. A 1 per cent solution of lignocaine is used, the block being carried out in two stages; the initial injection produces anaesthesia of the skin and subcutaneous tissues in the region of the nerve, then 5 minutes later a second injection of 5 or 6 ml close to the nerve anaesthetizes the median nerve territory in the hand. One may have to wait 10–15 minutes before achieving full anaesthesia. It is theoretically possible to block the median nerve at the elbow, but at this level there are other more effective ways of producing anaesthesia.

Ulnar nerve block (Fig. 7.11)

The ulnar nerve can be blocked at the wrist just radial to the tendon of flexor carpi ulnaris in a similar fashion to the median nerve, or it can be very easily located and blocked at the elbow, in the groove behind the medial epicondyle. A similar two-stage technique should be used.

Radial nerve block (Fig. 7.12)

There are occasional indications to block the radial nerve and this is best achieved by raising a subcutaneous weal of anaesthetic solution a few cm above the wrist on the radial aspect of the forearm, where the radial nerve breaks up into its terminal branches and lies in the subcutaneous tissues.

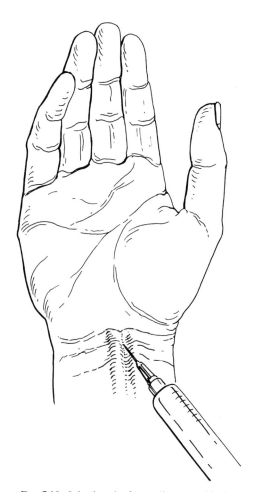

FIG. 7.10. Injection site for median nerve block.

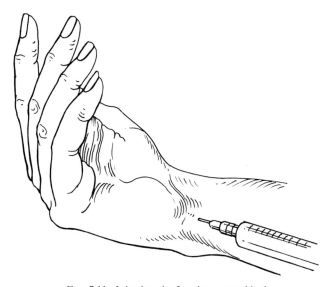

FIG. 7.11. Injection site for ulnar nerve block.

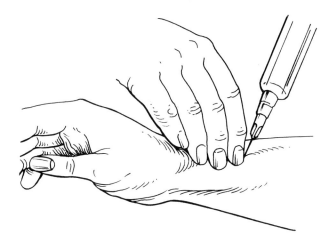

FIG. 7.12. Injection site for radial nerve block.

Intravenous block

Bier's technique [3–5] is extremely useful in hand surgery, its disadvantage being a time limit, usually of about 45 minutes, on the use of the tourniquet on the arm. This can be increased by use of the double tourniquet (see below). It precludes release of the tourniquet prior to closing the wound, as by then the zone of anaesthesia is often lost, unless it is combined with a block of the median and ulnar nerves at the wrist. However, it is a very safe and simple technique and requires no more skill than that required to do a good venipuncture, while the anaesthesia produced is immediate and the recovery rapid. A tourniquet (ideally a double tourniquet) is placed on the upper arm, over some wool padding, but not inflated at this stage. A small intravenous needle, preferably of the butterfly type, is inserted into a dorsal vein on the back of the hand and taped into position. The arm is then elevated and an Esmarch bandage used to exsanguinate the limb, taking care not to dislodge the intravenous needle. The tourniquet is inflated to a pressure of 300 mm mercury. If two tourniquets are being used, then the upper tourniquet only is inflated at this stage. The arm is now brought down to the horizontal and 40 ml of 0·5 per cent lignocaine (*without adrenalin*) injected slowly. The anaesthesia should affect the whole forearm and hand and is generally associated with a mottled appearance of the skin. It should occur immediately, and the operative or manipulative procedure can be started straight away. After some time,

and this varies somewhat with the age and personality of the patient, the tourniquet becomes uncomfortable, and if this occurs the lower tourniquet is inflated and the upper tourniquet deflated, and a further period of comfortable anaesthesia gained. This technique should not be used if surgery is likely to last for an hour or longer, as eventually the patient will begin to suffer significant pain at the tourniquet level. Release of the tourniquet at the end of the procedure should be carried out slowly, as a bolus of local anaesthetic solution suddenly entering the circulation can produce cardiac irregularity.

Brachial plexus block

It is possible to block the brachial plexus, either in the axilla or above the clavicle, and thereby produce anaesthesia and paralysis of the entire upper limb. These techniques are rather more difficult to learn than the simpler distal blocking ones but nevertheless repay some time and trouble taken in learning them. For more complicated hand surgery operations, lasting for 2 or 3 hours, a brachial plexus block, using a combination of lignocaine and bupivicaine can produce effective anaesthesia for up to 8 hours. A combination of 15 ml of 1 per cent lignocaine and 15 ml of 0·5 per cent bupivicaine produces effective anaesthesia within 10 minutes, and also has the long-lasting advantages of the bupivicaine.

Axillary approach

This technique is simple and safe, the only disadvantage being that one may not block the branches of the musculocutaneous nerve or the radial nerve. With the patient lying supine, and the arm abducted and externally rotated at the shoulder, the artery is palpated in the axilla as far proximally as possible. A small, 25 gauge needle, preferably on its own, without the syringe attached, is gently inserted near the axillary artery, the aim being to get the tip of the needle lying just anterior to the artery, and the hub of the needle should then jump up and down with the arterial pulse. Parasethesiae may be obtained at this stage, implying that one has touched one of the cords of the plexus. About half of the total solution is injected in this area, and the needle is then withdrawn and moved posteriorly so that its tip is lying just posterior to the axillary artery where the remaining half of the solution is injected. The aim of this technique is to flood the solution into the fibrous axillary sheath and thereby surround the cords and branches of the plexus with solution.

Supraclavicular approach

The brachial plexus can be blocked more proximally, as it crosses the first rib, by an injection above the clavicle, and this has the advantage that the musculocutaneous and radial nerves are more effectively blocked, thereby producing a more total anaesthesia of the upper limb. The patient should be lying supine, with a cushion placed behind the dorsal spine in order to bring the cervico-dorsal spine forward but allowing the appropriate shoulder to drop, and the head is turned to the opposite side. This stretches the brachial plexus and brings it near the surface. A small 25 gauge needle, again unmounted to begin with, is inserted through the skin approximately 2 cm above the mid-point of the clavicle, and gently inserted in a posterior, inferior and medial direction. As the needle is advanced in this direction paraesthesia is caused in the arm or hand, and if this occurs, the needle should be stopped and half of the anaesthetic solution injected. Ideally, paraesthesia should be produced in the hand, on both the radial and the ulnar aspect, to be quite certain of blocking the entire plexus. In some cases the appropriate paraesthesia is not produced, and it is then necessary to advance the needle to touch the first rib and inject the anaesthetic solution in a column back from the first rib towards the skin, thereby aiming to surround the trunks of the brachial plexus in this area. It is advisable to take some time with this procedure, as the main complication, if the needle is inserted too deeply or too medially, is to damage the apical pleura and cause pneumothorax. If the patient shows any signs of respiratory distress, the procedure should be terminated and a chest radiograph taken on inspiration.

Both these techniques of brachial plexus block require some skill to produce regular and good anaesthesia, but once mastered are of immense value in carrying out safe and effective hand surgery in many situations where general anaesthesia is impossible or difficult [1].

THE TOURNIQUET
J. CAMPBELL SEMPLE

Virtually all hand surgery should be carried out in a bloodless field below a pneumatic tourniquet. Many of

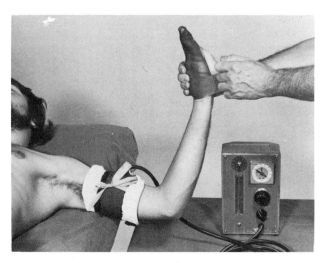

FIG. 7.13. A padded pneumatic tourniquet which is connected to a controlled pressure system. The forearm and hand are exsanguinated with steady pressure from a soft rubber bandage.

the advances of hand surgery in past decades would have been impossible were it not for the careful dissection which has been made possible by this technique. There are, however, some dangers involved in the use of tourniquets, and it is important to be aware of their limitations [6–10].

Tourniquets should always be of the pneumatic variety

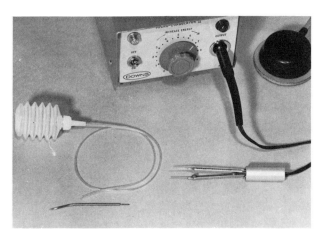

FIG. 7.14. A bi-polar coagulator unit (a) connected to a pair of fine bi-polar coagulation forceps, and (b) a small vacuum drainage system which is ideal for use in hand surgery.

(Fig. 7.13) and there should be an easily-read pressure gauge which should never be inflated above 300 ml mercury for the upper limb. The only safe method of assessing pressure is by a mercury manometer, and if an aneroid or other type of gauge is used, this should be checked regularly to make sure that it is reading accurately. A small, but steady, number of nerve palsies following the use of a tourniquet have been reported [11] and the most common reason is that the tourniquet has been in place for too long or at too high a pressure, the latter being due to an inaccurate gauge.

One of the more frustrating situations in hand surgery is for the tourniquet system to leak, with resulting bleeding, in the middle of a careful dissection in the hand. A mild ooze may occur from time to time, and this is generally held to be due to back pressure of venous blood through the bone marrow of the humerus, but a significant flow of blood is usually due to a leaking tourniquet system. It is, therefore, recommended that once a week the tourniquet systems in a hand surgery unit should be checked for leakage of the cuffs or tubing systems and for the accuracy of the pressure gauges.

With regard to the safe duration of tourniquet ischaemia [6], there is general agreement that 2 hours is probably a safe period, but the danger of nerve paralysis or other problems developing increases significantly after this time [12, 13]. If a further period of exsanguination is required, the tourniquet should be released and then re-inflated, although re-inflation should be delayed for 20–30 minutes, in order to allow the ischaemic muscles in the forearm to recover their normal biochemical balance. When the tourniquet is released finally it should be completely removed from the arm, as the tourniquet and its associated padding may well act as a partial venous tourniquet and increase the amount of bleeding in the limb in the post-ischaemic phase.

Haemostasis is obtained on the release of the tourniquet by compression and elevation and where this proves inadequate a bi-polar coagulation forceps is ideal (Fig. 7.14).

REFERENCES

[1] ERIKSSON E., Ed. *Illustrated Handbook in Local Anaesthesia.* Copenhagen, Munksgaard, 1969.

[2] CONNOLLY, W. B. AND BARRY, F. R. The place of peripheral nerve blocks in reconstructive hand surgery. *The Hand*, 1977, **9**, 157.

[3] ADAMS, J. P., DEALY, E. J. AND KENMORE, P. I. Intravenous regional anaesthesia in hand surgery. *Journal of Bone and Joint Surgery*, 1964, **46A**, 811.

[4] BELL, H. M., SLATER, E. M. AND HARRIS, W. H. Regional anaesthesia with intravenous lidocaine. *Journal of the American Medical Association*, 1963, **186**, 544.

[5] HOLMES, C. McK. Intravenous regional anaesthesia. A useful method of producing analgesia of the limbs. *Lancet*, 1963, **i**, 245.

[6] BRUNER, J. H. Tourniquet time, pressure and temperature factors for safe surgery of the hand. *The Hand*, 1970, **2**, 39.

[7] GRIFFITHS, J. C. Bio-mechanical effects of the tourniquet. *The Hand*, 1973, **5**, 113.

[8] PARKES, A. Ischaemic effects of external and internal pressure on the upper limb. *The Hand*, 1973, **5**, 105.

[9] SANDERS, R. The tourniquet, instrument or weapon. *The Hand*, 1973, **5**, 119.

[10] WARD, C. M. Oedema of the hand after fasciectomy with or without tourniquet. *The Hand*, 1976, **8**, 179.

[11] CALDERWOOD, J. W. AND DICKIE, W. R. Tourniquet paresis complicating tendon grafting. *The Hand*, 1972, **8**, 179.

[12] TOUNTAS, C. P. AND BERGMANN, R. A. Ultrastructural and histochemical observations of ischaemic human muscle and monkey muscle and nerve. *The Journal of Hand Surgery*, 1977, **2**, 31.

[13] WILGIS, E. F. S. Observations on the effects of tourniquet ischaemia. *Journal of Bone and Joint Surgery*, 1971, **53A**, 1343.

CHAPTER 8

General Principles of Management of the Injured Hand

J. I. P. JAMES

In the management of the injured hand, skilled primary care is the most important phase. A realization of this importance and the judicious application of the surgeon's skill at this stage can do more for the patient than at any other time. Details of sophisticated techniques in the repair of tendons and nerves and reconstructive procedures to alleviate loss of function are described in other sections of the book, but it must be stressed that the need for some of these procedures may be avoided by skilful early care of the injured hand. Moreover, where the reconstructive procedures will be necessary and be of great value, their application may be prevented because stiffness has developed in the hand, caused by simple errors in the initial management.

INITIAL ASSESSMENT

When a patient presents with an injured hand certain questions must be answered before examination and assessment of the damage. These include the time of injury, the exact mechanism of injury and what first-aid measures and medication were administered. In most injuries there is either cutting or crushing, although both may occur at the same time, with one predominating. A cutting injury, as by glass or a knife, usually means clean division of the structures and can, of course, be serious. Crushing and pulping injuries, as when hands are caught in moving machinery, causes such damage to the soft tissues that there is a great danger from haemorrhage and oedema in the tissue planes causing an immense

additional problem, even when the gross anatomical damage is not severe.

Other factors of importance are the patient's general health, age, occupation, whether it is the dominant hand which has been injured, and the precise use of the hand at work. Almost of equal importance are the patient's hobbies. A manual worker requiring no great skill may be an expert guitarist or involved in one of many other important leisure activities making great use of the hands. All these factors may determine decisions in initial management.

After obtaining this preliminary information a meticulous examination and assessment of the damage is necessary. Under sterile conditions and with the examiner masked, gloved and using sterile instruments, the first-aid dressings are removed to inspect the damage. In serious injuries, it is better not to remove temporary dressings until the patient is in the operating theatre but before the induction of anaesthesia. Bleeding may appear frightening to the inexperienced but is rarely serious and readily controlled by a pressure dressing. If the injury is confined to the hand, the patient is not shocked. The wound is then covered with a sterile dressing and an overall assessment of the function of the hand carried out to determine if deeper structures have been damaged. In addition to the usual tests for nerve and tendon function (see Chapters 5 and 6), an estimation of any skin damage or loss is made and the viability of tissues is assessed.

In this initial assessment, a prime factor is the viability of skin and digits. As a general rule, large, avulsed, distally based skin flaps will not be viable and should be

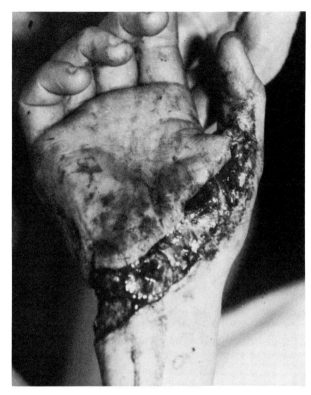

FIG. 8.1. A typical avulsed flap. Even in this young boy most of the skin was dead.

removed (Fig. 8.1). Flaps which are cyanosed, indicating poor venous return, are also not often viable. Pallor of a digit is usually ominous, particularly if it persists after any deformity is corrected, and a non-viable single digit, apart from the thumb, particularly if associated with crushing and skin damage, requires amputation. Where a significant loss of hand function can be anticipated from the loss of a digit, consideration should be given to the microsurgical repair of damage to vessels (see p. 148).

Severe injuries to the hand are commonly associated with damage to the skin which may be grossly lacerated, avulsed or burnt. Cuts and lacerations which cross flexion creases are likely to heal with later contracture. The importance of the viability of the skin has already been mentioned, but it is also important to assess whether there has been skin loss which will require replacement, or whether the skin may be closed by suture at the end of the primary wound excision (p. 126). This can often be assessed at the time of examination and appropriate

treatment planned before the operation is commenced.

The assessment of skin viability is not easy, particularly after crushing injuries and is the source of one of the most frequent errors of judgement in the management of hand injuries. Digits which have been degloved rarely justify attempts at preservation.

This initial examination to check viability, the state of the skin and nerve and tendon function can be very quick and precise, the findings being recorded in a detailed and accurate manner (p. 80). Not only does this allow a relevant plan of initial treatment, but will prove a valuable and necessary adjunct to any later reconstructive surgical procedures.

Anteroposterior and lateral radiographs of the hand are essential after injury. These are likely to show the gross details of any fracture or dislocation but may be inadequate in detail and more localized views may be required.

The assessment, management and planning of treatment of the more complex injuries requires considerable knowledge and experience of reconstructive procedures and is considered further in Chapter 35.

BASIC SURGICAL TREATMENT

Following the initial examination and assessment, wound excision can be carried out with a clear understanding of the damage which will be encountered. Correct primary treatment of any wound is by excision of the wound surfaces and is a basic essential of the management of hand wounds, no matter how complex the deeper injuries may be. Primary healing is expected with confidence after careful wound excision. If ignored or performed in a careless or perfunctory manner, sepsis is likely, is always serious and often totally disastrous. To avoid bacterial growth and spread into the tissues, wound excision should be done within 6–8 hours from the time of the injury. After this period the treatment is unfortunately that of an infected wound, fundamentally different from primary wound excision, and unsatisfactory in many instances.

Technique of wound excision (debridement)

It is recommended that wound excision should be carried out under general anaesthesia and with a pneumatic tourniquet applied to the upper arm after elevation (p. 114). It is very undesirable to embark on the repair of what was thought a simple laceration under a local anaesthetic and find a more complex injury requiring a general anaesthetic, good operating conditions and an experienced surgeon. A general anaesthetic is desirable in all except minor wounds of the skin. A brachial plexus or peripheral nerve block or Bier's technique are also very effective in appropriate circumstances (see Chapter 7). With the latter, as anaesthesia is lost when the tourniquet is deflated, it is impossible to check haemostasis and circulation of the skin before the wound closure, which is undesirable in all but minor injuries.

The hand and forearm are washed and thoroughly cleaned with cetrimide. A meticulous excision of the contaminated wound surfaces and removal of all non-viable tissue is then undertaken. The decision of what to remove may be difficult and the following clinical appearances are of help in the pre-operative assessment:

(1) Colour of the skin: pink skin indicates viability, blue congested skin impaired venous return, and grey skin deficient arterial blood supply and either of the latter suggest that the skin is likely to be non-viable; brownish discoloration of crushed skin indicates tissue death.

(2) Bleeding from the skin edges: red capillary bleeding is present in viable skin but is absent if the arterial inflow is deficient; profuse dark venous bleeding indicates venous congestion and is suggestive of non-viable skin.

(3) The capillary return after pressure on the skin: blanched skin returns to normal colour quickly when the blood supply is good but sluggishly when it is poor.

(4) The capillary return after release of the tourniquet: the speed with which flush of blood returns to the skin is a valuable guide to its blood supply; delay raises doubts about skin viability.

In addition to these four local signs, the patient's general circulatory state must be taken into consideration. The blood supply to the skin is markedly reduced in hypotension.

The viability of any damaged muscle must also be assessed. If muscle is pink, bleeding and contractile, it is certainly viable. If it is blue, friable and non-contractile, it is certainly dead and must be removed. Muscle that is non-contractile but is only minimally discoloured and has some capillary bleeding may recover and is worth preserving.

Various methods have been described to help in the diagnosis of tissue viability. The intravenous injection of disulphene blue or Kiton fast green stains all tissues with adequate blood supply [1]. Viable tissues fluoresce under ultra violet light in a blacked out theatre after the intravenous injection of fluorescin [2]. The blood supply to the skin can also be measured by recording the skin temperature at different sites with a thermocouple or by liquid crystallometry [3, 4, 5] by using thermography to measure the infra red radiation from the skin [6, 7, 8] or by measuring the radiation emitted after the intravenous injection of a radioactive tracer [9, 10]. All require experience in their use and judgement in their interpretation. They may be of value for research purposes but the experienced surgeon makes just as effective decisions on tissue viability clinically.

In the digits, only minimal skin edges can be removed to avoid subsequent difficulty in closure. The wound is extended where necessary to expose underlying structures, and a thin sheet of subcutaneous fat removed. Wound edges in the fascia are excised and where muscle is exposed and damaged, a surface layer of contaminated or dead tissue is removed (Fig. 8.2). Tendons, nerves and bones are cleaned as carefully as possible without further damage. Following this careful excision, the tourniquet is released and haemostasis secured. A check on viability of skin flaps and digits is again made at this stage. Where the skin can be approximated without tension, skin closure by suture is undertaken. Where skin has been lost or removed, skin grafts or flaps will be required (pp. 128–134).

In a hand which has been severely crushed and has become or will become grossly swollen, particularly if severely contaminated, there should be no hesitation in leaving the skin open for 48 hours followed by delayed primary suture or skin replacement. Leaving such a wound open is often much safer than to attempt primary suture. Skin flaps which have been traumatized may have a precarious blood supply and are more likely to die with the additional tension of the sutures. A wound which is heavily contaminated is much less likely to become infected if left open without tension rather than sutured.

Tetanus prophylaxis should be checked and boosted by active or passive immunization as required.

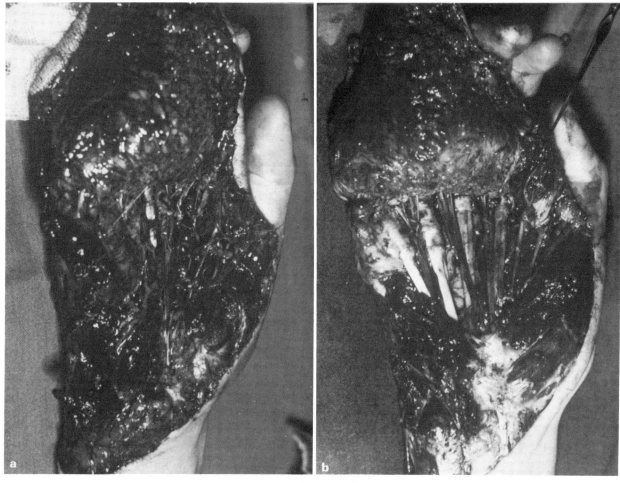

FIG. 8.2. An avulsed flap.

(a) A typical contaminated wound before excision. The flap is turned distally showing the cleavage plane between the tendons and digital nerves on the palmar aspect and the subcutaneous fat and skin superficially.

(b) After excision of the wound surfaces under tourniquet. Such a wound may be expected, after such meticulous excision of the contaminated surfaces, to heal primarily.

Repair of deep damaged structures

The management of injuries to bones, tendons and nerves is described in Chapters 13, 11, 12. At this stage of initial wound management, primary repair of these structures may be considered if the wound circumstances are satisfactory, such as a recent wound of a cutting nature and not grossly contaminated, but it should never be forgotten that the prime requisite of initial wound management is to obtain healing without infection or other complication. No harm can come from leaving the repair of deep structures at this stage and where the surgeon lacks experience, or the necessary facilities, wound excision alone should be carried out and the patient referred for elective reconstructive surgery to an experienced hand surgeon. An elective repair after 2–3 weeks with the necessary technical skill is much to be preferred to an inexpert attempt to repair the structures primarily because it was believed necessary. Though primary repair may be desirable, inept techniques in repairing nerves and tendons are disastrous.

POSTOPERATIVE MANAGEMENT

Antibiotics are rarely indicated if an adequate wound excision has been performed. They are no substitute for satisfactory primary wound care.

Bandaging the hand after injury or operation is rarely done satisfactorily without considerable experience and an appreciation of its importance. It may be as difficult as the operation itself and is certainly no less important. It is in this phase that many serious mistakes are made and irreparable damage done. To obtain the most successful and rewarding results, it is necessary for the surgeon to apply the dressings and bandage after any operation and to supervise personally the after care of patients. A basic problem with the hand is its vulnerability to stiffness and the great difficulty, and sometimes impossibility, of regaining mobility in a hand stiffened by mismanagement. The hand is a dextrous, supple and mobile tool, dependent upon a large number of small joints and on many tendons gliding over paths of considerable amplitude. When these supple movements are lost, so is function, even when the original anatomical damage was minimal.

There are three main causes of stiffening of the hand.

Infection

Severe infection of the hand leading to stiffening is now, fortunately, rare. As already stressed, a most important factor in the prevention of infection is adequate primary wound care. Where infection intervenes, excessive scarring develops which causes adhesions between the gliding structures.

Failure to prevent or control oedema and haemorrhage

In the crushed hand protein-rich oedematous fluid pours into the gliding planes of the digits and the hand (Fig. 8.3). Spreading haemorrhages also occur and may travel considerable distances along the gliding path of a tendon. If blood or fluid is allowed to accumulate and stay in the same place, fibroblasts grow into this excellent culture medium and in 3–4 weeks there is a fibroblastic 'gluepot' in which all the moving structures of the hand are stuck to each other, often with a catastrophic loss of function.

Dependency in the traditional sling (Fig. 8.4a) may be an additional factor aggravating swelling; where a sling

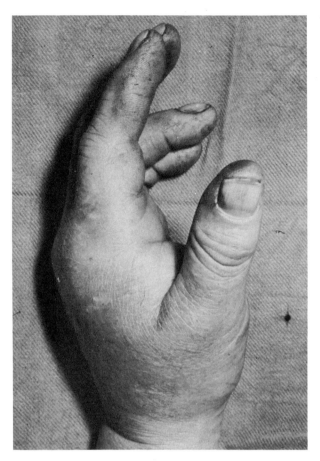

FIG. 8.3. A mildly crushed hand which was not elevated nor treated for oedema. This thick pudgy hand is typical of such cases after 2 or 3 days of neglect. The oedema pushes the finger straight at the metacarpophalangeal joint and tends to flex it at the interphalangeal joint, causing stiffness. Thumb abduction becomes limited. If the oedema is allowed to persist fibroblasts invade the serous fluid and the whole hand becomes a matted web of fibrous tissues.

is considered advisable, the high sling (Fig. 8.4b) is much more satisfactory. In the presence of oedema and swelling, elevation of the hand is essential, either within a roller towel (Fig. 8.5) or in a vacuum splint. A looped wrist bandage must be avoided as it itself may cause oedema by constricting the venous return at the wrist. Correct compression bandaging of the boxing glove type (p. 122, and Fig. 8.6) is of paramount importance in controlling the swollen hand.

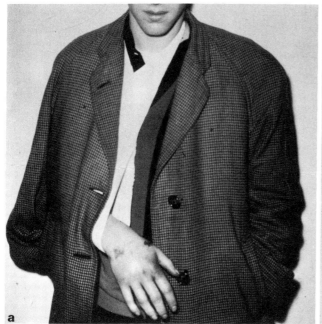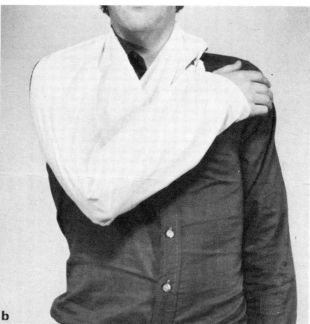

FIG. 8.4. The use of slings.

(a) The dependent sling so commonly used with disastrous consequences. The hand hangs down and over the edge of the sling to cause oedema. In many instances the thumb is pressed on the edge of the sling, adducting it. The metacarpophalangeal joints are extended and the fingers curl over the edge of the sling in flexion at the interphalangeal joints; all positions to be avoided.

(b) In contrast the high sling overcomes all of these positional problems, and if a sling has to be used it should always be as illustrated.

Errors in joint positioning

The metacarpophalangeal and proximal interphalangeal joints of the fingers are particularly vulnerable to stiffening if positioned wrongly. The joints of the thumb stiffen much less readily but an adductor or first web space contracture can be most disabling by limiting spread of the thumb.

The metacarpophalangeal joints of the fingers possess collateral ligaments which are lax in full extension but tautened in full flexion by the configuration of the metacarpal heads (p. 18, Fig. 1.30). The dangerous position for these joints to be immobilized is, therefore, in extension because the collateral ligaments may shorten permanently in this position, particularly in the presence of oedema, and in the course of 2–3 weeks, even in the young, may lead to irreversible contractures in extension,

thus limiting grasp. This constitutes a very serious deformity which may require a complete retraining of the function of the hand. Once the deformity becomes fixed, it is often permanent, as excision of the collateral ligaments (p. 275), though sometimes helpful, is unreliable particularly in the later stages. In contrast, the flexed position of the metacarpophalangeal joints is safe almost indefinitely as can be seen in Dupuytren's contracture where, after release, an immediate recovery of full extension at the metacarpophalangeal joint is usual even after years in the flexed position.

The proximal interphalangeal joints, in contrast, are in danger of stiffening in the flexed position and are much safer if immobilized in extension (p. 20, Fig. 1.34). The triangle of the capsular fibres anterior to the true collateral ligaments, situated between them and the pal-

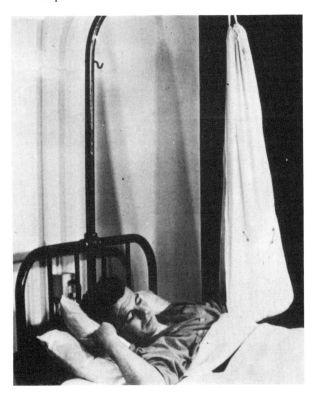

FIG. 8.5. The roller towel is a much better method for elevating a hand for the bedridden patient than suspension by a bandage round the wrist, which tends to constrict the wrist causing oedema. The patient can usually rig up something like this at home. A safety pin on either side of the hand, which can be seen in the photograph, prevents it from slipping out.

mar plate, have been shown to contract if the joints are held in flexion (pp. 20 and 278). If the proximal interphalangeal joints be immobilized in flexion for no more than three weeks, a flexion contracture is most likely to develop which is almost always irreversible or at least difficult and time-consuming to treat. If the finger should stiffen in extension, it will be found that the joint is usually mobile but that it is the extensor hood which has been damaged and is adherent proximally.

Correct joint positioning during immobilization

To avoid stiffness of the joints of the fingers, therefore, a safe position with the metacarpophalangeal joints flexed and the proximal interphalangeal joints extended should always be adopted whenever the hand is bandaged or splinted. In addition the thumb must be abducted in order to keep the first web structures stretched (Fig. 8.6a, b).

The technique of bandaging the hand

The hand should be immobilized in the following position:
    (1) the wrist slightly dorsiflexed;
    (2) the metacarpophalangeal joints flexed as near 90° as possible;
    (3) the interphalangeal joints extended; and
    (4) the thumb fully abducted.
This safe position of the hand is shown in Figure 8.6. The palmar concavity is filled with fluffed gauze or steel wool or plastic foam. It is advisable to insert gauze between the sides of the fingers. When the bandage is applied, it is put on firmly and the separation of the digits makes it more comfortable and less likely to cause pressure sores. With the hand placed in the correct position a roll of orthoband wool is applied and covered by a crepe bandage, first fixing it round the wrist. Looping it over the dorsum of the fingers to maintain the flexed position of the metacarpophalangeal joints the bandage is passed between the thumb and index finger to keep the thumb in abduction. The bandage is applied firmly enough to hold the correct position and to control oedema, but not too tightly as this may cause ischaemic contracture of the small muscles of the hand.

In a hand which has been severely crushed or is badly swollen, it may not be possible to obtain a satisfactory degree of flexion at the metacarpophalangeal joints, because if the joints are flexed fully, there may be some impairment of circulation. In these circumstances a degree of flexion less desirable than usual may have to be accepted. Further correction of the position can usually be obtained as the swelling subsides in a few days. On certain occasions, as after repair of cut extensor tendons on the dorsum of the hand, immobilization of the metacarpophalangeal joint in extension may be required.

A lack of appreciation of the importance of the metacarpophalangeal joint flexion (Fig. 8.7a) can often be seen in carelessly applied plasters for Colles' fractures

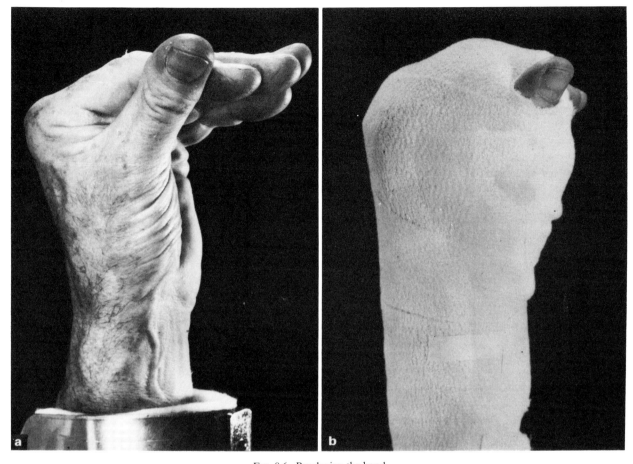

Fig. 8.6. Bandaging the hand.

(a) With the metacarpophalangeal joints flexed to 90°, the interphalangeal joints straight and the thumb abducted, the hand is safe from stiffening when immobilized even for a long time.

(b) The desired position and the appearance in a properly applied boxing-glove bandage.

and other injuries where the plaster extends in the palm beyond the distal crease preventing the metacarpophalangeal joints from flexing.

Flexion contractures of interphalangeal joints are still frequently seen due to errors in positioning of these joints (Fig. 8.7b). It is seldom that immobilization of the hand is required for longer than 3 weeks. On removal of the bandage or splintage, unless repair of tendon or nerve precludes this, active mobilization of the hand is the best way of dispersing oedema or preventing its return. An active muscle pump consisting of alternate digital extension and flexion is extremely

effective if done vigorously and frequently. When, because of pain or apprehension, the patient is reluctant to do this, supervision by a physiotherapist is necessary.

Oedema may occur for the first time when the compression bandage is removed. The development of this oedema must always be anticipated and watched for most carefully. In the early stages it may not always be obvious but is usually seen first on the dorsum of the fingers. If oedema develops and, with it, incipient stiffness following removal of the bandage, urgent admission to hospital for elevation and intensive hand exercises is required. A delay of even a few days may

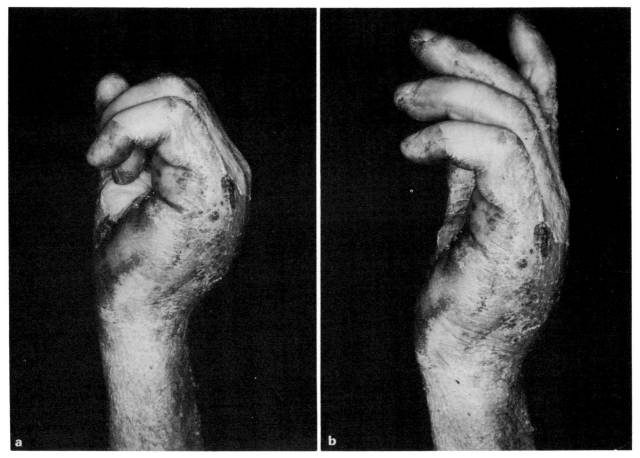

FIG. 8.7. Maximum flexion and extension after bandaging for 10 days with joints incorrectly positioned following a trivial injury.
(a) Flexion at the metacarpophalangeal joints.   (b) Extension at the proximal interphalangeal joints.

lead to irreversible and disabling loss of finger flexion. Prompt action in the way described, usually leads to quick recovery in about 48 hours.

As soon as fractures have healed and repaired nerves and tendons allow, the patient is encouraged to full hard use of the hand. Many are reluctant to do this as they feel they may do further damage, and it is important to give simple explanation and encouragement. In the early stages after injury, the tissues are often indurated and rather 'wooden' from haemorrhage, oedema and scarring. The quickest way to resolve these areas and to restore movement is the use of the hand in hard work. The patient should be instructed to 'massage the hand with a pick and shovel!'

REFERENCES

[1] TEMPEST, M. N. Use of intravenous dye techniques in assessment of tissue viability. *Journal of Bone and Joint Surgery*, 1960, **42B,** 646.

[2] LANGE, K. AND BOYD, L. J. Use of fluorescein to determine adequacy of circulation. *Medical Clinics of North America*, 1942, **26,** 943.

[3] FRESHWATER, M. F. AND KRIZEK, T. S. Liquid crystallometry: a new technique for predicting the viability of pedicle flaps. *Surgical Forum*, 1970, **21**, 497.

[4] HOEHN, F. AND BINKERT, B. Cholesterol liquid crystals: a new visual aid to study flap circulation. *Surgical Forum*, 1970, **21**, 499.

[5] WINSTEN, J., MANALD, P. D. AND BARSKY, A. J. Studies on the circulation of tubed flaps. *Plastic and Reconstructive Surgery*, 1961, **28**, 619.

[6] BLOOMENSTEIN, R. B. Viability prediction in pedicle flaps by infra red thermometry. *Plastic and Reconstructive Surgery*, 1968, **42**, 252.

[7] HACKETT, M. E. J. The use of thermography in the assessment of depth of burn and blood supply of flaps. *British Journal of Plastic Surgery*, 1974, **27**, 311.

[8] THORNE, F. L., GEORGIADE, N. G. AND MLADICK, R. The use of thermography in determining viability of skin flaps. *Archives of Surgery*, 1969, **99**, 97.

[9] BARRON, J. N., VEALL, N. AND ARNOTT, D. G. The measurement of the local clearance of radioactive sodium in tubed skin pedicles. *British Journal of Plastic Surgery*, 1952, **4**, 16.

[10] BRAITHWAITE, F., FARMER, F. T. AND HERBERT, F. I. Observations on the vascular channels of tubed pedicles using radioactive sodium. *British Journal of Plastic Surgery*, 1952, **4**, 38.

FURTHER READING

BOYES, J. H. *Bunnell's Surgery of the Hand*, 5th ed. Philadelphia, Lippincott, 1970.

JAMES, J. I. P. Traitment précoce des blessures de la main. *Revue de chirurgie orthopédique et reparatrice de l'appareil moteur*, 1960, **46**, 139.

JAMES, J. I. P. The early treatment of the injured hand. *Scottish Medical Journal*, 1960, **5**, 231.

JAMES, J. I. P. *The Proceedings of the Second Hand Club 1965–1967*, p. 504. London, British Society for Surgery of the Hand, 1975.

RANK, B. K., WAKEFIELD, A. R. AND HUESTON, J. T. *Surgery of Repair as Applied to Hand Injuries*, 4th ed. Edinburgh, Churchill Livingstone, 1973.

CHAPTER 9

The Skin

A. C. BUCHAN

Careful management of the skin is essential in the treatment of all open injuries of the hand. Many factors are involved in promoting wound healing but this chapter considers only the provision of skin cover, which is complementary to wound excision covered on p. 117.

The hand should be examined under sterile conditions in a good light and the assessment of movement, sensation etc., made on a conscious patient. A complete picture of the wound is made by combining the preoperative and operative findings. The surgeon has a precise assessment of the tissue damage and in particular, how much skin is lost and requires replacement (Fig. 9.1).

METHODS OF SKIN CLOSURE

It is usually desirable that all wounds have definitive skin repair at the time of wound excision, but there are a number of indications for the application of a dressing only after the wound excision and delay of skin closure for 2–5 days.

(1) To allow for an adequate late excision of a deep wound; this applies particularly to war wounds and those produced under similar circumstances.

(2) If the viability of the tissues, particularly of the skin, is in doubt; a delay of a few days after wound excision may make the situation clearer and perhaps indicate further removal of non-viable tissue.

(3) In extensive wounds where bleeding is difficult to control; premature closure of the skin may lead to a large haematoma or loss of skin grafts or flaps.

(4) In severe crush injuries where a skin flap is required, elevation and compression dressings for several days will reduce oedema before the skin flap is applied.

(5) Where there is a choice of alternative methods of treatment, delayed primary closure will give time for discussion with the patient and assessment of the co-operation that can be expected.

Approximation

Suture is only possible if there has been no skin loss and the skin edges can be approximated without tension. The skin is handled with care using fine non-crushing instruments. The wound edges are approximated accurately by 4/0 or 5/0 silk or nylon sutures that are not tied so tightly as to cause skin edge necrosis. Ragged wounds require careful piecing together inserting apical stitches where necessary; badly placed or excessive sutures can easily cause skin necrosis. On occasion the distal part of a digit is almost completely detached except for a neuro-vascular pedicle which provides an adequate blood supply. Preservation of the pedicle during debridement and careful suturing is required if viability of the distal segment is to be retained. Oedema may cause gaping of the wound edges even although there is no skin loss and the insertion of a skin graft is preferable to suturing under tension.

Trap-door types of wound must be sutured carefully to avoid the development of tension transversely across the flap, cutting off the distal blood supply and causing skin necrosis (Fig. 9.2). Skin flaps have a reduced blood supply and are far more sensitive to suturing under tension than normal skin.

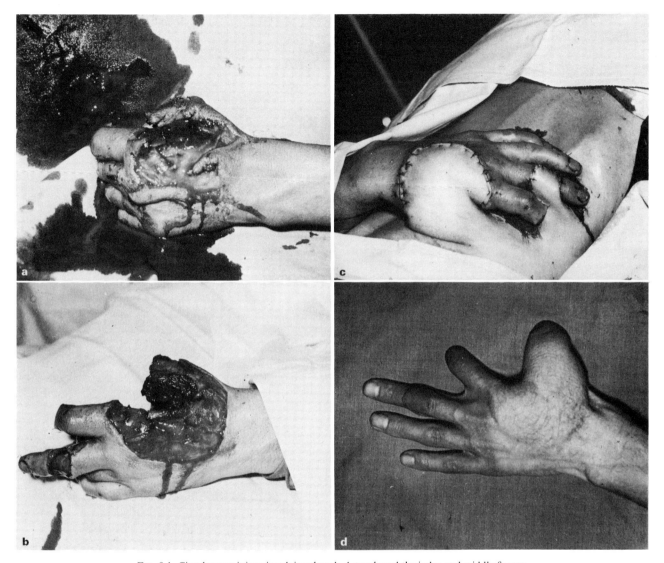

Fig. 9.1. Circular saw injury involving thumb, 1st web and the index and middle fingers.

(a) A complex wound before excision where it was difficult to be certain of the extent of the tissue damage.

(b) After excision when the nature of injury and the extent of the skin loss was known.

(c) Two abdominal direct flaps used to replace the skin loss.

(d) The end result.

Shortening of bone—Amputation

Part of an arm, hand or digit may be so badly damaged that there is no alternative to shortening the bone to obtain skin closure. The absolute indication for amputation is irreparable vascular damage but much can be salvaged now with microvascular surgery (p. 144). It may be possible to save the full length of a finger which has a complex injury involving tendon, nerve, bone or joint. However, if the end result is likely to be stiff, useless fingers which interfere with the function of the hand as a whole, the amputation of whole or part of one or even

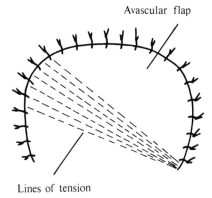

Avascular flap

Lines of tension

FIG. 9.2. Trapdoor type of wound showing tension lines across the flap resulting in necrosis in the distal part of the flap.

two fingers may be indicated. It is essential to preserve the full length of the thumb wherever possible.

There are occasions in which the skeletal structures have to be sacrificed but the skin that remains viable can be used to replace skin loss on adjacent fingers or areas on the hand.

Skin grafts

Skin grafts give a relatively simple method of replacing lost skin, but they provide skin only without subcutaneous tissues. They have no blood supply of their own, surviving on the tissue fluids from their new site until a capillary circulation is established. They will thus not survive on structures of relative avascularity such as bare bone without periosteum or tendon without paratenon. The absence of subcutaneous fat means that skin grafts will become adherent to, and may interfere with, the movement of underlying tendons, muscles or joints. This adherence may result in painful scars or instability of the skin leading to chronic ulceration. In addition, a healed skin graft cannot be undermined with safety, if subsequent reconstruction of deep structures is required.

Skin grafts are classified according to the thickness of the graft (Fig. 9.3).

Whole thickness (Wolfe) graft

This includes the whole thickness of the epidermis and

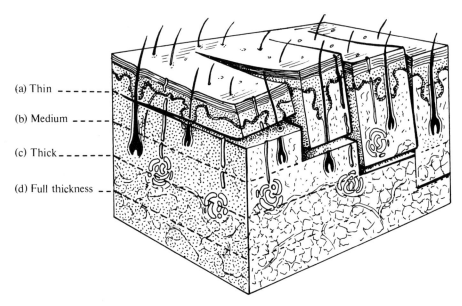

(a) Thin

(b) Medium

(c) Thick

(d) Full thickness

FIG. 9.3. Diagram of skin showing the proportion of dermis included in (a) thin, (b) medium and (c) thick split thickness grafts, and in (d) a full thickness graft. It will be noted that no epithelial structures are left in the donor site after removal of a whole thickness graft but are present after a split skin graft is cut. (Modified from McGregor, I. A., *Fundamental Techniques of Plastic Surgery*, 6th Ed. Edinburgh, Churchill Livingstone, 1975.)

dermis but without the subcutaneous fat. A pattern of the skin defect is made and the exact size of graft required is dissected by scalpel. The thin, non-hair-bearing skin in the groin medial to the anterior superior iliac spine is a very suitable donor site for the hand (Fig. 9.4a), but the flexure of the elbow or wrist is useful for smaller grafts. Some secondary thinning may be required and any loose areolar tissue is removed from the deep surface with fine curved scissors (Fig. 9.4b). The donor wound is sutured after undermining the surrounding skin (Fig. 9.4c). The Wolfe graft gives excellent quality skin re-

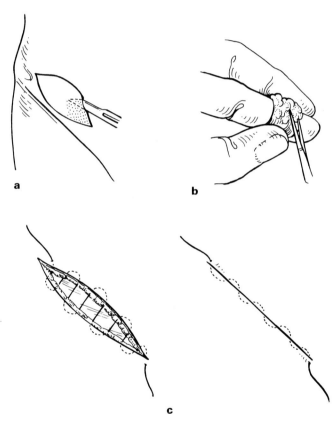

Fig. 9.4. Full thickness graft.

(a) A piece of skin of the exact size required cut by scalpel from the thin non-hairbearing area medial to the anterior superior iliac spine.

(b) Skin graft rolled over surgeon's finger and excess fat removed by fine scissors.

(c) Donor area skin defect closed by approximation using a continuous intradermal nylon suture.

placement and there is minimal shrinkage. It does not take easily and requires an exacting technique under optimal conditions which seldom apply in the immediate management of hand injuries. It is better reserved for the treatment of skin contractures, etc., where a good take can be expected and where the best possible skin replacement is required in small areas.

Split skin grafts

These include the whole thickness of the epidermis and a variable part of the dermis, being described as thin, intermediate or thick depending on how much of the dermis is included. Epithelial cells from the hair follicles, sebaceous glands and sweat glands are left behind in the donor site which heals by proliferation of these epithelial elements. A thin split-skin graft takes well even under difficult conditions and in the presence of infection. However, there is shrinkage of the graft up to half of its original size and in addition, the resulting texture and quality of the skin graft may be unsatisfactory. A thick split-skin graft contains a greater proportion of the dermis, its take is rather more uncertain than the thin graft but it shrinks less and gives better quality skin. This type of graft is used where conditions are favourable and where large sheets of good quality skin are required. An intermediate thickness graft has properties between those of a thin and a thick split-skin graft. The skin grafts used in the immediate treatment of hand injuries are usually of the intermediate or thick split-skin grade.

The thigh is a commonly used donor site for these grafts and large sheets of skin can be cut without difficulty but the donor area scars may be unacceptable. The lateral aspect of the buttock or the lower abdomen within the pantie area may be used where smaller grafts are required and the donor scars hidden as much as possible. The arm is a very convenient site but the scars that may be produced are unacceptable to some patients and the arm should never be used unless the patient's consent has been obtained [1]. Small razor grafts of hand skin for fingertip injuries may be taken from the hypothenar eminence [2].

The Bodenham, Braithwaite, Campbell or Watson modifications of the Humby skin grafting knife are very effective, generally available instruments (Fig. 9.5). After a little practice, large skin grafts can be cut without

Bodenham

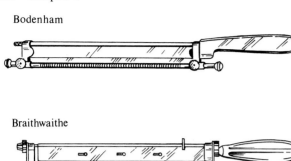

Braithwaithe

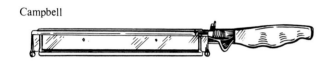

Campbell

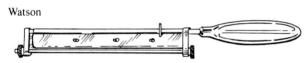

Watson

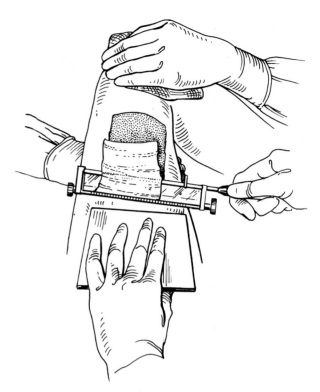

FIG. 9.5. Modifications of the Humby skin grafting knife. All have disposable blades. The Bodenham and the Braithwaite have a rotating oscillating depth guard. The Watson modification has a fixed and the Campbell an oscillating depth guard. Several other modifications of the Humby knife are available.

FIG. 9.6. The technique of cutting a split thickness skin graft. The skin grafting knife is held in the surgeon's dominant hand and the skin is stretched and flattened by a board held in his other hand. The assistant steadies the limb and supports the skin with one hand and stretches the skin with the other.

difficulty and these uncomplicated instruments are recommended for general use in hand injuries. All have disposable blades so that a sharp knife is always available and all have an adjustable roller in front of the cutting edge to regulate the thickness of the graft. The Watson modification has a smooth fixed roller but the others have a rotating roughened roller. The thickness adjustment markings on the knife should not be relied on without visually checking the clearance between the roller and the blade. A clearance of about 0·5 mm is likely to give a medium thickness graft but variations have to be made for individual surgeons and the thickness of the donor area skin. It is essential to have the skin well lubricated by either sterile liquid or soft paraffin so that the knife slides easily on the skin without puckering the skin. The outer surface of the blade should not be lubricated to avoid contamination of the deep surface of the graft with paraffin. The actual technique of cutting the graft is shown in Figure 9.6. It is important that the skin is stretched partly by an assistant and partly by a board held in the surgeon's left hand. The knife blade is angled slightly and pressed on the skin surface. The surgeon and his assistant must get into a comfortable position so that the knife is advanced smoothly and steadily with a gentle sawing movement without stopping to change position.

The Padgett-Hood or Reese drum dermatomes and the various modifications of the electric dermatome are more expensive complicated instruments which are seldom necessary in traumatic hand surgery, although a drum dermatome is required if the lower abdominal wall is used as a donor site.

Management of the graft

A whole thickness skin graft is cut to the size required and is sutured into position accurately edge to edge (Fig. 9.7a). A similar technique is used for a thick razor graft which is trimmed to the size of the skin defect but without overstretching the graft. The thin and intermediate thickness grafts are trimmed to overlap the surrounding skin and are held in position by a few sutures (Fig. 9.7b).

As haematoma is the commonest cause of graft failure, pressure dressings are commonly used to control blood collection under the graft which may interfere with its revascularization. Before applying the dressing, any blood or blood clots under the graft must be expressed and an inner layer of tulle gras is followed by a pad of fluffed wool impregnated with flavine emulsion or liquid paraffin. The wool must be applied carefully, building out any hollows in the graft bed and padding round bony prominences so that even pressure is obtained over the entire graft. Fluffed gauze or cotton wool give additional padding and are followed by the application of a firm crêpe bandage. The contiguous surfaces of the fingers must be separated by a layer of gauze to prevent maceration of the skin. This type of circumferential pressure dressing is usually very adequate for skin grafts on the hand but as an alternative, the standard tie over pressure dressing may be used. In this some of the sutures holding the graft in position are left long and are tied over an evenly applied bolus of flavine wool (Fig. 9.7c). The dressing is completed by the application of more wool or fluffed gauze and a crêpe bandage. Bulky compression dressings usually give enough immobilization but if necessary, a plaster of Paris or a metal splint may be incorporated in the dressings.

More grafts are now being left exposed without any dressing particularly in those areas in which it is difficult to apply an effective pressure dressing. This technique requires careful supervision to prevent the graft being floated off on blood clot or serum. In the hand, the exposure method is usually employed when there is no risk of bleeding as in delayed primary skin closure or in granulating areas. Any blood or serum that collects under the graft is expressed with a cotton bud through a small nick.

The first dressing is retained for 7 days, less if there is a risk of sepsis or haematoma and longer (10 or even 14

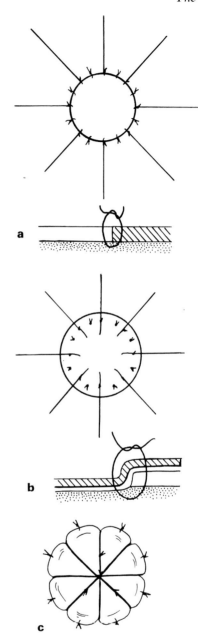

FIG. 9.7. Suturing of grafts.

(a) Whole thickness or thick split thickness grafts accurately sutured into position edge to edge.

(b) Thin razor graft sutured into position using overlapping technique.

(c) In both instances some sutures have been left long for a tie-over pressure dressing.

days) if a thick graft has been used. Extreme care is required in the removal of the dressings to avoid injuring the graft. The sutures are taken out and any crusting and loose or overlapping skin is removed. The whole area is carefully washed with 1 per cent cetrimide and dried. A pressure dressing is re-applied as protection and immobilization of the graft is required for the first 14 days. Further management and dressing will depend on how well the graft has taken and on the rate of wound healing. Any crusting, debris and loose epithelial scales, etc., are removed as they separate. A careful dressing technique and regular wound hygiene is very important at this stage.

Management of the donor site

This is extremely important, otherwise healing may be delayed for weeks. Profuse capillary bleeding follows the cutting of all split thickness grafts. A temporary dressing of fine mesh Vaseline impregnated gauze and a saline soaked pad is applied to control bleeding. At the end of the operation, the bleeding will have stopped and the superficial donor area dressings are removed leaving the innermost layer of Vaseline gauze undisturbed. A pad of dry gauze and a bulky wool dressing is held in position by a firm crêpe bandage. This dressing must be applied so that it does not slip and is left undisturbed for 2 weeks.

Serum exudes into the dressings and provision must be made for air to circulate round the dressings to allow evaporation of moisture and prevent formation of a sodden dressing which would encourage wound infection. Adhesive tape prevents evaporation and should not be used to prevent a dressing from slipping. Bed clothes must not be sealed round a leg donor site. A bed cradle and split bed clothes allows circulation of air and a Braun frame lifts the thigh off the mattress to allow a posterior thigh donor site to dry off. If there should be excessive soakage into the dressings during the forty-eight hours, the superficial part of the dressing is removed and replaced. On no account should the innermost layer of Vaseline gauze be disturbed. Provided the dressings remain dry and uninfected, they are left undisturbed for 14 days. The donor area from a thin graft will be healed but if a thicker graft has been cut, the dressings may still be adherent and cannot be removed

without stripping off the young healing epithelium. Adherent dressings must not be forcibly removed but any loose parts are cut away and a further dry dressing applied for another 3 or 4 days. It is better to retain adherent dressings until they separate on their own.

Recently, a plastic film (Opsite®) has been used on some donor sites, particularly where bandaging may be difficult. The plastic film, which should be adherent to the surrounding normal skin, may leak and require replacement. The technique can be very successful particularly in the smaller donor sites and the patients complain of less pain than with the conventional donor site dressing [3].

Skin flaps

Skin flaps have subcutaneous fat in addition to the whole thickness of the skin and as they have their own blood supply, can survive over avascular structures, thus preventing infection in exposed tendons or compound fractures. A skin flap does not shrink and because of its layer of subcutaneous fat it does not become adherent and can be undermined if reconstruction of an underlying tendon, bone, nerve, etc., is required later.

As survival of skin flaps is dependent on their retaining an adequate blood supply, great care is required in their design and execution. The blood supply is always reduced to some extent and perhaps to such a degree that the skin flap is only just viable. A skin flap is extremely sensitive to sutures tied too tightly, to tension or kinking in the pedicle or the presence of a haematoma, oedema or infection. In most instances of vascular insufficiency, adequate blood is entering the flap but there is venous congestion due to an impaired drainage. The blood supply of the skin varies greatly from one site to another and is at its poorest in the lower leg. In addition, it deteriorates with age and is affected by systemic disease such as diabetes or peripheral vascular disease. A preliminary delay operation may be required to make sure that a skin flap of doubtful viability is going to survive. The flap is partly raised dividing the vessels entering peripherally and from the deep surface but preserving carefully the vessels in the pedicle. The skin flap is sutured back in position and it is transferred 1–2 weeks later. Delayed flaps are not used in the *immediate* treatment of injuries.

CLASSIFICATION

Axial patterned flaps [4]

These are based on anatomically defined vessels with a recognizable cutaneous vascular territory. Examples that may be used in hand surgery include the deltopectoral

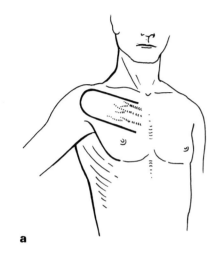

a

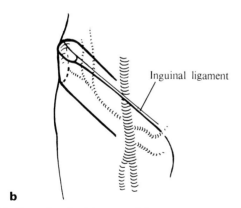

Inguinal ligament

b

FIG. 9.8. Examples of axial patterned flaps.

(a) Deltopectoral flap in which the pedicle is based on the lateral border of superior part of the sternum and includes perforating branches of the internal mammary vessels.

(b) Groin flap is based medially on the femoral artery and extends laterally over the anterior superior iliac spine. The medial part of the flap is raised under the deep fascia and contains the superficial circumflex iliac vessels. The dissection is not continued further than the medial border of the sartorius muscle.

flap based on the perforating branches of the internal mammary artery [5] (Fig. 9.8a), the groin flap based on the superficial circumflex iliac artery [6] (Fig. 9.8b) and the neurovascular island flap [7, 8] in which a skin flap from a finger pulp is transferred on a neurovascular pedicle to the pinch bearing area on the thumb (p. 503).

Recently, compound myocutaneous skin flaps have been introduced [9]. Skin, subcutaneous tissue and muscle are transferred as a unit with its blood supply from the muscle's vascular pedicle. The latissimus dorsi myocutaneous flap is an example that may be valuable in the arm as a motor unit. There are likely to be further developments in this rapidly expanding field.

Random patterned flaps

These are not based on any particular blood vessels and their vascular pattern is not anatomically defined. Most of the skin flaps used in the hand and arm belong to this group and when raised on the trunk or arm have a length breadth ratio of 1:1 or less.

Skin flaps may also be divided into three groups according to the way in which they are transferred from one site to another (1) local (2) direct or bridge and (3) distant. The latter are transferred using the arm as an intermediary and this method is not used in hand surgery.

Local flaps

Local flaps make use of skin in the immediate vicinity of the defect and can only be used when it is small. The larger the skin defect the further the flap has to be mobilized to give the tissue slide required. If the skin is advanced further than it should and particularly if it has already sustained even a minor degree of crushing, a vascular disaster in the flap is almost inevitable. Not only will the skin replacement fail but the size of the skin defect will be considerably larger than it was initially. Considerable judgement and skill are required in the manipulation of local skin flaps.

Palmar skin does not lend itself to local manoeuvres and most local flaps used on the hand are on the dorsum.

Many designs of local flap have been described. The V-Y advancement principle (Fig. 9.9) is used in the Kutler and

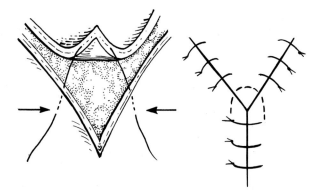

FIG. 9.9. V–Y advancement. The skin is incised as a V and sutured as a Y. The method of inserting the apical stitch to avoid necrosis at the apex of the V flap is also shown.

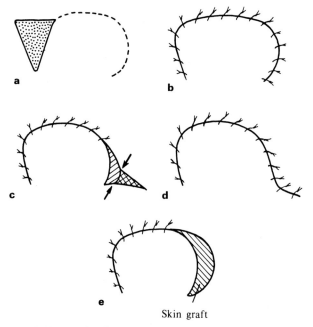

FIG. 9.10. Rotation flap.

(a) The skin defect is visualized as a triangle, and the flap is formed by projecting the base, the incision curving round towards the apex.

(b) The secondary skin defect may be closed by suturing the wound obliquely and distributing the skin defect along the whole length of the incision.

(c) and (d) By excising a triangle of skin

(e) or by inserting a skin graft.

The skin graft must be sutured through the skin and the deep fascia to avoid tension on the skin flap and possible disturbance of its blood supply.

Atasoy methods [10, 11] of finger-tip reconstruction described on pp. 238 and 239.

In a rotation flap, the skin defect is visualized and constructed as a triangle, and the base of the triangle is projected as a semicircular incision curving towards the apex of the triangle (Fig. 9.10a). If the defect is small and the skin lax, no back cut may be required and it may be possible to close the wound by inserting the sutures obliquely across the wound and distributing the skin defect along the entire length of the suture line (Fig. 9.10b). A back cut will be required if more skin advancement is necessary (Fig. 9.10c) and the secondary defect may be closed by approximation if the skin is lax (Fig. 9.10d), but more often in the hand, a skin graft will be necessary (Fig. 9.10e).

With a transposition flap in which the skin is slid laterally, the skin defect is also visualized as a triangle and the design of the flap is shown in the diagram (Fig. 9.11). This flap must be geometrically accurate, otherwise the tip of the flap cannot reach the furthest point of the skin defect. The flap usually has a 1:1 length breadth ratio and a skin graft is required to close the secondary skin defect.

Rotation and transposition flaps are useful methods of

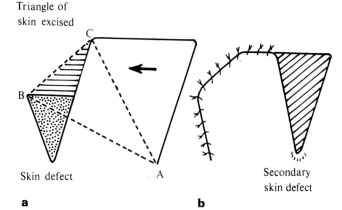

FIG. 9.11. Transposition flap in which the skin defect is visualized as a triangle. A rhomboidal shaped flap is designed. A is the hinge point round which the flap is transposed and the skin defect can only be covered by the skin flap if AB = AC. A triangle of excess skin is excised and the secondary skin defect is covered by a skin graft.

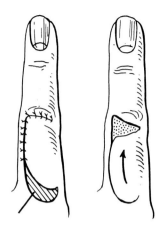

FIG. 9.12. Small rotation skin flap on dorsum of proximal phalanx used to cover exposed extensor tendon or a repair of the proximal interphalangeal joint.

replacing small areas of skin loss on the hand and digits (Figs. 9.12 and 9.13). Hueston [12] has described volar transposition flaps to cover digital amputation stumps to avoid any further shortening of the finger.

The Z plasty is one of the most useful and generally used local flaps in plastic surgery and involves the trans-

position of two or more triangular skin flaps (Fig. 9.14). It is commonly used in the correction of linear contractures that may occur over the flexure of joints but where there is little or no skin loss. It is also used to alter the line of a scar which may be in an undesirable position. The standard Z plasty has three limbs of equal length, the central one being in the line of the contracture. The other two incisions are placed at an angle of 60° at each end but on opposite sides of the central incision. When the flaps are transposed the central suture line is at right angles to the line of the original incision. In addition, the central limb is elongated at the expense of the transverse diagonal. Transverse lax tissue must be available to make a Z plasty possible and the method is most effective when a skin web is present. The design of a Z plasty may be altered by increasing or decreasing the apical angle of the triangular flaps or the length of the three incisions. A long contracture may be broken by a multiple Z plasty so that there is a maximal elongation in length without reducing the transverse axis to the same extent.

The Z plasty has a very limited place in the immediate treatment of injuries, owing to the risk of skin flap necrosis due to reduced viability of the skin in crushing injuries. There may very occasionally be a place for an immediate Z plasty in a longitudinal clean cut laceration

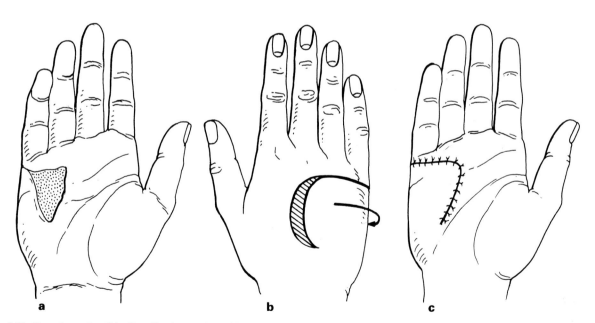

FIG. 9.13. Dorsal rotation flap (b) utilized to replace skin loss in ulnar part of palm (a). The secondary skin defect requires skin grafting.

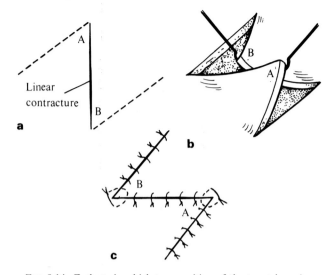

FIG. 9.14. Z-plasty in which transposition of the two triangular skin flaps results in the central part of the wound being at right angles to its original axis. The three incisions are of equal length and the outer incisions are at a 60° angle to the central incision. Apical sutures are inserted in the two apices of the triangular flaps.

on the volar aspect of a finger crossing the flexor skin creases. As a general rule, it is preferable to do the Z plasty on a badly placed scar or skin contracture as a late procedure when the wound has settled. Skin loss in both the longitudinal and transverse axis as occurs in burn contractures is not amenable to correction by a Z plasty, although it is sometimes useful to combine a Z plasty with a Wolfe graft. A Z plasty wound closure is a very satisfactory method of treating a single band Dupuytren's contracture with a significant flexion deformity (Fig. 32.12).

Direct or bridge flaps

Direct flaps involve the transfer of skin from distant donor sites by approximation of the donor and recipient areas. Many such flaps are described and are all basically two-stage procedures.

At the attachment stage, the flap is raised off the deep fascia, excess fat removed, the donor area defect grafted, a tie-over pressure dressing applied over it and the flap sutured into its new position. Immobilization with Elastoplast is used so that the pedicle of the flap is not kinked or under tension. The open undersurface of the skin flap where it bridges across from the donor to the recipient area is covered either by extending the skin graft on to the pedicle or by reflecting a skin flap from the recipient area to cover the open pedicle.

The detachment operation is usually done 3 weeks later when the flap has acquired enough blood supply from its new site to allow the pedicle to be divided with safety. Both ends are trimmed and sutured into position. The detachment operation may be complicated by a haematoma or sepsis and these wounds are often slow to heal.

Most flaps used in the hand and arm belong to this group and careful planning is essential for success. If possible, the whole of the skin defect should be covered by the skin flap at the attachment operation and the design of the flap should permit easy immobilization. It is obvious that the skin flap must be large enough, with an adequate blood supply and in a suitable position on the donor site to allow transfer. The method of *reverse planning* must be used working back from a pattern of the estimated skin defect, attaching a pedicle to it and then transferring the pattern to the most appropriate donor site (Fig. 9.15).

Care is required to avoid the pedicle becoming kinked or under tension. The flap is left exposed so that a haematoma can be easily recognized and evacuated. A tissue or sump drain may be required occasionally but the use of a closed suction drain is not possible, as the suture lines are not airtight.

If a flap becomes blue or congested, any kinking or tension in the pedicle is corrected, a haematoma is evacuated and sutures may be removed to allow drainage or to reduce tension. Elevation and gravity can help venous drainage and stagnant venous blood may be expressed by frequent gentle manual compression. Dextran has been advocated to prevent capillary sludging but there may be an added risk of bleeding. The metabolic requirements of a doubtfully viable flap may be reduced by cooling the flap and applying ice packs. Arterial blood flow into a flap can be encouraged by reflex vasodilatation or giving small regular doses of ethyl alcohol. Continuous supervision by experienced nursing staff during the first 24 or 48 hours may make the difference between success or failure.

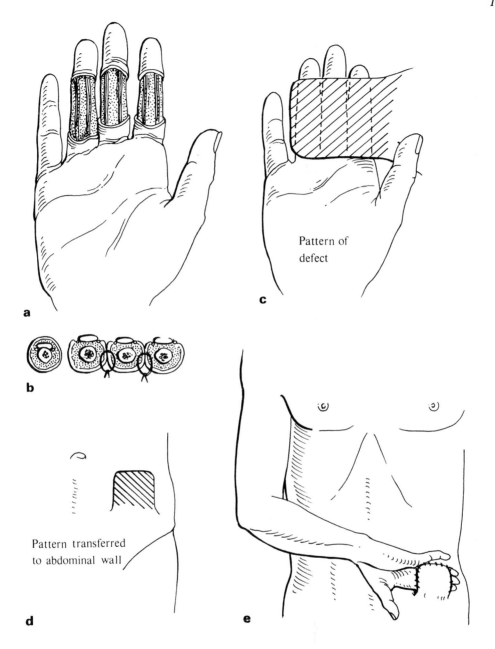

FIG. 9.15. Example of abdominal 'direct flap'. Skin defect on volar aspect of three fingers.

(a) Exposing the flexor tendons.

(b) By suturing the three fingers together, creating a surgical syndactyly, the three skin defects are converted into one.

(c) A pattern of the skin defect is made.

(d) The pattern is transferred to a suitable position on abdominal wall.

(e) Flap in position. The fingers are separated several weeks after the flap has been detached.

Varieties of direct or bridge flap in hand injuries

Cross finger flap (Fig. 9.16). This flap is particularly useful where there is a major loss of pulp tissue exposing the distal phalanx, when shortening of the finger is undesirable and when a skin graft would produce a painful, unstable, adherent scar. It is always raised on the dorsal aspect, care being taken to leave a layer of paratenon intact over the extensor expansion.

Thenar flap. Some surgeons have advocated the use of this flap for transverse amputations of the fingertips, but it is now used very infrequently and only in special circumstances for the following reasons:
(1) As the proximal interphalangeal joint requires 90° flexion to transfer the flap, the flexed joint may become permanently stiff,
(2) there is often excessive sweating from the palmar skin so that the flap tends to become moist and infected, and
(3) the palmar scar may become painful.

Cross arm flap (Fig. 9.16b). This flap is particularly useful for the replacement of multiple skin defects of the hand which can be draped round either the upper arm or forearm. The former allows more movement but even when one hand is fixed to the forearm, the other hand and both shoulders are left free and it is surprising how much most patients can do for themselves. The skin is very suitable for use on the hand but the donor area scars may not be acceptable to many patients.

Pectoral flaps. These flaps may be either random patterned with pedicles in any position or axial patterned based on the lateral border of the sternum and the perforating branches of the internal mammary artery to the second, third and fourth intercostal spaces (Fig. 9.8a). They provide excellent quality skin to replace large defects, but the donor area scars are not acceptable to most young women and to some men.

Submammary flaps. The submammary area is a useful alternative site for small skin flaps where cross arm or pectoral donor area scars are not acceptable. This donor site can usually be closed by undermining and approximation.

Abdominal flaps. The skin here is too thick and often with excess subcutaneous fat so that the flap on the hand is excessively bulky, requiring several thinning operations. However, the abdomen does provide large skin flaps and the donor area scars are covered by normal clothing. The flaps are random patterned in type and can be placed in any convenient position. Sandwich flaps (Fig. 9.17a, b) raised in form of an S or pocket flaps (Fig. 9.17c) may be used in circumferential skin loss in major injuries.

Groin flaps (Fig. 9.18). These are axial patterned flaps based on the superficial circumflex iliac artery [6]. The artery lies under the deep fascia 2.5 cm below the inguinal ligament and the anterior superior spine (see Fig. 9.8b). The deep fascia is raised with the flap to avoid injury to the vessels and it cannot be mobilized with safety any further than the medial border of the sartorius muscle. If it is necessary to extend the flap on to the buttock, this extension must be regarded as a random patterned flap, which will require a preliminary delay operation. The donor area can usually be closed by approximation after slightly flexing the hip even when the flap is 7–8 cm wide. The skin is very suitable for use in the hand and the donor area scar is inconspicuous. The laxity of the pedicle (Fig. 9.18) allows scope for finger and hand movement but as there may be excessive sweating in the area, the

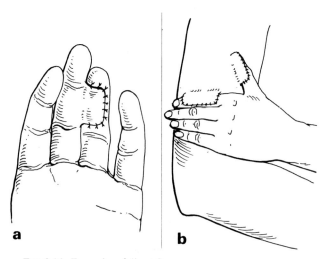

FIG. 9.16. Examples of direct flaps.
(a) Cross finger and
(b) Cross arm flaps to thumb and index finger.

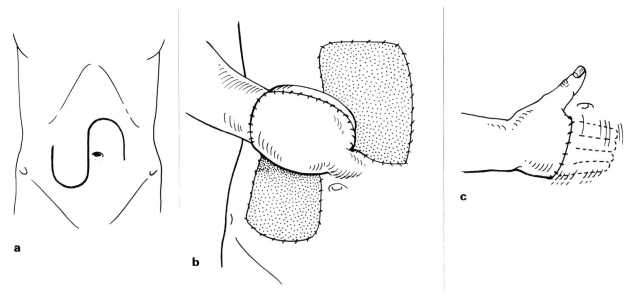

FIG. 9.17. Examples of abdominal flaps.

(a) 'Sandwich flap'. Raised in the form of an S, one flap being based superiorly and the other inferiorly.

(b) 'Sandwich flap'. The skin defect on the volar and dorsal aspects of the hand is covered by overlapping the two abdominal flaps.

(c) Pocket flap. Denuded digits may be buried in an abdominal subcutaneous pocket and the skin flap detached in stages three or four weeks later.

wound needs careful supervision. A preliminary division of the superficial circumflex iliac artery is necessary before the flap is completely detached.

Free skin flaps

The development of techniques for microvascular anastomosis has now made it possible to transfer an axial patterned flap by isolating the artery and vein feeding the flap, detaching the flap completely and suturing its artery and vein to appropriate vessels in the vicinity of the recipient area. At the present time free flap transfers have had little application to hand surgery as the simpler techniques of skin replacement can provide all the skin cover that is required.

The choice of method

Many factors must be considered in selecting the most appropriate method of treatment of the skin in any particular injury. In general, the simpler the method the better, provided there is no unnecessary sacrifice of function. There are often several alternatives and the decision is sometimes difficult. In the more complicated injuries with exposed bone or tendon, etc. grafts are likely to fail, producing further tissue loss and under these circumstances, skin flap closure is usually necessary.

The patient's work and hobbies have an extremely important bearing on treatment. A heavy manual worker requires a powerful hand with stable, hard, horny skin that will stand up to wear and tear. Finger length is of less importance and some reduction in the range of movement can be accepted. Skin grafts and direct flaps do not replace volar skin with the same characteristics as normal hand skin and their limitations must be taken into consideration. Precision workers require an effective pinch for the manipulation of small objects. A worthwhile pinch can be obtained from a good thumb and one or preferably two fingers. The pinch bearing areas must have stable skin with satisfactory sensation and be

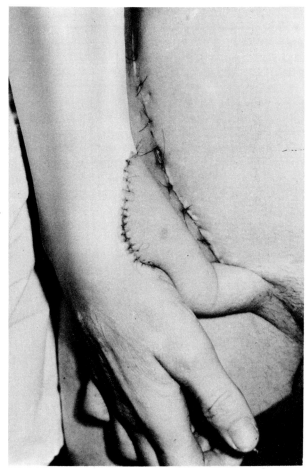

Fig. 9.18. Groin flap used to replace skin defect on volar aspect of the wrist. Donor area closed by approximation.

that might be available for later reconstruction should be left open.

It is important to make some assessment of the type of patient that is being treated. One group of patients is very well motivated, co-operating well with all treatment and making the maximum effort to develop as much function as possible in their injured hand. This type of patient can often overcome very considerable difficulties in learning how to make as much use as possible of what functional structures are left. In these patients, it is very much worth while undertaking any complicated method of treatment that may be indicated. At the other extreme are a group of patients who are unable to co-operate. Some are lazy and cannot be persuaded to work, others seem incapable of learning the simplest exercises and others cannot co-ordinate the action of different muscle groups. It is important to try to identify this group of patients in whom treatment should be simplified as much as possible. It can be disastrous to embark on complicated methods of treatment in a patient who either cannot or will not co-operate.

There is also a group of patients who are very prone to develop oedema and fibrosis as a response to injury. An awareness of this possibility and careful watching to prevent and control the oedema as much as possible is needed.

TREATMENT OF DIFFERENT TYPES OF INJURY

Cutting injuries

pain free. A reduced pinch or power grasp and stiff digits are often of less importance in clerical workers or housewives but finger length and appearance assumes much greater importance.

Age has also an extremely important bearing on treatment. The older age group patients have an increased risk of joint stiffness and immobilization of the hand by flaps is unwise. Their requirements so far as hand function is concerned are usually less than in the younger age groups and treatment should be simplified to the minimum necessary for useful hand function. In children, treatment should be very conservative and any options

In many of these wounds, as there is no skin loss, minimal wound excision is necessary and all that is required is accurate edge to edge suturing of the skin. The treatment of deeper lacerations in which nerves or tendons have been divided are discussed in Chapters 12 and 11. There is a group of slicing injuries produced by knives, planing or slicing machines, etc., in which skin and possibly underlying muscle or tendons are cleanly excised. Primary replacement of the skin loss by medium to thick split skin grafts is desirable. If important deep structures are exposed in the base of the wound, skin flap replacement by the appropriate method described above may be required.

Crushing and pulping injuries

Injuries produced by industrial presses, heavy weights, etc., carry a bad prognosis owing to the tissue damage and the thrombosis that is likely to occur in the blood vessels. Fat and crushed devitalized muscle may be extruded through bursting lacerations in the skin. The assessment of tissue viability may be very difficult, and it is often necessary to adopt a conservative line of treatment after an initial wound excision until tissue viability defines itself. In other patients, there may be no difficulty in deciding on the extent of tissue death and early skin closure usually by direct flaps can be undertaken with safety. Whatever method of treatment is used, oedema, fibrosis and stiffness are almost inevitable.

Severe injuries of this type are a challenging surgical problem in which there is often no perfect answer, but the critical point in their management is often related to the skin closure. Judicious reduction of hopelessly damaged fingers may reduce the skin problem so that skin grafts or small skin flaps are all that are required. The more the other fingers are damaged, the less desirable does amputation become and the greater the indication for skin flap replacement, possibly by a groin flap. In these difficult injuries it is again emphasized that there may be value in delaying skin closure as described in the introduction. At least one and preferably two fingers must be retained to act as a palmar post.

Thumb length must never be sacrificed unnecessarily. Treatment requires careful debridement, preservation of blood supply, fracture stabilization and skin closure by suture or a direct flap. If any major part of the metacarpal or proximal phalanx has been lost, the length of the thumb must be retained by some form of skeletal fixation or the insertion of a temporary silastic spacer until a bone graft in inserted after the wounds are healed. It may be possible to re-attach a completely amputated thumb using a microvascular repair (Chapter 10), skeletal stabilization and skin closure by suture, skin graft or flap according to circumstances. Alternatively, the skin may be excised from the detached part of the thumb which is then re-attached as a bone graft. The denuded thumb is then buried in a pectoral or groin flap which is tubed round the bone. The pedicle of this flap must be at least 9 cm wide. When the pedicle of the flap is divided 3 or 4 weeks later, a neurovascular island flap

(p. 503) is inset to give sensation in the pinch bearing area and to increase blood supply.

Degloving injuries

Large areas of skin and subcutaneous tissues may be stripped off the deep fascia when the hand and arm are caught between the rollers of powered wringers, paper-making machinery, conveyor belts, etc. If a finger ring is forcibly pulled distally, the skin may be avulsed and similar types of injury may occur in more proximal levels in the hand and arm. In many instances, the skin alone is involved but in others, muscles, tendons and nerves may be damaged. In most instances the avulsed skin flaps are distally based and part or whole of the avulsed skin is avascular. If it is sutured back, gangrene of the skin is almost certain to follow. In addition, the avulsed skin flap is almost always crushed at its distal end and its survival is even less likely.

There is no point in suturing back avulsed skin flaps in the hope that they will survive, and they must be trimmed back until good capillary bleeding is present at the cut edge. In many instances, the skin defect is suitable for replacement by skin grafts. Small areas of directly exposed tendons may be covered by suturing local soft tissues over the exposed areas with a few fine catgut sutures. There are occasions when important structures require cover by a direct skin flap possibly combined with a split graft in the less severely damaged areas.

The whole of a degloved thumb must be retained and the technique of burying the thumb skeleton in a one stage tube pedicle mentioned earlier gives a very satisfactory end result. A single degloved finger is usually better amputated except in very special circumstances. Skin grafts are not very successful and circumferential skin flap cover produces a finger that is much too fat even after several thinning operations and usually with a very restricted range of movement. If an attempt must be made to save the finger, the volar surface requires skin flap replacement by a cross finger, cross arm or groin flap and the dorsum by a split graft. A neurovascular island flap may well be required later to give sensation and durability in the pinch bearing area (p. 503). In very few patients is it justifiable to undertake treatment of this complexity for a degloved finger.

In very severe circumferential degloving injuries of the forearm, wrist and hand, the skin may be replaced by a skin graft which can give very adequate replacement in the forearm, wrist and hand but which may require considerable shortening of avascular digits until there is adequate blood supply for the graft to take. The alternative is to utilize a direct flap possibly of the abdominal sandwich or pocket flap type (Fig. 9.17) to cover and preserve the length of the avascular digits. The rest of the wound is covered by a split graft. This technique certainly preserves digital length but many operations are required to separate and thin the digits. The fingertips may be insensitive and subject to recurrent ulceration. In addition the appearance may not be acceptable. Unless the patient is young, co-operative and is fully aware of the time involved, the possible limitations and the likely end result, it is unwise to embark on such complex forms of reconstruction.

If the skin in a major degloving injury has not been crushed, it can be utilized as a skin graft. Conversion of the detached skin to a whole thickness graft by meticulous removal of the subcutaneous tissues on to the deep surface of the dermis has been advocated. This method is very time consuming and requires a very careful technique and a good vascular bed for success. It is now usually reserved for the highly specialized palmar skin which it is important to retain if possible. Other uncrushed areas of skin can be converted to a split graft using one of the skin grafting knives. Additional skin grafts from other donor sites are usually required.

The repair of hand injuries is fascinating and rewarding. In the more severe injuries, nothing should be sacrificed without first considering what might be possible in the later reconstructive phase after the wounds are healed and the hand has been mobilized. Very great scope exists for ingenuity in the management of these injuries.

REFERENCES

[1] XAVIER, T. S. AND LAMB, D. W. The forearm as donor site for split skin grafts. *The Hand*, 1974, **6**, 243.

[2] MOSHER, J. F. Split thickness hypothenar grafts for skin defects on the hand. *The Hand*, 1977, **9**, 45.

[3] JAMES, J. H. AND WATSON, A. C. H. The use of Opsite, a vapour permeable dressing, on skin graft donor sites. *British Journal of Plastic Surgery*, 1975, **28**, 107.

[4] MCGREGOR, I. A. AND MORGAN, G. Axial and random pattern flaps. *British Journal of Plastic Surgery*, 1973, **24**, 202.

[5] BAKAMJIAN, V. Y. A two stage method for pharyngo-oesophageal reconstruction with a primary pectoral skin flap. *Plastic and Reconstructive Surgery*, 1965, **36**, 173.

[6] MCGREGOR, I. A. AND JACKSON, I. T. The groin flap. *British Journal of Plastic Surgery*, 1972, **25**, 3.

[7] LITTLER, J. W. Neurovascular skin island transfer in reconstructive hand surgery. *Transactions International Society*

of *Plastic Surgeons, 2nd Congress*, pp. 175–179, Edinburgh, E. & S. Livingstone, 1959.

[8] TUBIANA, R. AND DUPARC, J. Restoration of sensibility in the hand by neurovascular skin island transfer. *Journal Bone and Joint Surgery*, 1961, **43B**, 474.

[9] MCGRAW, J. B., DIBBELL, D. G. AND CARRAWAY, J. H. Clinical definition of independent myocutaneous vascular territories. *Journal Plastic and Reconstructive Surgery*, 1977, **60**, 341.

[10] KUTLER, W. A new method for finger tip amputation. *Journal of American Medical Association*, 1947, **133**, 29.

[11] ATASOY, E., IOKIMIDIS, E., KASKAN, M. L., KUTZ, J. E. AND KLEINERT, H. E. Reconstruction of the amputated finger tip with a triangular volar flap; a new surgical procedure. *Journal of Bone and Joint Surgery*, 1970, **52A**, 921.

[12] HUESTON, J. T. Rotation flap to finger stumps. *Journal Plastic and Reconstructive Surgery*, 1966, **37**, 349.

FURTHER READING

BEASLEY, R. W. Principles of managing acute hand injuries, pp. 3000–3102. In: Converse, J. M. ed. *Reconstructive Plastic Surgery*, 2nd Ed., vol. 6. *The Hand and Upper Extremity*, Littler, J. W., ed. Philadelphia, Saunders, 1977.

CONVERSE, J. M., MCCARTHY, J. G., BRAUER, R. O. AND BALLANTYNE, D. L. Transplantation of skin grafts and flaps, pp. 152–239. In: Converse, J. M., ed. *Reconstructive Plastic Surgery*, 2nd ed., vol. 1. *General Principles*. Philadelphia, Saunders, 1977.

FLATT, A. E. *The Care of Minor Hand Injuries*. St. Louis, Mosby, 1977.

GRABB, W. C. AND SMITH, J. W., eds. Basic techniques of plastic surgery, pp. 3–105. In: *Plastic Surgery*, 2nd Ed. Boston, Little Brown, 1973.

MCGREGOR, I. A. *Fundamental Techniques of Plastic Surgery*, 6th Ed. Edinburgh, Churchill Livingstone, 1975.

RANK, B. K., WAKEFIELD, A. R. AND HUESTON, J. T. *Surgery of Repair as Applied to Hand Injuries*, 4th Ed. Edinburgh, Churchill Livingstone, 1973.

PULVERTAFT, R. G. ed. *The Hand*, pp. 33–73. In: *Operative Surgery*, Rob, C. and Smith, R. eds. London, Butterworth, 1977.

REID, D. A. C. Injuries—General principles—Skin injuries, pp. 65–79. In: Rob, C. and Smith, R. eds, *Clinical Surgery*, vol. 7, *The Hand*, Pulvertaft, R. G., ed. London, Butterworth, 1966.

CHAPTER 10

Injuries to Blood Vessels

INTRODUCTION

D. W. LAMB

Advances in the techniques of vascular repair have meant that major damage to the main artery to a limb is no longer necessarily an indication for amputation. With the development of the operating microscope and the use of fine instruments, the same now applies to injury to the smaller vessels of the hand. Reports of successful replantation of the hand and digits emerged from China in the 1960s, and this work has been developed by Buncke in the United States, O'Brien in Australia and Cobbett in Great Britain. There is now no doubt that the repair of small digital vessels and restoration of effective circulation is a practical proposition, and recent reports have indicated a success rate of over 90 per cent [1].

It must be realized that the expertise necessary for such success requires a great deal of preliminary practice to perfect the technique and ·constant use thereafter to maintain success. The time and facilities necessary for this are not readily available in most centres, as an emergency surgical team must be available over the 24 hours. This is very time consuming and once replantation or revascularization procedures are started an operating team and operating theatre are out of use for other purposes for many hours.

It is thus necessary to provide some guidelines for this procedure. It is still difficult to evaluate the indications fully, but it would seem that revascularization should only be attempted in clean cut wounds and the success rate will fall considerably if there is a crushing element present. There also seems no doubt that where the whole hand, or multiple digits or the thumb has been amputated, replantation should be attempted. Replantation of a single digit is less essential.

Another important factor is that while restoration of circulation can now be virtually guaranteed, the recovery of function of the other damaged tissues may be limited. This applies in particular to the quality of sensation.

It will be many years before a satisfactory evaluation of a sufficient number of successful cases of replantation can be made. Where revascularization alone is required, as distinct from total tissue replantation, there is no doubt of the success. The need for revascularization is about ten times more frequent than for replantation. Under normal temperature conditions the damaged part will remain viable for about 4 hours, but this can be extended to 10–12 hours by cooling.

BASIC TECHNIQUES IN MICROVASCULAR SURGERY

J. R. COBBETT

Although the techniques required had been worked out almost a decade earlier [2], the successful clinical application of microvascular surgery to the hand had to wait until 1965 when Susumu Tamai achieved the first successful replant of a totally amputated digit (a thumb) [3].

The first free composite graft involving microvascular techniques was in 1968 when one stage transfer of a toe to the hand was achieved [4], and free flaps for hand resurfacing were used from 1973 onwards [5].

In addition to replantation and transplantation, microvascular techniques have been used in the hand to deal with the rare condition of thrombosis of the ulnar artery and its branches in the palm [6].

Preliminaries

Surgical techniques cannot be learned from books, and indeed only a small amount can be picked up by personal tuition or observation. The vast majority of surgical techniques have to be self taught by constant practice. To the novice the use of the operating microscope and microsurgical instruments and sutures is extremely difficult. Time spent tying knots with microsurgical sutures in a piece of gauze under the microscope is well spent and needs no laboratory facility. Even this type of practice which helps the student to learn to drive the microscope, how to get the tips of his instruments into the field, and how to rest the ulnar borders of the hands as close to the field as possible, to damp down tremor, is unfortunately no substitute for animal work.

A minor irregularity on the intimal surface of a suture line, an inverted edge, an overtight suture can all spell thrombosis and disaster. It is only by work on animals that the operator can tell whether the technique is good enough to attempt small vessel surgery in the human. Furthermore, a clinical case, often at a difficult time of the day or night, with damaged vessels needing resection, with other structures requiring attention, is likely to present a far greater challenge to the microsurgical ability than an anaesthetized rat in the peace and calm of the laboratory when time seems unimportant.

The rat is a good animal for microsurgical practice as its blood vessels have a very similar diameter and toughness to those of the human hand. The abdominal aorta is readily available for the beginner to master, after which a small vessel such as the renal or femoral artery may be attempted. Once the surgeon is confident of getting a very high percentage of successful anastomoses on these vessels the first clinical case may be contemplated.

In the clinical situation the hand must be kept immobile by a combination of adequate anaesthesia and the use of a lead hand or similar fixation device. Most important, the exposure must be adequate and haemostasis complete. Blood in the wound not only obscures the view and makes instruments and sutures unmanageable but also constitutes a most vigorous vasoconstrictive agent.

The microscope

Despite the disadvantages of bulk, difficulties with sterilization and cost, an operating microscope is essential if optimal results are to be obtained. The type used will depend largely on the depth of the purchaser's purse as, on the whole, the more money spent the more useful the instrument. At one end of the scale is the table-mounted fixed-magnification binocular telescope, with or without its own lighting system, and giving a magnification of ×6–8. At the opposite end is the ceiling mounted machine with two or three separate heads, integral lighting, foot control of focusing and zoom magnification change with, as an added bonus, foot controlled electrically operated sideways and to and fro movement.

Integral lighting is truly shadowless; an assistant is only likely to be useful with a separate stereoscopic view, necessitating a separate microscope head; foot controls enable the hands to stay where they are needed; ceiling mounting cuts down microscope shake, and powered movements in a horizontal plane also are helpful. Any or all of these refinements can be dispensed with, but each helps to make what is a difficult procedure just that little bit easier and all are worthwhile if funds permit.

Instruments

A needle-holder, two pairs of scissors, one straight and one curved pair of jeweller's forceps and vessel clamps

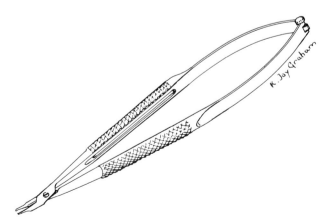

FIG. 10.1. O'Brien needle holder.

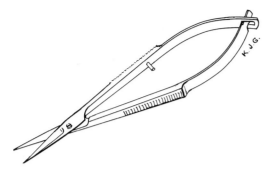

FIG. 10.2. Spring-handled scissors.

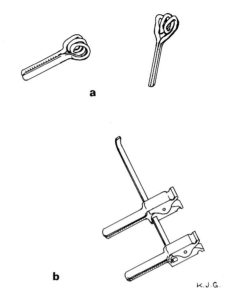

FIG. 10.4. Blood vessel clamps.
(a) Scoville-Lewis clip.
(b) Tamai clamp, (×2).

are all that are required. A multiplicity of instruments only causes confusion.

The needle-holder (Fig. 10.1) should have spring handles, not ring handles, which should be long enough to reach the first interdigital web when held with a pencil grip. There should be no lock. The tips must be fine enough to grip a 4 mm curved needle transversely without making it rotate between the jaws, so as to be parallel to them. A slight upward curve on the flat enables the angle at which the needle is held to be varied. There are several instruments of this type available, mostly modifications of the standard Barraquer. Jeweller's forceps (size 3) can be utilized as a needle holder.

Standard fine-spring scissors (Fig. 10.2) are useful for dissection and suture cutting. Angled de Wecke's scissors are handy in awkward situations; particularly in removing misplaced sutures.

Needlepoint jeweller's forceps size 5 (Fig. 10.3), straight and curved, are much cheaper than surgical equivalents and can be resharpened with emery cloth, or discarded if damaged.

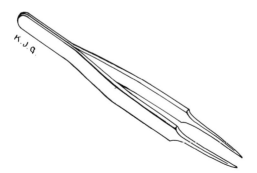

FIG. 10.3. Needlepoint jeweller's forceps.

There is a multiplicity of blood vessel clamps available. The simplest is a microsurgical Scoville-Lewis aneurysm clip (Fig. 10.4a) which needs forcible weakening before use. The Acland clamps incorporate two on a rigid frame with cleats for the stay sutures. The Millesi, O'Brien and Tamai (Fig. 10.4b) clamps, as well as one model of Acland clamp, possess some means of approximating the vessel ends and taking the strain off the sutures during the anastomosis. Some surgeons favour simplicity, but there are many who prefer the more complicated pieces of apparatus. Whatever clamps are chosen it is important that their force is only just enough to stop blood flow without crushing the vessel wall, and that they have a high resistance to slippage.

Sutures

10/0 nylon on round-bodied 4–6 mm needles are adequate for blood vessel suturing in all clinical situations. Finer suture material with electroplated ends forming a stiffened section which may be used as a needle are required for some fine animal work, and in the surgery of lymphatics.

Repair of a small blood vessel

Formal removal of the adventitial layers as previously practised is probably unnecessary, but it is as well to pull down a cuff of loose periadventitial tissue over the vessel end, and to cut it off.

At all times the vessel ends, particularly the intimal surface, should be kept moist with heparin saline solution of 1000 units to 100 ml. The intimal surface should be treated with great respect at all times. Ideally it should not be touched (or crushed) at all, the needle penetrating the vessel wall should be the only object to touch the endothelium.

The first suture is the most difficult. The adventitial and muscle layers only are picked up by straight forceps and the needle passed through the vessel wall, from without in (Fig. 10.5), about one and a half times the thickness of the vessel wall away from the cut end. If this manoeuvre proves to be too difficult the tips of the

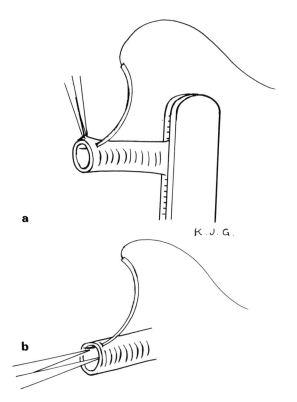

FIG. 10.5. Methods of passing the first suture, (a) Correct and (b) inadvisable, except for stay sutures (× 10).

forceps may be placed in the lumen as a counter-presser (or a special counter-presser may be purchased) but this intimal handling is to be avoided if possible. Having ensured that there is no rotational deformity at the junction, the needle is then passed from within out on the second side, and the suture tied.

A second suture is now placed about 120° around the circumference of the vessel (Fig. 10.6). One end of each of these two stay sutures is left long and gentle traction applied to them, perhaps by the weight of a small bull-dog clamp. This traction approximates the anterior vessel edges between the sutures, but the posterior edges, being longer, fall backwards away from the anterior suture line. This manoeuvre is known as 'eccentric biangulation' [7]. The anterior suture line is now completed, with interrupted sutures placed, in an artery, about 0·3 mm apart. That is to say a 1 mm diameter vessel, with a circumference of 3 mm will require about ten sutures in all. Somewhat fewer sutures may be used in a venous repair.

Having completed the anterior suture line, appropriate manipulation of the clamps and stay sutures will rotate the anastomosis and enable the posterior suture line to be completed. Care must be taken not to pinch the intima by picking up the whole thickness of the vessel wall and to avoid the only too easy error of suturing the back wall to the front. The end of one suture, held up, will often act as sufficient counter pressure for the passage of the next stitch.

Once the repair has been completed, the stay sutures are cut and gentle pressure with dry gauze is used to control the slight bleeding which occurs between the sutures once the clamps are removed. Any large leak may need reapplication of the vessel clamps and a further stitch, but once blood is allowed to be in contact with the area of the anastomosis it should not be allowed to remain stagnant for long as it may clot. It is better to remove an extra suture, wash out the area with heparin saline and then replace as many sutures as necessary at leisure.

A totally dry anastomosis on the removal of the clamps is more likely to be due to thrombosis than to watertight suturing. In the event of thrombosis, removal of a few sutures, local irrigation and resuture may establish a flow, but excision of the anastomotic area and a fresh start may be required.

Various alternative methods of small vessel repair have been described [8].

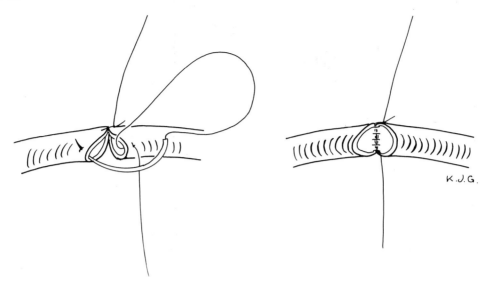

FIG. 10.6. Eccentric biangulation, (× 10).

REPLANTATION AND REVASCULARIZATION

G. D. LISTER

Quite apart from the need for microsurgical technique as described above, certain other factors play an important role in successful replantation and revascularization of severed parts.

Assurance of an adequate 'run-off'

Any vascular anastomosis requires for its success not only good surgical technique at the site of repair and a good head of pressure in the form of vigorous proximal flow, but also the absence of any increase in peripheral resistance, i.e. the presence of a good 'run-off'. Careful examination of the amputated part will give information in this respect. Evidence of a likely increase in peripheral resistance includes the following.

Avulsion of longitudinal structures

If a tendon or nerve shows considerable length dangling from the amputated part, the vessel will also have suffered longitudinal traction forces likely to have disrupted its branches. Such disruption will seriously impede or arrest flow.

Bruising of the skin along the line of the neurovascular bundle

This provides additional evidence of vascular disruption (Fig. 10.7). Referred to as the 'red streak' this sign of unsuitability for replantation was first described by the Chinese.

Injury to the amputated part

This will at least cause swelling with compromise of flow and at worst result in bleeding into tissues, intramural haemorrhage in the digital vessels and intravascular clotting. Replantation of severely crushed extremities is a futile exercise.

The repair of healthy vessels

Before re-attachment, adequate exposure of both vessel ends is obtained by longitudinal incisions along their line. In the finger these incisions are offset from one another. If bone shortening has to be performed subsequently, such offset incisions will later permit Z-plasty closure of the circumferential wound thereby eliminating subsequent constricting scar contracture and accommodating the excess of soft tissue resulting from the skeletal resection. The neurovascular bundles

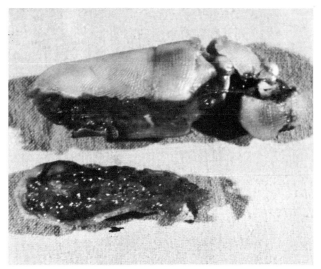

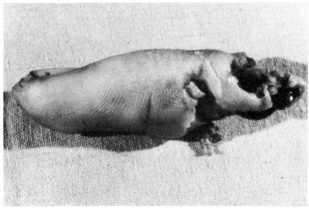

FIG. 10.7. This amputated digit is unsuitable for replantation not only because of the severe injury to one side but also because of the vascular disruption evidenced by the bruising of the other.

are dissected out under the microscope. The arteries are inspected under high magnification over at least 1 cm on either side of the amputation. Any portion which reveals bruising, thrombosis, disruption of branches or intimal damage, revealed by a relatively dark cross-striation at some point along its length, is excised. The superfluous adventitia is removed by pulling on it transversely in opposite directions with jeweller's forceps and excising it with scissors. This usually exposes the lumen which is then inspected for irregularity of the margin, intimal marking indicative of damage or atherosclerosis, and for intimamedia dissociation. When dissociation is

suspected, gentle traction on the intima may yield a long tubular cast of the vessel. The entire segment from which the intima came should be excised wherever possible. Atherosclerosis and intimamedia dissociation increases with age and must affect not only the visible vessel ends but also the proximal flow and the distal 'run-off'. This leads to a recognized higher incidence of failure after the fourth decade. Allied to the greater difficulty in achieving motion and the poorer results of nerve repair, this fact may influence the surgeon to forego replantation, especially in the single digit or distal multiple digit amputation. Having prepared the vessel ends, the presence of strong arterial flow should be established. The proximal part of the vessel, although healthy, may be in spasm over some distance. This spasm can be overcome by cannulation. The flow should be re-confirmed immediately before commencing anastomosis. Through a single midline dorsal incision as many veins as can be found are inspected in similar fashion. All vessels and nerves are tagged with distinguishing sutures of 8/0 nylon (Fig. 10.8). This tagging before re-attachment will greatly reduce frustration when the neurovascular structures are to be relocated later. Knowing *before* replantation the length of vascular

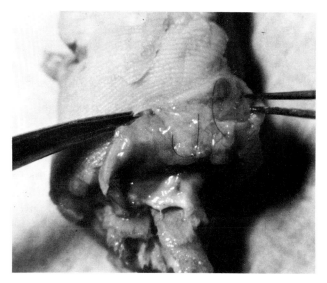

FIG. 10.8. The practice of tagging the neurovascular structures before re-attachment eliminates an irritating search when the time comes for microscopic repair. The double-end of 8/0 nylon forms a V representative of vessel, the single end marks the nerve.

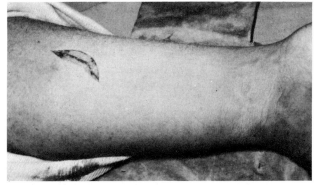

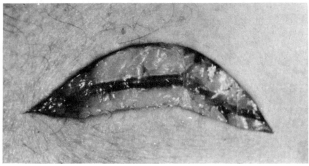

FIG. 10.9. The veins on the volar surface of the forearm yield grafts of ideal dimension for repairing defects in the digital artery.

resection necessary to ensure perfect vessel ends, and the skeletal level of amputation, the surgeon can decide whether judicious shortening of bone will permit tension-free vessel anastomoses or whether vein grafts will be necessary. If the latter, the grafts can be prepared from the volar surface of the forearm while the bone and tendon work of replantation is being done (Fig. 10.9).

Avoidance of tension

If vessels do not come together readily with one 10/0 monofilament nylon suture, then tension is present and its persistence will result in a leaking, unsatisfactory repair, reduction in flow and probable failure of re-plantation. Two anastomoses at either end of a reversed vein graft can be done more quickly and with greater success than one arterial repair under tension. It should be realized, however, that a vein graft is all too easily placed with torsion which seriously limits flow and that

vein grafts contract markedly after removal but extend marvellously when subjected to arterial flow. The arterial defect should be measured while holding the vessels under acceptable tension and the graft cut to size while still *in situ* in the forearm. Torsion can be prevented by placing aligning marking sutures on the graft before its transfer to the hand.

Multiplicity of vascular repairs

Despite all the precautions detailed above, a percentage of small vessel repairs fail. The more that are performed in any one replantation the greater the chance of survival of the replanted part. Thus in digital replantation, both arteries should be repaired together with as many veins as can be found. All repairs should be observed for 20 minutes after completion, during which time the adjacent digital nerve can be repaired, and then checked again for flow prior to skin closure.

Use of non-constrictive dressings

The success of a replantation should be assured before the patient leaves the operating room. A non-circum-ferential dressing of 1-inch plastic foam and plaster is applied. This is left undisturbed for 10–14 days except to ensure twice daily that no bloodsoaked gauze is adherent to the replanted part, for it will become constrictive as it dries no matter how it was applied.

Early re-exploration

A successfully replanted extremity should be pink and warm, with fast refill after compression and a good arterial pattern on Doppler studies as far as the tip. Any change in this situation indicates vascular occlusion with bluish congestion if on the venous side and pallor if on the arterial. Prompt re-exploration usually reveals a situation worse than expected and offers the best chance of salvaging the digit. This happens rarely with the straightforward replantation.

Observance of the above discipline has improved results to the extent that systemic heparin and dextran are used in the satisfactory replantation only for 20

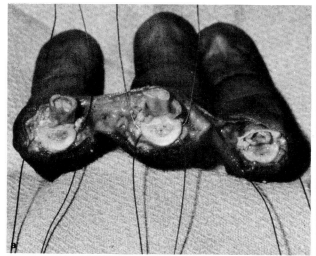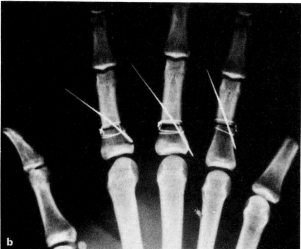

FIG. 10.10. Bony fixation.

(a) The preparation of the bone ends before re-attachment using intraosseous wires.

(b) In combination with oblique Kirschner wires which did not encroach on any joint, stable fixation was obtained which permitted early motion without preventing an early union.

minutes before and several hours after release of the vascular clamps. This has allowed the discharge of patients at the third day after replantation on aspirin alone. Indeed, two cases have been done recently as outpatients. Although this development is too new to permit analysis, at the time of writing the percentage success rate has remained identical to that being achieved on a more traditional regime of anticoagulants and prolonged hospital stay. With the increased rate of survival, the onus shifts more definitely from mere survival to restoration of good function [9]. As experience and confidence in the success of microvascular work increases, so the surgeon returns to more established considerations of hand surgery. Stable bony fixation is achieved by the use of Kirschner wires with intraosseous compression wiring (Fig. 10.10) [10]. This aids early union and allows early motion. When joints have been destroyed, arthrodesis is performed formally with due regard to the best functional position. The periosteum is repaired whenever possible. Tendon repair is always undertaken employing the technique described [11]. The tendon sheath is sutured wherever possible. Neurorrhaphy is done microsurgically (p. 192). Early active motion is encouraged. By these means it is hoped that replantation of an extremity will cease to be a seven day wonder and a lifetime impediment and become another technique employed in the restoration of the injured hand to full function.

REFERENCES

[1] WEILAND, A. J., VILLARREAL-RIOS, A., KLEINERT, H. E., KUTZ, J. E., ATASOY, E., AND LISTER, G. D. Replantation of digits and hands: analysis of surgical techniques and functional results in 71 patients with 86 replantations. *Journal of Hand Surgery*, 1977, **2**, 1.

[2] JACOBSON, J. H. AND SUAREZ, E. L. Microsurgery in anastomosis of small vessels. *Surgical Forum*, 1960, **11**, 243.

[3] KOMATSU, S. AND TAMAI, S. Successful replantation of a completely cut off thumb. *Plastic and Reconstructive Surgery*, 1968, **42**, 374.

[4] COBBETT, J. R. Free digital transfer. Report of a case of transfer of a great toe to replace an amputated thumb. *Journal of Bone and Joint Surgery*, 1969, **51B**, 677.

[5] DANIEL, R. K. AND TAYLOR, G. I. Distant transfer of an

island flap by microvascular anastomosis. *Plastic and Reconstructive Surgery*, 1973, **52,** 111.

[6] KLEINERT, H. E. AND VOLIANTIS, G. J. Thrombosis of the palmar arterial arch and its tributaries, etiology and newer concept in treatment. *Journal of Trauma*, 1965, **5,** 447.

[7] COBBETT, J. R. Small vessel anastomosis. *British Journal of Plastic Surgery*, 1967, **20,** 16.

[8] COBBETT, J. R. Microvascular surgery. *Surgical Clinics of North America*, 1967, **47,** 521.

[9] LISTER, G. D. Makro chirurgische probleme du replantation. *Hand chirurgie*, 1977, **9,** 45–50.

[10] LISTER, G. D. Intraosseous wiring of the digital skeleton. *Journal of Hand Surgery*, 1978, **3,** 427.

[11] LISTER, G. D., KLEINERT, H. E., KUTZ, J. E. AND ATASOY, E. Immediate controlled mobilisation following primary flexor tendon repair. *The Journal of Hand Surgery*, 1977, **2,** 441–455.

FURTHER READING

ACLAND, R. D. *Microsurgical Practice Manual.* St. Louis, Mosby, 1979.

O'BRIEN, B. McC., *Microvascular Reconstructive Surgery.* Edinburgh, Churchill Livingstone, 1977.

CHAPTER 11

The Cut Tendon

ANATOMICAL INTRODUCTION

K. KUCZYNSKI

The gross anatomy of the tendons of the hand and their sheaths is described on pages 9, 22–28, 46, 47.

Tendon is composed of collagen fibres in closely packed bundles separated by interfascicular connective tissue which contains the vessels and the living cells, tenocytes, concerned with maintenance of the tendon substance and which may take part in the process of repair [1]. Extracellular amorphous ground substance lies between the fibrillar elements. A delicate layer of loose connective tissue covering the tendon is called *epitenon* and continues into its interfascicular planes as *endotenon*. The tendon may lie in *paratenon* (Fig. 1.20, p. 10) or within a *synovial sheath* with parietal and visceral layers which are continuous through *mesotenon* (Fig. 11.1, p. 154).

Tendons have great tensile strength, and can be bent but resist stretching. The presence of elastic fibres in the tendon is postulated [2] as having a protective function by causing the increase in tension to be gradual, thus absorbing the first shock of contraction.

The basic function of a tendon is to transmit tension developed by the muscle. Additional advantages are that the muscle can act from a distance without encroaching by its bulk on the joint, its action is concentrated on a small area of the bone and can be applied to several joints. It also protects the muscle during an unexpected strain by buffer action of its elasticity [2].

Intratendinous structure

Collagen fibres may be arranged in a different manner in various tendons [3]. Its bundles run parallel to the long axis of the tendon, but in the long flexors they have a spiral arrangement near the insertion [4, 5]. This gives greater resistance to longitudinal splitting in the distal portion of superficialis which otherwise can be split longitudinally as readily as plantaris tendon. It is, however, quite resistant to lateral stretching which is so easy in plantaris and palmaris longus tendons probably due to the interweaving of the fibres. The fibres of profundus also have a distal spiral arrangement which may be associated with the considerable loads applied. Plantaris and palmaris longus tendons do not require spiral arrangement and interweaving of fibres as their loads are very much smaller. Interweaving of the tendon fibres helps to a wide spread in distribution of the pull over the tendon insertion. At the insertion itself the fibres fan out with the result that the change of the angle between the tendon and the bone during movement always finds some tendon fibres in the direct line of the pull.

The blood supply

Extensors are mostly without synovial sheaths and surrounded by paratenon in which vessels enter the tendon at frequent intervals [6].

In the proximal palm and the wrist the flexor tendons lie in the ulnar bursa (Fig. 1.43) invaginated into it from the radial side where the roots of the mesotenons are to be found; each superficialis tendon has an incompletely separated mesotenon. The flexor pollicis longus tendon lies in its own radial bursa. Vessels in the palmar bursae are continuous with those in the paratenon in the forearm proximally and in the midpalm distally.

In the digital flexor sheaths the vessels enter the tendon at both ends of the reflection of the sheaths, at the insertion and through vincula (Fig. 11.1).

The short vincula are particularly important to the long flexors, the long vinculum contributing only small vessels except for that which supplies the intermediate portion of the profundus tendon in the sheath [7]. The longitudinal channels, usually one artery and two veins, run on the dorsal aspect of the tendon of superficialis and are fed from the branches of the digital arteries destined for the proximal interphalangeal joint; they reach the tendon through the short vincula. Branches of digital arteries to the distal joint reach the tendon of the profundus by its short vinculum.

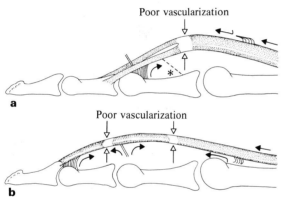

FIG. 11.1. The main blood supply of the flexor digitorum superficialis and profundus tendons within the digital sheath showing the critical, poorly vascularized segments between the separate vascular systems (shaded). The vascular inflow is indicated by black arrows. After Lundberg.

(a) The flexor digitorum superficialis tendon. There are two separated vascular systems. The proximal system originates from nutrient vessels in the proximal synovial reflexion, and from longitudinal intrinsic vessels from the palm region. The distal vascular system originates from the vinculum breva at the chiasma formation and the inconstant vinculum longum (*). Between these systems there is an apparently avascular segment.

(b) The flexor digitorum profundus tendon. There are three well defined vascular systems of different origin. A proximal system originates from nutrient vessels in the proximal synovial reflexion and from longitudinal intrinsic vessels from the palm region. An intermediate system originates from the vinculum longum at the proximal interphalangeal joint level. A distal vascular system originates from the vinculum breve at the tendon insertion.

Intratendinous vascular pattern

The interfascicular connective tissue separating the fibre bundles contains numerous vessels lying parallel to the fibres with frequent transverse anastomoses.

It is accepted that tendons receive blood vessels from the musculotendinous junction and from the insertion [8], while the intermediate portion is supplied in two different ways either (1) through paratenon, or (2) by synovial vincula, and that the vessels from both ends of the tendon are not able to nourish the middle portion if its own blood supply is interrupted. However, it has been suggested that tendons normally surrounded by paratenon show an open microcirculation throughout even after mobilization from the surrounding tissues along its whole length, and in addition after either the musculotendinous junction or distal junction was transectioned [9]. Recent observations suggest that inside the digital sheaths where the flexor tendons are stressed during activity against the pulleys, their palmar aspect is avascular and is probably nourished by the synovial fluid of the sheath [7]. Relatively avascular areas extending through most of the thickness of the tendon were found also: in the superficial tendon at the division into two slips and in the profundus tendon at both ends of the segment fed by the vinculum longum (Fig. 11.1).

Veins and lymphatics closely follow the arterial arrangement.

The nerve supply

This consists of perivascular sympathetic fibres and of relatively abundant free endings which are elaborated in some areas into Golgi tendon organs which together with Pacinian corpuscles in the tendon sheath provide a proprioceptive feedback to the central nervous system. A plexus of very fine nerve fibres present in the tendons and their sheaths is probably concerned with pain.

INJURIES OF THE FLEXOR TENDONS

D. W. LAMB

Wounds on the volar aspect of the wrist and hand are frequently associated with damage to the flexor tendons. With the exception of their passage through the carpal tunnel, the tendons lie superficially in the palm and digits. Following division of flexor tendons the affected digit tends to take up an abnormal posture relative to the remainder of the digits at rest and lies extended (Fig. 11.2). The presumptive diagnosis of the division

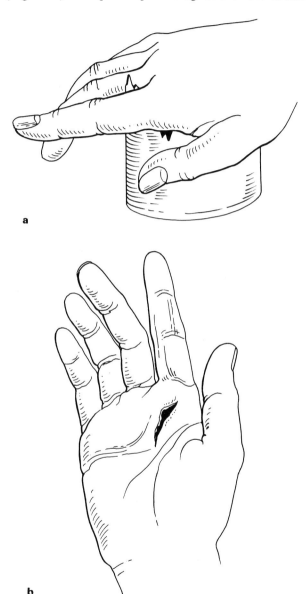

a

b

FIG. 11.2. Injury to flexor tendons showing (a) possible method of injury and (b) the posture of the index finger indicating that the flexor tendons are cut with the finger lying straight.

of the tendons can thus often be suspected by the posture of the hand at rest. The site of the skin wound does not always indicate the site of the tendon damage which will depend upon the direction in which the wounding implement has entered the hand and on whether the fingers have been flexed or extended at the time of injury.

The flexor tendons are unique in their structure (p. 153). For a considerable part of their course they are enveloped in synovial tissue which facilitates their essential gliding function and yet they have a limited blood supply. From full extension to full flexion of the digits the tendons have to move and glide over a distance varying between 5 and 7·5 cm. Following tendon division, the proximal end retracts and spontaneous healing in the complete division is rare. The ability of tendons to heal, even when coapted, is poor and a considerable amount of experimental work has shown that much of the tendon repair occurs from extratendinous sources. Potenza [10, 11, 12] reported that tendons healed by the fibroblastic response of surrounding tissue whose own integrity had been violated [13, 14, 15, 16, 17, 18, 19]. This tendon healing inevitably means adhesion to surrounding tissue with its adverse effect on the gliding so necessary for tendon function [20, 21]. Exclusion of this extratendinous source of the healing process is the reason for the poor results obtained when using a variety of materials in order to isolate the healing tendon and prevent its adhesion to surrounding tissues [16]. The need for this tendon healing process vitiates attempts at early free mobilization to encourage gliding following repair of tendons as was shown in the classical experiments by Mason and Allen [22].

Recent work [23, 24, 25] has shown that a tendon partially divided experimentally within its synovial sheath is capable of purely intratendinous repair if immobilized for long enough. This suggests that under ideal conditions the flexor tendons possess the ability to repair areas of injury without the ingrowth of adhesions.

Management of flexor tendon injuries

It is reasonable to assume that when a tendon is divided, the most satisfactory form of treatment is its immediate repair but unfortunately this is not always correct. There is well documented evidence that the result of primary repair of cut tendons, particularly where both flexor tendons are involved in the digital fibrous sheath, were extremely bad [26]. Serious adhesion of the tendon to the surrounding tissues was invariable and a stiff finger resulted. The function of the digit was so limited that amputation was often required, particularly if there was associated sensory impairment from digital nerve damage.

The first person to appreciate the significance of these results and to remedy the unsatisfactory state of affairs was Sterling Bunnell. He suggested that different lines of treatment might be advisable, dependent on which area was damaged. Divided tendons at the wrist or in the palm might do well with primary repair but in the restricted fibrous sheath between the metacarpal head and the superficialis tendon insertion, where two tendons were involved, the chances of success were much more remote. While appreciating that many factors might be involved in the quality of result obtained by repair, he advocated that in this area, to which he gave the name 'no man's land', primary healing of the skin wound was the main objective followed by later re-section of the damaged tendons and replacement by a tendon graft. Bunnell's influence in the management of flexor tendon injuries has been profound throughout the world over the past 30 years, and he was able to show that his own results and those trained by him were vastly superior to those obtaining previously. A large series of excellent functional results following tendon grafting have been reported [27, 28, 29, 30, 31, 32]. This method, however, requires a careful selection of patients, meticulous attention to operative detail and continuous postoperative care if results are to be satisfactory. This is not surgery for those inexperienced in the techniques of hand surgery and without the facilities and instrumentation required. The results of tendon grafting carried out as an occasional infrequent procedure are as bad as the older results of primary repair.

The techniques of tendon grafting are described on pp. 159–165, but before the institution of treatment for tendon injury factors which are known to affect the result must be assessed:

(1) the type of injury and the amount of scarring it has produced,
(2) the passive mobility of the joints,
(3) the sensory status of the digit,
(4) the age of the patient, and
(5) the patient's motivation.

Injuries associated with crushing or with fractures and joint damage invariably produce much fibrosis and a poor result. No tendon graft can function satisfactorily if it is carried out before there has been resolution of the tissues after injury and unless there is full passive mobility of the joints and good sensation in the finger. It has been shown that the results of tendon grafting after middle age are poor [27], and even in the young patient unless there is a proper motivation for full function and the necessary co-operation in postoperative management the results are inferior.

In view of the difficulties of tendon grafting, the inconsistency of results and the prolonged period off work often necessary, many surgeons have recently advocated and practised a return to primary repair of the cut flexor tendon even in 'no man's land'. Kleinert has said 'no man's land' is 'some man's land'. In view of the improved surgical technique possible with fine delicate instruments and non-reactive suture material on atraumatic needles for tendon repair, aided by operating magnifying loupes, there have been several series in recent years reporting good results from primary repair of flexor tendons [19, 25, 33, 34, 35, 36, 37]. However, this method is only justified in the clean lacerated wound performed by a surgeon trained in the atraumatic technique, and who has the necessary instruments and theatre facilities. Careful wound excision is required with a minimum of handling of the tendon and care should be taken that the vinculum is not damaged. A 5/0 monofilament wire suture is the best material for coapting the tendon satisfactorily. For many years the zig-zag suture (Fig. 11.3) has been used, but work on the tendon blood

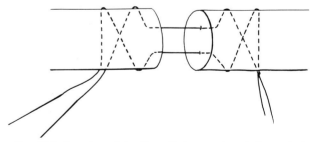

FIG. 11.3. Insertion of the Bunnell zig-zag wire stitch attached at each end to a straight needle. A pull-out wire is used in this illustration although this is seldom necessary.

supply suggests that this may strangle the intratendinous blood vessels [38, 39, 40, 41]; the most satisfactory current techniques are those which use the Kessler stitch [42] (Fig. 11.4), or the intratendinous method recently described [43]. By these techniques the tendon is sutured mainly on the volar or superficial aspect so that the main blood vessels running along the dorsal aspect of the tendon and entering on the deep aspect are not disturbed. A continuous 6/0 prolene suture is then used to hold the tendon ends accurately together (Fig. 11.4). The current practice is to attempt repair of both tendons where these are divided [34, 35] and to repair the fibrous flexor sheath if possible [25]. Any blood must be cleared from the sheath and careful haemostasis achieved before wound closure. Immobilization is required for a period of 3 weeks, but in order to prevent rigid adherence at the site of injury a technique whereby elastic traction is applied through the nail of the affected digit has been introduced [36]. On completion of surgery the wrist is immobilized with a dorsal plaster slab in a position of flexion sufficient to prevent any tension in the tendon with wrist and metacarpophalangeal joints about 30° flexed. The slab should extend to the tips of the fingers on the dorsum in such a way as to allow for full extension of the interphalangeal joints. The traction is then applied through a rubber band attached to the front of the wrist with enough tension to put the digit through a range of flexion but not so strong as to prevent the

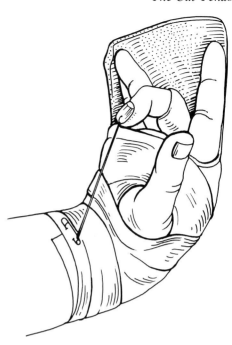

FIG. 11.5. Postoperative traction splintage (Kleinert) following flexor tendon repair. A posterior plaster slab is applied with the wrist and metacarpophalangeal joints flexed about 30°. The strength of the elastic must not prevent active extension against the plaster to avoid contractures of the proximal interphalangeal joint.

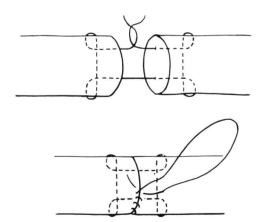

FIG. 11.4. Use of the Kessler stitch which grasps the tendon ends but is less likely to strangulate the blood supply than the zig-zag suture. The suture is tied to be buried. A circumferential 6/0 prolene suture is used to complete the repair.

digit extending to the limit allowed by the plaster (Fig. 11.5). Using these methods [36] excellent results in about 80 per cent of cases treated by primary tendon repair, even including 'no man's land', have been reported. Kleinert believes that such results can also be obtained by delayed primary suture up to 3–4 days from injury, and other reports have also suggested this [44]. The basic principles involved in primary flexor tendon repair are as follows.

(1) Complete anaesthesia and a careful and thorough wound excision under pneumatic tourniquet is necessary.

(2) Minimal extension of the wound using the zig-zag incision (Bruner [45]) (Fig. 11.6) may be required to expose the tendon for repair.

(3) Care is needed to avoid unnecessary surgical trauma by using fine surgical instruments, small needles and fine calibre (4/0 or 5/0) non-reactive suture materials. The tendons are held by their cut surfaces. If the tendon ends have been crushed, up to 1 cm can be

removed before repair and be compatible with a good result.

(4) Tissue dessication should be avoided by regular application of saline solution.

(5) Complete haemostasis is achieved at end of operation after releasing the tourniquet.

(6) Tension on suture line should be prevented and some controlled mobility allowed (Kleinert traction). Elastic traction is removed after $3\frac{1}{2}$ weeks. Any contracture of the proximal interphalangeal joint is stretched out by serial plaster casting.

In children elastic traction is not necessary but rigid immobilization is advisable in an above elbow plaster for 4 weeks.

Kleinert has reported the results of 360 primary tendon repairs in Zone II [34] (Fig. 11.7). The grading of results are:

(1) *excellent*, flexion within 1 cm of distal palmar crease with less than 15° loss of extension;

(2) *good*, flexion within 1·5 cm of distal palmar crease with less than 30° loss of extension;

(3) *fair*, flexion within 3·00 cm of distal palmar crease and between 30–50° loss of extension;

(4) *poor*, greater than 3·00 cm from distal palmar crease or more than 50° loss of extension or both.

Using these criteria the following results were obtained:

superficialis only cut and repaired: 100 per cent good or excellent,

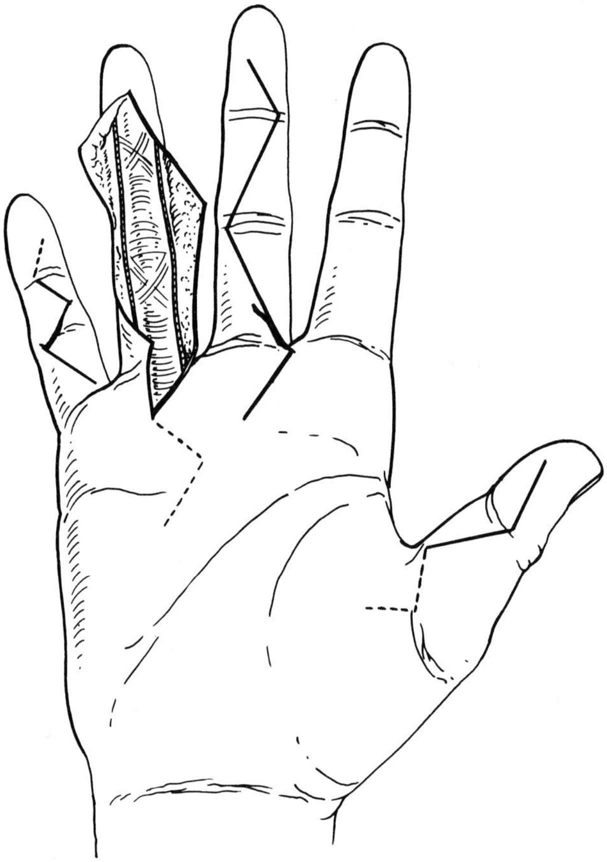

FIG. 11.6. Lacerations on the palm or digit can be extended by the volar zig-zag incision.

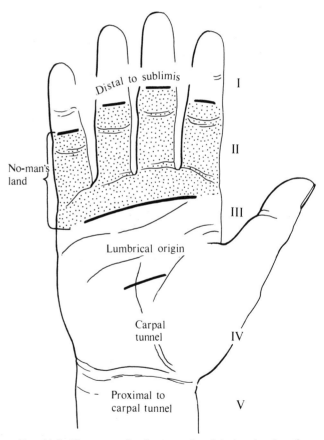

FIG. 11.7. Five zones for flexor tendon injuries showing the important zone is between the origin of the fibrous flexor sheath, and the superficialis insertion, the so-called 'no man's land'.

profundus only cut and repaired: 79 per cent good or excellent,

both tendons cut, profundus only repaired: 70 per cent good or excellent,

both tendons cut, both tendons repaired: 82 per cent good or excellent.

Where the result is poor to fair and improvement in movement has stopped, tenolysis should be considered but not until after 6 months from the repair. Comparable results using a different technique have also been described by Verdan who considered his results the same, if not superior, to those obtained by tendon graft [19,37]. As with the good results of tendon grafts however, it must be realised that these results from primary repair are being achieved by experts. In 10 years experience of primary repair by himself and associates Kleinert reported 87 per cent good to excellent results. In the same period on his teaching service 76 per cent poor results were obtained by untrained surgeons. Primary flexor tendon repair is not recommended for the inexperienced surgeon or where facilities are not of the best. Throughout the world most flexor tendon injuries are going to be received and treated in circumstances not conducive to good results for primary tendon repair. The young and inexperienced surgeon must realise that less harm is done to the patient by concentration on excision and primary healing of the wound than by careless tendon repair. Subsequent treatment can be carried out by the more experienced specialist surgeon.

Recommended management (based on the area affected (Fig. 11.7))

Clean laceration

Zone V. Primary repair of tendons and nerves with isolation of the nerve repair by silastic sheeting (p. 187).
Zone IV. Injuries within the carpal tunnel are rare and difficult to treat. As adhesion is common most surgeons recommend a secondary tendon graft to bridge the scarred area.

Kleinert recommends that primary repair of both superficialis and profundus be carried out. Synovium should be removed and part of the retinaculum left intact to prevent bow stringing.

Zone III. In the palm, primary repair of both tendons should be carried out (Fig. 11.8). The palmar fascia overlying the tendons should be excised. Any cut nerve is repaired at the same time.
Zone II. In 'no man's land', i.e. between proximal end of fibrous flexor sheath and superficialis insertion, minimal extension of the laceration either by mid-lateral (Fig. 11.9 and see Fig. 7.3–1) or Bruner's volar zig-zag incisions (Fig. 11.6) is undertaken to visualize the tendon ends.

Minimal handling of the tendons is necessary and both tendons repaired using the Kessler stitch (Fig. 11.4) with stainless steel wire or the zig-zag suture (Figs. 11.3 and 11.10). A circumferential stitch of the tendon ends with 6/0 nylon or prolene is inserted. The digital sheath is repaired if possible and careful haemastasis obtained. Postoperative immobilization as described by Kleinert is used. Any associated digital nerve damage is repaired primarily.

Zone I. In division of profundus tendon distal to superficialis insertion primary repair is carried out. If the proximal tendon has retracted into the palm, its retrieval and repair is difficult and the surgeon with little experience is advised not to attempt it.

Complicated injuries

In circumstances where the wound has been associated with crushing, extensively damaged tissues, wound contamination of several hours duration, associated skin loss, fracture of phalanx or joint injury, it is recommended that the wound should be excised and primary skin healing obtained. Later tendon repair or tendon graft as appropriate can be carried out.

Technique of tendon grafting

When it is thought inadvisable to carry out tendon repair or when this has failed, a tendon graft should be considered. The operation must not be carried out till the reaction to injury has settled and what Steindler called a 'tissue equilibrium' has occurred.

The divided tendon or tendons are removed and replaced by a tendon graft which spans the damaged area and is attached proximally and distally at sites

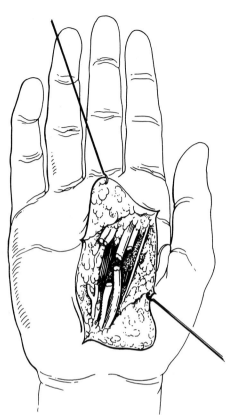
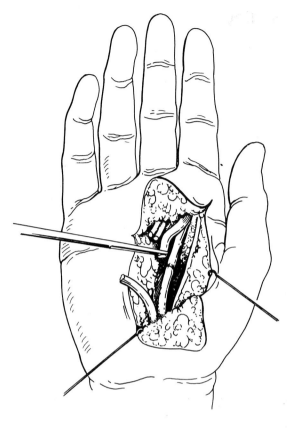

FIG. 11.8. Cut flexor tendons to the index finger of the right hand in the palm (Zone III). The nerve to the second cleft has also been divided. The nerve to the radial side of the index finger can be seen but is intact. The original laceration has been extended to give wide exposure.

(a)　The damage exposed.

(b) The profundus has been repaired by a Kessler wire stitch and circumferential interrupted 6/0 prolene. The ends of the cut superficialis can be seen.

where adhesion is less important. The instruments needed for this operation are shown in Fig. 11.11. The tendon is exposed by a midlateral digital incision (Fig. 11.9), joining up the posterior part of the flexion creases of the digit and extending proximally into the palm. An alternative incision is the volar zig-zag incision described by Bruner [45] (Fig. 11.12). This gives better exposure of the tendons and the neurovascular bundles in their entirety. If there has been extensive scarring of the skin at the site of injury, the lateral incision is more appropriate. A meticulous dissection of the tendons is carried out from the insertion of the profundus to the base of the palm at the site of the lumbrical attach-ment or, in the case of the thumb, to the musculo-tendinous junction of the flexor pollicis longus tendon. The fibrous flexor sheath must be dissected with great care in order to try and preserve a small portion of the intact sheath at two or three sites through which the tendon can be threaded and prevent a bow-stringing effect subsequently (Fig. 11.13). These pulley areas, best sited over the middle of the middle phalanx and near the base of the proximal phalanx, are obvious sites of potential adherence of the graft and should be no more than 2–3 mm in width. The remainder of the fibrous sheath is removed taking care to avoid damage to perio-steum, capsule and volar plate. If it has been some

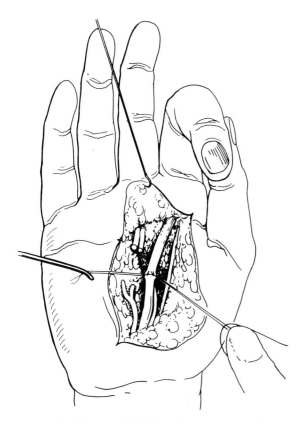

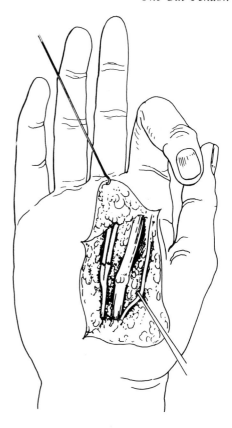

(c) Repair of the superficialis showing stay sutures being used to control the tendon to allow the insertion of the circumferential stitches.

(d) Completed repair of tendons and the repair of the cut digital nerves.

months since the injury, the pulleys and any remains of the fibrous flexor sheath over the metacarpophalangeal joint are likely to be stenosed and should be gently dilated by graduated bougies (Fig. 11.11). Where satisfactory pulleys cannot be prepared it is necessary to construct new pulleys. This is best done by using a strip of undamaged superficialis passing it deep to the neurovascular bundles in the digit and around the dorsum of the digit superficial to the extensor tendon.

In the thumb the tendon of extensor pollicis brevis can be used as a loop to form the pulley.

The profundus stump is split along its median raphe for the distal attachment of the graft. A flap of periosteum is elevated from the distal phalanx and a hole made through the distal phalanx with a bone awl directed to emerge at the tip of the finger just beyond the nail.

The looped end of a doubled piece of wire is passed through the eye of the bone awl and drawn into the finger.

Attention is now turned to the site of the free tendon graft. Donor tendons in order of preference are palmaris longus, plantaris and a long toe extensor. Palmaris is usually adequate in length and it should be removed through three short transverse incisions. It should be appreciated that there are anomalies of the palmaris in about 10 per cent of patients. Having been divided distally the tendon is withdrawn through the proximal incision (Fig. 11.14), and while still attached as the musculotendinous end a zig-zag wire stitch is inserted in the terminal part of the tendon. It is important that the tendon should not be handled in any way. There has been much controversy about the importance of removing intact paratenon together with the tendon.

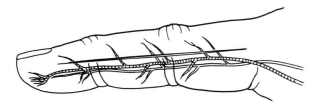

FIG. 11.9. Midlateral digital incision showing the volar flap which is elevated with the neurovascular bundle.

Some surgeons feel this is important in encouraging the revascularization of the tendon, but others feel that the paratenon is a potent factor in causing adhesions of the tendon in its new bed. It is more usual for the paratenon to be removed with the tendon and transposed.

The tendon graft is placed immediately in the digit and the ends of the wires are placed through the loop of the wire previously placed in the end of the finger. The looped wire is withdrawn distally through the tip of the finger and, in this way, the terminal part of the graft is guided underneath the small remaining stump of the profundus. The wire ends are tied over a dental roll placed over the tip of the finger and firm fixation secured (Fig. 11.15). Finally, the flaps of the profundus stump are attached to this distal end of the graft by interrupted 6/0 prolene suture. The graft is threaded proximally through the pulleys into the palm of the hand and prepared for proximal suture.

If the palmaris tendon is absent or inadequate a plantaris tendon is explored through a small vertical incision near the insertion of the tendo calcaneus on its medial side. The tendon is freed, dissected proximally by use of a Brand tendon stripper, and enucleated from the muscle belly in the upper part of the calf. This should be done gently and no great force is required. Sometimes there is an additional muscle belly attached to the mid-tendon and requires gentle freeing. Plantaris provides an excellent length of tendon where a long graft is required, e.g. when the proximal suture is above the wrist or in cases where more than one tendon graft is required at the same time. Where neither palmaris nor plantaris is available the 4th toe extensor is removed through a series of short transverse incisions on the dorsum of the foot. This is a more bulky tendon than either the palmaris or plantaris and is less satisfactory.

Before the proximal suture is carried out the tourniquet is released and all bleeding stopped, as any

blood clot will encourage adhesion formation. At this stage any associated digital nerve repair is carried out. If there is any tendency to hyperextension deformity at the proximal interphalangeal joint a slip of the superficialis which has been left for this purpose during the initial dissection of the tendon bed is sutured to periosteum proximally in order to hold the joint in about 10° of flexion. The skin wound of the finger is now closed.

The proximal suture presents a problem as a thin tendon graft is to be united with a more robust proximal profundus tendon and is best achieved by the smaller tendon being threaded through the larger tendon in two or three consecutive sites [30, 31] and held in place by fine 6/0 prolene mattress sutures. The junction is made in the vicinity of the lumbrical muscle and the stump of profundus is wrapped around the graft having been shaped into a fine fishtail (Fig. 11.16). The tension at which the proximal suture is carried out is a matter of

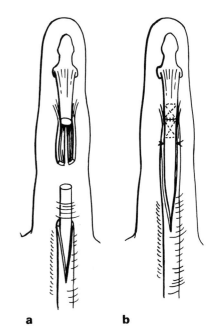

a   b

FIG. 11.10. Cut flexor tendons in the digit in Zone II in 'no man's land'.

(a) Both profundus and superficialis have been divided at a slightly different level.

(b) The profundus has been repaired by a Bunnell stitch and the superficialis by interrupted 6/0 prolene suture.

considerable importance and is best assessed by relating the posture of the finger to its fellows. Normally at rest the posture which the hand adopts is one of an increasing degree of flexion from the index to little fingers, and when the proximal suture has been carried out the affected digit should be lying in a slightly greater degree of flexion than would be its normal position of rest. In the case of graft in the thumb, the interphalangeal joint should be lying in about 30° of flexion with the wrist in slight dorsiflexion.

To allow the interweaving procedure to be carried out without undue handling of the tendon, a straight fine needle is passed through the lumbrical muscle to prevent the tendon from retracting. In order to prevent excessive adhesion around the proximal suture, three procedures may be used.

(1) The most satisfactory is to elevate a sleeve of synovium on the tendon before the interweaving procedure is carried out, and then slide the sleeve down over the suture line subsequently.

(2) The second procedure is to surround the tendon by the lumbrical muscle belly which is pulled distally before it is sutured.

(3) In the third technique, particularly applicable when plantaris has been used, the tendon graft can be stretched into a fascial layer [46] and wrapped round the suture line.

At the completion of operation a compression bandage is applied over fluffed gauze and wool holding the wrist in slight dorsiflexion, the thumb in abduction and the metacarpophalangeal joints flexed with the digits straight at the interphalangeal joints. The position is

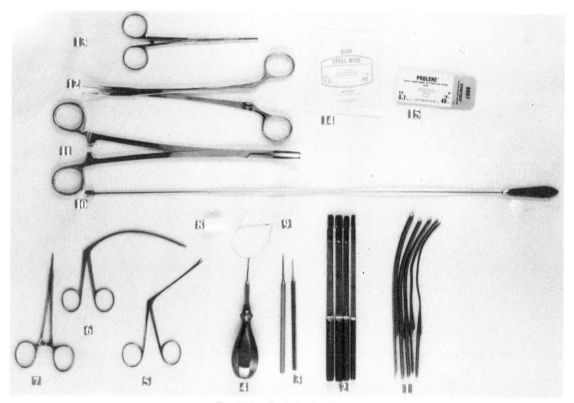

FIG. 11.11. Basic tendon tray.

(1) Hegar's dilators (size 1–5), (2) Echoff's tendon stripper, (3) Beaver handle with No. 62 blade, and 52M blade, (4) 5/32 bone awl threaded with 5/0 monofilament wire, (5) crocodile forceps, (6) Carroll tendon passing forceps, (7) goose-neck forceps (modified mosquito forceps), (8) dental roll, (9) straight round bodied needle, (10) Brand's tendon stripper, (11) and (12) Platt's tendon passing forceps, (13) Frischi tendon passing forceps, (14) monofilament steel wire with double-ended straight needles, (15) 6/0 prolene.

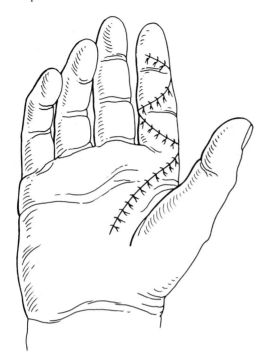

FIG. 11.12. Volar zig-zag incision for tendon graft in the right index finger.

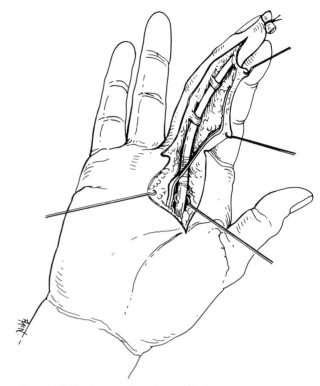

FIG. 11.13. Tendon graft by midlateral incision. The ulnar side is exposed because of nerve damage on that side. The neurovascular structures are retracted forwards in the anterior flap. Note placing of pulleys.

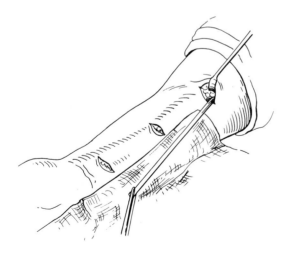

FIG. 11.14. The palmaris tendon is removed through three short transverse incisions. Before completing removal a zig-zag wire suture is inserted in the distal end. The tendon is then removed and inserted immediately into its new bed.

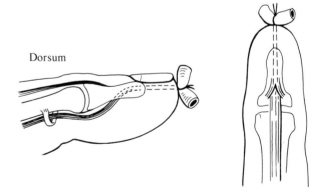

FIG. 11.15. Distal attachment of the tendon graft. The distal part of the palmaris is fixed under the stump of profundus to which it is attached by interrupted 6/0 proline sutures. The wires are taken through the drill hole in the phalanx and tied over a dental roll. The wire is easily removed 4 weeks after operation.

maintained for 3 weeks at which time the dressings and stitches are removed. The terminal wire suture is, however, left in situ for a further week.

A programme of mobilization and rehabilitation is carried out under the supervision of the physiotherapist (see Chapter 36). The patient is warned not to expect early functional movement of the digit and that a steady improvement in the range of movement should take place over several months. Usually after 3 months an assessment of the likely ultimate result is possible, but progress can continue for up to 12 months from operation. Good results are more likely in a young co-operative patient with an enthusiastic physiotherapist and close supervision by the surgeon.

Many methods have been introduced to assess the functional recovery after tendon grafting. Boyes has described classification into four grades: excellent, good, fair and poor [27]. Limitation of extension due to interphalangeal joint contracture or a short graft is judged by measuring the distance from the tip of the nail to the plane of the dorsum of the hand. The range of active flexion at the interphalangeal joints is assessed by goniometer and the overall range of flexion of the finger by estimating the distance from the terminal pulp to the distal palm. An excellent result is one where the finger extends fully and flexes to within a centimeter of the palm. A good result is consistent with contractures at

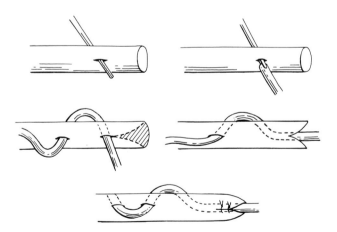

FIG. 11.16. The proximal suture of tendon graft (Pulvertaft technique). The smaller Palmaris is 'woven' through the profundus near its lumbrical attachment. The cut end of profundus is closed as a 'fishtail' around the palmaris.

the two interphalangeal joints limiting extension of up to 40° combined and a flexion deficit of 2·5 cm or less. In Boyes series 75 per cent came into these two categories.

Tenolysis

In those cases where there is an unsatisfactory range of movement consideration should be given to tenolysis. This should not be done until 9 months after operation. In a series of 220 grafts, Fetrow reported 60 where tenolysis was carried out [47]. Tenolysis consists of freeing the whole tendon graft from adhesion, followed by early mobilization. Results are disappointing as there is a strong tendency to bowstringing afterwards and occasionally rupture of the tendon follows interference with its blood supply. James has suggested that cortisone should be given to cover the period of tenolysis and postoperative mobilisation in order to lessen the inflammatory reaction [48].

The use of artificial tendons

Where considerable soft tissue damage has occurred following the injury and the bed is found to be badly fibrosed or where volar plate or periosteum has been damaged, a tendon graft is more likely to become adherent and the results are poor. In this type of case considerable advance has been made in recent years by the introduction of the technique of a temporary insertion of a silastic rod [49, 50, 51, 52, 53]. The judicious use of a silastic rod extending the length of the digit and palm can stimulate a satisfactory pseudo-synovium during a period of some weeks [54, 55, 56]. The injured tendons are removed and the bed in the digit is prepared in the same meticulous way as for a tendon graft. The largest size of rod which will fit comfortably into the digit and through the pulley is used. It is sutured distally but left free proximally at the wrist although lightly opposed to the proximal end of the tendon at the wrist. This does not interfere with early passive movement of the digit so necessary to prevent stiffness of the interphalangeal joints and helps to stimulate production of the smooth tunnel. An optimum period appears to be 10–12 weeks following which the rod is replaced by a plantaris graft. Two small incisions are all that is required, one over the distal part of the digit and the other at the wrist, and the tendon is threaded through the tunnel prepared by the silastic rod as the rod is withdrawn. It has been shown that significantly better gliding can occur after this procedure in the badly damaged digit than by primary grafting [52, 53, 55].

It must not be presumed, however, that this two stage procedure is simple or that all results are good. When performed in the digit which has been badly scarred, as recommended for its use, it must be considered as a salvage procedure and in these cases about one-third will have a poor result (Boyes classification). About 50 per cent of the total range of movement in the normal digit is an average result that can be anticipated.

A suggestion has been made that all tendon grafting should be preceded by silastic rod replacement, but at the present time there would appear to be no justification for this in the uncomplicated case. The use of a permanent artificial tendon [57] is a very attractive proposition, but there is a tendency for these tendons to break. Peacock [58, 59] and Hueston et al [60] have suggested the use of homografts of the whole flexor tendon system, but the lack of further communication

on the use of this interesting concept suggests that the results have been disappointing.

There is considerable debate about the management of the isolated profundus division in the presence of an intact superficialis [29, 61]. It cannot be stressed too much that there is never any justification for removing an intact superficialis to insert a graft. In general, the injury is left alone as the disability is slight (Fig. 11.17). On occasion and particularly in a young person who has need of a highly skilled function of the hand with active terminal joint flexion, there is a case for inserting a fine graft to replace the profundus while retaining the normal superficialis. This is a procedure which is not without danger and must be done very carefully, otherwise the tendon graft may become adherent at the decussation of the superficialis leading to deterioration of function. Honner [62] reports that a silastic rod inserted through the intact superficialis and followed by graft replacement will provide consistently satisfactory results.

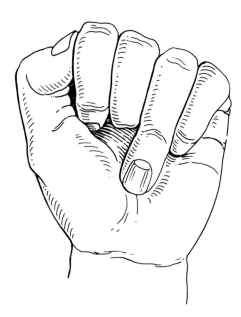

FIG. 11.17. An isolated profundus damaged gives only slight disability. Attempts to replace the profundus by a graft are inadvisable in the majority of patients.

Summary

The management of flexor tendon injuries is by no means as simple as it might appear to be. The results of primary repair before the advantage of modern delicate instrumentation and fine suture materials were so bad that there was a swing away from primary repair towards tendon grafting particularly in those injuries occurring in 'no man's land'. There is a current resurgence in the belief that primary repair properly performed in the right circumstances can give satisfactory results and it is likely that this will be the trend in the next few years. It cannot be stressed too strongly that no harm will come to the patient if the surgeon dealing primarily with the injury concentrates on skin healing and leaves the tendon surgery to someone more skilled and experienced in this type of surgery. If the incidence of successful primary repair increases there will be fewer indications for tendon grafting but this latter technique is still one in which all surgeons practising surgery of the hand to any extent must be confident and competent. In the more complicated cases the introduction of the silastic rod prior to grafting has given hope for improved results.

INJURIES OF THE EXTENSOR TENDONS

G. D. LISTER

The extensor tendons are subject to various injuries [63, 64, 65].

Rupture occurs most commonly at points of tendon attachment to bone [66]. By far the most frequent site is the extensor insertion into the distal phalanx, producing the characteristic mallet finger. Rupture at the insertion of the central slip into the middle phalanx results in flexion of the proximal interphalangeal joint and extension of the distal joint, the boutonnière deformity. Extensor tendons do rupture at sites other than their insertions. 'Drummer's palsy', is due to attrition rupture of the extensor pollicis longus. Such ruptures are uncommon except in the presence of another disorder, such as rheumatoid disease or a previous Colles fracture.

Traumatic dislocation of the extensor tendon, usually of the middle finger, results from a longitudinal tear of the radial fibres of the extensor hood at the metacarpophalangeal joint [65].

Avulsion may be a variant of tendon rupture, the mallet finger or boutonnière resulting from a traction fracture of the distal or middle phalanx respectively. In roller injuries of the upper extremity, by contrast, avulsion of the extensor tendons may occur proximally, the tendon being plucked from the muscle belly just proximal to the musculotendinous junction.

Loss of a significant section of tendon is much more common on the extensor than on the flexor surface of the hand. The loss may be immediate, as in abrasion injuries. These may be the consequence of roller injuries and involve the dorsum of the hand, but more commonly affect the fingers by contact with the road in automobile accidents. More than one digit is usually abraded over the proximal interphalangeal joint which is often laid open. Tendon loss may also arise as a primary feature or a secondary complication of necrosis of the overlying skin resulting from burns [67] or from crush or degloving injuries.

Simple lacerations, in contrast, may occur at any site and present few problems in management. For anatomical reasons, however, the diagnosis may be overlooked. Over the middle phalanx, the oblique retinacular ligament may remain intact although the tendon is divided. By tenodesis, the ligament may produce spurious extension and the mallet finger may not be apparent until some time after the injury. Over the proximal phalanx, the central slip may be completely divided but extension of the proximal interphalangeal joint is retained through the action of the lateral bands, a boutonnière deformity developing only as the lateral bands displace volarwards. Laceration over the metacarpophalangeal joint, that is distal to the intertendinous connections and proximal to the edge of the extensor expansion, does result in loss of extension of that joint. The injury may nonetheless be missed on examination since the patient can still fully extend the interphalangeal joints using his intrinsic musculature. Injury of an extensor to one finger alone proximal to the intertendinous connections may be masked by pull transmitted from an adjacent tendon through the connection. Lacerations of single tendons to the index or small fingers proximal to the metacarpophalangeal joints may also be overlooked, since there are two tendons to the index, extensor digitorum and extensor indicis, and three to the small, two from extensor digiti minimi and the intertendinous connection from the ring tendon of extensor digitorum. Thus the cut extensor tendon may be diagnosed only by exploration of all dorsal wounds under appropriate operating conditions [68].

Mallet finger

This deformity results from disruption of the extensor mechanism over the distal interphalangeal joint. The posture of the mallet finger is characteristic, with volar angulation of the distal phalanx of anything from 20–60°. In most cases, the proximal interphalangeal joint is hyperextended, producing a swan-neck deformity of the digit (Fig. 11.18). This is due to proximal movement of the extensor apparatus released from its distal insertion. This in turn increases the pull on the intact central slip insertion into the middle phalanx. In the early case the drooping of the distal joint is easily corrected passively. In later instances a fixed flexion contracture is superimposed.

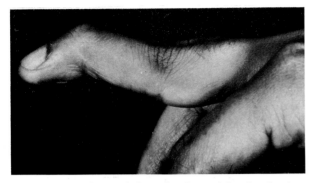

Fig. 11.18. A characteristic mallet finger deformity showing acute flexion at the distal interphalangeal joint. The hyperextension at the proximal joint resulting from increased traction of the central slip has produced a swan-neck deformity.

Closed injury

Lateral radiographs will determine whether avulsion of the dorsal lip of the distal phalanx or rupture of the tendon has occurred. Four different types of mallet finger may be identified [69]:

(1) Type 1 is a partial disruption of the extensor mechanism, in which there is an extension lag of between 20 and 25°.

(2) Type 2 is a complete avulsion of the extensor mechanism, often associated with a tear of the dorsal capsule, in which the lag will be between 45 and 60°.

(3) Type 3 is similar to Type 2, but associated with a small avulsion fracture at the base of the distal phalanx.

The mechanism of the injury is similar in these three groups and is usually a trivial flexion injury of the finger tip.

(4) Type 4 is a mallet deformity with separation of one-third or more of the dorsal margin of the distal phalanx, and may be associated with volar subluxation of the distal interphalangeal joint. The injury is usually caused by a forcible blow on the end of the extended digit.

Treatment

Many different types of treatment have been described for these injuries [63, 70, 71, 72, 73, 74], in some of which the morbidity and complication rate was more significant than the disability itself. The early literature recommended hyperextending the distal interphalangeal joint and flexing the proximal interphalangeal joint [72, 73, 75], thereby attempting to approximate the ends of the avulsed tendon. Immobilization of the proximal interphalangeal joint is seldom necessary and can result in a stiff interphalangeal joint while marked hyperextension can cause a skin slough over the dorsum of the distal interphalangeal joint. Open repair of the avulsed tendon [76], plaster immobilization of the entire digit [72], and percutaneous Kirschner wire fixation of the digit have been recommended.

Recently, a simpler approach has been advocated for these injuries, in which only the distal interphalangeal joint is splinted [69, 77, 78, 79, 80]. This method, using a simple plastic splint made in a range of sizes, has been found to be quite satisfactory for types 1 and 2 and for 3 except where the fragment is markedly displaced when, along with group 4, open reduction and internal fixation is indicated (Fig. 11.19a). A transverse incision directly over the joint may be extended for greater exposure by incisions along each mid-lateral line, creating an H. The fracture line may be difficult to locate unless the fragment is grossly displaced. The fragment attached to the tendon may appear misleadingly small on the radiograph, but when dissected out it is significantly larger. The discrepancy is due to the articular cartilage which makes up much of the fragment and is of course radiolucent. All haematoma must be meticulously cleaned from both fracture surfaces for no impediment to perfect reduction can be permitted (Fig. 11.19b). In most instances the fragment is large enough to be transfixed with a 0·028 inch Kirschner wire. In such cases the wire is passed first into the distal phalanx taking care to insert it as close to the dorsal cortex as possible to ensure maximum purchase later on the avulsed portion (Fig. 11.19c). The pin must be aimed somewhat volarwards in the distal phalanx to remain in the bone and avoid entering the nail matrix. The pin is withdrawn distally until only its proximal tip is to be seen protruding from the fracture surface. The surgeon then replaces the fragment and holds it firmly in place while hyperextending the distal interphalangeal joint. An assistant then advances the pin, impaling the fragment and passing on into the middle phalanx. Post-reduction films should then show perfect articular alignment (Fig. 11.19d).

Where the fragment is too small to take a Kirschner wire, it should nonetheless be retained, for it offers the

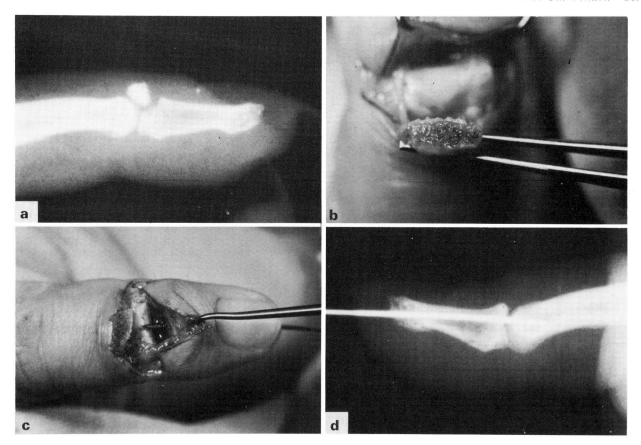

FIG. 11.19. (a). Intra-articular fracture of the distal interphalangeal joint produced by avulsion of the dorsal lip by the extensor tendon.

(b) The fracture has been exposed and here the fragment attached to the tendon is displayed and cleaned of haematoma.

(c) A 0·028 in K-wire has been driven out through the distal phalanx taking care to keep close to the dorsal cortex at the fracture site. It will be passed further into the phalanx until the small fragment shown in (b) can be held easily in position.

(d) The K-wire has been returned through the reduced fragment and into the middle phalanx immobilising the distal joint.

chance of bone to bone healing and maintains the end of the tendon in its proper configuration which simplifies secure fixation; a 3/0 or 4/0 monofilament wire suture mounted on two straight needles is passed through the tendon from side to side hard against the bony fragment. Each needle is then passed through the periosteum of the distal phalanx between the distal insertion of the collateral ligament and the proximal attachment of the lateral interosseous ligament of the distal phalanx. If the fragment is small, constituting less than two-thirds of the breadth of the base of the phalanx, the needles should be passed through holes previously drilled in a distal volar direction through the distal phalanx. By either method, the wire passes deep to the neuro-vascular bundles. The distal joint is then fixed in some hyperextension with a Kirschner wire and the fragment is reduced and secured by holding the two wires volarly under some tension with lead shot. The skin beneath the shot is protected by first passing the wire through a dental roll or similar soft padding. The monofilament wire is removed at 4 weeks and the Kirschner wire at 6 weeks.

Open laceration

Where both distal and proximal cut ends are adequate, repair should be effected using several figure-of-eight sutures, employing a synthetic non-absorbable suture. However, the tendon is more often divided at its insertion, precluding a simple end-to-end repair. Wound excision and splintage of the terminal joint as for the closed injury can give excellent results. If repair is elected, a 4/0 monofilament wire suture mounted on two straight needles is introduced into one or other margin of the cut proximal tendon end and passed in and out of that margin two or three times proceeding proximally. In the standard method the needle is then passed transversely through the tendon across to its opposite margin and there a matching weave is placed in that margin proceeding distally until the suture re-emerges from the tendon end permitting distal traction to be applied. However, such traction causes the tendon to bunch in an ugly manner. If two monofilament wires are employed, one to each of the distal bands, then the conjoined tendon maintains its normal configuration over the middle phalanx when distal traction is applied. The surgeon is then left with four needles. The two from each side are passed to the corresponding side of the distal phalanx through the periosteum distal to the attachment of the collateral ligament between bone and the lateral interosseous ligament to emerge 5 mm volar to the nail and 5 mm from the midline (Fig. 11.20). A Kirschner wire is inserted to immobilize the joint, the pull-out wires are drawn out to advance the tendon to its insertion and fixed with lead

shot as previously described. The pull-out wires should be removed at 4 weeks and the Kirschner wire at 6 weeks.

Complicated cases

Where the tendon injury is accompanied by extensive bony and articular damage or by skin loss, the management of the tendon is often determined by the repair selected for skeleton or skin. Where there is extensive joint damage primary arthrodesis is indicated. The tendon should nevertheless be repaired by simple suture to prevent later hyperextension of the proximal interphalangeal joint.

When skin and tendon are both lost over the distal two phalanges, the distal joint is often severely damaged and arthrodesis beneath flap cover is appropriate. However, where the joint is good and it is decided to try to maintain motion, a tendon graft as described below should be inserted primarily beneath the flap, thus minimising the necessary period of immobilisation.

Reconstruction of late mallet deformity

Extension lags of 15–20° are seldom disabling and rarely require surgery. Where treatment is requested, the choice lies between arthrodesis and reconstruction of the tendon. If there is a fixed flexion contracture, an unstable joint, scarred, ulcerated or adherent skin or osteoarthritic changes, then arthrodesis is the procedure of choice. Where these conditions do not exist, reconstruction is indicated. The results are often disappointing as scarring may limit flexion at the joint. At operation it is usually possible to distinguish the greyish white scar tissue from normal tendon. The scar should be excised and the tendon end will be revealed as identifiable bundles as opposed to the glassy homogeneity of scar tissue. Rarely, it is possible to advance the tendon as in an acute laceration. In most cases a graft of palmaris, plantaris or fascia lata is inserted. Two longitudinal holes 8–10 mm apart are drilled through the dorsal lip of the base of the distal phalanx, firstly with an 0·28 in Kirschner wire and then with a 1/16 in or 3/32 in drill. The graft is passed proximally through one and back distally through the other hole—a large bore hypodermic needle will facilitate this difficult manoeuvre, passing the needle through the hole

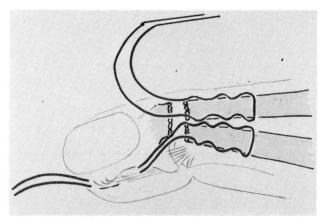

FIG. 11.20. This diagram illustrates the technique of repairing an extensor tendon divided too close to its insertion to allow simple interrupted suturing. A 4/0 monofilament wire is passed along both edges of each of the two conjoined tendons. Both wires are then passed out through the pulp and fixed with lead shot.

in the bone, placing the graft in the needle which is then withdrawn swiftly. The two ends are woven into the two tendons of the extensor apparatus gauging the correct tension by observing the distal joint with the wrist flexed, when the joint should be extended fully, and with the wrist extended, when the joint should be flexed a little less than its radially adjacent finger. A Kirschner wire is inserted to fix the joint in extension and removed after 4 weeks.

Boutonnière deformity [81]

A traumatic boutonnière results most commonly from a cut dividing the central slip either completely or to such an extent that later use results in rupture or from a closed avulsion of the central slip [82]. The proximal displacement of the central slip is accompanied by an increase in pull through the lateral bands causing hyperextension of the distal joint—the corollary of the swanneck deformity of mallet finger. The deformity, easily corrected passively in the early stages, becomes progressively more fixed (Fig. 11.21). The fixed deformity is very disabling requiring difficult reconstructive surgery which is often unsuccessful.

In order to make the diagnosis early and institute effective treatment, one must have a complete knowledge of the history of the lesion. The initial injury is an avulsion of the central slip from the base of the middle

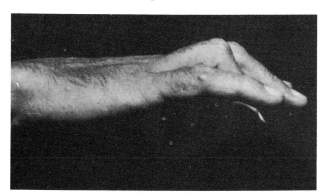

FIG. 11.21. A wound over the proximal interphalangeal joint six weeks previously has produced inability to extend the ring finger, a boutonnière deformity was developing with hyperextension of the distal joint. (This illustration also appeared in Lister, G. O. *The Hand: Diagnosis and Indications*, Edinburgh, Churchill Livingstone, 1977.)

phalanx, usually resulting from a flexion force against the fully extended digit [83]. Initially the patient presents with a swollen joint with dorsal tenderness, but may have little or no proximal interphalangeal joint extension lag. Both patient and physician may minimize the significance of this injury but a potential boutonnière deformity should be suspected. If a lateral X-ray shows an avulsion from the base of the middle phalanx, the diagnosis is confirmed.

The proximal interphalangeal joint is splinted in extension for five to six weeks [83, 84], encouraging motion in the distal joint. After this time, dynamic splinting is used and flexion is restored gradually to avoid stretching the healed extensor mechanism.

Many boutonnière deformities are seen late—from two weeks to many months after the injury. If the deformity can be corrected passively, then splinting as described for the acute injury is begun [69]. An alternative to splintage in all except the most minor degrees of deformity is open repair.

The joint is approached through a midline dorsal incision to expose the extensor expansion for one centimetre distal and proximal to the joint. In an avulsion fracture, the joint is fixed in ten degrees of flexion by a transarticular 0·035 inch Kirschner wire and then fixation of the avulsed fragment to the middle phalanx is undertaken separately. Occasionally the fragment can be held in firm position by a single 0·028 inch wire passed through it into the middle phalanx, but the purchase of such a wire is not good and rotation of the fragment and movement along the pin often causes loss of reduction. In such a situation the fragment is held by 2/0 monofilament stainless steel wire passed through two holes drilled in the fragment with a 0·028 in Kirschner wire. The corresponding holes in the middle phalanx can be placed in two situations, either laterally on each side of the finger, or dorsally. The latter is more difficult to achieve and carries some risk of breaking off a further cortical fragment but has the advantage that the wires when passed can be twisted on each other like the intraosseous wiring employed in facial fracture fixation. This applies compression, speeding union. The ends of the wire can then be turned into a third hole in the cortex, thus burying it permanently beneath the skin. Employing this method motion has been permitted as early as 10 days after operation with good results. Using the more orthodox technique, the K-pin is removed at 4 weeks, motion commenced and the laterally situated wires removed 2 weeks later.

When rupture close to the insertion precludes simple repair, a marginal weaving suture along the central slip is used. A 3/0 or 4/0 non-absorbable synthetic suture on a curved needle is employed. Two holes are then drilled in the dorsal lip of the base of the middle phalanx 5–8 mm apart passing volarwards, distally and towards the midline to converge. Using a hypodermic needle which has been bent to shape the suture is passed from one hole to the other and tied down, thereby relocating the central slip. The joint should be transfixed with an 0·035 in Kirschner wire.

Complicated cases

Motion in the proximal interphalangeal joint is so much more important to hand function than movement at the distal joint that greater effort should be made to avoid arthrodesis. Where extensor tendon injury is accompanied by multiple articular fractures therefore, these should be reduced and fixed as best as possible and extensor tendon repair or reconstruction performed. Where skin cover has been lost, the same considerations apply and reconstruction of the extensor apparatus should be attempted.

Reconstruction

If the patient has a fixed deformity when seen, then attempts should be made to stretch out the contracture with dynamic splinting in the form of a Capener splint during the day and a joint jack at night. If the contracture persists then capsulectomy is necessary at the time of reconstruction.

Primary or secondary reconstruction of the central slip to correct a boutonnière deformity is one of the procedures in hand surgery in which it is most difficult to achieve consistent success. This fact is attested to by the multiplicity of procedures described in the literature [83]. These include advancement of the central slip [85], dorsal plication of the lateral bands [86, 87], transposition of the lateral bands [88], replacement of the central slip with the flexor digitorum superficialis passed through the middle phalanx [89] or with a lateral band retrieved from an adjacent finger [90], the use of a

distally based flap of central slip [91] and free tendon grafting [92] as described above for reconstructing a mallet finger. In all, the difficulty lies in adjusting the tension of the reconstruction in such a way as to give maximum extension while not losing full flexion [93]. The relative importance of flexion and extension differs according to digit and occupation. Full flexion of the index finger, while desirable, is not as important as full extension. The converse becomes more true as one progresses ulnarwards across the digits.

Whatever method is adopted, removal of fixation should be followed by the use of dynamic splintage which assists extension while permitting flexion. Regular measurements of joint range should be made and the splint retained until its removal causes no increase in extensor lag.

Where there is extensive scarring around the proximal interphalangeal joint due either to the original injury or to several attempts at correction and if the passive range is acceptable, correction of the boutonnière deformity may be most simply achieved by tenotomy of the conjoined tendon at the distal joint [94], taking care to preserve the oblique retinacular ligaments.

The extensors proximal to the metacarpophalangeal joint

Multiple lacerations

Division of single tendons at sites other than those which result in mallet finger and boutonnière deformities present no difficulties, good results following repair with non-absorbable synthetic sutures. The number of tendons which will be found at the wrist is quite unpredictable [95]. The author has encountered as few as five and as many as fourteen finger extensors. When several have been lacerated, some problem in matching ends may present. However, the angle of the cuts are usually dissimilar and, as no two tendons are of identical size or shape, will ensure correct approximation. Where the laceration has occurred beneath the extensor retinaculum, this should be repaired, for ugly bowstringing on wrist extension and painful dislocation on pronation and supination may otherwise result. After any extensor tendon repair the hand should be splinted for 4 weeks with the wrist in full extension and the metacarpophalangeal joints in like flexion. Thus the straight fingers are parallel to the forearm.

Reconstruction

Where repair has not been undertaken within the first three weeks after injury or where abrasion, burns or debridement have resulted in loss of sections of the extensors, there are three possibilities available for reconstruction.

(1) Attaching the distal end to an intact digital extensor.

(2) Tendon graft

(3) Tendon transfer

As a general rule, one digital motor can extend two fingers with acceptable efficiency. It is desirable, however, that the index finger and thumb are capable of independent extension. It follows therefore that loss of extension of any one of the ulnar three fingers can be corrected by weaving the distal end into one of its intact neighbours. Loss of two ulnar extensors requires reconstruction by transfer or graft. If either the extensor indicis or the extensor digit minimi remains intact and the tendon to that digit from extensor digitorum is also unharmed, then transfer is preferable. If the proximal end of the cut tendon lies proximal to the wrist and has done so for more than 6 weeks, it can be assumed to have lost its motor power, and a transfer is preferable.

Tendon graft

The following pre-requisites are necessary for a tendon graft when this is indicated:

(1) Stable union of all associated fractures.

(2) Full passive range of motion in the joints on which the graft is to act.

(3) The provision of a scar-free bed with stable, mobile skin cover. Any of the following tendon sources may be used in the order of preference: palmaris longus, plantaris, extensor digitorum longus of toes, 2, 3 or 4 or fascia lata.

The damaged tendon ends should be exposed through separate incisions, the path for the graft being prepared by tunnelling with a blunt-nosed instrument. The proximal tendon end should be grasped with tissue forceps and steady traction applied for some ten minutes to overcome any shortening. The graft is woven through both ends of the tendon for it is the strongest of all repairs. 4/0 non-absorbable synthetic figure-of-eight sutures are placed one on either side of each of three weaves, each bite taking both the edge of the slit through which the tendon was passed, and the tendon itself. All free tendon ends should be buried within the tendon. The tension is judged by adjusting the position of the wrist. Wrist flexion should produce balanced finger extension with the metacarpophalangeal joints held at neutral. Extension of the wrist should permit full flexion of the fingers. All extensor repairs, excepting under the retinaculum, should be splinted for four weeks postoperatively with the wrist dorsiflexed and the metacarpophalangeal joints flexed to a degree which brings the extended fingers in line with the forearm to limit the likelihood of contracture of the collateral ligaments.

Tendon transfer

In selecting the tendon to be transferred, certain well-established rules should be observed (see Chapter 35).

The tendons commonly selected for transfer to digital extensors are: extensor indicis proprius, extensor digiti minimi, flexor carpi radialis, flexor carpi ulnaris, flexor digitorum superficialis of ring and middle and palmaris longus.

When both tendons of extensor digiti minimi are used, adequate extension of the small finger by the extensor digitorum must be assured. The intertendinous connection from the ring finger, which invariably represents the contribution of extensor digitorum to the small finger, should be inspected. If it is short and broad its extensor action will be relatively weak. It should then be split off the ring tendon and shortened sufficiently to give balanced extension. Although flexor carpi ulnaris and flexor digitorum superficialis are not synergistic with the finger extensors they provide good transfers provided early training is given. The two superficialis tendons, passed around the ulna or through the interosseous membrane are employed when all five digits require motors, one being taken to the thumb and index extensors, the other to those of the middle, ring and small fingers.

The tension of transfers to the fingers should be

judged in the same fashion as previously described. By contrast, transfers to the extensor pollicis longus require

to be made under greater tension as the only problem seen with such a transfer is weakness of thumb extension.

REFERENCES

[1] MATTHEWS, P. AND RICHARDS, H. The repair reaction of flexor tendon within the digital sheath. *The Hand*, 1975, **7**, 27.

[2] ELLIOT, D. H. Structure and function of mammalian tendon. *Biological Reviews*, 1965, **40**, 392.

[3] ENNA, C. D. AND DYER, R. F. Tendon plasticity—a property applicable to reconstructive surgery of the hand. *The Hand*, 1976, **8**, 118.

[4] WILSON, W. F. AND HUESTON, J. T. The intratendinous architect of the tendons of Flexor digitorium profundus and Flexor pollicis longus. *The Hand*, 1973, **5**, 33.

[5] SHREWSBURY, M. M. AND KUCZYNSKI, K. Flexor digitorum superficialis tendon in the fingers of the human hand. *The Hand*, 1974, **6**, 121.

[6] BROCKIS, J. S. Blood supply of the flexor and extensor tendons of the fingers in man. *Journal of Bone and Joint Surgery*, 1953, **35B**, 131.

[7] LUNDBORG, G., MYRHAGE, R. AND RYDEVIK, B. The vascularization of human flexor tendons within the digital synovial sheath region—structural and functional aspects. *The Journal of Hand Surgery*, 1977, **6**, 417.

[8] PEACOCK, E. E. JR. A study of circulation in the normal tendon and healing grafts. *Annals of Surgery*, 1959, **149**, 415.

[9] LUNDBORG, G. The microcirculation in rabbit tendon. In vivo studies after mobilisation and transection. *The Hand*, 1975, **7**, 1.

[10] POTENZA, A. D. Tendon healing within the flexor digital sheath in the dog. An experimental study. *Journal of Bone and Joint Surgery*, 1962, **44A**, 49.

[11] POTENZA, A. D. Prevention of adhesions to healing digital flexor tendons. *Journal of the American Medical Association*, 1964, **187**, 187.

[12] POTENZA, A. D. The healing of autogenous tendon grafts within the flexor digital sheath in dogs. *Journal of Bone and Joint Surgery*, 1964, **46A**, 1462.

[13] LINDSAY, W. K. The fibroblast in flexor tendon healing. In Proceedings of the American Society for Surgery of the Hand. *Journal of Bone and Joint Surgery*, 1964, **46A**, 909.

[14] LINDSAY, W. K. Tendon Healing—A Continuing Experimental Approach Prepared for edition of the *Monographies du Groupe d'Etude de la Main*, Paris, 1970.

[15] MAYER, L. The physiological method of tendon transplantation. *Surgery, Gynecology and Obstetrics with International Abstracts of Surgery*, 1916, **22**, 298.

[16] MAYER, L. AND RANSOHOFF, N. Reconstruction of the digital tendon sheath. *Journal of Bone and Joint Surgery*, 1936, **18**, 607.

[17] PEACOCK, E. E. Some problems in flexor-tendon healing. *Surgery*, 1959, **45**, 415.

[18] PEACOCK, E. E. Tendon repair. Some aspects of wound healing affecting restoration of gliding function. *Journal of Bone and Joint Surgery*, 1964, **46A**, 909.

[19] VERDAN, C. E. Primary repair of flexor tendons. *Journal of Bone and Joint Surgery*, 1960, **42A**, 631.

[20] SMITH, J. W. AND CONWAY, H. La dynamique du glissement du tendons normaux et graffes. *Revue de Clinique Orthopedique*, 1966, **52**, 185.

[21] VAN DER MUELEN, J. S. Healing and repair of tendons. *The Hand*, 1969, **1**, 108.

[22] MASON, M. L. AND ALLEN, H. S. The rate of healing of tendons. An experimental study of tensile strength. *Annals of Surgery*, 1941, **13**, 424.

[23] LUNDBORG, G. Experimental flexor tendon healing, without adhesion formation—a new concept of tendon nutrition and intrinsic healing mechanisms. *The Hand*, 1976, **8**, 235.

[24] MATTHEWS, P. AND RICHARDS, H. The repair potential of digital flexor tendons. *Journal of Bone and Joint Surgery*, 1974, **56B**, 618.

[25] RICHARDS, H. J. Hunterian lecture. *Annals of the Royal College of Surgeons of England*, 1975.

[26] BUNNELL, S. *Surgery of the Hand*, 5th ed., Philadelphia, J. B. Lippincott, 1956.

[27] BOYES, J. H. Flexor-tendon grafts in the fingers and thumb. An evaluation of end results. *Journal of Bone and Joint Surgery*, 1950, **32A**, 489.

[28] COLVILLE, J. Tendon graft function. *The Hand*, 1973, **5**, 152.

[29] PULVERTAFT, R. G. Repair of tendon injuries of the hand. *Annals of the Royal College of Surgeons of England*, 1948, **3**, 3.

[30] PULVERTAFT, R. G. Tendon grafts for flexor tendon injuries in the fingers and thumb. A study of technique and results. *Journal of Bone and Joint Surgery*, 1956, **36B**, 175.

[31] PULVERTAFT, R. G. Flexor tendon grafting, p. 297. In, Flynn: *Hand Surgery*, Baltimore, Williams and Wilkins, 1966.

[32] TUBIANA, R. Technique of flexor tendon grafts. *The Hand*, 1959, **1**, 108.

[33] BOLTON, H. The problem of the primary tendon repair. *The Proceedings of the Second Hand Club*, p. 54–55. British Society for Surgery of the Hand, 1975.

[34] KLEINERT, H. L. AND STORMO, A. Primary repair of flexor tendons. Orthopedic Clinics of North America, 1973, **4**, 865.

[35] KLEINERT, H. L. Symposium on tendon surgery in the hand, p. 91. American Academy of Orthopedic Surgeons. Philadelphia, C. V. Mosby. 1975.

[36] LISTER, G. D., KLEINERT, H. E., KUTZ, J. E. AND ATASOY, E. Immediate controlled mobilisation following primary flexor tendon repair. *The Journal of Hand Surgery*,

[37] VERDAN, C. E. Half a century of flexor tendon surgery. Current status and changing philosophies. *Journal of Bone and Joint Surgery*, 1972, **54A**, 472.

[38] GONZALEZ, R. I. The blood supply of tendons with injury and repair (discussion). *Journal of Bone and Joint Surgery*, 1965, **47A**, 631.

[39] PEACOCK, E. E. A study of the circulation in normal tendons and healing grafts. *Annals of Surgery*, 1959, **149**, 415.

[40] SMITH, J. W. The blood supply of tendons with injury and repair. In Proceedings of the American Society for Surgery of the Hand. *Journal of Bone and Joint Surgery*, 1965, **47A**, 631.

[41] SMITH, J. W. Blood supply of tendons. *American Journal of Surgery*, 1965, **109**, 272.

[42] KESSLER, I. The 'grasping' technique for tendon repair. *The Hand*, 1973; **5**, 253.

[43] TSUGE, K., YOSHIKAZIN, I. AND MATSUSHI, Y. Intra-tendinous tendon suture in the hand. *The Hand*, 1975, **7**, 250.

[44] SALVI, V. Delayed primary suture in flexor tendon division. *The Hand*, 1971, **3**, 181.

[45] BRUNER, J. M. The zig-zag volar-digital incision for flexor tendon surgery. *Plastic and Reconstructive Surgery*, 1967, **40**, 571.

[46] BRAND, P. Principles of free tendon grafting including a new method of tendon suture. *Journal of Bone and Joint Surgery*, 1959, **41B**, 208.

[47] FETROW, K. O. Tenolysis in the hand and wrist. A clinical evaluation of two hundred and twenty flexor and extensor tenolyses. *Journal of Bone and Joint Surgery*, 1967, **49A**, 667.

[48] JAMES, J. I. P. The value of tenolysis. *The Hand*, 1969, **1**, 118.

[49] BASSETT, C. A. L. AND CARROLL, R. E. Formation of tendon sheath by silicon-rod implants. *Journal of Bone and Joint Surgery*, 1963, **45A**, 884.

[50] HELAL, B. Silastics in tendon surgery. *The Hand*, 1969, **1**, 120.

[51] HUNTER, J. Artificial tendons—early development and application. *American Journal of Surgery*, 1965, **109**, 325.

[52] HUNTER, J. M. Artificial tendons. *Journal of Bone and Joint Surgery*, 1965, **47A**, 631.

[53] LEONARD, A. G. AND DICKIE, W. R. Observations on the use of silicone rubber spacers in tendon graft surgery. *The Hand*, 1976, **8**, 66.

[54] HUNTER, J. M. AND SALISBURY, R. E. Use of gliding artificial implants to produce tendon sheaths. Techniques and results in children. *Plastic and Reconstructive Surgery*, 1970, **45**, 564.

[55] RAYNER, C. R. W. The origin and nature of pseudo-synovium appearing around implanted silastic rods. *The Hand*, 1976, **8**, 101.

[56] URBANIAK, J. R., BRIGHT, D. S., GILL, L. H. AND GOLDNER, J. L. Vascularisation and the gliding mechanism of free flexor tendon grafts inserted by the silicone rod method. *Journal of Bone and Joint Surgery*, 1974, **56A**, 473.

[57] SARKIN, T. L. The plastic replacement of severed flexor tendons of the fingers. *Journal of Surgery*, 1956, **44**, 232.

[58] PEACOCK, E. E. Morphology of homologous and heterologous tendon grafts. *Surgery, Gynecology and Obstetrics with International Abstracts of Surgery*, 1959, **109**, 735.

[59] PEACOCK, E. E. Restoration of finger flexion with homologous composite tissue tendon grafts. *American Journal of Surgery*, 1969, **26**, 564.

[60] HUESTON, J. T., HUBBLE, B. AND RIGG, B. R. Homografts of the digital flexor tendon system. *Australian and New Zealand Journal of Surgery*, 1967, **36**, 269.

[61] REID, D. A. C. The isolated flexor digitorum profundus lesion. *The Hand*, 1969, **1**, 108.

[62] HONNER, R. The late management of the isolated lesion of the flexor digitorum profundus tendon. *The Hand*, 1975, **7**, 171.

[63] KAPLAN, E. B. Anatomy, injuries and treatment of the extensor apparatus of the hand and digits. *Clinical Orthopaedics and Related Research*, 1959, **13**, 24.

[64] TUBIANA, R. Surgical repair of the extensor apparatus of the fingers. *Surgical Clinics of North America*, 1968, **48**, 1015.

[65] KETTLEKAMP, D. B., FLATT, A. E. AND MOULDS, R. Traumatic dislocation of the long finger extensor tendon. A clinical, anatomical and biomechanical study. *Journal of Bone and Joint Surgery*, 1971, **53A**, 229.

[66] MASON, M. L. Rupture of tendons of the hand. With a study of the extensor tendon insertion in the fingers. *Surgery, Gynecology and Obstetrics*, 1930, **50**, 611.

[67] MAISELS, D. O. The middle slip or boutonnière deformity in burned hands. *British Journal of Plastic Surgery*, 1965, **18**, 117.

[68] KELLY, A. P. Primary tendon repairs. A study of 789 consecutive tendon severances. *Journal of Bone and Joint Surgery*, 1959, **41A**, 581.

[69] GREEN, D. P. AND ROWLAND, S. Chapter 6 in Rockwood and Green. *Fractures*, Vol. I. Philadelphia, J. B. Lippincott. 1972.

[70] MCFARLANE, R. M. AND HAMPOLE, M. K. Treatment of extensor tendon injuries of the hand. *Canadian Journal of Surgery*, 1973, **16**, 366.

[71] FOWLER, F. D. New splint for treatment of mallet finger. *Journal of the American Medical Association*, 1959, **170**, 945.

[72] SMILLIE, I. S. Mallet finger. *British Journal of Surgery*, 1937, **24**, 439.

[73] WILLIAMS, E. G. Treatment of mallet finger. *Canadian Medical Association Journal*, 1947, **57**, 582.

[74] LEWIN, P. A simple splint for baseball finger. *Journal of the American Medical Association*, 1925, **85**, 1059.

[75] BUNNELL, S. *Surgery of the Hand*. Philadelphia, J. B. Lippincott, 1944.

[76] BOYES, J. H. *Bunnell's Surgery of the Hand*, 5th Ed. Philadelphia, J. B. Lippincott, 1930.

[77] ABOUNA, J. M. AND BROWN, H. The treatment of mallet finger. *British Journal of Surgery*, 1968, **55**, 653.

[78] BROOKS, D. Splint for mallet fingers. *British Medical Journal*, 1964, **2**, 1238.

[79] MASON, M. L. Mallet finger. *Lancet*, 1954, **266**, 1220.

[80] STACK, H. G. Mallet finger. *The Hand*, 1969, **1**, 83.

[81] SOUTER, W. A. The problem of boutonnière deformity. *Clinical Orthopaedics and Related Research*, 1974, **104**, 116.

[82] MILFORD, L. The Hand. In *Campbell's Orthopaedics*, 5th Ed. St. Louis, C. V. Mosby, 1971.

[83] SOUTER, W. A. The boutonnière deformity. *Journal of Bone and Joint Surgery*, 1967, **49B**, 710.

[84] MCCUE, F. C. AND ABBOTT, J. L. The treatment of mallet finger and boutonnière deformities. *Virginia Medical Monthly*, 1967, **94**, 623.

[85] KILGORE, E. S. AND GRAHAM, W. P. Operative treatment of boutonnière deformity. *Surgery*, 1968, **64**, 999.

[86] LITTLER, J. W. AND EATON, R. G. Redistribution of forces in the correction of the boutonnière deformity. *Journal of Bone and Joint Surgery*, 1967, **49A**, 1267.

[87] SALVI, V. Technique for the buttonhole deformity. *The Hand*, 1969, **1**, 96.

[88] MATEV, I. Transposition of the lateral slips of the aponeurosis in treatment of long-standing 'boutonnière deformity' of the fingers. *British Journal of Plastic Surgery*, 1976, **57**, 455.

[89] STACK, H. G. Buttonhole deformity. *The Hand*, 1971, **3**, 152.

[90] SNOW, J. W. A method for reconstruction of the central slip of the extensor tendon of a finger. *Plastic and Reconstructive Surgery*, 1976, **57**, 455.

[91] SNOW, J. W. Use of a retrograde tendon flap in repairing a severed extensor in the PIP joint area. *Plastic and Reconstructive Surgery*, 1973, **51**, 555.

[92] NICHOLS, H. M. Repair of extensor tendon insertions in the fingers. *Journal of Bone and Joint Surgery*, 1951, **33A**, 836.

[93] HARRIS, C. AND RUTLEDGE, G. L. The functional anatomy of the extensor mechanism of the finger. *Journal of Bone and Joint Surgery*, 1972, **54A**, 713.

[94] DOLPHIN, J. A. Extensor tenotomy for chronic boutonnière deformity of the finger. *Journal of Bone and Joint Surgery*, 1965, **47A**, 161.

[95] SCHENCK, R. R. Variations of the extensor tendons of the fingers. *Journal of Bone and Joint Surgery*, 1964, **46A**, 103.

CHAPTER 12

The Cut Nerve

. . . it is important to realize that the peripheral nervous system is an extension of the central nervous system, that neither can function in absence of the other, and that together they are responsible for integrating all the activities of the body.'

G. J. Romanes in *Cunningham's Textbook of Anatomy*

ANATOMY

K. KUCZYNSKI

The peripheral nerves lie outside the brain and the spinal cord and consist of nerve fibres (axons with their cellular sheath) and their connective tissue coverings. The cell bodies of these axons may lie outside or within the central nervous system and by their central connections form one functional unit with the latter.

The structural unit of the nervous system is *the neurone,*

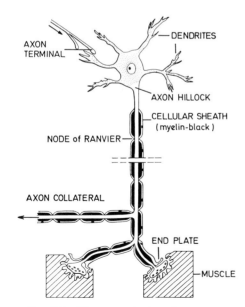

FIG. 12.1. Diagrammatic view of a neurone.

i.e. the nerve cell with its processes (Fig. 12.1). The cell body (perikaryon) and the dendrites contain Nissl substance but the axon does not. This substance contains ribose nucleic acid (RNA) which is concerned with the protein synthesis and may be transformed into a more active form during so-called 'chromatolysis' in the process of repair following injury. The axoplasm, surrounded by the cell membrane called axolemma, is in the form of a viscous fluid in which a bi-directional flow takes place. At the nodes of Ranvier the axons may give rise to the branches, i.e. collaterals (Fig. 12.1). This is why a motor cell may innervate 200 or more muscle fibres when only a relatively gross movement is required as in the large muscles of the limb; the number of the muscle fibres in a motor unit at the extremity of the limb is probably small. The number of axons present in any peripheral nerve is considerably in excess of what is required for normal function. Loss of a great percentage of axons is required before there is any significant deficit [1–3]. In clinical practice it is common to find hemitransection of a peripheral nerve or even subtotal division while distally there is clinical normality or only minimal neurological loss.

There are *two varieties of the nerve fibres* distinguished by the relative amount of myelin present in the cellular sheath. Those which have no compact myelin sheath are called *non-myelinated fibres* (Fig. 12.2) while those with a myelin layer are known as *myelinated fibres* (Fig. 12.3). Most of the peripheral nerves contain a mixture of both varieties. Both types of fibres are surrounded by a chain of Schwann cells arranged end to end. In the case of non-myelinated fibres, one Schwann cell may

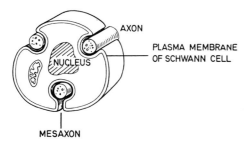

FIG. 12.2. Arrangement of the unmyelinated nerve fibres in relation to the Schwann cell and the mode of formation of the mesaxon.

accommodate parts of many axons, while in the mye-linated variety each axon is associated with only one Schwann cell at any one level. In the latter case, the membrane of the Schwann cell is wrapped spirally around the axon thus producing a sheath of alternating layers of lipid and protein, the myelin sheath [71].

Figure 12.3 shows in greater detail the organization of the myelinated fibre. The Schwann cells, separated from the endoneurial tube by a basement membrane, lie end to end meeting at the node of Ranvier where their finger-like processes interdigitate. There is a space between these processes which allows the extracellular ions to reach the axon, while the internodal part of the axon is insulated from these ions by the cellular sheath (Schwann cell and myelin sheath). This is important in saltatory propagation of the impulse from node to node.

The peripheral nerve trunks in the limbs are composed of motor, sensory and sympathetic nerve fibres enclosed in three connective tissue coats. On functional grounds the fibres are considered as either efferent or afferent. The efferent fibres are of three varieties: (1) large fibres to the extrafusal muscle fibres, (2) small fibres to the muscle spindles which alter their contraction and control their sensitivity, and (3) postganglionic sympathetic fibres (vasomotor, pilomotor and sudomotor). The afferent fibres consist of the peripheral processes of the sensory nerve cells of the spinal ganglia which are dis-tributed to the sensory endings.

Nerves to the muscles carry not only efferent fibres (α, γ and vasomotor) but also sensory fibres to the muscles and often also to the adjacent tendons, bones and joints. Cutaneous nerves are not exclusively sensory to the skin and subcutaneous tissue but also contain efferent sympathetic fibres. In some cases (e.g. the digital nerve) sensory fibres to the joints, ligaments and bones may also be present.

The nerve fibres are not distributed in a uniform pattern throughout the cross-section of the trunk but are collected into separate bundles called funiculi or fasciculi, invested with a cellular connective tissue sheath of peri-neurium. Usually these funiculi contain motor, sensory and sympathetic fibres but this is not always so. Each funiculus repeatedly divides and its branches unite with those of the other funiculi to form a plexus along the length of the nerve (Fig. 12.4). However, some parts of the plexus may remain as separate bundles for a considerable distance, particularly in the distal part of

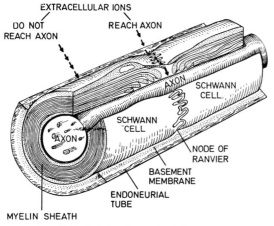

FIG. 12.3. Details of a myelinated nerve fibre.

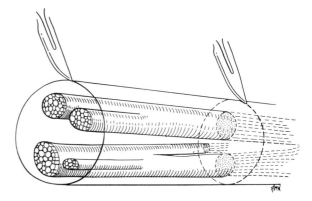

FIG. 12.4. The exchange of fibres in the funicular plexus and difference in the pattern of two cross-sections.

the limb. This results in rapid changes in the funicular pattern and in variation in size and content of the funiculi at different levels. It should be remembered that the funicular pattern is subject to such a wide range of variation that its precise arrangement can be only established at the time of operation. Anatomical textbooks refer to the usual distribution of the peripheral nerve supply in the upper limb.

In clinical practice there is considerable variation and anomalies of motor and sensory distribution are extremely common. Variation in the true autonomous zones of each of the major nerves is considerable [1, 4–8].

These factors must be borne in mind during examination following suspected nerve injury and are of importance during subsequent surgery. In addition, it is believed that interconnections may be present between the main nerves in the forearm [1, 9–11] which are almost certainly responsible in part for the relatively small intrinsic loss which may follow complete division of one or other of these nerves.

The connective tissue of the peripheral nerve trunk is made up of three layers. *Epineurium* consists of areolar connective tissue which separates the funiculi and is condensed on the surface of the nerve trunk to form an investing layer (Fig. 12.5). This layer is only loosely attached to the surrounding structures and thus the nerve enjoys considerable mobility except in those areas where the branches are given off and where the nutrient arteries enter the trunk. *Perineurium* invests each funiculus of nerve fibres. It is a relatively thin but dense multilayered sheath of fibrous tissue containing a compact network of collagen and elastic fibres (Fig. 12.5). These fibres are arranged in 6–12 concentric laminae separated by clefts lined by mesothelial cells (perineurial spaces). The inner layer of perineurium forms a membrane composed of one or two layers of flattened cells, which is called perilemma which is of critical importance in maintaining function in the intact peripheral nerve. Damage to this layer determines the degree of dysfunction which may follow injury of all types including stretching injuries, division, and perhaps even ischaemia. There is some evidence suggesting that the intrafunicular contents communicate with the subarachnoid space via mesothelial clefts. The perineurium is considered to be a diffusion barrier, is thought to maintain the intrafunicular pressure, to provide mechanical protection against stretching and to be resistant to infection. *Endoneurium* is the connective tissue inside the

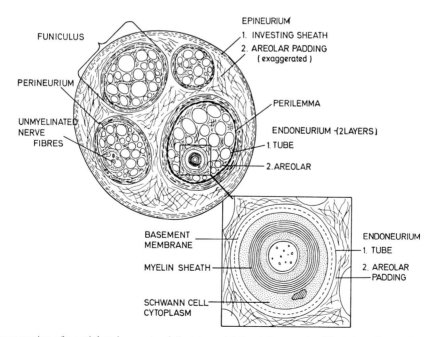

FIG. 12.5. Cross-section of a peripheral nerve trunk (not to scale). Inset shows a simplified view of a myelinated nerve fibre.

funiculus. Immediately outside each nerve fibre the collagen is organized to form a thin limiting membrane which is called endoneurial tube. It contains the Schwann cell, the myelin sheath in myelinated fibres, and the axon.

Vascular supply

With the exception of the median artery, the blood vessels of the peripheral nerve trunks of the upper limb consist of numerous small neutrient vessels providing a very good blood supply. Arteriae nervorum enter the nerve and do not leave it, terminating intraneurally. The number and size of these small arteries are variable from subject to subject and even on the two sides of the same individual. In some regions a nerve may not receive a nutrient artery for a considerable distance, the circulation being maintained by the intraneural vessels, e.g. median nerve between the axilla and elbow. The nutrient arteries divide into anastomotic branches at some distance from the nerve trunk (Fig. 12.6) and it is important to ligate these vessels as far from the nerve as possible in order to preserve their anastomosis. From the nutrient arteries an intraneural vascular net is formed which extends the length of the nerve so that a nerve can be mobilized or freed over fairly long areas without detriment to the blood supply. There are four longitudinal systems recognized in this framework: (1) surface chains, (2) interfunicular chains, (3) perineurial channels and (4) intrafunicular capillary net. The venous system corresponds to the arterial arrangement. Lymphatic vessels are limited to the epineurial tissues.

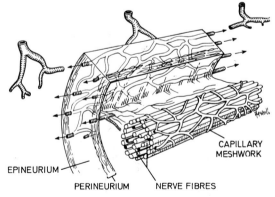

FIG. 12.6. The blood supply of the peripheral nerve trunk. After Bateman.

Afferent nerve endings in the hand consist of (1) cutaneous group (touch, pressure, pain, vibration, warmth and cold), and (2) proprioceptive group found in striated muscle, tendons, ligaments and joints, which provides automatic feedback to the central nervous system.

Stimulation of the cutaneous receptors evokes a complex response with spatial and temporal summation of impulses from many different endings. An axon of a peripheral sensory neurone may end in several receptors while one receptor may be supplied by many nerve fibres. Information from the periphery is thus scrambled and has to be sorted out by central activity.

Some endings adapt rapidly to a sustained stimulus and become silent while others continue to discharge and are called slowly adapting.

The nerve fibres reach the cutaneous receptors by piercing the deep fascia and entering into formation of the subcutaneous plexus of vessels and nerves. From there the fibres gain the dermal nerve plexus where they intermingle with the sympathetic fibres. From this plexus fibres run into papillary layer of the dermis to form the subepidermal plexus from which axons continue to a great variety of receptors.

Cutaneous receptors

Only most characteristic are given.

(1) Meissner's corpuscles (Fig. 12.7a) are most numerous ($50/mm^2$) in the palmar aspect of the digital skin. An outer connective tissue capsule contains horizontally stacked laminar cells which are interleaved with terminal nerve branches derived from several axons. They are rapidly adapting and probably report movement and vibration.

(2) Pacinian corpuscles (Fig. 12.7b) are rapidly adapting too and are thought to be concerned with vibration. They are abundant in deep structures such as joints, tendons, periosteum, dermis and subcutaneous tissue. Again they are most numerous in the digits. A single axon enters the base of the corpuscle and becomes surrounded by the cells of the inner bulb. The outer bulb consists of a series of concentric lamellae.

(3) Merkel's discs (Fig. 12.7c) are probably concerned with tactile sensibility and pressure. They are slow adapting. They are found in the deep layers of epidermis, closely applied to clear, spherical epidermal cells; they can be regarded as expanded nerve terminals.

CAPILLARY MESHWORK

EPINEURIUM

PERINEURIUM   NERVE FIBRES

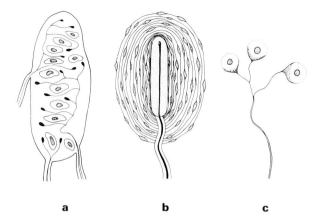

FIG. 12.7. (a) Meissner's corpuscle showing axons entering the capsule and running between the lamellar cells. (b) Pacinian corpuscle showing the axon terminal surrounded by concentric lamellae. (c) Merkel's endings showing disc-shaped terminals applied to epidermal cells. Not to scale.

(4) Nerve endings embedded in the external root hair sheath, which are rapidly adapting and probably subserve touch and vibration.

(5) Dermal plexus, intermingled with sympathetic fibres and those fibres which are destined for the free endings in the epidermis. Some are slowly some rapidly adapting and are thought to be concerned with deep pressure, pain and temperature. There is extensive overlap in their distribution.

Proprioceptive receptors

Coordinated activity of the muscles of the hand relies on the information fed to the central nervous system from the following afferent receptors:

(1) Free endings in the connective tissue sheaths and round individual muscle fibres.

(2) Pacinian corpuscles in the deep fascia and aponeuroses.

(3) Muscle spindles, which are numerous in the hand and which report on the extent and rate of stretching of the muscle.

(4) Tendon organs which are terminals of nerve fibres found amongst the collagen fibres of the bundles of tendon.

(5) Joint receptors.

ELECTROPHYSIOLOGICAL TECHNIQUES

K. KUCZYNSKI

Stimulation of sensory receptors and nerve fibres results in movements of ions across the nerve cell membrane which are associated with a change in the local electrical potential. This change is called an *action potential* and is transmitted along the axon. In unmyelinated fibres the conduction is continuous and uniform, and at much slower velocity than in myelinated fibres in which the conduction is saltatory, the action potential jumping from one node of Ranvier to the next one.

The conduction velocity is related to the size of the fibre and the internodal distance, and can range from less than 2 to more than 100 m/sec.

Recording of the action potential of a single nerve fibre presents considerable technical difficulties and in clinical practice use has been made of a *compound action potential* (CAP), i.e. the total potential recorded from the nerve trunk and resulting from excitation of its constituent fibres by an electrical stimulus (Fig. 12.8).

The action potential passing along a nerve trunk provides a considerable amount of information about the nerve condition. Recent electrophysiological techniques provide objective means of functional assessment of the peripheral nerves and may lead to a profound influence on the degree and quality of the functional recovery following a nerve repair [12]. These techniques show whether the potential is present or absent, whether it is of a smaller amplitude (measured in millivolts) when compared with that of a normal fibre, whether the conduction velocity is lower than normal and if there is considerable change in the shape of its wave.

Accurate localisation of any nerve damage and its extent to the actual area of failed conduction as defined by the *absence of CAP*, is of importance as this may

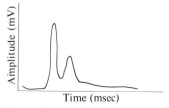

FIG. 12.8. Recording of a compound action potential.

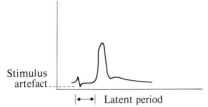

Stimulus artefact

|←→| Latent period

FIG. 12.9. Latency of compound action potential.

indicate the scope and possible benefit of surgical intervention, e.g. in neurolysis or decompression.

The amplitude of the CAP, as compared with the normal, gives information about the *functional state of the axons*, particularly when combined with the information regarding the *conduction velocity*, which normally depends on the diameter of the fibres, being slowest in the small ones. The speed of conduction can be calculated from the *latency* of the CAP (Fig. 12.9), which is the interval between the stimulus and the onset of the action potential, the distance between the site of the stimulus and recording point being known. The speed can also be measured by comparing responses to a stimulus recorded from two different sites; the time taken by the nerve impulse to travel between the two recording sites and the distance separating them, are used to calculate the conduction velocity. *Diseased or regenerating axons* can be identified by their lower speed of conduction.

The shape of the CAP wave normally has a smooth outline and shows two or three peaks (Fig. 12.8). *The diseased nerve* may have an *irregular outline, broadening of the CAP* and its *transformation into multiple peaks* as the potentials of the still active individual fibres become separate in time and cannot combine to produce the compound potential.

Clinical uses of compound action potentials

Study of motor function is usually carried out in conjunction with electromyography. Stimulation of the median and ulnar nerves through the skin and recording response by EMG can be used to obtain information on conduction velocity, number of active fibres and synchronization of the action potentials; this may help in differentiation of nerve disease from muscle pathology.

Study of sensory function can be carried out by percu-

taneous recording of the median and ulnar nerves at the wrist, stimulating ring electrodes applied around the digits. This technique may be used also to monitor regeneration in these nerves.

Assessment at operation of nerve damage. The CAP provides better information with regard to function and the precise site of injury than the external appearance of the nerve. Application of this technique to *neuromas in continuity* allows for a decision whether neurolysis would be sufficient or resection and suture is required. Recently single fascicular recordings have been used for this purpose [13]. Electrophysiological techniques are also used to map out the *intraneural disposition of fasciculi* and to differentiate between motor and sensory ones by stimulation of the distal stump and recording the motor response, while stimulation of the proximal stump causes subjective response from the patient thus identifying the fascicle as sensory [14].

PHYSIOLOGY
W. M. McQUILLAN

The physiology of cutaneous sensibility is complex and no general agreement exists. The specific theory of Müller [15], the concepts of von Frey [16], the writings of Head [17], and more recently the pattern theory [18] all have their devotees. The complexity of the phenomenon of normal cutaneous sensibility, however, is all too often rather glossed over with the somewhat simplistic concept referred to by Sinclair as that 'rigid Victorian concept of the nervous system, likened to a telephone exchange' [18]. The belief that specific nerve endings subserve specific functions still lingers on in the minds of many surgeons. From this belief stems the concept that the more accurately nerves or fascicles are co-apted the greater will be the quantity and quality of successful re-innervation of distal endoneural tubes.

This may be so, but the fundamental changes which lead to recovery of nerve function may not be based upon such factors, and the concept that improved results will accrue from more complex surgery is unsupported by evidence. The weight of evidence demands that the basic biological processes although not fully understood be given due consideration. Much research is required, e.g. are nerve endings reinnervated or regenerated *de novo*?

Restoration of motor function after nerve repair relies upon the establishment of new pathways either by the functional take-over of pathways which are anatomically present but functionally dormant or alternatively by axonal regeneration establishing new motor function. Trick movements are common, and may fool all but the most experienced. The ratio of axon to motor unit innervation is important in determining the prognosis. In relatively unimportant motor function, e.g. wrist extension, finger extension, the ratio of axon to motor unit is extremely low [1]. In the intrinsic muscles of the hand this ratio is very much higher and hence the quality of regeneration which is required to restore intrinsic function in the hand must be very much greater than that required to restore wrist extension after section of the radial nerve [4, 19–21]. Although it is possible that establishment of a reconnection to pre-existing motor endplates does occur the fundamental basis of motor regeneration may consist in the formation of new motor endplates [22].

The rate of regeneration following nerve division is commonly given as 1 mm/day or 1 in/month [3].

These figures are very approximate and do not obtain when the injury is part of a serious wound, when recovery may be very much slower. In children and young adults the rate of recovery may be accelerated. There is some evidence that increased temperature of the affected part may result in increased rate of regeneration [23, 24]. Where extensive mobilization is required to achieve nerve repair, e.g. anterior transposition to facilitate ulnar nerve repair, the rate of motor recovery is much slower.

Restoration of sensation

The best clinical model for studying return of cutaneous sensibility is the clean transection of the median nerve in the forearm. Following successful repair there is a latent period during which there are no significant clinical changes.

After 2–3 weeks the patient often begins to experience painful paraesthesia radiating into the median nerve distribution, while as soon as six weeks after successful surgery the patient experiences painful paraesthesiae in the fingers. Delayed conduction is obvious by a visible delay between stimulation with a pin prick and the patient's response. The patient finds this to be an un-pleasant experience but in the early stages cannot localize it [25].

This is akin to the protopathic level of response described by earlier writers [26–28]. In time the quality of sensory recovery improves, first an awareness of pin prick, then sensibility becomes more acute with accurate localization developing. Crude restoration of temperature awareness occurs next [29] while last of all comes the ability to differentiate between shape, size and texture [30].

Following successful median nerve repair improvement in the quality of sensory recovery often continues for some 2–3 years after injury [31, 32] and in good quality sensory recovery tactile appreciation is clear. To improve the usefulness of the hand sensory retraining [33] is vital. The central connections of sensory nerves are often not given sufficient thought nor is retraining of the awareness of cutaneous sensibility, a routine part of rehabilitation following nerve injuries. Recent studies suggest that this is a most important part of rehabilitation following nerve injury where cutaneous sensibility is an important function [34]. Vibro-tactile sensibility is an important technique which gives a more accurate measure of sensory loss and may lead to a better understanding of the value of different methods of repair [32–35].

NERVE DIVISION

W. M. McQUILLAN

The results of repair of divided nerves are at best imperfect, and frequently disappointing. It is right that new methods should be tried, and research pursued to find improved techniques.

In this biomechanical age the emphasis is too often on the mechanical without sufficient understanding of the biological. Surgical training and practice tend to encourage a mechanistic and occasionally simplistic approach to the problems resulting from injury. Such an attitude may have some relevance in the management of fractures but may lead to serious failure of understanding when applied to the problem of the divided peripheral nerve. Peripheral nerves are highly complex structures with considerable physiological resilience but are readily damaged by injury and by chemical change.

The effects of nerve division

Pathological changes in the nerve

At the site of injury there is haemorrhage, the extent of which is dependent on a number of factors, not least the size of the longitudinal blood supply of the individual nerve. The median artery can be of some size [36] and the haemorrhage can be considerable. In addition to haemorrhagic changes within the nerve, proximal and distal damage can be extensive particularly when the nerve has been subjected to stretching or to severe violence, e.g. in gun shot wounds [37–43]. Following complete division, retraction of the nerve ends always takes place resulting in the formation of a gap.

In all degenerative nerve lesions certain changes occur. Even in injuries associated with minimal tissue damage there is always damage to the nerve on both sides of division. Within the nerve there is degeneration of the individual axons, degradation of myelin and the invasion of the distal nerve by round cells and macrophages. Proliferation of fibroblasts and Schwann cells begins within a few days [43–46] and the axon distal to the site of injury rapidly undergoes Wallerian degeneration [47, 48]. Proximally some axonal degeneration takes place, which may be minimal in clean transections and extend only as far as the first node of Ranvier. Where the violence of the injury has been more severe the degeneration proximally may extend for many centimetres.

In addition to these changes within the nerve fibres, there are always changes within the cell body [49, 50]. Cell death may occur with loss of mitochondria in the nerve cell body, but more frequently chromatolysis is seen which may be an index of the increased metabolic demands following axonal degeneration distally. In addition to changes within the cell body there may be changes within other neurones which have synaptic connections with the parent cell [51, 52].

Following injury the inevitable inflammatory response produces hyperaemia, exudation and cellular migration. There is fibroblastic activity, round cell invasion while macrophages are also in evidence. The Schwann cell may act as a macrophage but Schwann proliferation is the more common response [47, 53]. The combined effects of these changes is to produce dissolution of the gross architecture of the nerve proximally and distally from the site of the nerve division (Fig. 12.10). This affects the connective tissue of the nerve but more importantly the inner layer of the neuroectoderm, the perilemma is also affected.

At the site of division an area of considerable cellularity develops in which there are no natural anatomical barriers. In clinical practice nerve division rarely occurs in isolation, and the common injuries also produce damage to muscle or tendon. The body

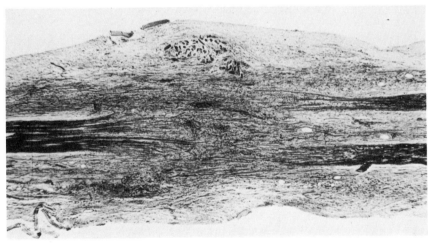

Fig. 12.10. Experimental nerve division in the intercostal nerve of the sheep. This nerve was exposed atraumatically, divided with a scalpel and resutured *in situ*. The dissolution of the nerve architecture is clearly seen.

response to tendon or muscle damage is an intensive proliferative fibroblastic reaction in which the paratenon [54] and the epineurium are involved. This response is almost certainly mediated by humoral factors [54, 55]. Thus when nerve and tendon injury co-exist proliferation of the fibroblasts within the structure of the nerve is inevitable.

In experiments on the median nerve of the rabbit studies were carried out to assess the degree of fibrosis and neuroma formation within a divided nerve, when the nerve injury was an isolated phenomenon and when it was part of a more complex injury [56]. In the first experiment the median nerve alone was divided cleanly. In half of the cases the nerve was isolated by silastic material (see p. 187). There were no significant histological differences between the two groups. In a second experiment muscle and tendon at the site of nerve division were also cleanly divided. In half of the cases, the nerve was isolated by silastic. Where nerve isolation was carried out, neuroma formation was minimal, but in the absence of isolation it was considerable. This suggests that a co-existence of muscle and tendon injury with nerve division results in a greater proliferation of the connective tissue within the nerve than occurs if nerve isolation is used or if the nerve injury is the only lesion. In clinical practice it is probably wise to separate 'in time' definitive surgery on tendon or muscle and on nerve. Nerve isolation (see p. 187) provides a useful technique to achieve this aim.

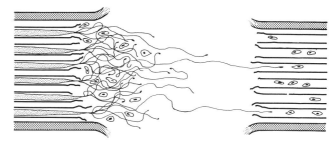

FIG. 12.11. Diagrammatic representation of regeneration in one nerve bundle.

upon chemotaxis than upon mechanical and anatomical factors alone [1, 2]. In laboratory animals nerve regeneration proceeds much more satisfactorily and successfully than in primates, and in some, e.g. the rodents, nerve regeneration may occur where a large gap has been created or where nerve ends are turned through 180° [57–60]. Thus, species difference has to be recognized [60] and in man regeneration will not occur unless the nerve ends are in close apposition. The factors which determine the distal route of a regenerating axon are, as far as is known entirely haphazard. Important factors in nerve regeneration are the degree and extent of tissue damage, the gap between the nerve ends, the amount of reaction which is created by the presence of foreign material while the oxygen tension at the site of injury may be of fundamental importance [61]. The quality of function is influenced also by the ultimate diameter achieved by the successful neurite.

Regeneration

For regeneration to occur certain important conditions must obtain. Firstly the proximal axons must be capable of sprouting or neurite formation (Fig. 12.11). Cell death is much more common in stretching injuries or avulsion injuries than in clean divisions. Where death of the cell body occurs regeneration is not possible. The mechanism of violence, therefore, is of importance in determining the prognosis (see p. 186). Neurite formation or axon sprouting normally begins 4–5 days after injury. The axon sprouts proceed in all directions and one may become invested by a Schwann cell [2, 4, 52, 53]. Continuous investment with Schwann cells may guide a neurite across into the distal neural tube, but the probability of this happening is thought to be based more

Prognosis after nerve injury

The nature of the pathological changes following the nerve lesion is of fundamental importance in prognosis. Nerve division has the poorest prognosis of all, and following division of a major nerve in an adult entirely normal function is seldom regained. A neurological deficit of some degree can usually be identified in children but the functional deficit may be small. Apart from the type of nerve injury, the factors which determine the quality of recovery are as follows:

Age of the patient

The younger the patient, the better the prognosis. In elderly patients it is often futile to embark upon prolonged surgery on the nerve, and other reconstructive procedures should be considered from the outset.

The severity of the injury

The priorities in the treatment of nerve injury relate to the severity of wounding, and in extensive wounds, high velocity gunshot wounds etc., primary attention to nerve division has a low priority. Limb viability, basic wound care and prevention of infection are the first considerations [62, 63]. In a high velocity wound nerves may be injured over a considerable length and the prognosis following repair is poor. Where the wounds are simple in type, i.e. transections with sharp instruments, the priority of the surgical treatment of the nerve injury becomes much higher. In civilian practice the commonest nerve injury is division of median and/or ulnar nerves in the forearm as a result of incised or lacerated wounds when nerve repair is given high priority.

The level of the lesion

The more distal the lesion the better the prognosis.

Type of nerve

Nerves have different prognoses according to their function and extent of distribution (see p. 31). In the upper limb the radial nerve has the best prognosis for repair, while the ulnar nerve has the poorest.

State of the injury

The presence of a gap between the nerve ends, tissue loss, wide retraction of the nerve ends, all affect the prognosis adversely. Closure of gaps in nerves either by lengthy nerve mobilization or by grafting invariably results in a poorer outcome than when the nerve can be repaired easily with one suture line.

Management of the divided nerve

The question as to whether divided nerves should be repaired primarily or secondarily has long been a subject of controversy [1, 4]. Until a prospective controlled surgical trial has been carried out this will remain an exercise in advocacy. The management of any particular case of nerve division must depend upon a number of factors.

The severity of the injury must be given primary consideration. Delay between the receipt of the wound and the person arriving for definitive treatment must not be excessive. In recent clean division the options are: (1) primary nerve repair, (2) secondary repair, or (3) delayed nerve repair using nerve isolation [56, 64–66].

Primary nerve repair

In the author's own case material the largest single group of failures are those on whom primary nerve repair has been carried out, often by relatively inexperienced surgeons. Many young surgeons, particularly those who have recently acquired a specialist qualification, cannot resist the temptation to suture a divided nerve which they find in an operative field. Indeed any suggestion that they should not do this is considered to be a slur on their technical competence. It is not. What one does suggest is to make a plea for recognition that regeneration is dependent upon the complex biological processes referred to above.

The disadvantages of primary nerve repair are as follows:

(1) The surgeon has no knowledge of the extent of the nerve injury proximal and distal to the site of division.

(2) The epineurium is tenuous and does not readily facilitate repair.

(3) The procedure is being carried out under adverse circumstances when wound infection is always a probable risk.

(4) Extensive exploration both proximal and distal to the site of injury is necessary to achieve satisfactory identification of the lesion. The haemorrhagic effects of the wounding make microscopically assisted nerve repair futile if one believes that fascicular suture is preferable to epineural repair.

Those who advise primary nerve repair often fail to understand that such repairs may be carried out by inexperienced surgeons through an incision which is inadequate for the purpose and whose surgery results in considerable additional tissue damage because of the amount of suture material which is inserted around and through the nerve structure. In distal lesions of major nerves, and in digital nerves, primary nerve repair is advised but only when the circumstances of operating conditions, experience and facilities are optimal.

Secondary nerve repair

It was formerly taught that secondary nerve repair always gave results superior to primary nerve repair [4]. The disadvantages are that the procedure is time consuming because of fibrosis and the changes proximal and distal to the site of division invariably result in considerable neuroma which must be resected. This produces a gap which can only be closed by mobilization of a nerve over a prolonged distance or by grafting. Despite the disadvantages it is the method of choice when nerve injury is part of a complex problem.

Nerve isolation

This technique is quite different from nerve wrapping. Nerve wrapping at the time of definitive repair has been attempted over the years and many materials suggested [67].

Nerve isolation obtains the best conditions for definitive nerve repair without the disadvantages of definitive primary repair or classical secondary suture. Silastic tubing* or an alternative is used to provide an investing sheath around the nerve at primary surgery of the wound. Secondary nerve repair is carried out when circumstances allow [63] and exploration is simple as the tissue changes at the site of nerve injury are minimal.

The concept of isolation of the peripheral nervous system from the musculoskeletal system has long been a subject of debate [68, 69]. This essentially simple method of producing isolation of a peripheral nerve from the associated environment has been found in practice to be a very simple adjunct and to have great value in dealing with nerve division. This method enables results which seem superior to those formerly obtained using ordinary primary or secondary nerve suture. Thus, in the author's opinion the indications for primary nerve repair are few, as follows.

(1) In children with recent clean nerve divisions as the biological responses influencing recovery are more advantageous than in older persons.

* Silastic tubing is distributed by Messrs Dow Corning in U.S.A. and elsewhere, and by Dunlop Precision Rubber—England.

(2) Self-inflicted wounds which form a considerable number of nerve divisions. Because of the psychiatric state, primary nerve repair with silastic isolation should be carried out. This does not preclude the possibility of definitive secondary nerve repair if no recovery has occurred within an acceptable period.

Technique of nerve repair

The nerve must be exposed by an incision sufficient to display normal nerve proximal and distal to the site of injury.

Epineural suture is the commonly employed method. Fine suture material is used (see p. 191). The site of nerve repair is mobilized so that the nerve ends can be brought together without tension. Healthy nerve is exposed on both sides by formal resection. Multiple incisions across the nerve should be avoided. Where possible one clean transection is best. Healthy nerve bundles 'pout'.

The nerve is orientated by lining up superficial vessels and matching its shape (most nerves are oval-shaped). Two lateral sutures are inserted and the nerve ends brought together as these stay sutures are tightened simultaneously and their ends are held in bulldog clamps. An anterior suture is inserted and the nerve rotated as the lateral sutures are passed to the contra-lateral side, one in front and the other behind. A posterior suture is then inserted.

When primary nerve repair is carried out the epineurium is tenuous—and it is tempting to insert many sutures, which is a mistake. Epineural repair is easiest when the epineurium has proliferated, i.e. in 2–3 weeks after injury.

Management of the patient

While controversy may continue as to the best techniques of nerve repair there is no argument that fundamental principles of patient management cannot be ignored.

Significant nerve injury produces paralysis and anaesthesia. All joints in the affected limb must be put regularly through a full passive range of movement. Development of contractures by failure to pay attention to this basic principle is a serious mistake.

Anaesthetic skin is readily injured and the loss of vaso-motor control makes the healing of burns and trophic ulcers somewhat protracted. Patients must always be instructed in the management of anaesthetic skin.

Individual nerves

The median nerve

The median nerve is the major sensory nerve of the upper limb and has been referred to as 'the eyes of the hand' [70]. Division of the median nerve above the elbow joint results in loss of flexion of the thumb, index and long fingers together with paralysis of the thenar muscles and anaesthesia of the radial side of the hand.

The median nerve is commonly injured in wounds of the forearm particularly where it becomes superficial in the distal third and is often accompanied by division of

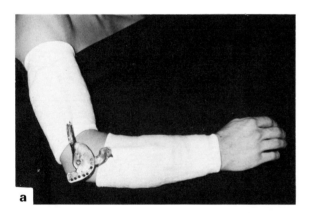

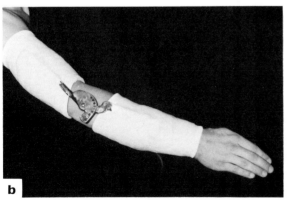

Fig. 12.12. A turnbuckle splint.

flexor tendons to the wrist and hand. Anomalies in distribution of the median nerve are common [1] (see Chap. 1). Variations in the motor supply to the thenar musculature have been described at length [8], and the surgeon must always be aware of the possibility of such variations. When nerve division is accompanied by tendon division, primary tendon repair, nerve isolation and delayed nerve suture offers the best prospect of a satisfactory result.

At the time of definitive nerve repair tension at the suture line can be avoided by flexion of the joint furthest from the site of division. In clinical practice flexion of the elbow joint is the best manoeuvre. In divisions in the distal forearm closure by flexion at the wrist often results in a traction lesion of the distal nerve when the joint is subsequently allowed into a neutral or extended position. In certain cases re-routing the nerve anterior to pronator teres may facilitate suture without tension.

In all cases where length has to be made up by elbow flexion, the joint should be slowly straightened using a turnbuckle splint (Fig. 12.12). Injuries in the forearm always result in proliferative changes in the paratenon and in the connective tissues generally which can produce nerve compression in the carpal tunnel. Decompression of the carpal tunnel is always indicated at the time of definitive repair of the distal portion.

The ulnar nerve

This provides the greater proportion of the intrinsic supply to the hand and its loss produces a significant functional deficit because of the lack of control at the metacarpophalangeal joints. This consists of loss of an adequate span of the hand both in extension and abduction of the fingers, and in gripping as the metacarpophalangeal joints hyperextend.

The results of repair of the ulnar nerve are disappointing and normal intrinsic recovery is achieved infrequently. Anterior transposition of the nerve at the elbow is frequently necessary in order to achieve satisfactory ulnar nerve repair, and should always be carried out if there is any tension in the ulnar nerve either above or below the elbow joint (see p. 405). The nerve should be transposed deep to the common flexor origins as superficial transposition results in a troublesome neuritis, and impairs functional recovery.

The radial nerve

The radial nerve has the best prognosis for repair and its loss is the easiest to substitute by tendon transfer (see p. 509) should motor recovery not take place. Its course in the upper arm may render direct suture difficult, particularly close to the spiral groove.

The nerve may branch very markedly above the elbow and repair at this level is sometimes difficult. Terminal branches of the posterior interosseous nerve may be divided accidentally or occur at the time of surgical exploration. Repair of the posterior interosseous nerve should always be attempted but functional recovery may depend eventually on tendon transplantation.

The musculocutaneous nerve is not commonly injured but if divided repair should always be considered. Failure to restore elbow flexion can be compensated for by tendon transplantation (see p. 507).

Digital nerves

Wounds of the hand and finger often involve digital nerves and/or flexor tendons. Primary treatment should normally involve apposition of the digital nerves. Definitive repair may be necessary as a secondary procedure carried out separately or at the time of tendon graft. The autonomous zone of one digital nerve is very small and overlap may result in a minimal deficit even if surgical repair is not carried out. Troublesome neuroma formation is common after digital nerve division and repair is the best prevention of such an irritating complication.

Partial nerve division

Partial nerve division poses problems in management. In the initial stages the divided portion of the nerve retracts while the intact portion remains in its normal position. This results in the formation of a gap which is wider towards the periphery than at the intact portion of the nerve (Fig. 12.13a).

Attempts to suture the divided portion of the nerve directly will commonly produce an entrapment neuropathy of the intact portion of the nerve. A number of partial nerve lesions left without suture, develop no important functional deficit. In the author's view partial

nerve lesions should be treated by simple isolation of the whole nerve using Silastic sheeting without any surgery to the divided portion of the nerve in the first instance. The disability can be subsequently evaluated and exploration carried out as necessary.

Where a functionally significant portion of a nerve remains intact no surgical treatment may be necessary provided fibrosis and entrapment is prevented at the site of injury. Silastic isolation will achieve this object. The higher the level of the lesion the better the result.

Later exploration of partial nerve injuries is often best limited to a simple neurolysis with resection of lateral neuroma (Fig. 12.13b). Loop suture was formally advised [4] but the results are at best uncertain. The intact portion of the nerve will frequently carry sufficient function to eliminate most of the usual deficit which one would expect with any specific nerve lesion. There may be a place for loop suture in distal lesions, but the risk is of an entrapment neuropathy of the intact portion (Fig. 12.13c).

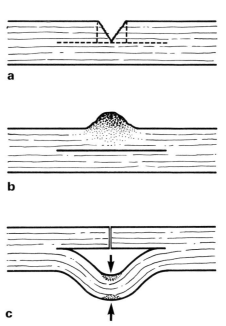

FIG. 12.13. (a) The effects of incomplete nerve division with the dotted lines indicating the incisions necessary to achieve any repair of the divided portion.

(b) The lateral neuroma which results whatever is done.

(c) A standard loop suture with the resultant probable effects on the intact portion of the nerve.

Aids to peripheral nerve surgery

Nerve stimulator. A nerve stimulator is an essential adjunct in the management of cases of nerve division. It facilitates identification of motor nerves and helps to identify anomalous branches and their function. A nerve stimulator is vitally important when dealing with secondary exploration of partial nerve lesions and many models are available.

Nerve markers. Where there is any suspicion of tension in the suture line (tension should be avoided wherever possible) radio-opaque nerve markers are useful. Three markers are inserted as shown (Fig. 12.14), the first two on the proximal end. Subsequent radiological examination will show whether nerve disruption has taken place by an increase in the distance between the second and third markers. If this does occur re-exploration is essential.

Magnification. There is a vogue at the present time for peripheral nerve surgery to be carried out with the operating microscope as described later (p. 192). As yet there is no evidence in clinical practice nor in recent experimental work [80] that such magnification gives improved results. Its application is still an experimental technique which is time consuming and should be restricted to those who have considerable experience of the technique (see p. 193). Simple magnification ×2–4, e.g. with a loupe, facilitates peripheral nerve surgery in a

technical sense. This is particularly useful for those who are becoming afflicted by presbyopia.

Suture material. Over the years many suture materials have been described [72–74]. Those which are unsatisfactory include cat-gut, silk, human hair. Nylon and prolene are available in fine diameters, e.g. 6/0–8/0 and such material is satisfactory. In the ideal nerve repair four sutures are all that are necessary. If more sutures become necessary it is likely that excessive tension exists at the suture line which can only be overcome by further nerve mobilization or grafting.

Post-operative care

Following any nerve repair, protection of the suture line by a simple plaster splint is essential for three weeks. Where extensive mobilization of the nerve has been necessary and nerve length made up by joint flexion, this joint position should be corrected gradually by the use of turnbuckle splintage (Fig. 12.12).

Failure of recovery

Following definitive nerve repair there are times when the surgeon is posed with the problem of lack of recovery within an expected period. If there is no clinical or electromyographic evidence of recovery within six to eight months of definitive nerve repair, the options which are open are re-exploration of the nerve or reconstruction by using tendon transplantation and/or neurovascular skin island flaps (see p. 503). Where repair has been carried out by an experienced surgeon re-exploration is probably only worthwhile if one is prepared to resect over a considerable distance and insert nerve grafts.

Nerve grafting using magnification is a technique which is gaining greater acceptance at the present time (see p. 193). It may be that such methods will give satisfactory results but as yet there is not sufficient evidence to recommend this method for routine use. Standard grafting using saphenous, sural or cutaneous nerves of the forearm will give a measure of protective sensibility. Few of such grafts provide satisfactory motor recovery and should be reserved mainly for those cases where protective sensibility is required. Motor loss is best treated by tendon reconstruction (see p. 513).

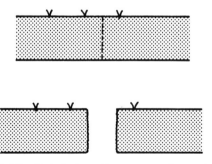

Fig. 12.14. The effect of using radio-opaque markers to determine the subsequent disruption of the suture line. It can be seen that if the markers are inserted as shown above, should disruption of the suture line take place, it will be immediately apparent radiologically that there is a greater gap between the two sutures to the right than between the two in the intact proximal portion of the nerve.

Injuries of the brachial plexus

Closed injuries of the plexus are frequently the result of traction. With the increasing use of both motor cycle and crash helmet the incidence of *traction injuries* to the plexus appears to be on the increase and is the commonest cause of damage in our experience.

They may be classified according to the roots damaged.

(1) Upper lesions affecting C5/6/7 roots.
(2) Lower lesions affecting C8 and T1 roots.
(3) Complete lesions affecting the whole plexus.

The level of nerve injury is also important and is classified as:

(a) *Pre-ganglionic*, where the injury occurs proximal to the posterior root ganglion.

(b) *Post-ganglionic*, where the injury occurs distal to the ganglion.

To diagnose the level of the lesion the intact axon reflex may prove of value. Bonney's test [4, 75] is still useful but not totally reliable because the plexus injury may be both pre- and post-ganglionic.

Cervical myelography is important in identifying pre-ganglionic avulsion of the nerve root from the cord. When this has happened the myelogram will usually show a meningocoele at the site of root disruption (Fig. 12.15). This finding means that the prognosis for recovery of that root is nil.

In a small percentage there is no myelin degeneration and recovery will take place fairly rapidly. In this group recovery even in the small muscles of the hand is a clear probability and frequently occurs.

By far the larger group have degenerative changes, where recovery of intrinsic function in the hand is highly improbable. The management of these lesions of the brachial plexus can be an extremely difficult problem. If there is clear evidence on cervical myelography of avulsion of certain roots, nerve repair is not possible and other types of surgical treatment can be considered at an early stage.

Where the lesion is in the upper roots arthrodesis of the shoulder offers the patient a prospect of a more useful functioning limb. Where the lower roots (i.e. C8 and T1) are alone involved amputation through the forearm may be advisable. Where the entire plexus is involved amputation above elbow has to be considered, and the choice for the patient is between amputation and accepting a useless and insensitive limb. Where myelography is negative and the lesion is thought to be post-ganglionic it has usually been considered advisable to adopt a conservative and expectant attitude with the hope of assessing the degree of recovery later, while concentrating on the prevention of joint contractures. This, however, commits the patient to a very long and protracted period of up to 2 years with no guarantee that there will be a useful limb at the end of that time. This is an unattractive prospect both for the patient and for the surgeon, prolonged delay in definitive treatment making the former depressed and apathetic.

At the present time therefore a much more aggressive

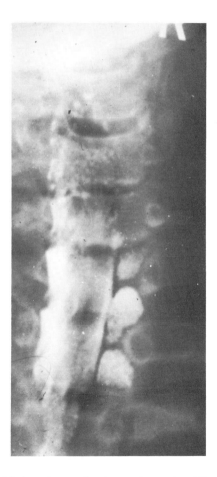

FIG. 12.15. A myelogram showing meningocoeles at the roots of the brachial plexus.

policy is being adopted in some centres towards the treatment of post-ganglionic traction lesions of the plexus [76].

Patients are being submitted to detailed investigation and surgical treatment consisting of neurolysis, nerve grafting or in some cases nerve transfers [77]. A problem which the surgeon faces here is to temper enthusiasm for new methods and for helping patients, by the awareness that nerve grafting may vitiate the possibilities of spontaneous recovery. Nerve grafting for post-ganglionic lesions may have a place but this remains a highly experimental technique, the results of which can only be seen after a number of years.

Open wounds of the brachial plexus are uncommon in the Western world but are seen frequently in areas where knife fighting is a method of settling disputes. Such divisions are worthy of exploration and repair although the surgical problems which result may be formidable.

In gunshot wounding, i.e. *high velocity wounding*, direct surgical treatment of the plexus lesion is probably unwise and a conservative approach is likely to be more rewarding.

MICROSURGERY IN NERVE REPAIR

G. D. LISTER

The median nerve at the wrist contains some 10 000 axons. To suggest, therefore, that microsurgical repair restores normal intraneural anatomy would be not only arrogant but display ignorance of nerve structure. Magnification gives the surgeon a better opportunity to do all that is at present humanly possible to align fascicles accurately without any impediment to regrowth of the axons down the distal sheaths. The benefit of magnification is demonstrated by inspecting with the microscope repairs done with the naked eye. This often demonstrates fascicles protruding from the epineurium or turned back upon themselves, interposition of epineurium or adjacent soft tissue between the nerve ends, distortion of fascicles by sutures or other factors likely to impede growth. Simple alignment of fascicles, however, does not ensure that proximal axons will eventually arrive at the appropriate endings.

Setting up the microscope for the procedure is im-

portant and the surgeon must be comfortably seated, his arms supported as far as the ulnar border of his hands. The instruments must be in good condition which can only be achieved if they are always kept separately in their own rack and are cleansed by the surgeon personally or by a trusted aide. The hand must be kept immobile by adequate anaesthesia combined with the use of a lead hand or similar fixation device. The exposure must be adequate and haemostasis complete. The microscope must be correctly focussed for both surgeon and assistant and the lighting must be bright even at high magnification.

Primary fascicular repair

Whatever the injury or nerve involved inspection under the microscope will often reveal that the fascicles in the cut end are obscured by fat globules adherent to the epineurium, Pacinian corpuscles and epineurium itself. The fat and Pacinian corpuscles should be trimmed away and, if pulling the epineurium in opposite directions does not reveal the fascicles, the last millimetre or two of the nerve end should be cut off by sharp section using either microscissors or a fresh knife with the nerve laid on a firm surface. Pulling again on the epineurium will reveal the fascicular ends as white, hemispheral structures which bulge out of their surrounding perineural sheaths. The fascicles differ in size and in grouping and a map of the ends of the nerve should be drawn by the surgeon, noting epineural blood vessels, fascicular size and groupings. The median nerve at the wrist contains an average of twenty identifiable fascicles arranged in four to six groups and by using the map, the correct orientation can usually be seen.

The development of stains which distinguish sensory from motor nerves by a differing concentration of acetyl cholinesterase bodes well for the future [78], although the necessary delay of 24 hours makes it presently impractical. Advocates of simple epineurial repair have reported good results and analysis of the outcome of different techniques of nerve repair has resulted in conflicting conclusions [79, 80]. However personal inspection of epineurial repairs reveals that the fascicles are often irregularly arranged or that there is a dead space separating the fascicular ends filled with blood clot. Organization of the clot might be expected to increase the scar between the fascicular ends. Also it has been shown that accurate fascicular suture ensures that the maximum number of axons remains within the fascicle, the only channel by which a significant number can proceed distally [81].

With this in view using the previously prepared map, the groups of fascicles are approximated using 10/0 nylon. The needle is passed through the perineurium. which lies behind the hemispherical bulge of axons, and is a difficult suture to place, for the fascicular end 'wriggles'. It is facilitated by holding the fascicle on a firm support while placing the stitch. Two such sutures should be placed in each group of fascicles ensuring that their correct alignment is obtained. On completion, the fascicles should be well aligned, with no ends protruding and no bulging at the site of repair. The epineurium need not be repaired but it might be reasonably supposed to buttress the fascicular repair against disruption and its repair is usually performed with interrupted or continuous 8/0 or 9/0 nylon. Where any tension is encountered in placing these microsutures, the surgeon should not hesitate to resort to grafting using the lateral cutaneous nerve of the forearm which offers a convenient source of graft [82].

Secondary grafting procedures

A group of workers in Vienna, under the direction of Dr. Hanno Millesi, has been responsible for the introduction of the present technique of interfascicular nerve grafting [83], based on original experimental work, conducted in cats and rabbits under carefully controlled conditions. The following is a summary of their conclusions.

(1) Regenerating axons can be damaged to the point of degeneration by shrinkage of scar tissue.

(2) The amount of surrounding scar tissue is directly related to the degree of tension on the suture line.

(3) The proliferating connective tissue which binds the nerve ends together is derived mainly from the epineurium.

(4) Microsurgical repair gives better results than conventional nerve suture.

Their technique of interfascicular nerve grafting described below eliminates tension and gives, in the secondary nerve reconstruction, results at least as good as those obtained by primary epineural suture and better than those after neurorrhaphy under tension.

The deleterious effects of tension in nerve repair have been further shown in nerve conduction studies at the fascicular level [84].

The indications for exploration before a possible nerve graft are as follows.

(1) When no primary nerve repair was carried out:

(a) A nerve injury was recognized at primary exploration *but not repaired*. The secondary procedure should be performed 10 days to 4 weeks after injury, the timing being determined by the nature of trauma and the healing of other structures damaged.

(b) Absence of recovery 6 weeks after *an unexplored injury* which was associated with sensory and motor loss.

(2) After nerve repair was carried out:

(a) The *presence* of a cripplingly painful neuroma.

(b) *Absence* of an advancing Tinel's sign three months after repair.

(c) The presence of Tinel's sign persistently less strong however, than that elicited at the site of repair.

It now appears that secondary nerve grafting can be of value even years after the original injury. Millesi has reported cases of recovery from atrophy and return of protective sensation following interfascicular grafting in median nerve repair 20 years after injury. This does not imply that such delay is acceptable; the earlier the graft procedure, the better the outcome.

The exposure of the nerve should be generous, as all dissection should proceed from normal tissue to scar, thus aiding identification and avoiding injury to intact fascicles. Having carefully dissected out the nerve proximally and distally and isolated the neuroma from surrounding scar, the microscope is then used. The epineurium is split longitudinally proximally and distally from the points at which the nerve appears of normal dimension and consistency. Incisions are best made with a knife and require to be surprisingly deep to penetrate the thickened epineurium. The fascicles are then revealed and further dissection proceeds towards the neuroma, the epineurium being held apart by surgeon and assistant.

The groups of fascicles can be dissected out with ease using a small knife, the planes of separation being readily achieved. The epineurium can be dissected off the bundles right around the nerve in some instances,

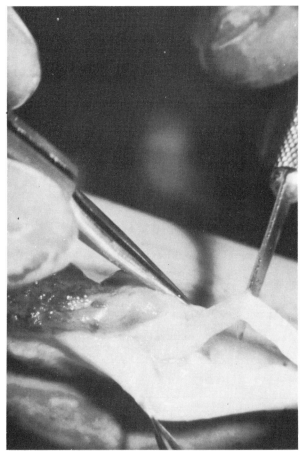

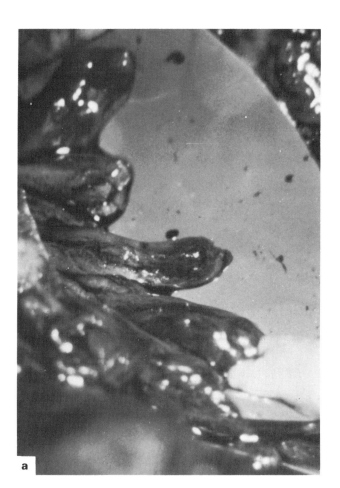

FIG. 12.16. This dissection of the median nerve 6 months after injury shows some points in technique. The nerve is stabilized by surgeon and assistant holding the epineurium with jeweller's forceps. One fascicular group has been dissected out as far as the neuroma and is being transected at a healthy level using a scalpel.

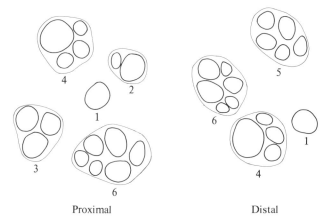

Proximal   Distal

FIG. 12.17. (a) Five transected fascicular groups in a median nerve await placement of interfascicular grafts. The size and number of the fascicles in each group is obscured except in that second from the top.

(b) A plan has been prepared both proximally and distally to aid in matching. The proximal 4 corresponds to the second-top group in (a). The proximal 3 and 2 were joined to the distal 5.

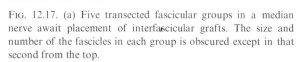

such as the median in the forearm. In other sites, including the ulnar nerve in the forearm, the epineurium gives off septa which separate one fascicular group from another. This should be recognized, otherwise some smaller fascicles may be overlooked in the investing epineurium. As dissection proceeds towards the neuroma, a point will be reached at which the surrounding scar increases in bulk and fascicular separation becomes more difficult.

Each fascicle should be pursued into and through the scar. This is a laborious process requiring retraction of the scar by surgeon and assistant and gentle sharp dissection of the fascicles keeping the knife blade close by but parallel to the fascicle. If fascicles deteriorate into strands of scar they can be sacrificed, transection being performed where scar first becomes evident along the nerve (Fig. 12.16). The level of transection should be staggered somewhat to avoid coincident suture lines (Fig. 12.17a).

As each group is cut it should be turned up towards the microscope and the number and relative size of the fascicles it contains should be drawn on a map of the two ends of the nerve (Fig. 12.17b). Where doubt exists regarding the integrity of any fascicle it should be retained. The development of microelectrodes for intra-operative recording of nerve conduction promises to eliminate the guesswork from this aspect of peripheral nerve microsurgery [85].

Once all dissection and mapping is completed, the scar and epineurium between the proximal and distal sites of fascicular transection may be excised. Alternatively they can be retained in continuity as a useful splint for the nerve ends, to be removed on completion of the interfascicular grafting. With all joints relaxed the gap between the nerve ends is measured. The nerve map is then studied and the closest matching of fascicular groups selected (Fig. 12.17b).

This aspect of nerve grafting causes most criticism. With the knowledge that cross-connections exist within peripheral nerves how can such matching be other than guesswork? Such interchanges exist between fascicles in the upper arm certainly and can be seen during internal neurolysis of the ulnar nerve at the elbow. In the fore-arm and wrist, however, where the majority of nerve grafts are performed, such connections between fascicles have ceased, a fact which can be confirmed by the surgeon while dissecting the nerve proximal and distal

to the neuroma. Less confidence is felt at present in deciding which fascicles form a group and which groups correspond but the size and arrangement of the fascicles is usually distinctive.

Having determined the number of fascicular groups to be grafted and the length of the gap, the total length of graft required is known and should now be obtained. All microscopic work requires a dry field and haemostasis should be achieved after release of the tourniquet while the grafts are being removed. Once the grafts are in the field, suction should be avoided for a graft can disappear into the suction nozzle.

The usual source of grafts is the sural nerve which in the adult can yield over 40 cm of uninterrupted length (Fig. 12.18). It is located midway between the posterior aspect of the lateral malleolus and the Achilles tendon.

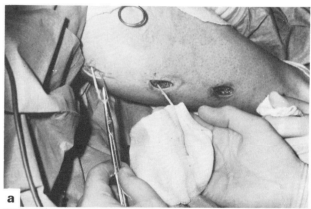

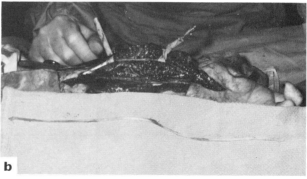

FIG. 12.18. (a) A sural nerve graft is taken, usually from the contralateral leg so that two teams can work simultaneously.

(b) Here a 35 cm graft is laid beside the wrist from which the median nerve destroyed by an extensive electrical burn has been dissected.

Once isolated its course is determined by gentle distal traction. It is then removed through a series of small transverse incisions, care being taken at each to define and divide small branches, rather than avulse them in the process of withdrawing the main trunk proximally. Where a lengthy gap is to be bridged or where multiple nerves are being repaired, as in brachial plexus injuries, both sural nerves may not suffice, and other sources of graft are as follows.

(1) The lateral cutaneous nerve of thigh.

(2) The saphenous nerve.

(3) The lateral and medial cutaneous nerves of forearm.

(4) The intercostal nerves.

(5) The cutaneous branches of the cervical plexus.

Where possible the suture lines and the graft itself should be laid in a well-vascularized bed away from scar tissue. This can often be achieved by re-routing the nerve, for example by placing the superficial terminal branch of the radial nerve on the volar aspect of the wrist alongside the radial artery or by carrying a grafted median nerve along the course of the uninjured ulnar neurovascular structures (Fig. 12.19). The grafts

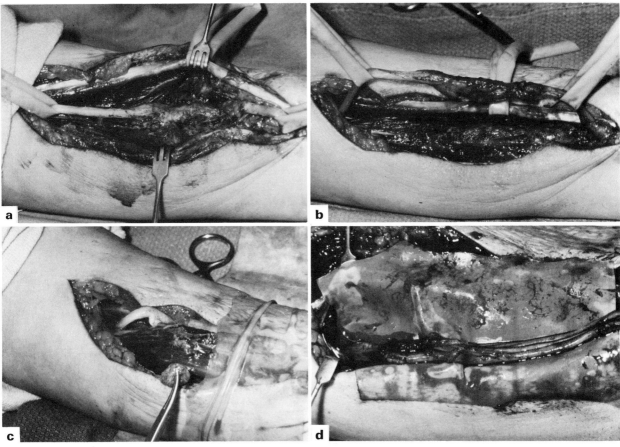

FIG. 12.19. (a) The heavily scarred bed of a non-functioning median nerve following a gunshot wound before dissection of the nerve.

(c) To avoid laying the graft in such a bed, the neuroma is transected and passed beneath flexor digitorum superficialis to lie alongside the uninjured ulnar neurovascular bundle.

(b) A lengthy neuroma elevated from the scar.

(d) After dissection, four interfascicular grafts are inserted.

are laid in position with a slight excess for each interfascicular defect. Not only does this ensure complete lack of tension but it permits later re-operation on the distal suture line if nerve growth should fail to proceed beyond it. This proves necessary in approximately one case in ten, the excess graft allowing resection and re-suture of the distal repair without tension.

The grafts and nerve fascicles tend to adhere within minutes and this adhesion has been shown by Millesi to be adequate attachment under experimental conditions. Subsequent wound closure may dislodge the grafts, however, and therefore the epineurium of each graft in turn is sutured to the perineurium of the corresponding fascicular groups using 9/0 or 10/0 nylon. One suture would suffice but orientation is more securely maintained by two. Postoperatively, the arm is splinted to protect the suture lines and the patient encouraged to exercise the fingers. The donor leg is bandaged with a firm elastic bandage and walking encouraged from the first postoperative day.

Millesi [86] has reported that after interfascicular grafting 57.9 per cent of median nerve injuries and 56.4 per cent of ulnar nerve injuries regained sensation to grade S3 or better, that is, they regained tactile sensibility and pain sensation. Motor function recovered to grade M3 or better in 81.7 per cent of median nerve and 79.5 per cent of ulnar nerve grafts, that is, they showed contraction against resistance. An additional benefit which can be confidently anticipated after this procedure is elimination of neuroma pain. The factors which adversely affected the outcome were increased age, increased length of the defect and delay between injury and graft.

REFERENCES

[1] SUNDERLAND, S. *Nerves and Nerve Injuries*, pp. 2–68. Edinburgh, Livingstone, 1972.

[2] OLIVECRONA, H., TONNIS, W., AND KRENKEL, W. *Handbuch der Neurochirurgie*. Peripheres und Sympathisches Nervensystem. Berlin, Springer-Verlag, 1974.

[3] SHERRIN, J. *Injuries of Nerves and their Treatment*. New York, Wood, 1907.

[4] SEDDON, H. *Surgical Disorders of the Peripheral Nerves*. Edinburgh, Churchill Livingstone, 1972.

[5] APPLETON, A. B. Case of abnormal distribution of the N-musculocutaneous with complete absence of the ramus cutaneous N-radialis, *Journal of Anatomy*, 1911, **46,** 89.

[6] KERR, A. T. The brachial plexus of nerves in man, the variations in its formation and branches. *American Journal of Anatomy*, 1918, **23,** 285.

[7] ROWNTREE, T. Anomalous innervation of the hand muscles. *Journal of Bone and Joint Surgery*, 1949, **31B,** 505.

[8] LANZ, H. Anatomical variations of the median nerve in the carpal tunnel. *The Journal of Hand Surgery*, 1977, **2,** 44.

[9] GRUBER, W. Uber die verbindung des nervus medianus mit dem nervus ulnaris am unterarme des menschen und der saugethiere. *Archives of Anatomy and Physiology*, 1870, **37,** 501.

[10] PIERSOL, G. A. *Human Anatomy*, 3rd Edition. Philadelphia, Lippincott, 1907.

[11] MANNERFELT, L. Studies on the hand in ulnar nerve paralysis. A clinical experimental investigation in normal and anomalous innervation. *Acta orthopaedica Scandinavica*, 1966, Suppl. 87.

[12] TERZIS, J. K., DYKES, R. W. AND HAKSTIAN, R. W. Electrophysiological recordings in peripheral nerve surgery: A review. *The Journal of Hand Surgery*, 1976, **1,** 52.

[13] WILLIAMS, H. B. AND TERZIS, J. Single fascicular recording: an intraoperative diagnostic tool for management of peripheral nerve lesions. *Plastic and Reconstructive Surgery*, 1976, **57,** 562.

[14] HAKSTIAN, R. W. Funicular orientation by direct stimulation. An aid to peripheral nerve repair. *Journal of Bone and Joint Surgery*, 1968, **50A,** 1178.

[15] MÜLLER, J. *Handbuch der Physiologie des Menschen*, 2nd Edition. Coblenz, 1838.

[16] FREY, N. Von. Beitrage zur sinnesphysiologie des haut. *Ber. Sachs, Ges, Win, math-phys*, 1895, **47,** 166.

[17] HEAD, H. *Studies in Neurology*, p. 837. London, 1920.

[18] SINCLAIR, D. *Cutaneous Sensation*. London, Oxford Medical Publications, 1967.

[19] WEIR MITCHELL, G. *Injuries to Nerves and their Consequences*. Philadelphia, Lippincott, 1872.

[20] ZACHARY, R. B. Results of nerve suture. In *Peripheral Nerve Injuries*, Ed. Seddon, H. J. Special Report Service, Medical Research Council. No. 282. London, H.M.S.O., 1954.

[21] TEIGS, O. W. Innervation of voluntary muscle. *Physiological Reviews*, 1953, **33,** 90.

[22] SORBIE, C. AND PORTER, T. L. Reinnervation of paralyzed muscles by direct motor implantation. *Journal of Bone and Joint Surgery*, 1969, **51b,** 156.

[23] GOLDBY, J. H. A. AND GAMBLE, H. J. The effect of temperature on the maturation of regenerating peripheral nerves in the rat. *Journal of Anatomy*, 1959, **93,** 436.

[24] HAFTEK, J. Influence of heat on the regeneration of sensory nerve fibres. *Neurologia, Neurochirurgia: Psychiatria Polska*, 1967, **1,** 239.

[25] SUNDERLAND, S. Rate of regeneration of sensory nerve fibres. *Archives of Neurology and Psychiatry*, 1947, **8,** 1.

[26] HEAD, H., RIVERS, W. H. R. AND SHERRAN, J. The cutaneous nervous system from a new aspect. *Brain*, 1905, **28,** 96.

[27] HEAD, H. AND SHERRAN, J. The consequences of injury to peripheral nerves in man. *Brain*, 1905, **28,** 116.

[28] TROTTER, W. S. AND DAVIES, H. M. Experimental studies in the innervation of the skin. *Journal of Physiology*, 1909, **38,** 134.

[29] SHARPEY-SCHAEFFER, E. The permanent results of denervation of a cutaneous area. *Quarterly Journal of Experimental Physiology*, 1930, **20,** 95.

[30] MCEWAN, L. E. Median and ulnar nerve injuries. *Australian and New Zealand Journal of Surgery*, 1962, **32,** 89.

[31] MCQUILLAN, W. M. Sensory recovery after nerve repair. *The Hand*, 1970, **2,** 19.

[32] MCQUILLAN, W. M., NEILSON, J. M. M., BOARDMAN, A. K. AND HAY, R. L. Sensory evaluation after median nerve repair. *The Hand*, 1971, **3,** 101.

[33] WYNN-PARRY, C. Personal communication, 1978.

[34] MCQUILLAN, W. M. Recovery of sensibility following nerve injury. Combined Meeting British-American Society for Surgery of the Hand, Edinburgh, 1977.

[35] NEILSON, J. M. M., BOARDMAN, A. K., MCQUILLAN, W. M., SMITH, D., HAY, R. L. AND ANTHONY, J. K. F. Measurement of vibro-tactile threshold in peripheral nerve injury. *Lancet*, 1969, 669.

[36] SUNDERLAND, S. Blood supply of the nerves of the upper limb in man. *Archives of Neurology and Psychiatry*, 1945, **53,** 91.

[37] PUCKETT, W. O., GRUNDFEST, H., MCELROY, W. D. AND MCMILLEN, J. H. Damage to peripheral nerves by high velocity missiles without direct hit. *Journal of Neurosurgery*, 1946, **3,** 294.

[38] HARVEY, E. N. AND MCMILLEN, J. H. An experimental study of shock waves resulting from impact of high velocity missiles on animal tissues. *Journal of Experimental Medicine*, 1947, **85,** 321.

[39] MEDICAL RESEARCH COUNCIL. *Peripheral Nerve Injuries.* Special Report Service Medical Research Council No. 282. London, H.M.S.O., 1954.

[40] FORRESTER-BROWN, M. Peripheral nerve injuries in civil practice. *Medical Press*, 1940, **203,** 246.

[41] BUNNELL, S. The surgery of nerves of the upper extremity. *American Journal of Orthopaedic Surgery*, 1956, **13,** 101.

[42] BANG-RASMUSSEN, K. Peripheral nerve lesions in the upper extremity. *Journal of Bone and Joint Surgery*, 1962, **44B,** 443.

[43] NOBEL, W. Peroneal palsy due to haematoma in the common peroneal nerve after distal torsional fractures and inversion ankle sprains. *Journal of Bone and Joint Surgery*, 1966, **48A,** 1484.

[44] SCHWANN, T. H. *Mikroskopische Untersuchungen über die Uebereinstimmung in der Struktur und dem Wachsthum der Thiere und Pflanzen.* Berlin, G. E. Reimer, 1839.

[45] CAUSEY, G. *The Cell of Schwann.* Edinburgh, Livingstone, 1960.

[46] ABERCROMBY, M. AND JOHNSON, M. L. Quantitative histology of Wallerian degeneration. 1. Nuclear population in rabbit sciatic nerve. *Journal of Anatomy*, 1946, **80,** 37.

[47] YOUNG, J. S. The functional repair of nervous tissue. *Physiological Reviews*, 1942, **22,** 374.

[48] WOODHALL, B. AND BEEBE, G. W. *Peripheral Nerve Regeneration.* Washington, U.S. Government Printing Office, 1956.

[49] BRATTGORD, S. O., EDSTRÖM, J. E. AND HYDEN, H. Chemical and structural changes in nerve regeneration. In *Metabolism of the Nervous System*, Ed. Richter, Oxford. Pergamon, 1957.

[50] MACKEY, E. A., SPIRO, D. AND WIENER, J. A study of chromatolysis in dorsal tract ganglia at the cellular level. *Journal of Neuropathology and Experimental Neurology*, 1964, **23,** 508.

[51] ROMANES, G. J. Motor localization and the effects of nerve injury on the ventral horn of the spinal cord. *Journal of Anatomy*, 1946, **80,** 117.

[52] MATTHEW, M. R., COWEN, W. M. AND POWELL, T. P. S. Transneuronal cell degeneration in the lateral geniculate nucleus of the macaque monkey. *Journal of Anatomy*, 1960, **94,** 145.

[53] GUTH, L. Regeneration in the mammalian peripheral nervous system. *Physiological Reviews*, 1956, **36,** 478.

[54] PEACOCK, E. F. AND VAN WINKLE, W. Tendon healing and repair. In *Surgery and Biology of Wound Repair.* Philadelphia, Saunders, 1970.

[55] WEBSTER, M. E. AND PIERCE, J. V. The nature of the kallidins released from human plasma by kallikreins and other enzymes. *Am. N.Y. Acad. Sci.*, 1963, **104,** 91.

[56] MCQUILLAN, W. M. Nerve isolation techniques. An adjunct to secondary nerve repair. *Journal of Bone and Joint Surgery*, 1967, **46B,** 186.

[57] FORRESTER-BROWN, M. Personal communications, 1965.

[58] INGEBRITSEN, R. A contribution to the biology of the peripheral nerves in transplantation. *Journal of Experimental Medicine*, 1916, **23,** 251.

[59] KLINE, D. G., HAYS, G. J. AND MORSE, A. S. A comparative study of response of species to peripheral nerve injury. II. Crush and Severance with Primary Suture. *Journal of Neurosurgery*, 1964, **21,** 980.

[60] SUNDERLAND, S. The capacity of regenerating axons to bridge long gaps in nerves. *Journal of Comparative Neurology*, 1953, **99,** 481.

[61] MCCULLOUGH, A. W. Studies of peripheral nerve regeneration. *Journal of Comparative Neurology*, 1959, **113,** 471.

[62] NOLAN, B. AND MCQUILLAN, W. M. Traumatic limb ischaemia. *British Journal of Surgery*, 1965, **52,** 559.

[63] MCQUILLAN, W. M. AND NOLAN, B. Ischaemia complicating injury. *Journal of Bone and Joint Surgery*, 1968, **482,** 492.

[64] MCQUILLAN, W. M. Origin of fibrosis after peripheral nerve division. *Lancet*, 1965, 1220.

[65] MCQUILLAN, W. M. Nerve repair—the use of nerve isolation. *The Hand*, 1970, **2,** 7.

[66] McQuillan, W. M. Peripheral nerve injuries. In *Operative Surgery*, ed. Smith & Rob, pp. 150–158. London, Butterworths, 1977.

[67] Boyes, J. In *Bunnell's Practice of Hand Surgery*. Philadelphia, Lippincott, 1974.

[68] Trotter, W. The insulation of the nervous system. In *The Collected Papers of Wilfred Trotter, F.R.S.* London, Oxford University Press, 1941.

[69] Lorente De No. Endothelial lining in ruptured nerve is altered basically in structure and function. The ineffectiveness of the connective tissue sheath of nerve as a diffusion barrier. *Journal of Cellular and Comparative Physiology*, 1953, **35**, 195.

[70] Moberg, E. Objective methods for determining the functional value of sensibility in the hand. *Journal of Bone and Joint Surgery*, 1958, **40B**, 454.

[71] Kuczynski, K. Functional microanatomy of the peripheral nerve trunks. *The Hand*, 1974, **2**, 1.

[72] Naffziger, H. C. Methods to secure end to end suture of peripheral nerves. *Surgery, Gynaecology and Obstetrics*, 1921, **32**, 193.

[73] Guttmann, L. Experimental study on nerve suture with various suture materials. *British Journal of Surgery*, 1943, **30**, 370.

[74] Sunderland, S. and Smith, G. K. The relative merits of various suture materials for the repair of severed nerves. *Australian and New Zealand Journal of Surgery*, 1950, **20**, 185.

[75] Bonney, G. The value of axon responses in determining the site of lesion in traction injuries of the brachial plexus. *Brain*, 1954, **77**, 588.

[76] Millesi, H. Surgical management of brachial plexus injuries. *The Journal of Hand Surgery*, 1977, **2**, 367.

[77] Narakas, A. Personal communication, 1979.

[78] Gruber, H., Freilinger, G., Holle, J. and Mandl, H. Identification of motor and sensory funiculi in cut nerves and their selective reunion. *British Journal of Plastic Surgery*, 1976, **29**, 70.

[79] Grabb, W. C., Bement, S. L., Koepke, G. H. and Green, R. A. Comparison of methods of peripheral nerve suturing in monkeys. *Plastic and Reconstructive Surgery*, 1970, **46**, 31.

[80] Cabaud, H. W., Rodkey, W. G., McCarroll, H. R., Mutz, S. B. and Niebauer, J. J. Epineurial and perineurial fascicular nerve repairs: A critical comparison. *The Journal of Hand Surgery*, 1976, **1**, 131.

[81] Hudson, A. R., Morris, J., Weddell, G. and Drury, A. Peripheral nerve autografts. *Journal of Surgical Research*, 1972, **12**, 267.

[82] McFarland, R. M. and Mayer, J. R. Digital nerve grafts with the lateral antebrachial cutaneous nerve. *The Journal of Hand Surgery*, 1976, **1**, 169.

[83] Millesi, H., Meissl, G. and Berger, A. Interfascicular nerve grafting of the median and ulnar nerves. *Journal of Bone and Joint Surgery*, 1972, **54A**, 727.

[84] Terzis, J., Faibisoff, B. and Williams, H. B. The nerve gap: Suture under tension vs. graft. *Plastic and Reconstructive Surgery*, 1975, **56**, 166.

[85] Williams, H. B. and Terzis, J. K. Single fascicular recordings: An intraoperative diagnostic tool for the management of peripheral nerve lesions. *Plastic and Reconstructive Surgery*, 1976, **57**, 562.

[86] Millesi, H., Meissl, G. and Berger, A. Further experience with interfascicular grafting of the median, ulnar and radial nerves. *The Journal of Bone and Joint Surgery*, 1976, **58A**, 209.

CHAPTER 13

Fractures

D. W. LAMB

These are among the most common of injuries, may be difficult to treat and, unless special care is taken, poor results often follow. Angulation, displacement and rotational deformity, even if slight, may lead to important impairment of hand function.

It is equally important to realise that fractures of the hand can be overtreated just as easily to the detriment of the hand as a whole.

These fractures may occur as isolated injuries or be part of more extensive trauma to the hand complicated by skin loss and tendon, nerve and vessel damage (see Chapter 18).

The principles of management described here are essentially those for uncomplicated fractures, but are usually valid, even when complicated by other tissue damage; where management differs, modifications will be given.

The initial step in management is to determine whether the fracture should be considered to be stable or unstable and thus whether immobilization is indicated. This requires a combination of clinical examination, study of the radiographic appearances and recognition of the basic type of fracture. Experience is of great value in this assessment, but certain practical points in guidance for those lacking this can be laid down. For example, isolated fractures of the metacarpal shafts tend to be stable [1], because the interosseous muscles and other soft tissue attachments to adjacent bones provide natural splintage. Fractures of the metacarpal necks with less than 25° volar angulation, the common deformity, are often stable and can be left unsplinted [1, 2]. Crack fractures of phalanges, particularly of the

middle and distal phalanx are usually stable. In contrast, fractures of the base of the first metacarpal (Bennett's type) and fifth metacarpal bones, multiple fractures of metacarpals, fractures of the metacarpal necks with marked displacement, transverse fractures of the proximal and middle phalanges and fractures involving joints are usually unstable [3].

Fractures which are assessed as *stable do not require immobilization*; early active movement of the fingers and use of the hand is encouraged.

A fracture which is assessed as *unstable requires immobilization* either by *external splintage* or by *internal fixation*.

External immobilization

In the presence of multiple fractures and particularly in crushing injuries where oedema is evident or anticipated, very satisfactory treatment is obtained by use of the *boxing-glove bandage* (Chapter 8, Fig. 8.6) and elevation. This method controls oedema and splints the joints in a 'safe' position, which can be maintained without risk for at least 3 weeks during which the fractures are likely to heal.

In isolated fractures, when there is often little general swelling of the hand, a most effective form of external immobilization has been found to be *the foam covered metal splint* which is recommended for general use (Fig. 13.1). During application it is important to see that no joint should be immobilized unless it is absolutely necessary to control the fracture and quite often only a

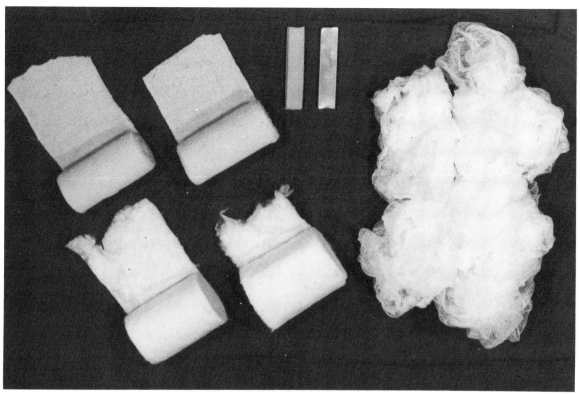

Fig. 13.1. Fluffed gauze, orthoband and 3″ crepe bandages are used for application of the boxing-glove compression bandage. Two short portions of metal splinting are shown. Various lengths of this foam covered aluminium splinting have been found to be very suitable for splinting minor fracture of the fingers.

single digit requires splintage. The splint should be applied to the volar aspect to avoid pressure over the vulnerable dorsal knuckle skin and great care is taken that the metacarpophalangeal joint is flexed as fully as possible and that the proximal interphalangeal joint is nearly straight (Fig. 13.2). It is important that the splint should be bent to the required angles to fit the individual hand before it is applied. Commercial splints of this kind are often too malleable to maintain the correct position and, therefore, the edges of the splint should be turned and flared by a pair of pliers to produce the required rigidity. Alternatively, a stronger splint can be made in the hospital workshop. The splint is fixed firmly, not too tightly, to the digit and hand by strapping (Fig. 13.2) which is reinforced by a bandage to maintain the desired position. This type of splintage usually leaves unaffected digits free to enjoy a full range of movement. If it is necessary to immobilize

the wrist, this should be done in some degree of dorsiflexion; otherwise the flexed position of the metacarpophalangeal joints is impossible to maintain. In order to obtain full flexion of the metacarpophalangeal joints the splint should be bent proximal to the distal transverse palmar crease. To avoid rotatory deformity the digit should point towards the tuberosity of the scaphoid and the nails should be seen to lie in parallel.

Illustrations in some articles and books show the position of immobilization of phalangeal fractures with the metacarpophalangeal joints almost straight and the proximal interphalangeal joints flexed to 90°, a position most likely to produce contractures at these joints which may be permanent.

Plaster of Paris is seldom necessary, apart from the management of fractures of the thumb, though there is no great objection to its use. However, its incorrect and careless application is often seen to immobilize

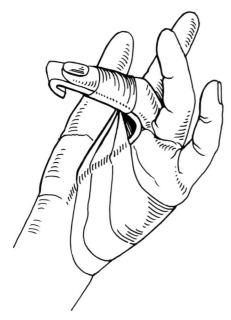

FIG. 13.2. Application of foam-covered metal splint to volar aspect of middle finger with metacarpophalangeal joint flexed to 90° and proximal interphalangeal joint in 10–15° flexion.

unnecessarily uninjured parts of the hand which may become affected by protracted joint stiffness so that serious impairment of hand function results from the treatment of what was initially a relatively minor injury.

It cannot be overemphasized that uninjured digits should be freely and actively moved from the beginning, and that the period of necessary immobilization should be made on clinical grounds only.

Internal fixation [4]

This should be considered in fractures difficult or impossible to control by external splintage or in which splintage might be detrimental to the restoration of function. Continuous traction of any type is not recommended in the treatment of fractures of the hand. The most useful and simple method of internal fixation is by means of Kirschner wires introduced percutaneously, where possible, cut off subcutaneously and removed as soon as their purpose is achieved. The ease of insertion of the wire is greatly enhanced by the use of a power drill. The finer gauges of Kirschner wire are used.

As a general rule the finest wire should be used that will provide stability, particularly where a joint has to be crossed. The calibre of wire for this purpose is in the ranges of 0·035, 0·045 and 0·0625 in (0·9, 1·1, 1·6 mm). While these can be introduced on a hand drill, such as the Bunnell drill, this requires two hands and, therefore, an assistant has to hold the fracture reduced or the surgeon does this and the assistant drills the wire. It is much easier to use a power drill so that the reduced fracture can be held stabilized in one hand while the wire is inserted with the other.

There are many directions in which the wire may be introduced but in general these resolve into either (1) longitudinal insertion along the line of the shaft of the bone affected, or (2) by transverse fixation.

Longitudinal wiring

On occasion it is impossible to avoid transfixion of the articular surface to get secure fixation, and the smallest gauge wire which will control the fracture should be used. Where possible, however, it is inadvisable to transgress the articular surface and the wire should be passed obliquely across the shaft of the bone from one corner to the opposite cortex. This will give good fixation and this technique can be used for unstable fractures of the metacarpal shafts or for the phalanges (Fig. 13.3).

Where there is a severe fracture involving a joint surface which is obviously irremediable and unlikely to result in joint movement, primary arthrodesis is indicated. The use of longitudinal or obliquely orientated Kirschner wires for this is very satisfactory.

A useful technique is to insert a longitudinal wire directly across the joint holding it in the desired degree of flexion and correct rotation (see Fig. 35.2). Two obliquely inserted wires are passed across the joint ensuring that the bone surfaces are in firm apposition. The central wire is then removed.

Transverse wiring

The wires are inserted percutaneously at right angles to the shaft which is a very excellent method of fixation of unstable metacarpal shaft fractures [5] (see Fig. 13.6).

The same method may be used for long oblique fractures of the shafts of the phalanges if these are impossible to control conservatively (see Fig. 13.9). Following introduction of Kirschner wires they should be cut off immediately subjacent to the skin but leaving them sufficiently projecting from the bone to ensure easy removal.

It is seldom that the wires require to be left in for

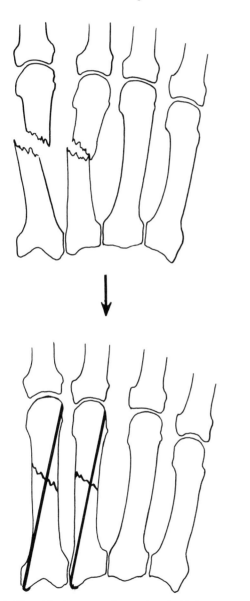

FIG. 13.3. Unstable fractures of second and third metacarpal shafts controlled by oblique longitudinal wires.

more than 3–4 weeks following which they should be removed. Provided they have been firmly fixed at the time of insertion, it is unusual for them to loosen or back out during this period and infection is extremely uncommon. Where it is impossible to reduce the fracture satisfactorily by closed manipulation, open reduction will be required, followed by insertion of the Kirschner wire. This simple method is usually fully applicable, even in open fractures.

Occasionally, in multiple severely displaced fractures more rigid fixation is required and the small A.O. plate and screws [6] or other micro-bolts and screws [7] may be considered. The use of small plates, bolts and screws has been introduced in recent years for the fixation of unstable fractures of the hand. This technique is more difficult than the use of Kirschner wires and requires considerably more soft tissue dissection and **exposure of the fragments. This encourages greater tissue** reaction, swelling and possible fibrosis but has the advantage of giving more rigid fixation. However, this method of treatment is very rarely required and should be reserved for those occasions when the simpler Kirschner-wire technique is found inadequate.

Another simple method which can be kept in reserve for those fractures which are difficult to control by the Kirschner wiring is the technique of intraosseous wiring [8]. A hole is drilled in each bone fragment with a fine drill. Gauge 32 wire is passed through these holes and tightened till firm compression of the fragments is obtained. The end of the wire is buried in a small hole drilled in bone adjacent to the fracture which prevents fraying of soft tissues over the wire end. While this method may be of value in the occasional fracture it is of particular value in maintaining the position of bone fragments after corrective osteotomy.

Non-union of fractures of the hand is rare, while malunion followed by limitation of motion is only too common. Prolonged immobilization of the hand is never justified and inevitably leads to joint stiffness. The secret of success in the treatment of fractures of the hand lies in the use of the most simple appropriate method [2]. Where immobilization is required it should be ensured that the joints are in the recommended safe position, that unnecessary immobilization of uninjured parts is avoided, that oedema is controlled and that the period of immobilization does not exceed three or four weeks.

Anaesthesia in the treatment of hand fractures

Where there are multiple fractures and in particular where they are associated with soft tissue injuries which require wound excision these fractures are best dealt with under general anaesthesia and with an arm tourniquet.

Where manipulation, open reduction or internal fixation of a single fracture is required this can be done readily using the technique of intravenous regional analgesia [9] (see Chapter 7).

Treatment of isolated special fractures

Metacarpal fractures

Bennett's fracture [10, 11]

This involves the base of the first metacarpal (Fig. 13.4a); it is not particularly common, but it is usually unstable. This instability is difficult to control by external splintage although Pollen reported success with his method [12], and Kaplan has recommended immobilization of the thumb in opposition which he finds a stable position [13]. However, there is a tendency for the fracture to slip, and while this can be counteracted by

continuous traction it is uncomfortable and not advised. The displacement can be reduced easily by manual traction and should be then stabilized in the corrected position by a percutaneous Kirschner wire introduced by the other hand of the operator using a power drill and fixing the first metacarpal shaft preferably to the adjacent second metacarpal or into the carpus (Fig. 13.4b) [14, 15]. Such an excellent fixation is usually obtained that no external splintage is required. The wire is removed after 4 weeks. Other more complicated methods of internal fixation of the fragments have been described [16, 17, 18], but they are seldom required.

Fracture of the base of the fifth metacarpal [19]

This is similar to the Bennett's fracture and is unstable with the same tendency of the metacarpal to slip proximally off the hamate. Following reduction by manual traction, internal immobilization by percutaneous transverse fixation with Kirschner wires to the fourth metacarpal shaft is advocated (Fig. 13.5).

Fractures of the metacarpal shaft

There are two main varieties: the long oblique fracture, and a short transverse one (Fig. 13.3). Both varieties can usually be left unsplinted, active movement of the digits being encouraged, as they all tend to be stable being supported by soft tissues and adjacent meta-

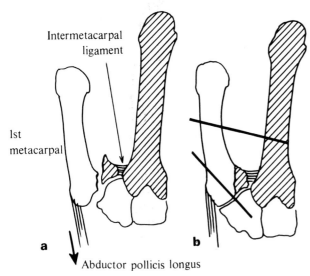

Fig. 13.4. Bennett's fracture. (a) Showing displacement. (b) Reduction by manual traction. Maintained by Kirschner-wire drilled percutaneously into 2nd metacarpal or carpus.

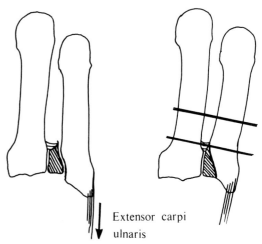

Fig. 13.5. Characteristic displacement of fracture of base of fifth metacarpal. Internal fixation by transverse K-wires.

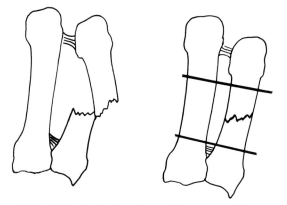

FIG. 13.6. Widely displaced and unstable transverse fracture of fifth metacarpal shaft. Stabilized by two transverse Kirschner-wires inserted percutaneously into each fragment and into the fourth metacarpal.

carpals. If angulation occurs, it tends to be slight and angled dorsally. In fractures of the metacarpal shafts which are markedly displaced and likely to be unstable, transverse percutaneous Kirschner wiring to intact metacarpals has proved very effective (Fig. 13.6) and allows early active finger movements [5].

In the long spiral fracture angulatory deformity occurs seldom, but it is important to ensure that no shortening occurs as it may result in an unsightly retraction of the metacarpal head. If there is any sign of such sliding displacement and shortening, transverse Kirschner wire fixation in the corrected position with the finger pulled out to length is very effective.

Fractures of the metacarpal shaft of the thumb, other than the Bennett's type, commonly result from a blow or fall on the thumb while it is in the adducted position.

There is usually an adduction deformity at the fracture, and this can be readily reduced and remains stable if the thumb is abducted and maintained in a scaphoid type Plaster of Paris cast for 4 weeks.

Fractures of the metacarpal necks

Fractures of the neck of the fifth metacarpal are by far the commonest of all metacarpal fractures [20]. They are usually caused by a blow with a clenched fist, the characteristic angulation being forwards (Fig. 13.7). In the fifth metacarpal angulation up to 25° or even 30° is acceptable as it seldom leaves any permanent deformity or deficiency of function; the finger should be used

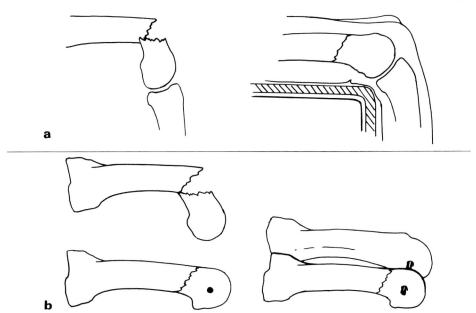

FIG. 13.7. Fracture of neck of metacarpal with characteristic volar angulation and displacement of metacarpal head.

(a) Treated by reduction and external immobilization on volar splint.

(b) Treated by reduction and internal immobilization by transverse Kirschner-wire to adjacent metacarpal head.

actively without reduction or splintage. In the middle three metacarpals, which are much less frequently damaged, this degree of angulation is unacceptable as the head of the metacarpal causes a prominence in the palm which is painful on gripping. Reduction is usually easy; the finger can be immobilized on a volar applied metal foam-backed splint (Fig. 13.7a). Alternatively, after correction a transverse Kirschner wire fixing the reduced head to the adjacent metacarpal head will control the deformity adequately (Fig. 13.7b).

Fractures of the phalanges

Fractures of the proximal and middle phalanges tend to be of similar type and require the same management. Fractures of the shaft of the proximal phalanx are among the more common hand fractures, and they are considered generally to be difficult to treat both because of the tendency for displacement to recur and also because of the difficulty in restoration of good finger movements particularly at the proximal interphalangeal joint.

There are two distinct types of fracture of these phalanges: (1) those involving the shaft of the bone which can be managed usually by conservative splintage, and (2) those involving the ends of the bone which are commonly associated with displacement of fragments bearing articular surfaces; these require open reduction and internal fixation more frequently.

Fractures of the proximal phalanx (Fig. 13.8)

These can be subdivided into fractures of the head, shaft and base.

Fractures of the head. These injuries are fortunately not common; they involve usually the joint surface with separation and displacement of an articular fragment, sometimes with its rotation by ligamentous attachments. It is important that these fragments should be accurately reduced. Sometimes this is possible by manual traction and closed manipulation the reduction being stable enough to be maintained by external splintage (Fig. 13.2). In most cases, however, in order to obtain accurate reduction of the articular surface and to prevent re-displacement, it is necessary to fix the fragments by open reduction using a Kirschner wire.

Fractures of the shaft. These may be of diverse kinds but there are two distinct types.

(1) The *transverse* or slightly oblique fracture near the middle of the shaft (Fig. 13.8c) is a very characteristic fracture of this bone which results usually in a typical volar angulation with the proximal fragment flexed and the distal one hyperextended (Fig. 13.8c, d). The displacement is due to the pull of the intrinsic muscles; relaxing this pull by flexion of the metacarpophalangeal joint results usually in correction of

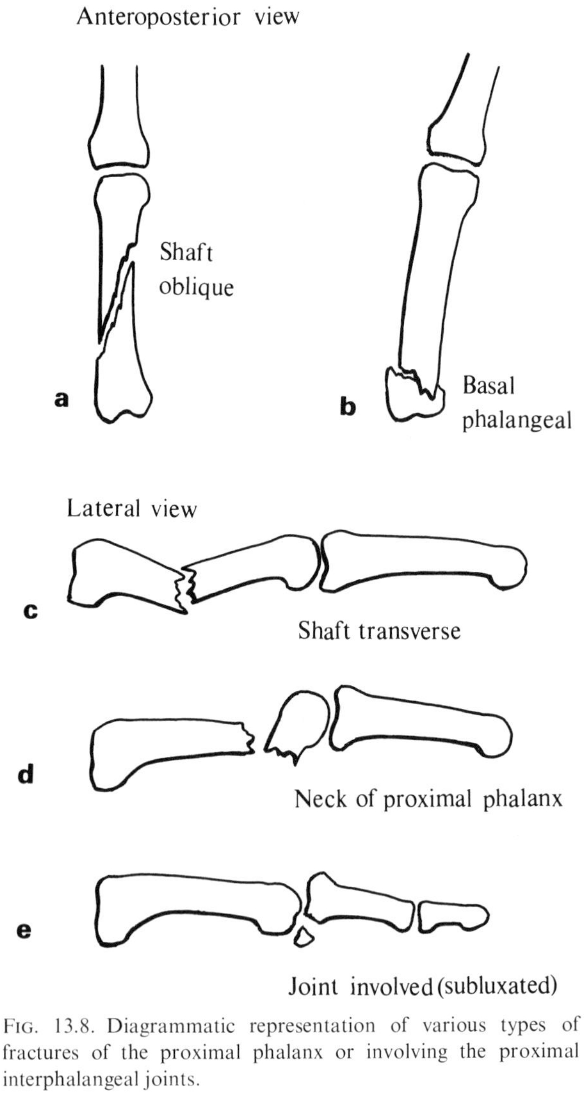

FIG. 13.8. Diagrammatic representation of various types of fractures of the proximal phalanx or involving the proximal interphalangeal joints.

the displacement and stabilization of the fracture. The reduction is maintained by the application of a metal splint along the volar aspect of the hand and finger, with the metacarpophalangeal joint fully flexed and the proximal interphalangeal joint flexed not more than 10–15° (Fig. 13.2). In most cases, the fracture is clinically stable after 3 weeks, when the splint can be removed and the finger mobilized [21].

Limitation of movement is liable to follow this fracture for two main reasons: (a) stiffness of the proximal interphalangeal joint (p. 209) and (b) adherence of the tendons at the fracture site (p. 517). Risk of both these sequelae is increased by immobilization; every effort should be made to avoid prolonging it for more than 3 or 4 weeks.

A particularly serious form of this injury is seen not infrequently in coal miners when the finger is crushed by a fall of stone or coal. It results commonly in an open fracture with a wound on the dorsum of the finger and division of the extensor tendon. The combination of these injuries leads commonly to adherence of the tendon and poor movement in the proximal interphalangeal joint.

If displacement of the transverse type of fracture cannot be controlled by splintage, internal fixation [22] with a long oblique Kirschner [23] wire inserted from one corner of the bone to the opposite corner obliquely across the fracture is indicated (Fig. 13.3).

(2) The other fracture which may occur in the shaft is the *long oblique variety* (Fig. 13.8a). It is usually stable and can be immobilized on a splint, but occasionally the fragments slide on each other with rotational

deformity. Under these circumstances the fracture can be easily controlled by percutaneous insertion of two short transverse Kirschner wires, cut off subcutaneously (Fig. 13.9).

Fractures of the base. These are not common apart from that involving the base of the phalanx of the little finger at the metaphyseal area of the adolescent hand (Fig. 13.8b). It results commonly in an abduction deformity requiring traction and manipulation to correct alignment. Immobilization by stirrup strapping to the adjacent digit (Fig. 13.10) is usually all that is required. Early active movement is encouraged.

Fractures of the middle phalanx

These resemble those of the proximal phalanx, but are less common. The treatment is similar. The angulation of the shaft is less pronounced and the fracture can usually be easily managed on a metal splint. Fractures of the base affect commonly the articular surface and are associated with avulsion of articular fragments which lie either on the dorsal or volar aspect of the joint (Fig. 13.8e). In the former they are commonly avulsion fractures caused by the pull of the central slip of the extensor apparatus, on the volar aspect they are associated with avulsion of the distal attachment of the volar plate. These displacements may be associated with subluxation of the joint at the time of injury or it becomes evident subsequently [24]. The fragments may involve a third or more of the articular surface and as the displacement is often difficult to control by splintage, the fragment should be pinned back in place with a Kirschner wire. This procedure usually stabilizes the fragments to such an extent that no external immobilization is needed, early active movements of the joint being encouraged.

Fractures of the distal phalanx

These are commonly caused by crushing injuries to the tip of the digit and are associated with comminution of the bone. These injuries are quite different from those of the proximal and middle phalanges and the management is discussed fully in chapter 16. The problems which arise from these injuries are more likely to be

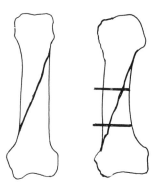

FIG. 13.9. Long oblique fracture of proximal phalanx fixed by transverse K-wires.

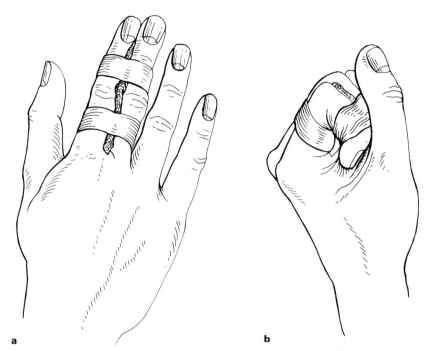

Fig. 13.10. (a) 'Stirrup' strapping to adjacent intact digit. The joints are not impeded. (b) Stirrup strapping showing range of flexion.

due to the crushing of soft tissue rather to the bone injury itself. Pain and tenderness of the pulp and the sequelae of damage to the nail and its bed are not infrequent.

Compound and multiple fractures

The management of compound fractures differs little from that of the simple fracture. The principles of careful wound excision take priority and the fracture subsequently is treated on its merits.

Where there has been severe crushing of the hand and there is doubt about the viability of the skin, or where skin replacement has been required, the use of internal fixation by the Kirschner wire technique is preferred to external immobilization.

As a general rule where there have been multiple fractures, in the presence of skin damage, or where there is concern for the circulation, firm internal skeletal fixation is recommended.

Provided there has been thorough wound excision and a careful assessment of skin viability, and replace-

ment of skin where necessary, it is seldom that infection supervenes in compound fractures of the hand.

In the badly crushed hand with multiple fractures and the probability of severe swelling a most suitable method of treatment, as has already been mentioned, is the use of the 'boxing glove' dressing applying firm compression and immobilising the joints in the correct safe position (Fig. 8.6). Elevation for 48–72 hours is recommended (Fig. 8.5).

Complications of fractures of the hand

Non-union

Non-union of fractures of the hand is extremely uncommon. If associated with pain or loss of function bone grafting is carried out. The most satisfactory method is an intramedullary graft taken either from the iliac crest or from the subcutaneous border of the upper ulna. If the rigidity of fixation is inadequate this can be supplemented by a longitudinal K wire (see also Chapter 35).

Mal-union

Mal-union of fractures of the hand is not uncommon, but in many cases it does not lead to any loss of function. The deformities which must be anticipated and prevented where possible may be angulatory, rotatory or shortening.

As a general rule minor degrees of *angulatory deformity*, particularly in the metacarpals, does not lead to loss of function. What is acceptable in the metacarpals, however, is often not suitable for phalangeal fractures which require a much greater degree of anatomical reduction.

Rotary deformity is particularly difficult to anticipate, and it is important, particularly when applying external splintage, that flexed fingers should point towards the tuberosity of the scaphoid and that the nails of the digits should be lying parallel. If these precautions are not taken it is embarrassing to find that what may only be 2 or 3° of rotary deformity may lead to difficulty and impingement of the digit against others when the fingers are being flexed. If this should occur and lead to functional impairment it is necessary to do a corrective osteotomy [25] through the site of the fracture, with a careful derotation of the correct amount, and this position is maintained by splintage, Kirschner wire fixation or by intraosseous wiring which is most appropriate [8] (see also Chapter 35).

Shortening may occur by sliding at the fracture site and occurs particularly in long oblique fractures of the shaft. In most cases this is not of importance and produces little cosmetic or functional disturbance. On occasion, however, particularly with the central metacarpals, sufficient shortening occurs to lead to recession of the metacarpal head which may cause distress due to its appearance. This has to be assessed as a hazard in the initial management of this type of fracture and if there is evidence of this shortening occurring internal fixation with Kirschner wire would be indicated.

Restriction of digital movement

The initial aim of management of all fractures of the hand is to restore full function. In certain cases damage to joints precludes this goal. In too many cases, however, joint stiffness results from unnecessary or excessive joint immobilization.

The joint which is most likely to become stiff is the proximal interphalangeal joint and particularly following fractures of the proximal phalanx. Careful anatomical reduction of these fractures and early movement of the joint is necessary.

Evidence of joint stiffness is manifest by the restricted passive range of movement. Specific exercises to mobilise these joints will often be successful in restoring good mobility (see Chapters 22 and 36).

Where the active range of joint movement is less than the passive the presence of tendon adherence should be suspected and is a common cause of limited joint movement.

In metacarpal fractures this seldom affects the flexor tendons but adherence of the extensor tendons to the fracture is not uncommon. There is a strong tendency for this to improve spontaneously and it is seldom that tenolysis is required. The effects of this adherence are much less likely where early active movements of the digits is encouraged and, where this has not been possible, immobilization of the metacarpiphalangeal joints in the flexed position.

Tendon adherence occurs most commonly following fractures of the proximal phalanx and may affect both the extensor and flexor tendons. This complication is sometimes impossible to prevent but its effects are mitigated by avoiding joint immobilization for more than the 3 or 4 weeks necessary.

There is a strong tendency for tendon adherence to improve spontaneously by encouraging active use and mobilization exercises. So long as there is improvement in the active range of joint movement the treatment should continue to be conservative. Once all improvement has stopped, and if there is a significant impairment of active joint movement but good passive movement, then tenolysis of the tendons is indicated (see Chapter 35).

Summary

A plea is made for a simple approach to the management of fractures of the hand. An early assessment of the type of fracture and decision as to whether it requires any immobilization is important. The stable fractures should be treated by early active use of the hand [20].

Where the fracture is assessed to be unstable external splintage is recommended as the method of management.

Where splintage does not control the fracture, where there are multiple fractures, where there are compound fractures associated with crushing and skin loss, and where there is anxiety about the distal circulation internal fixation is recommended. Unstable fractures at the base of the first and fifth metacarpals and fractures involving the joints with articular fragments are also best treated by internal fixation. The simplest method is the use of the Kirschner wire. Intraosseous wiring has an occasional place, but it is seldom that there is any justification for use of plates, bolts or screws.

REFERENCES

[1] JAMES, J. I. P. Fractures of the phalanges and metacarpals. *The Proceedings of the Second Hand Club (1956–1967).* British Society for Surgery of the Hand, 1975.

[2] FURLONG, R. *Injuries of the Hand.* London, J. & A. Churchill, 1957.

[3] LEE, M. L. H. Intra-articular and peri-articular fractures of the phalanges. *Journal of Bone and Joint Surgery,* 1963, **45B,** 103.

[4] STARK, H. H. Use of internal fixation for closed fractures of phalanges and metacarpals. *Journal of Bone and Joint Surgery,* 1968, **46A,** 1365.

[5] LAMB, D. W., ABERNETHY, P. A. AND RAINE, P. A. M. Unstable fractures of the metacarpals. A method of treatment by transverse wire fixation to intact metacarpals. *The Hand,* 1973, **5,** 43.

[6] SIMONETTA, C. The use of A.O. plates in the hand. *The Hand,* 1970, **2,** 43.

[7] IKUTA, Y. AND TSUGE, K. Micro-bolts and micro-screws for fixation of small bones in the hand. *The Hand,* 1974, **6,** 261.

[8] LISTER, G. D. Intraosseous wiring of the digital skeleton. *Journal of Hand Surgery,* 1978, **3,** 427.

[9] HOLMES, C. McK. Intravenous regional analgesia. *Lancet,* 1963, **i,** 245.

[10] BENNETT, E. H. On fracture of the metacarpal bone of the thumb. *British Medical Journal,* 1886, **3,** 12.

[11] BILLING, L. AND GEDDA, K-O. Roentgen examination of Bennett's fracture. *Acta Radiologica,* 1952, **38,** 6.

[12] POLLEN, A. G. The conservative treatment of Bennett's fracture—subluxation of the thumb metacarpal. *Journal of Bone and Joint Surgery,* 1968, **50B,** 91.

[13] KAPLAN, L. The treatment of fractures and dislocations of the hand and fingers. *Surgical Clinics of North America,* 1940, **20,** 1695.

[14] JOHNSON, E. C. Fracture of the base of thumb: a new method of fixation. *Journal of American Medical Association,* 1944, **126,** 27.

[15] WAGNER, C. J. Method of treatment of Bennett's fracture dislocation. *American Journal of Surgery,* 1950, **80,** 230.

[16] BADGER, F. C. Internal fixation in the treatment of Bennett's fractures. *Journal of Bone and Joint Surgery,* 1956, **38B,** 771.

[17] MOBERG, E. Technique of operation for Bennett's fracture. *Journal of Bone and Joint Surgery,* 1958, **40B,** 362.

[18] SPANGBERG, D. AND THOREN, L. Bennett's fracture. A method of treatment with oblique traction. *Journal of Bone and Joint Surgery,* 1963, **45B,** 732.

[19] PETRIE, P. W. R. AND LAMB, D. W. Fracture-subluxation of base of fifth metacarpal. *The Hand,* 1974, **6,** 82.

[20] BUNNELL, S. *Surgery of the Hand.* 5th Ed. Philadelphia, J. B. Lippincott, 1970.

[21] WRIGHT, T. A. Early mobilisation in fractures of the metacarpals and phalanges. *Canadian Journal of Surgery,* 1968, **11,** 491.

[22] PRATT, D. R. Exposing fractures of the proximal phalanx of the finger longitudinally through the dorsal extensor apparatus. *Clinical Orthopaedics,* 1959, **15,** 22.

[23] JOSHI, B. B. Percutaneous internal fixation of fractures of the proximal phalanges. *The Hand,* 1976, **8,** 86.

[24] WILSON, J. N. AND ROWLAND, S. A. Fracture-dislocation of the proximal inter-phalangeal joint of the fingers. *Journal of Bone and Joint Surgery,* 1966, **48A,** 493.

[25] REID, D. A. C. Corrective osteotomy in the hand. *The Hand,* 1974, **6,** 50.

CHAPTER 14

Joint Injuries

L. H. MILLENDER

Injuries of the soft tissues supporting the joints are among the most frequent of the hand. Regrettably they are often considered minor and are relegated to a junior surgeon who, when radiography is negative, discharges the patient with a diagnosis of a simple sprain when there may be a complete ligamentous tear.

This chapter presents a rational approach to the diagnosis and treatment of acute soft tissue injuries to the joints of the hand and stresses the complications which can result from delay or inadequate treatment (see Chapter 15 for injuries of the wrist).

Diagnosis

The surgeon must ascertain which anatomical structure is damaged and to what extent [1].

(1) Is it a partial or complete tear of a collateral ligament?

(2) Is the volar plate or the extensor apparatus partially torn or completely ruptured?

(3) Does the swollen joint represent oedema due to contusion or haemarthrosis from intra-articular fracture?

If the history and examination are considered from an anatomical standpoint, the approach becomes rational, the examination easily and quickly performed, giving meaningful results [2].

History

Inquiries are made regarding the nature of the injury, and the direction and magnitude of the force. If the proximal interphalangeal joint was forced laterally, a collateral ligament injury is likely; whereas if there was hyperextension, the volar plate could have been torn [3]. Direct jamming may result in a cartilaginous impaction fracture negative on radiographic examination. If, however, the direct compression had a lateral, volar or dorsal component, there may be both cartilaginous and ligamentous damage. In contrast, a crushing injury may cause no fracture and no ligamentous tear, but be significant because of soft tissue bleeding, oedema and synovitis. The magnitude of the force gives some indication of the severity of the injury.

Physical examination

Physical examination must be careful and gentle. *No information and no good can come from a rough, painful examination.* Important points are: observation of the amount and site of swelling, active and passive range of movement, areas of maximum tenderness and stability to stress [1, 2, 3, 4, 5].

Immediately after injury *swelling* is minimal, and the severity of the injury might not be appreciated. However, after 8–10 hours, if the swelling is slight it suggests the injury is minor. The site of the swelling is important. At an early stage, the joint is usually swollen diffusely; if seen after the general swelling has subsided, the swollen area may be localized to the site of maximal damage. In old injuries swelling represents permanent periarticular fibrosis and scarring often associated with a healed ligament.

The active and passive range of *movement* should be

carefully evaluated. Active range reveals the condition of the musculotendinous apparatus and also some idea about joint stability [2, 4, 6, 7]. If there is a volar instability, the proximal interphalangeal joint subluxes on full extension. Important information regarding the intra-articular structure is obtained by feel of the joint on passive movement.

Assessment of joint stability and areas of *tenderness* confirms one's impression. Although the entire joint is painful, *the area of maximal damage consistently reproduces most discomfort on direct pressure.*

The stress test for ligamentous instability confirms the diagnosis, and if seen early, or there is major instability, can be carried out easily without anaesthesia. But if there is pain or muscle spasm a local anaesthetic block should be used. Lateral stress should be performed both in full extension (Fig. 14.1) and in about 30° of flexion, as the joint may be stable in full extension if the volar plate is intact, while instability can be demonstrated in flexion. This is especially true in injuries of the ulnar collateral ligament of the metacarpophalangeal joint of the thumb. Examination of the contralateral joint for comparison is advisable.

Radiographs should include anteroposterior and true lateral views of the involved joint [1]. A subluxation or fracture-subluxation of the proximal interphalangeal joint may be missed without a true lateral radiograph. Chip fractures represent avulsion of tendons or ligaments and confirm clinical diagnosis. Stress radiography confirms instability already anticipated by feeling the joint.

Partial ligamentous injuries

Most soft tissue injuries are partial tears with anatomical continuity maintained. Included also are crushing type injuries which cause periarticular oedema, haemarthrosis and synovitis. The complications include persistent swelling and a feeling of stiffness especially in the morning and in cold weather [8], which commonly lasts for 6–12 months in the more severe partial tears and there may be some degree of permanent swelling secondary to periarticular fibrosis. The periarticular structures are intricate and easily scarred [5, 8], resulting in restriction of joint movement and additional adhesions can form around the tendons checking their excursion. Permanent limitation of movement may occur in neglected cases or in patients who do not exercise properly [6].

The aim of treatment is to:
(1) resolve swelling and pain,
(2) allow time for soft tissue healing, and
(3) institute exercises at the proper time and of correct type to restore full function.

Immobilization is the basic treatment for these injuries [1, 2, 4, 9, 10]. It allows the acute reaction and oedema to resolve and alleviates pain. For moderately severe injuries a well-moulded volar plaster splint to support the entire hand is appropriate. An aluminium splint for an isolated digit can be used for the minimal injury. In a mild injury swelling and pain usually subside after a few days when exercises are instituted. For the more severe injuries immobilization is necessary for 10–14 days. The period of immobilization can be estimated from the initial swelling and its response to immobilization.

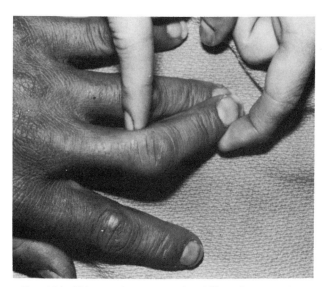

FIG. 14.1. This test demonstrates instability of the proximal interphalangeal joint secondary to tear of the radial collateral ligament.

Complete ligamentous injuries

Collateral ligaments

Complete discontinuity of the collateral ligament results from a forceful lateral deviation of the digit. Because

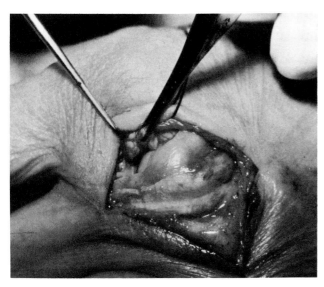

Fig. 14.2. Collateral ligament injuries of digital metacarpophalangeal joints. The collateral ligament which has been avulsed from the proximal phalanx is seen to be held in the forceps. This is only demonstrated after the capsule has been opened.

the collateral ligaments are strong, tough thick structures [11], complete tears require substantial force which may cause complete lateral dislocation, particularly in the proximal interphalangeal joint. Injuries of the proximal interphalangeal joints and of the metacarpophalangeal joint of the thumb are more common than those of the metacarpophalangeal joints of the fingers. These two former injuries are frequent in athletic activities, such as baseball and American football, and rugby [9]. Skiing is also a common cause of injuries of the ulnar collateral ligament of the thumb. Recently there have been reports of collateral ligament avulsions (Fig. 14.2) and avulsion fractures in the metacarpophalangeal joint of the long finger associated with finger wrestling.

Proximal interphalangeal joints

Some authorities feel that where there is full active movement without lateral subluxation, the joint can be treated with 3 weeks of splinting with resulting healing [4, 10, 12]. Others have advocated open repair [9, 13, 14]. The author has used both methods and considers conservative management preferable in most cases. The

indications for operation would include: (a) associated avulsion of a large bony fragment; (b) lack of normal joint congruity on radiography suggesting an interposition of soft tissues; (c) significant instability on the stress test; and (d) persistent pain, tenderness and instability after a three week period of splinting. Surgery can be done under regional anaesthesia; the joint is inspected, irrigated and the ligament returned to its normal bed with a pull-out wire technique or by direct suture. The digit is immobilized for 3 weeks when active movements are started. Full range is usually obtained in approximately 3 weeks.

Metacarpophalangeal joint of the thumb

Injuries of the collateral ligament of the thumb are usually seen on the ulnar side (Fig. 14.3a) and are associated with a forceful radial stress. Although Coonrad and Goldner have suggested a trial of conservative treatment [15], most authors recommend exploration and repair. Stener [16] pointed out how the adductor aponeurosis may become interposed between the bone and the ruptured ligament (Fig. 14.3b), which is thus displaced from its bed and unable to heal. It is felt that all acute complete ligamentous tears of the thumb should be repaired. The adductor aponeurosis is partially incised to expose the ligament which is usually detached distally [17], but may also be detached proximally or torn across its substance thereby precluding healing without lengthening. Direct suture or pull-out wire technique is used. The thumb is immobilized for 5–6 weeks when exercises are begun.

In chronic cases with pain and instability the choice of procedure depends on many factors. If degenerative arthritis has developed arthrodesis is best and provides a painless, stable and functional thumb. Without degenerative changes various reconstructive procedures have been suggested. Neviaser recommends distal advancement of the scarred ligament left attached proximally [18]; the adductor is then detached from its sesamoid and advanced distally and dorsally by 10 mm which provides dynamic stability. Other ligamentous reconstructive procedures have been advocated [19, 20].

Metacarpophalangeal joints of the fingers

Injuries of these ligaments are uncommon because there is normally lateral mobility at this level which absorbs some of the force [5]. When seen immediately or within the first few days, splinting with the joint in extension allows the ligament to heal. Because of the cam effect

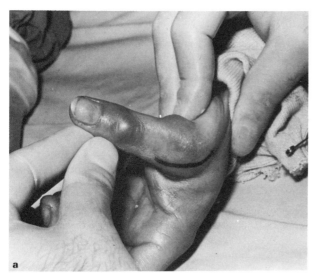

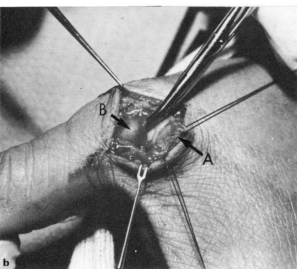

FIG. 14.3. Collateral ligament tear from metacarpophalangeal joint of thumb.

    (a) A complete tear of the ulnar collateral ligament demonstrated on stress test.

    (b) Ruptured ulnar collateral ligament: A shows avulsed retracted end of ligament from the phalangeal attachment, B shows adductor aponeurosis which traps the ligament after it has retracted.

of the metacarpal head (p. 18) placing the joint in extension relaxes tension in the collateral ligament and thus healing is more likely to occur.

These injuries are often not diagnosed initially and are seen from weeks to months after injury. Patients complain of pain, swelling and lateral deviation of the finger.

For chronic tears of these ligaments, exploration is indicated. A dorsal longitudinal incision is made, the sagittal fibres of the expansion divided and the extensor apparatus retracted. Surprisingly often there is no tear of the capsule. The collateral ligament, which is intra-articular and deep to the capsule, is found avulsed from either its proximal or distal attachment (Fig. 14.2) and usually must be repaired with a pull-out wire. The joint is splinted in mid-position, keeping the collateral ligament slightly relaxed for four weeks.

Volar plate injuries

Proximal interphalangeal joints

These injures are frequently seen [2] and are caused by a hyperextension force against the fully extended finger. The tear may occur at the distal cartilaginous attachment with or without an avulsion fracture [9], or at the junction of the cartilaginous and membranous parts or at the proximal attachment.

Acute volar plate injuries are often not recognised as significant, as the pain and swelling may not be severe. Patients may not be treated adequately with resulting chronic lesions of the plate in which the most important problem is the symptomatic swan-neck deformity. Even if this does not develop spontaneously, the patient complains of pain and stiffness after minimal hyperextension stress (Fig. 14.4).

As treatment of the acute volar plate injury is simple and chronic lesions can be troublesome, any suspected acute tear should be treated. Simple splinting in 30–35° of flexion is often advised [10, 21]. Immobilization of the finger in flexion for 2 weeks followed by an extension block for additional 1 or 2 weeks is adequate. In older symptomatic tears with or without swan-neck deformity and no proximal interphalangeal joint arthritis, volar plate repair (Fig. 14.5) with or without flexor digitorum superficialis tenodesis is recommended [2, 12, 22, 23].

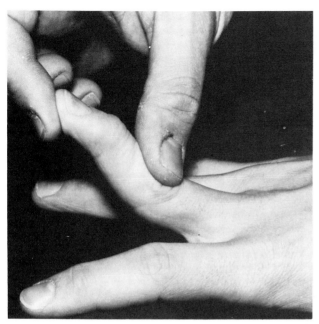

FIG. 14.4. Test illustrating the instability on the volar aspect of the proximal interphalangeal joint secondary to a chronic volar plate tear and with resultant swan-neck deformity.

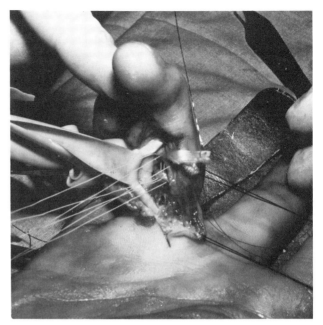

FIG. 14.5. Operation to repair complete tear of volar plate. The plate is being repaired with non-absorbable sutures. The flexor tendons have been retracted with a rubber loop. Note that one slip of flexor digitorum superficialis has been sectioned proximally and is to be utilised to reinforce the volar plate repair.

Metacarpophalangeal joint of the thumb

These are relatively common due to the frequency of hyperextension stresses which occur in the thumb. Similarly to the proximal interphalangeal injuries, examination may be relatively unrevealing, unless there is a major ligamentous disruption which results usually in a dislocation. History of a hyperextension stress is important and various degrees of volar tenderness, ecchymosis, swelling and pain are demonstrated. Pain on passive hyperextension implies a volar plate tear and treatment should be instituted [7]. Because the flexor pollicis brevis and adductor pollicis insert into the volar plate through the sesamoid bones, the torn ends of the plate can become separated by the pull of these muscles, precluding healing [7] and in view of this, open repair is recommended by some. Most authorities, however, feel that in uncomplicated tears (joints with good lateral stability) splinting in flexion for 3–4 weeks results usually in healing [1, 2]. This conservative approach has been found successful especially in cases treated early. However, in neglected cases or in cases with persistent hyperextension in-

stability and pain on stress, exploration is indicated [12, 23]. The plate is approached through a volar zigzag incision. After the tendon sheath is incised and the flexor pollicis longus tendon retracted, the ruptured plate is exposed. The rupture occurs usually proximally at the metacarpal attachment, although it may be distal or there may be a displaced sesamoid fracture with the tear through the mid-portion of the plate. Repair is carried out by direct suture or with a pull-out technique; the thumb is splinted in flexion for four weeks when exercises are begun. This procedure results in a pain-free stable joint.

Dislocations

Dislocation represents the end stage in soft tissue injury and may be seen in any digital joint [2, 9], the most frequent being the proximal interphalangeal joints and the metacarpophalangeal joint of the thumb. The injury is due to hyperextension or lateral force, and is often associated with sport. Dislocation of the distal joint is frequently combined with crushing injury, and is commonly open. Dislocation of metacarpophalangeal joints of the fingers is quite uncommon and is almost exclusively confined to the two marginal fingers. Dislocations of the carpometacarpal joints of the fingers are also uncommon and are associated with crushing injuries. Whereas true dislocation of the carpometacarpal joint of the thumb occurs, the more common injury is an avulsion fracture of the metacarpal beak, the well-known Bennett's fracture–dislocation (see Chapter 13).

Proximal interphalangeal joints

The displacement of the proximal interphalangeal joint in order of frequency is: dorsal, lateral and much less common, anterior. The common *dorsal* dislocation is often associated with sport and due to forceful hyperextension. This is always combined with a tear of the volar plate [9, 10], which may be represented by a small avulsion fracture of the base of the middle phalanx. In true dorsal dislocation, the collateral ligaments remain intact.

Diagnosis of these injuries is easy from the obvious distortion of the digit, which may rarely compromise circulation. Even when the diagnosis is clinically apparent, radiographic confirmation is required prior to reduction.

Closed reduction is usually easily carried out by traction and manipulation and when seen immediately may be possible without anaesthesia. However, when pain and swelling are present, a metacarpal or wrist block will provide adequate anaesthesia [4]. After closed reduction the joint is carried through a full range of movement and lateral stability is checked. Post-reduction anteroposterior and true lateral radiographs are mandatory to confirm reduction and to exclude associated fracture which may not be apparent before reduction. In stable dorsal dislocations, splinting of the metacarpophalangeal joint in moderate flexion and the proximal interphalangeal joint in 25 or 30° of flexion for a few days allows pain and swelling to subside. After this the proximal interphalangeal joint alone is splinted in 25 or 30° of flexion for a total of two and a half weeks. Thereafter a dorsal block splint is applied, allowing flexion, but preventing extension for an additional week.

This allows further healing of the volar plate and provides at the same time early movement [2, 4, 5, 10].

Surgical intervention is indicated when (1) the dislocation is combined with an open injury; wound excision should precede reduction; (2) interposition of volar plate or flexor tendons prevents closed reduction; incomplete closed reduction must be looked for carefully. It is more commonly seen in lateral dislocations. This can be easily carried out through a volar zigzag incision which readily exposes the lesion.

Morbidity from simple dorsal dislocations is not insignificant. Prolonged stiffness with swelling and permanent pericapsular thickening are common; morning stiffness or discomfort in inclement weather may persist for 6–12 months. In older patients or in those reluctant to exercise, permanent limitation of movement may result.

Lateral dislocations in these joints always result in a complete tear of the collateral ligament and a major portion of the volar plate [8]. These injuries are easy to reduce but may not be stable after reduction. Post-reduction films are mandatory in order to confirm completeness of reduction. If the soft tissues are interposed within the joint, the anteroposterior radiograph shows a gap or offset. These are best treated like complete collateral ligament tears by open fixation.

In contrast to the usual dorsal dislocation which is due to a pure hyperextension stress, the *fracture-dislocation* is associated with a combined hyperextension and longitudinal compression force. Size and amount of comminution are related to the proportion of the longitudinal versus the hyperextension force. In order to assess accurately the amount and degree of comminution, true lateral radiographs are mandatory.

Treatment is difficult and depends upon the size and comminution of the fracture. Usually the joint can be reduced by traction and manipulation, but if the fragment is large the joint is often unstable. If the fragment is small and reduction is satisfactory, the joint should be immobilized in 20–30° flexion for approximately 9 days; a dorsal extension block splint should then be applied to allow flexion but prevent full extension [1]. If the fragment comprised 30 per cent or more of the joint surface the preferred method of treatment is open reduction through a volar zigzag approach, using a small Kirschner wire to transfix the fragment, and if necessary, a percutaneous transarticular wire to hold the joint in the reduced position [1].

Distal interphalangeal joints

Dorsal dislocations of this joint are frequently compound due to the tight, soft tissue envelope surrounding the joint and to the associated crushing injury. Because of a very short lever arm to the distal joint, forceful indirect injuries usually result in dislocations of the proximal interphalangeal joint. Dislocations of the distal joint are treated similarly to the proximal interphalangeal joint. However, sometimes they are unstable, and if so, should be held in reduced position with a percutaneous Kirschner wire [1, 2, 4, 5]. Some permanent limitation of movement should be expected after these injuries but is rarely of any functional significance.

Metacarpophalangeal joints of the fingers

Dorsal dislocations of these joints are quite uncommon, being seen five times less frequently than dislocation of the metacarpophalangeal joint of the thumb [4]. Unless associated with multiple injuries they are always confined to the two border fingers. Kaplan has described the pathological anatomy and showed why the complex dislocations are irreducible by closed methods [24]. The metacarpal head herniates through the ruptured volar plate which becomes displaced dorsally and locked between the proximal phalanx and the metacarpal head. The head is trapped between the long digital flexors, displaced radially, and the lumbrical displaced ulnarwards. The fourth structure completing the Japanese finger trap, thereby making the dislocation irreducible, is the superficial transverse ligament of the palm (natatory), which crosses transversely anterior to the metacarpal [24].

Diagnosis is obvious from appearance and radiographs, but an attempt should be made to distinguish the simple, usually reducible, dislocation from the complex, irreducible one. In the simple dislocation the proximal phalanx is displaced dorsally at a 90° angle to the metacarpal, while in the complex dislocations the two bones are parallel and overriding. This can be appreciated on radiographs, and if the sesamoids are also seen within the joint, this suggests complex dislocation.

Treatment

Simple dislocations can be reduced by closed means. McLaughlin [25] pointed out that one can convert the simple dislocation into a complex one by attempting to reduce the joint by straight traction, which can pull the volar plate into the widened joint space. Proper reduction entails hyperextending the proximal phalanx and applying dorsal pressure as the proximal phalanx is manipulated into a reduced position.

Complex dislocation requires open reduction; however, it is justifiable to attempt one closed manipulation after anaesthesia is instituted [1]. A zigzag volar incision is used. The radial neurovascular bundle of the index finger and the ulnar neurovascular bundle of the little finger are quite superficial and care must be observed to avoid damaging them. After the flaps are formed and retracted, the metacarpal head is seen herniated between the flexors and lumbrical. Reduction is achieved by dividing the superficial transverse ligament of the palm and extracting the volar plate from the joint. After reduction, the plate is re-attached to the site of its avulsion from the metacarpal.

Recently a dorsal approach in order to reduce these dislocations has been described [26]. The author has no experience with this method but in rare cases which cannot be reduced by volar procedure, a combined approach may be necessary.

The hand is immobilized for 2–3 weeks when flexion exercises are begun.

Carpometacarpal joints of the fingers

These are uncommon and are caused by major force injuries to the base of the hand [27]. Because of the marked ligamentous stability, especially of the second, third and fourth joints, these injuries are associated with significant soft tissue disruption [27]. Dislocations of the three above joints are almost always dorsal (Fig. 14.6), and probably are due to a direct dorsal blow to the hand [1], while the fifth carpometacarpal joint, being more exposed and having a range of 20–30° of movement, may present differently [28, 29]. Two types of dislocation of the fifth joint have been described:

(1) a volar radial dislocation in which all soft tissues are avulsed from the metacarpal, the base of which is

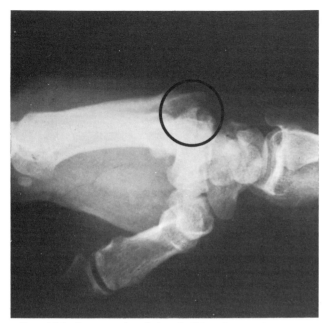

FIG. 14.6. An example of dorsal dislocation at the carpometacarpal joint.

found to lie volar to the third or fourth carpometacarpal joint; open reduction is necessary.

(2) the base of the fifth metacarpal is displaced ulnarwards and there are enough soft tissue attachments remaining to allow closed reduction [30].

Diagnosis of these injuries is difficult, frequently missed, thus delaying and complicating treatment. Because of marked swelling clinical diagnosis is not apparent, and radiographs difficult to interpret especially if one is not considering this diagnosis. Good lateral, oblique and cone-down views of the joint are helpful. These dislocations can occur in association with metacarpal fractures and both must be considered in any injury of this area.

Closed reduction of acute carpometacarpal dislocations, especially of the second, third and fourth are usually easy if good anaesthesia and longitudinal traction are applied. After length has been regained, reduction is obtained by direct pressure over the base of the metacarpal. Percutaneous fixation is recommended as there is a tendency to redislocation. In the volar and radial dislocation of the fifth joint, open reduction and Kirschner wire fixation is generally needed.

In chronic cases, arthrodesis of the involved joint alleviates the pain and restores the grip strength without loss of function [31]. Even after fusion of the fifth carpometacarpal joint no functional disability has been noted.

Carpometacarpal joint of the thumb (Fig. 14.7)

Pure dislocations of this joint are uncommon. The mechanism is a longitudinal force transmitted along the shaft of the metacarpal when the carpometacarpal joint is in flexion.

Closed reduction is easy but quite unstable and resubluxation is frequent [4]. Most surgeons recommend that after reduction is carried out, percutaneous

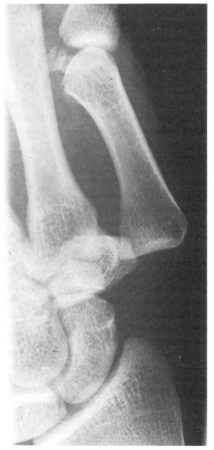

FIG. 14.7. Dislocation of the carpometacarpal joint of the thumb.

Kirschner wire fixation is used if there is any tendency towards resubluxation [32, 33].

Eaton has pointed out that most will eventually require surgical stabilization, because the deep ulnar ligament will heal in a lengthened position, rendering the joint unstable.

Eaton described a surgical procedure in which a strip of the flexor carpi radialis tendon, left attached to its metacarpal, is passed through a hole drilled perpendicularly through the base of the first metacarpal to reconstruct the stretched out deep ulnar ligament. This is an excellent surgical procedure for the symptomatic unstable carpometacarpal joint.

Metacarpophalangeal joint of the thumb

Dorsal dislocation of this joint must be associated with a major disruption of the ligaments. With tears of the volar plate and accessory collateral ligament, the proximal phalanx can hyperextend 90°, but for a complete dislocation (bayonet type) with the proximal phalanx lying dorsal and parallel to the metacarpal, there must in addition be a complete tear of the major portion of the collateral ligament [7]. The metacarpal head is herniated volarly between the flexor pollicis brevis and adductor pollicis, and the volar plate becomes interposed between the bones. Lateral radiographs confirm the diagnosis, and show the sesamoid dorsal to the metacarpal head, indicating the position of the volar plate.

These dislocations can usually be reduced by closed manipulation [1]. Because of spasm of the intrinsic muscles around the joint, regional anaesthesia is preferable to simple wrist block. Reduction is accomplished by traction and gentle manipulation, and the joint must be checked for stability and completeness of reduction. If there is marked lateral instability, or reduction is unstable, repair of the disrupted lateral and volar structures should be performed through a volar zigzag incision [1].

The metacarpal head is seen as soon as the skin and subcutaneous tissues are opened, care being taken to avoid the radial digital nerve crossing the flexor tendon sheath. The flexor pollicis longus will seem to be displaced ulnarwards. Usually the volar plate which is displaced dorsally between the bones prevents reduction which is accomplished as soon as it is released. Lateral stability is assessed, and generally major tears of the collateral ligament can be demonstrated. Repair of ligaments and volar plate is carried out with pull-out wire technique or by direct suture and the joint is immobilized for 4 weeks. A stable, pain-free joint usually results but symptoms tend to persist for a minimum of 6 months.

Traumatic dislocation of extensor tendon

This injury, a tear of the sagittal fibres of the extensor apparatus at the metacarpophalangeal joint is caused by forceful flexion against a fully extended joint, with the extensor tendon slipping into the intermetacarpal valley. This relatively uncommon injury is analogous to the more common deformity in rheumatoid arthritis. Initially the patient may be able to flex and extend the joint but the extensor tendon will snap as it dislocates and relocates on flexion and extension. Later, no active extension is possible, but the tendon relocates on passive extension. In time, however, the tendon becomes fixed in the dislocated position and passive extension is impossible.

Treatment is usually surgical. If seen early, healing will probably occur if the metacarpophalangeal joint is splinted in extension, but surgical repair is preferable. The lesion can be easily exposed by a longitudinal incision over the metacarpophalangeal joint, and the torn sagittal fibres repaired. When seen late, the repair is not only necessary, but the contralateral contracted sagittal band should be released. In older and more fixed cases the oblique fibres will have to be released additionally in order to relocate the tendon.

Avulsion fractures

Most of the soft tissue injuries discussed can be associated with avulsion of bony fragments torn away with the ligament or tendon [2]. The mechanism of injury is the same as that described for the soft tissue injuries. Avulsion fractures are seen with injuries of the collateral ligaments, volar plates and with mallet and boutonnière lesions (see Chapters 11 and 16).

The fracture confirms the diagnosis and gives information regarding the displacement of the ligament. When the fragment is large it represents a significant intra-articular lesion and must be treated by accurate open reduction and internal fixation. As the fragment is actually pulled from the bone and not crushed,

100 per cent anatomical reduction is usually possible. Small fragments, however, are excised usually when the ligament or tendons are repaired, because they may not unite and be a source of tenderness and joint irritation.

REFERENCES

[1] ROWLAND, S. A. AND GREEN, D. P. Fractures and dislocations of the hand. In Rockwood, C. A. and Green, D. P., eds, *Fractures*, Vol. I. Philadelphia, J. B. Lippincott, 1975.

[2] NALEBUFF, E. A. AND MILLENDER, L. H. Skeletal and ligamentous injuries of the hand. In Cave, E., Burke, J. and Boyd, R., eds, *Trauma Management*. Chicago, Year Book Medical Publishers, 1974.

[3] FLATT, A. E. *The Care of Minor Hand Injuries*. St. Louis, C. V. Mosby, 1959.

[4] EATON, R. G. *Joint Injuries of the Hand*. Springfield, Charles C. Thomas, 1971.

[5] WEEKS, P. M. AND WRAY, R. C. *Management of Acute Hand Injuries*. St. Louis, C. V. Mosby, 1973.

[6] CURTIS, R. Capsulectomy of the interphalangeal joints of the fingers. *Journal of Bone and Joint Surgery*, 1954, **36A**, 1219.

[7] STENER, B. Hyperextension injuries to the metacarpophalangeal joint of the thumb—rupture of ligaments, fractures of sesamoid bones, rupture of flexor pollicis brevis. *Acta Chirurgica Scandinavica*, 1963, **125**, 583.

[8] FLYNN, J. E. *Hand Surgery*. Baltimore, Williams and Wilkins, 1975.

[9] McCUE, F. C., HONNER, R., JOHNSON, M. C., JR., AND GIECK, J. H. Athletic injuries of the proximal interphalangeal joint requiring surgical treatment. *Journal of Bone and Joint Surgery*, 1970, **52A**, 937.

[10] MOBERG, E. Fractures and ligamentous injuries of the thumb and fingers. *Surgical Clinics of North America*, 1960, **40**, 297.

[11] KUCZYNSKI, K. The proximal interphalangeal joint: anatomy and causes of stiffness in the fingers. *Journal of Bone and Joint Surgery*, 1968, **50B**, 656.

[12] MILFORD, L. The hand. In Crenshaw, A. H. ed. *Campbell's Orthopaedics*, 5th ed. St. Louis, C. V. Mosby, 1971.

[13] FLATT, A. E. Athletic injuries of the hand. *Journal of the Louisiana State Medical Society*, 1967, **119**, 425.

[14] REDLER, I. AND WILLIAMS, J. T. Rupture of a collateral ligament of the proximal interphalangeal joint of the finger following trauma. *Journal of Bone and Joint Surgery*, 1967, **49A**, 322.

[15] COONRAD, R. W. AND GOLDNER, J. L. A study of the pathological findings and treatment in soft-tissue injury of the thumb metacarpophalangeal joint. *Journal of Bone and Joint Surgery*, 1968, **50A**, 439.

[16] STENER, B. Displacement of the ruptured ulnar collateral ligament of the metacarpophalangeal joint of the thumb. *Journal of Bone and Joint Surgery*, 1962, **44B**, 869.

[17] LAMB, D. W., ABERNETHY, P. J. AND FRAGIADAKIS, E.

Injuries of the metacarpo-phalangeal joint of the thumb. *The Hand*, 1971, **3**, 164.

[18] NEVIASER, R. J., WILSON, J. N. AND LIEVANO, A. Rupture of the ulnar collateral ligament of the thumb (gamekeeper's thumb): correction by dynamic repair. *Journal of Bone and Joint Surgery*, 1971, **53A**, 1357.

[19] ALLDRED, A. J. Rupture of the collateral ligament of the metacarpo-phalangeal joint of the thumb. *Journal of Bone and Joint Surgery*, 1955, **37B**, 443.

[20] FRYKMAN, G. AND JOHANSSON, O. Surgical repair of rupture of the ulnar collateral ligament of the metacarpo-phalangeal joint of the thumb. *Acta Chirurgica Scandinavica*, 1956, **112**, 58.

[21] BORGESKOV, S. Conservative therapy for fractures of the phalanges and metacarpals. *Acta Chirurgica Scandinavica*, 1967, **133**, 123.

[22] ADAMS, J. P. Correction of chronic dorsal subluxation of the proximal interphalangeal joint by means of a criss-cross volar graft. *Journal of Bone and Joint Surgery*, 1959, **41A**, 111.

[23] BOYES, J. H. *Bunnell's Surgery of the Hand*, 4th ed. Philadelphia, J. B. Lippincott, 1964.

[24] KAPLAN, E. B. Dorsal dislocation of the metacarpophalangeal joint of the index finger. *Journal of Bone and Joint Surgery*, 1957, **39A**, 1081.

[25] McLAUGHLIN, H. L. Complex 'locked' dislocation of the metacarpophalangeal joints. *Journal of Trauma*, 1965, **5**, 683.

[26] BECTON, J. L., CHRISTION, J. D., JR., GOODWIN, H. N. AND JACKSON, J. G. III. A simplified technique for treating the complex dislocation of the index metacarpophalangeal joint. *Journal of Bone and Joint Surgery*, 1975, **57**, 695.

[27] WAUGH, R. L. AND YANCEY, A. G. Carpo-metacarpal dislocations. *Journal of Bone and Joint Surgery*, 1948, **30A**, 397.

[28] BUZBY, B. F. Palmar carpo-metacarpal dislocation of the fifth metacarpal. *Annals of Surgery*, 1934, **100**, 555.

[29] KER, H. B. Dislocation of the fifth carpometacarpal joint. *Journal of Bone and Joint Surgery*, 1955, **37B**, 254.

[30] NALEBUFF, E. A. Isolated anterior carpometacarpal dislocation of the fifth finger: classification and case report. *Journal of Trauma*, 1968, **8**, 1119.

[31] WATSON-JONES, R. *Fractures and Joint Injuries*, 4th ed. Edinburgh, E. & S. Livingstone, 1956.

[32] WAGNER, C. J. Method of treatment of Bennett's fracture dislocation. *American Journal of Surgery*, 1950, **80**, 230.

[33] WIGGENS, H. E., BUNDENS, W. D., JR. AND PARK, B. J. A method of treatment of fracture-dislocations of the first metacarpal bone. *Journal of Bone and Joint Surgery*, 1954, **36A**, 810.

CHAPTER 15

Injuries to the Wrist

J. H. DOBYNS and R. L. LINSCHEID

'Practice' suggests practical, and so it shall be in this tourist guide to an old familiar region, which yet has many unexpected paths and byways. The root words for wrist mean bend, turn or twist, and such are the unique, functional characteristics of the area. The distal radio-ulnar, radiocarpal and midcarpal joints, with associated carpometacarpal joints, cooperate so skillfully, that normal action in one system alone without participation of the others is unknown. In addition to the transverse orientation of the joint systems, there are columnar or longitudinal functional units [1]. The radial column supports the multiple, positional needs of the thumb; the central column supports the flexion–extension needs of the hand; the ulnar column permits and assists the vital rotational needs of the entire unit, and all three of these interrelate with one another. Also the radius pivots around the distal ulna, and the carpus is slung from the distal radius. Not only are these characteristics interesting, but they permit a better understanding of the many types of injury to which the wrist is susceptible.

Another concept is critical in understanding wrist problems. The proximal carpal row is an intercalated segment, dynamically unsupported in a link system [2–4]. Link systems tend to collapse in a Z-configuration when under pressure and not balanced by either static or dynamic forces. This is true of the wrist, whose principle support is the static one of an intact scaphoid with its intact ligamentous attachments (see p. 15). With disruption of the usual stabilizing elements (such as a scaphoid fracture (Fig. 15.1a), a scapholunate dissociation (Fig. 15.1b), or other less well-defined ligament damage) the wrist will assume one of the two possible Z-collapse configurations [5], either a dorsiflexion collapse pattern (Fig. 15.1c), or a palmar flexion collapse pattern (Fig. 15.1d). Some degree of this abnormal articular alignment is compatible with good wrist function, but all such abnormal stresses lead to increasing joint deterioration [6].

The use of the hands in a protective and supportive fashion results in a high incidence of wrist injury, mostly to deeper structures. This chapter is devoted only to skeletal and articular structures and their support elements. Within this group the relative incidence of injury in various studies [7–9] is fairly consistent except for sprains. If all ligament [10] injuries, small fragment fractures and impingement syndromes were included, sprain would probably be the most common wrist injury. Specific identification of the sprain patterns are covered in this chapter. Equally frequent are the various fractures of the distal radius, which usually have associated injuries to the distal ulna, or its ligaments. Almost as common are scaphoid fractures and the sprain, subluxation and dislocation injuries of the distal radioulnar joint. Next are the dislocations and fracture dislocations of the carpus itself. Injuries to the lunate bone are relatively common if one assumes Kienbock's disease to be a post-traumatic condition. Statistics are poor for the frequency of other carpal bone fractures, but the frequency probably follows this order: triquetrum, hamate, trapezium, capitate, pisiform and trapezoid. Injuries are considered from the distal border of pronator quadratus to include the finger carpometacarpal and intermetacarpal joints [11–13].

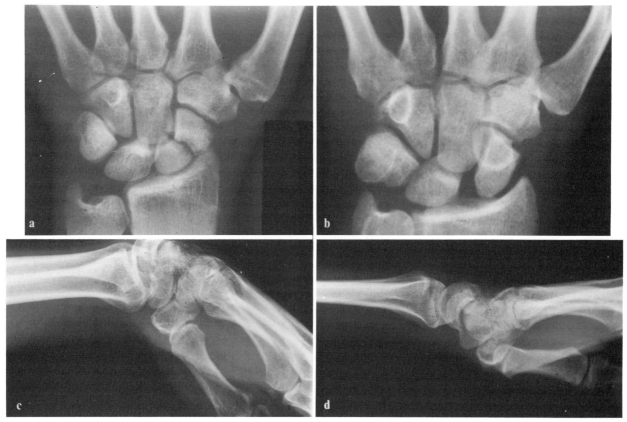

FIG. 15.1. The precise and disciplined alignment of forearm, wrist and hand depends upon an intact bone and/or ligament system. With scaphoid fracture (a) or with ligament damage only, the usual patterns of collapse are: (b) Scapho-lunate dissociation, (c) dorsi-flexion instability and (d) palmar flexion instability. As in (c) dorsal translocation is often a compensatory alignment for a malunited Colles' fracture. Scapho-lunate dissociation as seen in (b) may occur with any of those patterns.

Diagnosis

That a specific diagnosis is useful to the physician should be obvious, since it provides him with a key to management and prognosis. It is equally important to the patient, whose peers and supervisors dismiss a sprained wrist as of no consequence, but will honour necessary treatment and restrictions if a specific name is given to the problem. History is a key point in diagnosis. Most useful is an assessment of the forces applied and the direction in which the wrist was stressed. If in doubt, it can be assumed that the wrist was forced into extension with compression and impingement stresses dorsally and tension stresses volarly. However, there is some rotation or torque in most injuries, and they may be principally rotary in nature, as when the hand is caught in a spinning steering wheel. Flexion of the wrist with compression and impingement stresses volarly and tension stresses dorsally may occasionally occur. Typical of this are many motorcycle injuries, particularly when the hand continues to grip the steering bar. Angulatory stresses with radial or ulnar deviation are seen occasionally. Also seen are direct crush injuries which may be lateral, but are usually anteroposterior in direction, and tend to flatten out the carpal arch by fracture, tissue-tearing or both. It is difficult to elicit facts of trivial or repetitive wrist injury, but the painful push-up, the duffed golf shot, the erratic tennis stroke and many others have all been specifically incriminated. It is well-known that fractures of the scaphoid do not show on early radiographs, but it is not so well-known that similar fractures in all the carpal bones and the distal radius also may not be readily seen.

Gross swelling, deformity, and abnormal motion are easily identified, but in most wrist injuries the findings are much more subtle. Often variability in the range of motion, the grip strength, the endurance or the various combinations of joint laxity, subluxation and clicking may be the significant clues. Almost any involved bone or joint can be palpated, and many areas are quite prominent including both radial and ulnar styloid, the head of the ulna, Lister's tubercle, the distal radioulnar joint, the dorsal surface of the proximal scaphoid, the adjacent tuberosities of scaphoid and trapezium with the scaphotrapezial trapezoidal joint between them, the pisiform, the hook of the hamate, and the margins of the carpometacarpal joints of the fingers. Many of the tendons which cross the wrist and even some of the vessels and nerves can be easily palpated or even inspected.

With so many landmarks there should be no difficulty of accurate description, nor of defining accurately the most useful and consistent diagnostic finding of localized tenderness. There may be generalized tenderness, but usually only when there is generalized pathology. There may be multiple areas of specific tenderness, or multiple structures spanned by one area of tenderness. In such cases there is usually some ancillary finding which will discriminate. Joint surface, ligament, musculotendinous unit may be separately stressed. The use of local anaesthesia may be of value to assess the depth of the lesion and may relieve pain dramatically. Tenderness is best elicited by a palpating digit. The cause and location of pain produced by movement or simple compression can be important diagnostically.

Testing of wrist laxity should be a part of every examination. The most difficult part of this examination is to obtain muscular relaxation. The examination consists of moving the carpus in either a dorsal–volar plane or a radioulnar plane, with the forearm stabilized. There is great variability in normal wrist laxity during these manoeuvres, but for diagnostic purposes *pain* produced by such manoeuvres is most important. Abnormal alignments (subluxations) of the carpal bones or 'clicks' should also be noted. The normal wrist may click, but clicking with pain has been noted in tears of the triangular fibrocartilage or the adjacent meniscoid and also in

scapholunate dissociations, triquetrolunate tears and triquetrohamate tears.

Radiographic examination of the wrist is vital in making a diagnosis [14] since most post-traumatic wrist conditions of significance will have some abnormal radiographic finding. A fundamental problem is recognizing the normal radiography of the wrist where both the static and the dynamic positioning show variations. Changes in shape and number of the bones in this region are common in congenital problems. Coalitions are seen and accessory bones are common, though the type described most often in the literature (bipartite scaphoid) probably does not exist [15]. Many of the angles created by the intersecting bones are of special importance in diagnosis as are the distances between bony margins. Typical of this is scapholunate dissociation where the scapholunate angle on the neutral lateral exceeds the normal mean of $47°$ and the scapholunate gap generally exceeds the normal average of 2–3 mm [5, 16]. The most important need of radiological diagnosis is the requirement for superb quality radiographs. Fractures with serious consequences may appear as small lines of condensation or radiolucency. Radiographs are often of insufficient quality to demonstrate fractures. Another problem is the irregular contour and the common overlap of wrist bones. Special views often help [7, 17, 18]; for instance carpal tunnel views [19, 20], carpal bridge views [21], the ulnar-deviated, supination, oblique view to show the scaphoid [22] and the $45°$, supination, oblique for the hamate hook [23]. A supination postero-anterior view often shows a scapholunate dissociation that is not obvious on the anteroposterior [1]. Similarly, dynamic stress, such as fist compression, often demonstrates such instabilities as the scapholunate dissociation [24]. For clarity, giant views and xerograms may be useful, and, the most useful technique for showing subtle changes in the bones is the trispiral tomogram [24, 25]. Careful monitoring is required since the cuts may not be thin enough (usually 3 mm cuts are taken), or they may not include the suspect area. Cineradiography is a useful technique [26], particularly in suspected instability, attempting to record the instability dynamically. Arthrography is used to locate leaks between the various joint compartments [27]. A dye leak between radiocarpal and midcarpal joint at the triquetrohamate joint may suggest this as the most significant problem in a clinical situation where the entire ulnar side of the carpus and the distal radioulnar joint had been under suspicion. Radiography may show findings which are not relevant to the current problem and must, therefore be interpreted in conjunction with the other data. The place of thermography, radioactive scans, EMI scanning etc. is not yet established in the day-to-day diagnosis of the injured wrist.

Sprains of the wrist [28]

Only specific lesions are considered, though circumstances may still warrant use of 'wrist sprain', wrist pain syndrome, possible fracture, etc. The conditions, discussed in order of frequency, are dorsal avulsion and shear fractures, scapholunate sprain, impingement sprain, triquetrolunate and triquetrohamate sprains, finger carpometacarpal sprain, thumb carpometacarpal sprain, distal radioulnar sprain, pisotriquetral sprain and hamate hook sprain. Many of these conditions overlap with more significant subluxation, dislocation, or fracture–dislocation problems. Occasionally, small chip fractures and some late cases of impingement sprain will show marginal exostoses.

Dorsal avulsion and shear fractures [7, 29]

These probably can occur from volar-flexion stress with the dorsal radiotriquetral ligament pulling off a bone fragment, but they are seen most commonly after dorsiflexion stress due to impingement and shearing of bone and ligament. Though painful, these injuries respond well to simple support.

Scapholunate sprain

Any injury accompanied by tenderness over the scapholunate junction just distal to Lister's tubercle should be considered a scapholunate sprain with potential for dissociation.

Dissociation can be demonstrated clinically by clicking or subluxation or unusual prominence [6, 30–33]. A scapholunate gap, increased scapholunate angle, subluxation during motion or a scapholunate leak during arthrography are all convincing radiological criteria [3, 24, 34]. The dissociation should be reduced by closed manipulation (usually by pushing dorsally on the scaphoid tuberosity and volarly on the proximal end of the scaphoid), and held in a cast which inhibits compressive stresses for 6 weeks. If reduction cannot be held, percutaneous Kirschner wires are used to hold position. If the reduction cannot be obtained or maintenance requires undue force, open reduction followed by percutaneous Kirschner wire fixation and possibly by ligament reconstruction is warranted [7]. In addition to the manoeuvre described to reduce the scaphoid, it may also be necessary to apply pressure over the dorsum of the capitate, pushing it volarward in the lunate cup and thereby realigning the lunate which has usually slipped under the capitate and is rotated. At least two Kirschner wires are needed to maintain this position, one through the radial styloid across scaphoid and into capitate, the other through the radius across lunate and into capitate or hamate. Occasionally a Kirschner wire across scaphoid into lunate is helpful also. In late cases, it may be necessary to clear fibrous tissue from the scapholunate interval and to reconstruct the scapholunate ligament. At the very least, any ligament remnants present should be reapproximated and the dorsal capsule tightened. Such cases should be held 8 weeks before the wires are removed and another 4 weeks before support is discontinued. Even then, a mild recurrence of instability may occur, but sufficient stability for good wrist function is usual [24].

Impingement sprain

Impingement and shear stresses are also seen in repetitive trauma with the wrist constantly forced into dorsiflexion. The classic instance of this occurs in gymnasts who develop both acute and chronic symptoms, and on occasion may have to stop performance or even undergo surgery for relief. At surgery, the findings are fibrosis and thickening of the synovium, stripping of local ligaments, denuding of contact articular cartilage, and sometimes marginal exostosis formation.

Triquetrolunate sprain

Triquetrolunate tears are sustained usually from dorsiflexion stresses similar to those giving scapholunate tears, and the two may occur together. Dissociation is difficult to determine and clinical findings plus positive arthrography are often the major clues to this injury. It usually can be treated satisfactorily with wrist support for 6 weeks, if the diagnosis is made early.

Triquetrohamate sprain

Triquetrohamate tears are similar except that the injuring stress is often rotational. Treatment is similar to that for triquetral lunate tears. However, in either case, if the diagnosis is made late, ligament reconstruction or even localized intercarpal fusion may be needed.

Finger carpometacarpal sprain

Carpometacarpal sprains are common. Though injury may be from direct impaction or dorsiflexion, a surprisingly common mechanism is palmar flexion stress or even angulatory or rotational stress. Early diagnosis and support are sufficient, but delayed treatment or chondral surface damage may result in persistent and chronic pain [35].

Thumb carpometacarpal sprain

A similar problem occurs at the thumb carpometacarpal and/or scaphotrapeziotrapezoidal joints. Causative stress is usually dorsiflexion. Early identification and treatment with a thumb spica support are important in preventing persisting problems.

Distal radioulnar sprain

The most common area for sprain problems is possibly the distal radioulnar joint [36–39]. Ligament injuries are sustained in dorsiflexion stress and are also common in rotatory stress situations. Ligament damage, unless very mild, is usually associated with injury to the triangular fibrocartilage and often with a small fracture of the ulnar styloid or a portion of it. These injuries are best managed by early diagnosis and 6 weeks of support with the forearm supinated. If the diagnosis is made late or the disruption is marked, open repair should be considered since extremely late treatment of this problem is difficult, short of distal ulnar excision.

Pisotriquetral sprain

Joint capsule (pisotriquetral), adjacent bones (triquetrum and hamate) and flexor carpi ulnaris tendon are all attached to the pisiform [40] and these fibres may be damaged acutely by impact, dorsiflexion stress and flexor carpi ulnaris contraction or by repetitive stresses. Rest and protection usually suffice, although osteochondral damage may result.

Hamate hook sprain

Excessive contact stresses in the palm may apply force to this area through the carpal ligaments or directly to the soft tissues over the hook [41, 42]. In either case, stopping the activity is curative.

Distal radius injuries [5] (Fig. 15.2)

Perhaps even more common than the undetected scaphoid fracture is the undiagnosed fracture of the distal radius. The same rule prevails. If history is suggestive and local tenderness is present, treat. Time will show positive radiographic changes and the position of the fracture line or the collapse tendency will provide one of three types:

(1) The Colles' type [8, 43–47], includes all fractures distal to the pronator quadratus, which tend to collapse into dorsiflexion.

(2) The Smith group [48–50] includes all those fractures in the same area, which tend to collapse into volar flexion.

(3) The articular margin fractures, which have a potential for subluxation or even dislocating along with the carpus. This group includes those fractures commonly known as Barton's fracture [51–53], reverse Barton's fracture, radial styloid fracture [54, 55], etc.

Colles' fracture (Fig. 15.2a)

This often has the additional deformities of supination, shortening, and radial displacement. It is frequently comminuted, particularly in demineralized bone with the more common comminution in the dorsal cortex. Bone contact and stability are frequently good in the deformed position and healing may be quite rapid if the subsequent mechanical and cosmetic deformities are acceptable.

Treatment may be simply that of comfortable support and early rehabilitation. This can be a particularly appealing concept for the older age group with diminished functional needs and intractable osteoporosis. However, for active individuals with skilled or demanding requirements for hand function, this is a poor choice since both cosmesis and function do correlate with anatomic restoration, particularly in terms of restored and well aligned joint surfaces.

All Colles' fractures can be reduced to a near normal position, usually by the simple application of effective traction, perhaps with some ancillary manipulation after traction has restored full length and alignment. The problem is maintaining this position, particularly the full length and the normal inclination of the distal radial articular surface, since the comminution of the dorsal cortex permits shortening and dorsal tilt so readily. The usual manner of doing this is to use 15° of flexion and 20–30° of ulnar deviation to produce tension in the dorsal soft tissues and periosteum which is maintained by a

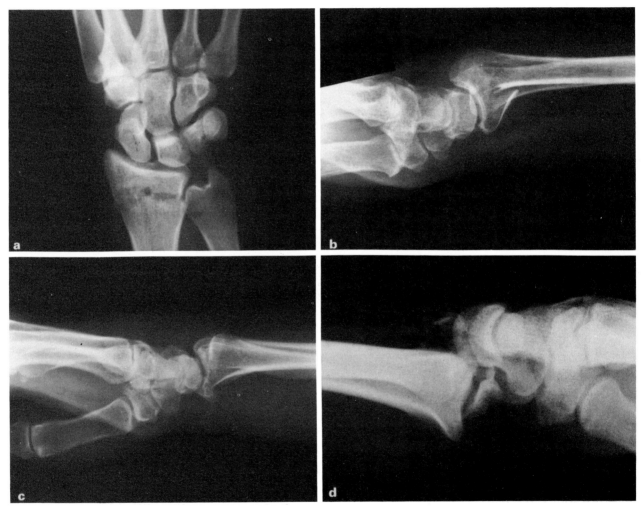

Fig. 15.2. Fractures of the distal radius e.g. (a) Colles' fractures tend to collapse into dorsiflexion or (b) volar flexion (Smith fractures). A group of margin fractures may dislocate with the associated carpus. (c) Usually, these fractures involve the volar lip. (d) Dorsal lip fractures are also seen. The frequent instability is demonstrated by (c) subluxation and (d) dislocation. Radial styloid involvement alone or with volar lip or dorsal lip fractures (d) is common.

dorso-radial plaster slab [56, 57]. The position, however, may aggravate nerve entrapment tendencies volarly and increase tension in the digit extensors dorsally, and its extremes should never be used.

Alternative methods for retaining the reduced position are known. They include open reduction and internal fixation [7, 57], but more commonly the various techniques of percutaneous pin fixation with the pins supported either by plaster (pin and plaster technique) [58–64] or by external rod fixation devices (Roger–Anderson apparatus [7] or Hoffman apparatus). These techniques do not guarantee immunity from the common complications of injuries to the distal radius, but these can be treated efficiently while the late complications due to malalignment are avoided. Occasionally, instability of the distal ulna, an unattached articular fragment of the distal radius, or the overall relationship of carpus to distal radius will require added percutaneous fixation wires to control the position.

It should be noted that these techniques which in essence maintain some distraction in order to restore normal anatomy, do not shorten the healing time. They may, in fact, prolong it, since new bone consolidation to support the deficient areas takes more time. The usual fixation time needed for percutaneous pins and their supporting apparatus is 8 weeks or longer.

Smith fractures (Fig. 15.2b)

These are much less common and are usually more stable after reduction [48, 50]. Also, the usual post-reduction positions of neutral or slight dorsiflexion at the wrist permit better function. Good reduction is needed. When it cannot be achieved by closed methods percutaneous pin fixation or open reduction and internal fixation are indicated [50]. The volar lip of radius fracture, usually included with Smith fractures, is placed in the third group as an articular margin fracture with potential dislocation.

Articular margin fractures

The common trio of articular margin fractures are volar lip, radial styloid and dorsal lip fractures in order of frequency. Combinations of these three and a combination including all or part of the ulnar margin of the radius are common. In addition to the distortion of joint surfaces common to all, they have the potential for subluxation (Fig. 15.2c) or occasionally overt dislocation of the carpus along with the marginal fracture fragments (Fig. 15.2d). It is well known that after reduction, positioning should be such that the compressive stresses exerted by the carpus fall against the major intact radial fragment and not against the smaller marginal fragment [48]. If the margin fragments do not remain snugly reduced, thus restoring an intact joint line, they should be fixed by percutaneous pin or if necessary by open reduction and internal fixation [52]. Intercarpal malalignment may be seen in any distal radial fractures, but particularly in this group, and external support should be continued until sound healing is present. The need for smooth, well-aligned joint surfaces and wrist stability is much greater than the need for a full range of wrist motion.

Distal ulna fractures and dislocations

Damage to the distal ulnar complex, both ligamentous and bony, is probably very common in the group of distal radial fractures [45, 65–67]. No significant distortion of the distal radius is possible without damaging some element of the distal ulna. Usually the only requirement is to ensure that the distal ulna is congruous with the ulnar notch of radius after reduction of the radial fracture. This congruity is best demonstrated and maintained in supination, and occasionally requires percutaneous pin fixation of ulna to radius. Occasionally, as in open injuries, there is an opportunity to return the detached ligament support (usually triangular fibrocartilage with or without an ulnar styloid fragment) to its position. This should also be considered when open reduction of distal radius fractures is carried out since it adds an element of stability. Because ulnar styloid fractures near the base represent loss of the strongest support between the two bones (the triangular fibrocartilage), this injury should be treated by support in supination until healing is demonstrated. If the styloid fracture is old or is merely through the distal half, symptomatic treatment only is sufficient. Fractures of the articular portion of the distal ulna should be reduced and supported until healed. If not well reduced, open reduction should be considered since articular incongruity at the distal radioulnar joint is painful and interferes with rotation. Fractures of the neck require similar treatment, their importance depending principally upon whether there is sufficient deformity to alter the articular relationship of the ulnar head. In late cases where there is such deformity distal ulna excision is preferable [68–70]. Instability of the distal ulna occurs as an isolated injury, the usual tendency being for dorsal subluxation or volar dislocation [71–75]. A history of injury and the clinical finding of tenderness and swelling are the most reliable guides to this injury. A true lateral radiograph shows dorsal or volar malalignment of the distal ulna, though the degree is often slight. There may be difficulty in obtaining a true lateral particularly with the volar dislocation group, some of which present with the distal ulna locked under the radius, thus inhibiting normal rotation. Both groups should be treated by manipulative reduction and in some instances this may require open reduction, particularly if the injury is seen late. If joint surfaces are intact, the forearm should be placed in the most stable position (usually supination) and if necessary fixed in that position by transfixing Kirschner wires.

Scaphoid fractures

Though much the best known and most common of carpal fractures, the scaphoid fracture still presents many problems [4, 76–81], principally due to delayed diagnosis and treatment. In biomechanical test situations, it can be produced consistently by dorsiflexion stress applied to a wrist in 90° extension and about 7° of radial deviation [82] whereas the Colles' fracture is produced with a lesser degree of dorsiflexion. Both of these positions are common support positions for the falling body and with slight variations of point of impact, angulation and torque, all of the many varieties of wrist fracture and ligament injury can be reproduced. Though there are many other specific, diagnosable injuries in the carpus, the scaphoid fracture remains the most common serious injury and must be excluded in the presence of snuffbox area pain and tenderness, even without a history of trauma. Special views, such as trispiral tomography, usually reveal the fracture even if early and not displaced but are generally unnecessary. The amount of padding in the support dressing depends upon the local swelling, but the minimum firm support should include the forearm, wrist and thumb and is also the maximum support

used by one of us (R.L.L.). If a fracture is confirmed, it is the other author's practice to apply a lightly padded long arm cast for the first 6 weeks with all digits included in a similar but more extensive way than that recommended by Dehne *et al.* [83]. Though many heal with less support than this [84, 85], it is unknown for a scaphoid fracture with minimal displacement to fail to heal when diagnosed early, and thus supported. At the present time such support is only used for those fractures (about 20 per cent) which are unstable because of extensive comminution with angulation of 20° or more between the fragments, displacement of more than 2 mm between the fragments, or a collapse pattern of the carpus (either dorsiflexion or volar flexion instability). Special problems in the acute fracture include the proximal pole which is almost always deprived of circulation (even the common mid-waist fracture may produce ischaemia of the proximal half of the scaphoid). Nevertheless, if a fracture with ischaemic fragments is diagnosed early and treated adequately, it heals satisfactorily and the ischaemic portion usually revascularizes, though the overall treatment course is somewhat extended. Only in comminuted fractures or long delayed union is fragmentation seen. A displaced scaphoid fracture (the displaced portion is usually the proximal fragment) occasionally heals in malposition if there is approximately 60 per cent contact. However, union is slow and there is some distortion of joint surfaces. If displaced fractures cannot be manipulated into a near normal position and maintained there, it is usual practice to carry out open reduction and internal fixation [86, 87]. In comminuted fractures this may require a volar bone graft to restore scaphoid length. Healing is then similar to the undisplaced scaphoid fracture.

Another problem in acute scaphoid fractures is the articular fracture at the distal end which should be treated with respect even though it may resemble the simple, easy healing scaphoid tuberosity fracture. Any fracture involving the articular surfaces of the scaphotrapeziotrapezoidal joint should be protected until soundly healed. If the articular surfaces are considerably distorted and cannot be restored, open reduction should be considered.

Delayed union, nonunion and malunion are all possibilities with scaphoid fractures [88–95]. Many of these problems stem from delayed diagnosis or inadequate early treatment. Delayed union at any stage is probably worth a trial of cast treatment unless there is a gap or displacement of more than 1 mm, considerable angulatory deformity of the scaphoid (nearly always volar collapse and dorsal angulation), displacement of one of the fragments or definite evidence of a nonunion. If there is evidence of healing activity cast treatment should be continued. Otherwise the delayed union is probably best treated by open reduction, internal fixation and bone graft. Signs of nonunion are sclerosis at the fracture margins, rounding of the corners and definite evidence of motion between the fragments, and may occasionally warrant excision of the pseudarthrosis and graft of the two bone fragments. This is to be considered more often for delayed union. Some scaphoid fractures unite in the angulated, deformed position just described and most delayed union cases have some of this collapse. If open reduction is performed on such an angulated scaphoid, it is preferably treated by restoring its normal contour which usually means opening out the volar fracture line, closing the dorsal gap and fixing the position, often with the additional aid of a volar graft to fill in the gap. Fractures healing in the angulated position leads to mild progressive deterioration of the adjacent joint surfaces.

Other problems inherent in scaphoid fracture management are those of ischaemia, fragmentation and arthrosis. Ischaemia is seldom a problem unless there is early comminution or late fragmentation. The chief problem is comminution since the intact ischaemic fragment, if of reasonable size, usually remains unfragmented for years. While fracture comminution may occur after ischaemia, it is more frequent for simultaneous comminution and ischaemia to lead to the cystic changes and ultimate absorption, known as Preiser's disease [96]. Once fragmentation and ischaemia have reached a certain level of deformity and absorption it is unlikely that union or reconstitution is possible. The secondary reconstructive techniques utilized in post-traumatic arthrosis of this area are variable and ingenious, but beyond the scope of this chapter. The most common area of painful arthrosis develops between the distal scaphoid fragment and the adjacent radial styloid. This is often such that a partial radial styloid excision should be considered at the time of an open procedure for delayed union. Open reduction and internal fixation are either done through the styloid interval (snuffbox approach) [97–100] or by volar approach (Matti and Russe) [101, 102]. If internal fixa-

tion is used, Kirschner wires or small compression screws are both popular [103, 104]. Where carpal malpositioning has developed and is to be corrected at the same time, the additional use of Kirschner wires to maintain alignment of radius, scaphoid and other carpal bones may be considered. Bone graft may be applied successfully by a variety of techniques with the principle being that the bone graft should cross the fracture line into both fragments with minimal articular injury. Successful union does not end all problems. Articular surface changes and subsequent damage due to deformity or abnormal motion patterns of the scaphoid may result in sufficient arthrosis for the wrist to remain symptomatic.

Other carpal bone fractures

These are easy to miss whether there are single or multiple fracture lines through the body of the bone. Radiography should be repeated and special views undertaken, such as trispiral tomograms [105]. Even with these, fractures are missed because the cuts were either too thick (3–4 mm is average), were in the wrong plane (sometimes anteroposterior and lateral tomograms are necessary) or were not carried far enough.

Lunate fractures

Lunate fractures [106, 107] are either fairly common or quite rare depending upon whether Kienbock's disease [106–111], lunate cysts [112, 113], etc. are included in this group. However, there are certain lunate fractures which do not have significant ischemic findings. The most common is the avulsion or shear fracture of the dorsal lunate horn. If not associated with other injury, it can be treated quite simply with support until symptoms subside. Fractures through the lunate body occur in certain patterns [113, 114]. One is a three-part fracture with two fracture lines, dividing the lunate into three roughly equal parts; dorsal, middle, and volar. Another pattern is a fracture midway between the two articular surfaces of the lunate. Compression or short oblique fractures are seen, usually at the ulnar proximal corner of the lunate. These and other fractures are seen with and without obvious ischemia [115]. The little experience available with early identification and early treatment of these fracture types suggests that many of them heal if identified early and treated adequately with a support which inhibits compressive stresses. Even delayed union, when not ischemic, may heal with such treatment. Unfortunately, many such fractures are identified only after ischemia develops and these respond poorly to treatment though they do sometimes heal in a deformed configuration.

Triquetral fractures

The triquetrum is the carpal bone most involved in dorsal chip fractures (Fig. 15.3a) [7, 116]. Unless there is associated injury, these may be treated symptomatically.

Fractures of the triquetral body [117–119] also occur and must be identified and treated early by cast.

Hamate fractures

Fractures of the body (Fig. 15.3b) [120, 121] occur and may involve the midcarpal articular surfaces. They heal well if identified early and treated adequately, though secondary joint arthrosis is seen. An interesting and surprisingly common hamate fracture is that of the hook (Fig. 15.3c) [122, 123]. This may occur anywhere from junction of body and hook to tip of hook. Stress over

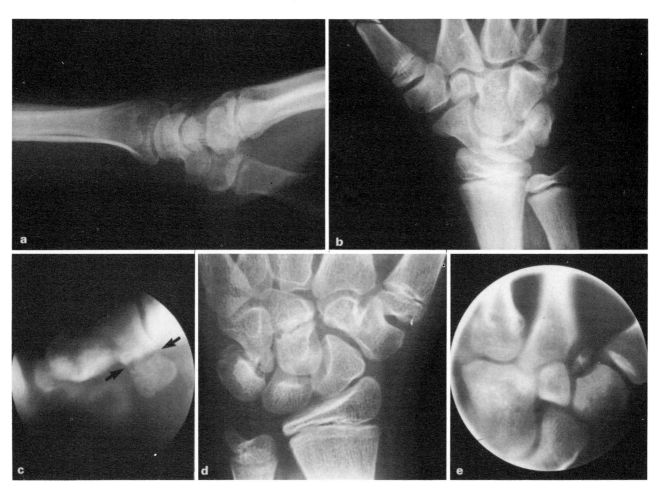

FIG. 15.3. Fractures of the carpus, other than scaphoid, are not as uncommon as is believed, but they are often difficult to identify. Representative examples are (a) triquetral dorsal chip, (b) the hamate articular fracture, (c) the hamate hook fracture, (d) capitate body delayed union and (e) trapezial lateral wall fracture.

the carpal ligaments seems to be a common cause with the greatest group of current cases involving sportsmen who are gripping clubs, bats or rackets. The pain is related to the causative manoeuvre (such as a duffed shot in golf) and associated with discrete pain to pressure over the hook of the hamate. So few of these have been identified early and treated adequately that it is not known whether they heal. They heal with open reduction and internal fixation. However, current literature suggests that excision of the hook of the hamate is equally effective.

Capite fractures

Capitate fractures (Fig. 15.3d) [124, 125] are rare, but may be seen in all parts of the bone and nonunion may develop [7]. A fracture of particular interest involves the proximal articular surface, and may occur with or without peri-lunar dislocation [7] or associated scaphoid fracture [126, 127]. In either instance the small fragment, mostly articular cartilage covered, may displace and rotate. If a normal position cannot be obtained, open reduction is needed. Though ischaemic, the fragment will heal and revascularize.

Trapezial, trapezoidal, pisiform fractures

These are all seen (Fig. 15.3e) [9, 128] but have the usual problems of identification. They will heal if treated early and adequately by appropriate splintage. They all may be associated with early fracture-dislocation or late arthrosis of their related joints.

Dislocations and fracture dislocations (Fig. 15.4)

The intricate alignment of the carpal bones [129, 130] may be altered by any of the injuries previously discussed, but the incidence of persisting instability is highest in this group. Ligament injuries are difficult to identify accurately and treat effectively. Most difficult are the localized ligament tears, often intra-articular, which provoke little tissue reaction and heal slowly, if at all, in the joint fluid environment.

The most common group of dislocations affecting the carpus are those of the perilunate type [9, 131, 132]. The lunate is central, well protected and strongly anchored at least on its volar surface. It and various groupings of its neighbours are, therefore, usually left behind while other parts of the carpus sublux or dislocate around it. Usually stress is in dorsiflexion and radial deviation so tearing of the carpus from the lunate usually begins on its radial side and may extend completely around, eventually isolating the lunate from all its carpal neighbours. The traumatic rent thus produced involves an area of ligament weakness [11, 133] lying between lunate and capitate. Transscaphoid-perilunate dislocation is most common (Fig. 15.4a) [9, 134–137]. Perilunate dislocations (Fig. 15.4b) and radial styloid fractures with perilunate dislocations (Fig. 15.4c) [137, 138] are also common, and other types of fracture-dislocation such as transscaphoid-transcapitate perilunate dislocation (Fig. 15.4d) [138–140] are seen. Fracture identification is easiest from a radiograph made during the traction stage of the reduction manoeuvre. Lunate dislocation is usually the end stage of the perilunate injury [23, 141]. The carpus usually dislocates dorsally, then rebounds and pushes the lunate volarly until the capitate is better aligned with the radius than is the lunate. The radiograph suggests a lunate rather than a perilunate dislocation. The lunate may be rotated into the carpal tunnel, but is still attached to the radius by the volar radiolunate ligament and still has some blood supply. Even this may strip away and the lunate lies free of soft tissue but despite this the lunate, if not fractured, should be replaced. This applies also to any associated bone such as half the scaphoid, the triquetrum, etc. When closed reduction is possible and near anatomical alignment can be maintained, closed treatment is still preferable. Neutral positioning of the wrist with forearm in midposition and elbow and digits included in the support dressing is advised. As the support loosens, gentle maintenance pressure may be needed. For instance, a three-point pressure system may be devised to translocate the distal carpal row volarward into the cup of the proximal row. Frequently, alignment cannot be maintained by these methods. Open reduction and internal fixation is then recommended, preferably with both dorsal and volar approaches [7, 24]. Kirschner wires are sufficient to maintain fracture fixation and radiocarpal, midcarpal and scapholunate alignment. Through the dorsal approach the joint surfaces can be inspected and osteocartilaginous debris removed. Through the volar approach the median nerve may be inspected and decompressed and the capsular tear repaired; sometimes it is also possible to identify and repair some of the large intracapsular ligament fascicles.

Radiocarpal dislocation without fracture is rare [142, 143], but it is more common with fractures of the dorsal, volar or styloid margins of the radius. All are unstable, and closed reduction, if stable, should be maintained for 6–8 weeks. In the perilunate dislocation group, the sign of the unstable carpus is often a gap appearing between scaphoid and lunate [5, 131, 132, 144]. This may be seen in the radiocarpal dislocation group also, but a more common sign of instability is translocation of the entire carpus ulnarward so that the lunate comes to lie distal to the ulna (Fig. 15.4e). If either sort of instability is noted and cannot be controlled, open reduction and internal fixation is certainly indicated and quite possibly

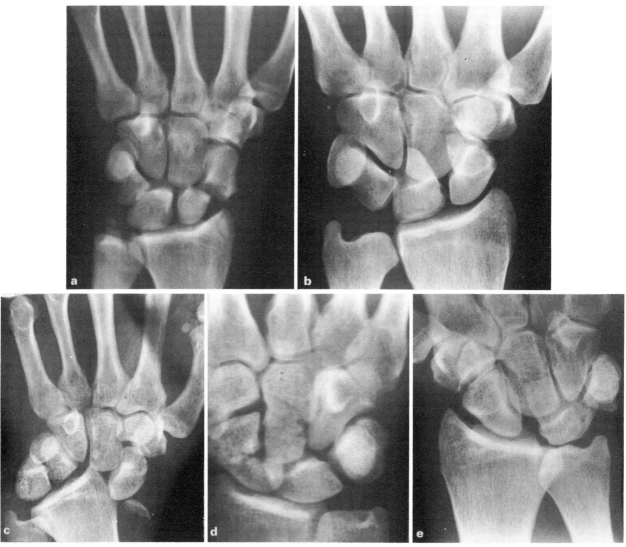

Fig. 15.4. Typical dislocations are the (a) trans-scaphoid perilunate, (b) perilunate, (c) trans-styloid perilunate, and (d) trans-scaphoid trans-capitate perilunate. (a) and (d) are radiographs taken in traction with the dislocation no longer obvious but the fractures much better visualized, (e) shows severe ulnar trans-location.

repair or reconstruction of the principal ligaments (usually radioscapholunate or volar radiolunate).

Midcarpal and isolated carpal bone dislocations occur [145–148], but are rare and difficult to identify. Reduction is necessary and should be followed by prolonged support if it can be maintained; open reduction and internal fixation if it cannot. Isolated scaphoid dislocation [149–153] is a variant of the perilunate dislocation group usually occurring when the carpus returns to the neutral position, but leaves the scaphoid behind trapped against the dorsal radius.

Various types of axial dislocations and fracture dislocations are seen, usually with extreme trauma [7], when one or more digits and the associated carpus are disrupted from the remainder. Thumb, trapezium and scaphoid or ring and little finger with hamate and triquetrum may be displaced from their digital and carpal associations. Often soft tissue damage or neurovascular injury take precedence over the skeletal problem in these injuries though reduction and fixation are usually needed.

Carpometacarpal dislocations and fracture dislocations occur in each digit [154]. Those of the thumb are considered in Chapters 13 and 14. A cause of this problem at the finger carpometacarpal joints is the motorcycle injury with volar flexion stress. Similar mild stress may result in osteochondral fractures or subluxations which may develop dorsal exostoses or painful arthrosis. The overt dislocations and fracture dislocations are easily identified and demand reduction, either closed or open. In many cases, fixation is needed since dislocation in this area is often unstable. With severe instability or joint involvement, open reduction should be considered.

Conclusion

Injuries of the wrist area are neither as simple as history makes them out to be nor so complex that they cannot be understood, identified and treated. Much unnecessary disability persists because of insufficient awareness regarding the varied problems of the wrist exposed to single or repetitive trauma.

REFERENCES

[1] TALEISNIK, J. The ligaments of the wrist. *Journal of Hand Surgery.* St Louis, The C. V. Mosby Company, 1976.

[2] LANDSMEER, J. M. Studies in the anatomy of articulation. I. The equilibrium of the 'intercalated' bone. *Acta morphologia Neerlands—Scandinavia,* 1961, **3,** 287.

[3] LANDSMEER, J. M. Les Coherences spatiales et l'equilibre spatial dans la region carpienne. *Acta anatomica,* 1968, **70** (suppl. 54) 1.

[4] GILFORD, W. W., BOLTON, R. H. AND LAMBRINUDI, C. The mechanism of the wrist joint: with special reference to fractures of the scaphoid. *Guys Hospital Reports,* 1943, **92,** 52.

[5] LINSCHEID, R. L., DOBYNS, J. H., BEAUBOUT, J. W. AND BRYAN, R. S. Traumatic instability of the wrist: diagnosis, classification, and pathomechanics. *Journal of Bone and Joint Surgery,* 1972, **54A,** 1612.

[6] SEBALD, J. R., DOBYNS, J. H. AND LINSCHEID, R. L. The natural history of collapse deformities of the wrist. *Clinical Orthopedics,* 1974, **104,** 140.

[7] DOBYNS, J. H. AND LINSCHEID, R. L. Fractures and dislocation of the wrist. In Rockwood, C. A. and Green, D. P. eds. *Fractures.* Philadelphia, Lippincott, 1975.

[8] BÖHLER, L. *The Treatment of Fractures,* 4th ed. Baltimore, William Wood, 1942.

[9] SPEED, K. *Traumatic Injuries of the Carpus, including Colles' Fracture.* New York, Appleton, 1925.

[10] MAYFIELD, J. K., JOHNSON, R. P. AND KILCOYNE, R. F. The ligaments of the human wrist and their functional significance. *Anatomical Record,* 1976, **186,** 417.

[11] KAPLAN, E. B. *Functional and Surgical Anatomy of the Hand,* 2nd ed. Philadelphia, Lippincott, 1965.

[12] LEWIS, O. J., HAMSHERE, R. J. AND BUCKNILL, T. M. The anatomy of the wrist joint. *Journal of Anatomy,* 1970, **106,** 539.

[13] LEWIS, O. J. The hominoid wrist joint. *American Journal of Physical Anthropology,* 1969, **30,** 251.

[14] DESTOT, E. *Injuries of the Wrist.* London, Ernest Benn, 1925.

[15] LOUIS, D. S. et al. Congenital bipartite scaphoid—fact or fiction. *Journal of Bone and Joint Surgery,* 1976, **58A,** 1108.

[16] SERRAFIAN, S. K., MELAMED, J. L. AND GOSHGARIAN, G. M. Study of wrist motion in flexion and extension. Corr 126: 153–159, July–August 1977.

[17] KÖHLER, A. AND ZIMMER, E. A. *Borderlands of the Normal and Early Pathology in Skeletal Roentgenology.* Based on 11th German ed. New York, Grune and Stratton, 1968.

[18] KRIEUN, M. E. AND EDEIKEN, J. *Roentgenologic Atlas of the Hand and Wrist in Systemic Disease.* Baltimore, Williams & Wilkins, 1973.

[19] WIOT, J. F. AND DORST, J. P. Less common fractures and dislocations of the wrist. *Radiological Clinics of North America*, 1966, **4**, 261.

[20] HART, V. L. AND GAYNOR, V. Roentgenographic study of the carpal canal. *Journal of Bone and Joint Surgery*, 1941, **23**, 382.

[21] LENTINO, W., LUBETSKY, H. W., JACOBSON, H. G. AND POPPEL, M. H. The carpal–bridge view: a position for the roentgenographic diagnosis of abnormalities in the dorsum of the wrist. *Journal of Bone and Joint Surgery*, 1957, **39A**, 88.

[22] ROTHBERG, A. S. Fractures of the carpal navicular: importance of special roentgenography. *Journal of Bone and Joint Surgery*, 1939, **21**, 1020.

[23] STARK, W. A. Recurrent perilunar subluxation. *Clinical Orthopedics*, 1970, **73**, 152.

[24] DOBYNS, J. H. *Traumatic Instability of the Wrist*. Instructional Course Lectures—American Academy of Orthopedic Surgeons. Chapter 11, vol 182–199, St Louis, Mosby, 1975.

[25] JOHNSON, C. M. The role of tomography in the evaluation of carpal injuries. *American Journal of Roentgenology and Radiation Therapy* (in press).

[26] ARKLESS, R. Cineradiography in normal and abnormal wrists. *American Journal of Roentgenology Radium Therapy and Nuclear Medicine*, 1966, **96**, 837.

[27] KESSLER, I AND SILBERMAN, Z. An experimental study of the radiocarpal joint by arthrography. *Surgery, Gynecology and Obstetrics*, 1961, **112**, 33.

[28] LINSCHEID, R. L. AND DOBYNS, J. H. Wrist sprains. In Tubiana, R. ed., *The Hand*. Philadelphia, Saunders (in press).

[29] FAIRBANK, T. J. Chip fractures of the os triquetrum (carpal cuneiform). *British Medical Journal*, 1942, **2**, 310.

[30] ARMSTRONG, G. W. D. Rotational subluxation of the scaphoid. *Canadian Journal of Surgery*, 1968, **11**, 306.

[31] ENGLAND, J. P. S. Subluxation of the carpal scaphoid. *Proceedings of the Royal Society of Medicine*, 1970, **63**, 581.

[32] VAUGHAN-JACKSON, O. J. A case of recurrent subluxation of the carpal scaphoid. *Journal of Bone and Joint Surgery*, 1949, **31B**, 532.

[33] HOWARD, F. M., FAHEY, T. AND WOJCIK, E. Rotatory subluxation of the navicular. *Clinical Orthopedics*, 1974, **104**, 134.

[34] CRITTENDEN, J. J., JONES, D. M. AND SANTARELLI, A. C. Bilateral rotational dislocation of the carpal navicular: case report. *Radiology*, 1970, **94**, 629.

[35] CURTISS, P. H., J. R. The hunchback carpal bone. *Journal of Bone and Joint Surgery*, 1961, **43A**, 392.

[36] SNOOK, G. A., CHRISMAN, O. D., WILSON, T. C. AND WIETSMA, R. D. Subluxation of the distal radio-ulnar joint by hyperpronation. *Journal of Bone and Joint Surgery*, 1969, **51A**, 1315.

[37] VESELY, D. C. The distal radio-ulnar joint. *Clinical Orthopedics*, 1967, **51**, 75.

[38] COLEMAN, H. M. Injuries of the articular disc at the wrist. *Journal of Bone and Joint Surgery*, 1960, **42B**, 522.

[39] WEIGL, K. AND SPIRA, E. The triangular fibrocartilage of the wrist joint. *Reconstructive Surgery and Traumatology*, 1969, **11**, 139.

[40] WESTON, W. J. AND KELSEY, C. K. Functional anatomy of the pisi-cuneiform joint. *British Journal of Radiology*, 1973, **46**, 692.

[41] STARK, H. H. et al. Fracture of the hook of the hamate in athletes. *Journal of Bone and Joint Surgery*, 1977, **59A**, 575.

[42] O'DONOGHUE, D. H. *Treatment of Injuries to Athletes*. Philadelphia, W. B. Saunders, 1962.

[43] ANDERSON, R. AND O'NEIL, G. Comminuted fractures of the distal end of the radius. *Surgery, Gynecology and Obstetrics*, 1944, **78**, 434.

[44] BACORN, R. W. AND KURTZKE, J. F. Colles' fracture: a study of two thousand cases from the New York State Workmen's Compensation Board. *Journal of Bone and Joint Surgery*, 1953, **35A**, 643.

[45] FRYKMAN, G. Fracture of the distal radius including sequelae–shoulder–hand–finger syndrome, disturbance in the distal radio-ulnar joint, and impairment of nerve function: a clinical and experimental study. *Acta orthopaedica Scandinavica*, 1967, **108** (suppl), 1.

[46] GARTLAND, J. J., Jr. AND WERLEY, C. W. Evaluation of healed Colles' fractures. *Journal of Bone and Joint Surgery*, 1951, **33A**, 895.

[47] COLLES, A. On the fracture of the carpal extremity of the radius. *Edinburgh Medical Journal*, 1814, **10**, 182.

[48] ELLIS, J. Smith's and Barton's fractures: A method of treatment. *Journal of Bone and Joint Surgery*, 1965, **47B**, 724.

[49] SMITH, R. W. A Treatise on Fractures in the Vicinity of Joints, and on Certain Forms of Accidental and Congenital Dislocations. Dublin, Hodges & Smith, 1854.

[50] THOMAS, F. B. Reduction of Smith's fracture. *Journal of Bone and Joint Surgery*, 1957, **39B**, 463.

[51] BARTON, J. R. Views and treatment of an important injury to the wrist. *Medical Examiner*, 1838, **1**, 365.

[52] DEOLIVEIRA, J. C. Barton's fractures. *Journal of Bone and Joint Surgery*, 1973, **55A**, 586.

[53] AUFRANC, O. E., JONES, W. N. AND TURNER, R. H. Anterior marginal articular fracture of distal radius. *Journal of the American Medical Association*, 1966, **196**, 788.

[54] EDWARDS, H. C. Mechanism and treatment of backfire fracture. *Journal of Bone and Joint Surgery*, 1926, **8**, 701.

[55] FITZSIMONS, R. A. Colles' fracture and chauffeur's fracture. *British Medical Journal*, 1938, **2**, 357.

[56] CAROTHERS, R. G. AND BOYD, F. J. Thumb traction technique for reduction of Colles' fracture. *Archives of Surgery*, 1949, **58**, 848.

[57] CHARNLEY, J. *The Closed Treatment of Common Fractures*, 3rd ed. Baltimore, Williams & Wilkins, 1961.

[58] BATE, J. T. Apparatus for use in reduction and fixation of fractures of distal radius. *Clinical Orthopedics*, 1969, **63**, 190.

[59] BRADY, L. P. Double pin fixation of severely comminuted fracture of the distal radius and ulna. *Southern Medical Journal*, 1963, **56**, 307.

[60] COLE, J. M. and OBLETZ, B. E. Comminuted fractures of the

distal end of the radius treated by skeletal transfixion in plaster cast: an end-result study of thirty-three cases. *Journal of Bone and Joint Surgery*, 1966, **48A**, 931.

[61] DE PALMA, A. F. Comminuted fractures of the distal end of the radius treated by ulnar pinning. *Journal of Bone and Joint Surgery*, 1952, **34A**, 651.

[62] DOWLING, J. J. AND SAWYER, B., Jr. Comminuted Colles' fractures: evaluation of a method of treatment. *Journal of Bone and Joint Surgery*, 1961, **43A**, 657.

[63] GREEN, D. P. Pins and plaster treatment of comminuted fractures of the distal end of the radius. *Journal of Bone and Joint Surgery*, 1975, **57A**, 304.

[64] MARSH, H. O. and TEAL, S. W. Treatment of comminuted fractures of the distal radius with self-contained skeletal traction. *American Journal of Surgery*, 1972, **124**, 715.

[65] HYMAN, G. AND MARTIN, F. R. R. Dislocation of the inferior radio-ulnar joint as a complication of fracture of the radius. *British Journal of Surgery*, 1940, **27**, 481.

[66] LIPPMAN, R. K. Laxity of the radio-ulnar joint following Colles' fracture. *Archives of Surgery*, 1937, **35**, 772.

[67] MCDOUGALL, A. AND WHITE, J. Subluxation of the inferior radio-ulnar joint complicating fracture of the radial head. *Journal of Bone and Joint Surgery*, 1957, **39B**, 278.

[68] DARRACH, W. Partial excision of lower shaft of ulna for deformity following Colles' fracture. *Annals of Surgery*, 1913, **57**, 764.

[69] DINGHAM, P. V. C. Resection of the distal end of the ulna (Darrach operation): an end-result study of twenty-four cases. *Journal of Bone and Joint Surgery*, 1952, **34A**, 893.

[70] LUGNEGARD, H. Resection of the head of the ulna in post-traumatic dysfunction of the distal radio-ulnar joint. *Scandinavian Journal of Plastic and Reconstructive Surgery*, 1969, **3**, 65.

[71] ALBERT, S. M., WOHL, M. A. AND RECHTMAN, A. M. Treatment of the disrupted radio-ulnar joint. *Journal of Bone and Joint Surgery*, 1963, **45A**, 1373.

[72] DAMERON, T. B., Jr. Traumatic dislocation of the distal radio-ulnar joint. *Clinical Orthopedics*, 1972, **83**, 55.

[73] HEIPLE, K. G., FREEHAFER, A. A. AND VANT HOF, A. Isolated traumatic dislocation of the distal end of the ulnar or distal radio-ulnar joint. *Journal of Bone and Joint Surgery*, 1962, **44A**, 1387.

[74] ROSE-INNES, A. P. Anterior dislocation of the ulna at the inferior radio-ulnar joint: case reports with a discussion of the anatomy of rotation of the forearm. *Journal of Bone and Joint Surgery*, 1960, **42B**, 515.

[75] VESELY, D. C. The distal radio-ulnar joint. *Clinical Orthopedics*, 1967, **51**, 75.

[76] FISK, G. R. Carpal instability and the fractured scaphoid. *Annals of the Royal College of Surgeons of England*, 1970, **46**, 63.

[77] LINDGREN, F. Some radiological aspects on the carpal scaphoid and its fractures. *Acta chirurgica Scandinavica*, 1949, **98**, 538.

[78] LONDON, P. S. The broken scaphoid bone: the case against pessimism. *Journal of Bone and Joint Surgery*, 1961, **43B**, 237.

[79] ROTHBERG, A. S. Fractures of the carpal navicular: importance of special roentgenography. *Journal of Bone and Joint Surgery*, 1939, **21**, 1020.

[80] STEWART, M. J. Fractures of the carpal navicular (scaphoid): a report of 436 cases. *Journal of Bone and Joint Surgery*, 1954, **36A**, 998.

[81] VERDAN, C. Fractures of the scaphoid. *Surgical Clinics of North America*, 1960, **40**, 461.

[82] WEBER, E. R. AND CHAO, E. Y. C. An experimental approach to the mechanism of scaphoid wrist fractures. *Journal of Hand Surgery*, 1978, **3**, 142.

[83] DEHNE, E., DEFFER, P. A. AND FEIGHNEY, R. E. Patho-mechanics of the fracture of the carpal navicular. *Journal of Trauma*, 1964, **4**, 96.

[84] GOLDMAN, S., LIPSCOMB, P. R. AND TAYLOR, W. E. Immobilization for acute carpal scaphoid fractures. *Surgery, Gynecology and Obstetrics*, 1969, **129**, 281.

[85] MAZET, R., Jr. AND HOHL, M. Fractures of the carpal navicular: analysis of ninety-one cases and review of the literature. *Journal of Bone and Joint Surgery*, 1963, **45A**, 82.

[86] MCLAUGHLIN, F. L. Fracture of the carpal navicular (scaphoid) bone: some observations based on treatment by open reduction and internal fixation. *Journal of Bone and Joint Surgery*, 1954, **36A**, 765.

[87] MCLAUGHLIN, H. L. AND PARKES, J. C., II. Fracture of the carpal navicular (scaphoid) bone: gradations in therapy based upon pathology. *Journal of Trauma*, 1969, **9**, 311.

[88] AGERHOLM, J. C. AND LEE, M. L., II. The acrylic scaphoid prosthesis in the treatment of the ununited carpal scaphoid fracture. *Acta orthopaedica Scandinavica*, 1966, **37**, 67.

[89] AGNER, O. Treatment of ununited fractures of the carpal scaphoid by Bentzon's operation. *Acta orthopaedica Scandinavica*, 1963, **33**, 56.

[90] AGNER, O. Treatment of non-united navicular fractures by total excision of the bone and the insertion of acrylic prostheses. *Acta orthopaedica Scandinavica*, 1963, **33**, 235.

[91] DWYER, F. C. Excision of the carpal scaphoid for ununited fracture. *Journal of Bone and Joint Surgery*, 1949, **34B**, 572.

[92] MAZET, R., Jr. AND HOHL, M. Conservative treatment of old fractures of the carpal scaphoid. *Journal of Trauma*, 1963, **1**, 115.

[93] PEREY, O. A re-examination of cases of pseudarthrosis of the navicular bone operated on according to Bentzon's technique. *Acta orthopedica Scandinavica*, 1954, **23**, 26.

[94] SMITH, L. AND FRIEDMAN, B. Treatment of ununited fracture of the carpal navicular by styloidectomy of the radius. *Journal of Bone and Joint Surgery*, 1956, **38A**, 368.

[95] BENTZON, P. G. K. AND RANDLØV-MADSEN, A. On fracture of the carpal scaphoid. *Acta orthopaedica Scandinavica*, 1946, **16**, 30.

[96] PREISER, G. Eine typische post-traumatische und zur Spontan-fraktur fubrende Ostitis des Navicular Carpi. *Fortschritte auf dem Gebiete der Röntgenstrahlen und der Nuklearmedizin*, 1910, **15**, 189.

[97] MAZET, R., Jr. AND HOHL, M. Radial styloidectomy and

styloidectomy plus bone graft in the treatment of old ununited carpal scaphoid fractures. *Annals of Surgery*, 1960, **152**, 296.

[98]   MURRAY, G. Bone graft for non-union of the carpal scaphoid. *British Journal of Surgery*, 1934, **22**, 63.

[99]   MURRAY, G. Bone graft for non-union of the carpal scaphoid. *Surgery, Gynecology and Obstetrics*, 1935, **60**, 540.

[100]   MURRAY, G. End results of bone grafting for non-union of the carpal navicular. *Journal of Bone and Joint Surgery*, 1946, **28**, 749.

[101]   RUSSE, O. Fracture of the carpal navicular: diagnosis, non-operative treatment, and operative treatment. *Journal of Bone and Joint Surgery*, 1960, **42A**, 759.

[102]   UNGER, H. S. AND STRYKER, W. C. Non-union of the carpal navicular: analysis of 42 cases treated by the Russe procedure. *Southern Medical Journal*, 1969, **62**, 620.

[103]   GASSER, H. Delayed union and pseudarthrosis of the carpal navicular: treatment by compression–screw osteosynthesis: a preliminary report of twenty fractures. *Journal of Bone and Joint Surgery*, 1965, **47A**, 249.

[104]   MAUDSLEY, R. H. AND CHEN, S. C. Screw fixation in the management of the fractured carpal scaphoid. *Journal of Bone and Joint Surgery*, 1972, **54B**, 432.

[105]   JOHNSON, C. M. The role of tomography in the evaluation of carpal injuries. *American Journal of Roentgen and Radiation Therapy* (in press).

[106]   PERSSON, M. Causal treatment of lunatomalacia: further experiences of operative ulna lengthening. *Acta chirurgica Scandinavica*, 1952, **100**, 531.

[107]   STAHL, F. On lunateomalacia (Kienbock's disease): a clinical and roentgenological study, especially on its pathogenesis and the late results of immobilization treatment. *Acta chirurgica Scandinavica*, 1947, **126** (suppl), 1.

[108]   DORMAN, A. The results of treatment in Kienbock's disease. *Journal of Bone and Joint Surgery*, 1949, **31B**, 518.

[109]   KIENBOCK, R. Uber traumatische Malazie des Mondbeins und ihre Folgezustande: Entartungsformen und Kompressionsfrakturen. *Fortschritte auf dem Gebiete der Röntgenstrahlen und der Nuklearmedizin*, 1910, **16**, 78.

[110]   NAHIGIAN, S. H., Li, C. S., RICHEY, D. G. AND SHAW, D. T. The dorsal flap arthroplasty in the treatment of Kienbock's disease. *Journal of Bone and Joint Surgery*, 1970, **52A**, 245.

[111]   TILLBERG, B. Kienbock's disease treated with osteotomy to lengthen ulna. *Acta orthopaedica Scandinavica*, 1968, **39**, 359.

[112]   BROLIN, I. Post-traumatic lesions of the lunate bone. *Acta orthopaedica Scandinavica*, 1964, **34**, 167.

[113]   RODHOLM, A. K. AND PHEMISTER, D. B. Cyst-like lesions of carpal bones, associated with fractures, aseptic necrosis, and traumatic arthritis. *Journal of Bone and Joint Surgery*, 1948, **30A**, 151.

[114]   BROLIN, I. Post-traumatic lesions of the lunate bone. *Acta orthopaedica Scandinavica*, 1964, **34**, 167.

[115]   LEE, M. L. H. The intraosseous arterial pattern of the carpal lunate bone and its relation to avascular necrosis. *Acta orthopaedica Scandinavica*, 1963, **33**, 43.

[116]   FAIRBANK, T. J. Chip fractures of the os triquetrum (carpal cuneiform). *British Medical Journal*, 1942, **2**, 310.

[117]   BARTONE, N. F. AND GRIECO, R. V. Fractures of the triquetrum. *Journal of Bone and Joint Surgery*, 1956, **38A**, 353.

[118]   BONNIN, J. G. AND GREENING, W. P. Fractures of the triquetrum. *British Journal of Surgery*, 1944, **31**, 278.

[119]   DURBIN, F. C. Non-union of the triquetrum: report of a case. *Journal of Bone and Joint Surgery*, 1950, **32B**, 388.

[120]   BOWEN, T. L. Injuries of the hamate bone. *Hand*, 1973, **5**, 235.

[121]   MILEH, H. Fracture of the hamate bone. *Journal of Bone and Joint Surgery*, 1934, **16**, 459.

[122]   ANDRESS, M. R. AND PECKAR, V. G. Fractures of the hook of the hamate. *British Journal of Radiology*, 1970, **43**, 141.

[123]   TORISU, T. Fracture of the hook of the hamate by a golfswing. *Clinical Orthopedics*, 1972, **83**, 91.

[124]   REIDER, J. J. Fractures of the capitate bone. *United States Armed Forces Medical Journal*, 1958, **9**, 1513.

[125]   ADLER, J. B. AND SHAFTAN, G. W. Fractures of the capitate. *Journal of Bone and Joint Surgery*, 1962, **44A**, 1537.

[126]   FENTON, R. L. The naviculo-capitate fracture syndrome. *Journal of Bone and Joint Surgery*, 1956, **38A**, 681.

[127]   STEIN, F. AND SIEGEL, M. W. Naviculo-capitate fracture syndrome: a case report; new thoughts on the mechanism of injury. *Journal of Bone and Joint Surgery*, 1969, **51A**, 391.

[128]   CORDREY, L. J. AND FERRER-TORELLS, M. Management of fractures of the greater multangular: report of five cases. *Journal of Bone and Joint Surgery*, 1960, **42A**, 1111,

[129]   MACCONAILL, M. A. The mechanical anatomy of the carpus and its bearings on some surgical problems. *Journal of Anatomy*, 1941, **75**, 166.

[130]   WRIGHT, R. D. A detailed study of movement of the wrist joint. *Journal of Anatomy*, 1935, **70**, 137.

[131]   CAMPBELL, R. D., Jr., LANCE, E. M. AND YEOH, C. B. Lunate and perilunate dislocations. *Journal of Bone and Joint Surgery*, 1961, **46B**, 55.

[132]   CAMPBELL, R. D., Jr., THOMPSON, T. C., LANCE, E. M. AND ADLER, J. B. Indications for open reduction of lunate and perilunate dislocations of the carpal bones. *Journal of Bone and Joint Surgery*, 1965, **47A**, 915.

[133]   POIRIER, P. AND CHARPY, A. *Traite' d'Anatomie Humaine*, tome I, pp. 226–231. Paris, Masson, 1911.

[134]   DE QUERVAIN, F. *Clinical Surgical Diagnosis for Students and Practitioners*. 4th ed. New York, William Wood, 1913.

[135]   RUSSELL, T. B. Inter-carpal dislocations and fracture-dislocations: a review of fifty-nine cases. *Journal of Bone and Joint Surgery*, 1949, **31B**, 524.

[136]   BOHLER, L., TROJAN, E. AND JAHNA, H. Behandlungsergebnisse von 734 frischen einfachern Bruchen des Kahnbeinkorpers der Hand. Weiderherstell, Chir Traumatol, 1954, **2**, 86–111.

[137]   WAGNER, C. J. Fracture–dislocations of the wrist. *Clinical Orthopedics*, 1959, **15**, 181.

[138]   FAHEY, J. H. Fractures and dislocations about the wrist. *Surgical Clinics of North America*, 1957.

[139]   WESELEY, M. S. AND BARENFELD, P. A. Trans-scaphoid,

transcapitate, transtriquetral, perilunate fracture–dislocation of the wrist: a case report. *Journal of Bone and Joint Surgery*, 1972, **54A,** 1073.

[140] RUSSELL, T. B. Inter-carpal dislocations and fracture–dislocations: a review of fifty-nine cases. *Journal of Bone and Joint Surgery*, 1949, **31B,** 524.

[141] WAGNER, C. J. Perilunar dislocations. *Journal of Bone and Joint Surgery*, 1956, **38A,** 1198.

[142] ROSADO, A. P. A possible relationship of radio-carpal dislocation and dislocation of the lunate bone. *Journal of Bone and Joint Surgery*, 1966, **48B,** 504.

[143] WEISS, C., LASKIN, B. S. AND SPINNER, M. Irreducible radio-carpal dislocations: a case report. *Journal of Bone and Joint Surgery*, 1970, **52A,** 562.

[144] WATSON-JONES, R. *Fractures and Joint Injuries*, 4th ed., vol. 2. Edinburgh, Churchill Livingstone, 1955.

[145] DUKE, R. Dislocation of the hamate bone: report of a case.

[146] IMMERMANN, E. W. Dislocation of the pisiform. *Journal of Bone and Joint Surgery*, 1948, **30A,** 489.

[147] LEWIS, H. H. Dislocation of the lesser multiangular: report of a case. *Journal of Bone and Joint Surgery*, 1962, **44A,** 1412.

[148] SEIMON, L. P. Compound dislocation of the trapezium: a case report. *Journal of Bone and Joint Surgery*, 1972, **54A,** 1297.

[149] KUTH, J. R. Isolated dislocation of the carpal navicular: a case report. *Journal of Bone and Joint Surgery*, 1939, **21,** 479.

[150] GORDON, S. L. Scaphoid and lunate dislocation: report of a case in a patient with peripheral neuropathy. *Journal of Bone and Joint Surgery*, 1972, **54A,** 1769.

[151] WHITFIELD, G. A. Recurrent dislocation of the carpal scaphoid bone (abstr). *Journal of Bone and Joint Surgery*, 1962, **44B,** 963.

[152] TAYLOR, A. R. Dislocation of the scaphoid. *Postgraduate Medical Journal*, 1969, **45,** 186.

[153] WALKER, G. B. W. Dislocation of the carpal scaphoid reduced by open operation. *British Journal of Surgery*, 1943, **30,** 380.

[154] WAUGH, R. L. AND YANCEY, A. G. Carpometacarpal dislocations: with particular reference to simultaneous dislocation of the bases of the fourth and fifth metacarpals. *Journal of Bone and Joint Surgery*, 1948, **30A,** 397.

CHAPTER 16

Injuries to the Fingertip

B. H. HELAL

The finger tips have highly developed sensory and manipulative functions (p. 4). Their importance is shown by the size of the sensory and motor areas devoted to them in man's brain. The highest expression of their functional capacity is seen in the extraordinary skills of a master violinist or guitarist and of those using Braille. These qualities cannot be reproduced by grafted tissues.

Applied anatomy (see pp. 6, 7, 14 and 40)

Injuries to the pulp

The pulps are very vulnerable to injury, especially in persons in close contact with fast moving mechanical devices (Fig. 16.1). The injuries are basically of two varieties: crushing or bursting and incised or slicing.

The treatment should be as conservative of pulp as possible and excision should be confined to trimming away the protruding fat with sharp pointed scissors. Suture is often unnecessary but if there is a wide gaping wound a few plain collagen catgut sutures suffice. It is sometimes worth delaying repair for twenty-four hours in order to elevate the hand, which may remove much of the swelling and pouting of the subcutaneous tissue. Avulsed skin is worth preserving and repositioning, especially in children. Split skin (Thiersch) grafts should be kept away from the apex of the pulp. It should be covered by a mobile local skin advanced distally, by either a V-Y plasty [1], a local neurovascular island flap [2], or Kutler procedure [3, 4] (Fig. 16.2) in this order of preference.

The V-Y plasty

The base and apex of the triangle are defined by a V-incision. Careful superficial dissection of the two limbs must be carried out in order to avoid denervation, then the triangle of skin is moved distally to allow its base to be sewn over the amputated finger tip (see also Fig. 17.2). The area left proximally by distal migration is

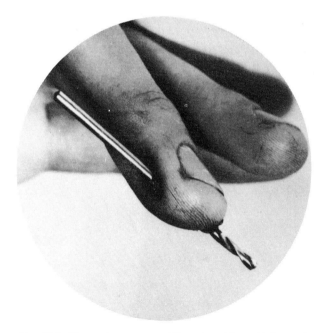

FIG. 16.1. Finger tips are especially vulnerable to high speed mechanical devices. This is a typical drillbit injury.

238

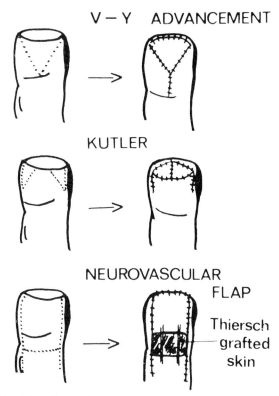

V – Y ADVANCEMENT

KUTLER

NEUROVASCULAR FLAP

Thiersch grafted skin

FIG. 16.2. Three techniques to produce immediate cover of finger tip amputations.

sewn together as a short vertical limb below the apex, the suture line now being Y-shaped.

Local neurovascular island flap

Midlateral incisions are made and connected by a transverse volar incision. The neurovascular bundle is dissected out and the flap of skin and subcutaneous tissue distal to the transverse limb of the incision dissected free with its nerve and blood supply preserved and advanced to cover the amputated finger tip. The exposed area left proximally is covered by a split skin graft.

The Kutler technique

Triangular flaps are created on each side of the stump and swung together over the apex of the stump, the two bases meeting in the midline. The areas vacated by the apices of the triangles are sewn together to form the lower limb of a Y. Care must be taken not to undermine the triangles as this may lead to their necrosis.

Cross finger, thenar or hypothenar flaps (see Chapter 9) are not recommended as the finger joints may stiffen in flexion and the functional results of grafting skin poor in sensory endings to the apex of the pulp are disappointing. In small children the potential for healing is great and methods of skin cover are seldom needed.

In the *traumatic apical pulp amputations*, if the detached part is available it is usually worth reattachment particularly in children as it seems to act as a good dressing and although it does not usually survive, if left alone will eventually separate, leaving a perfectly epithelialized pulp as the normal pulp skin is pulled distally by contracting scar tissue (Fig. 16.3). This result is often better than after a skin graft which has inferior sensitivity with the added disadvantage of

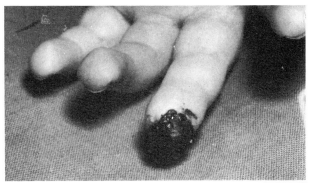

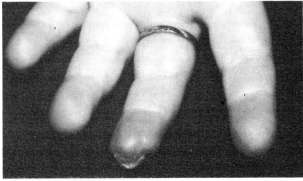

FIG. 16.3. Result of preservation and re-attachment of apex of pulp. Contracting scar tissue has drawn the normal volar skin over the apex of the pulp. Function was normal.

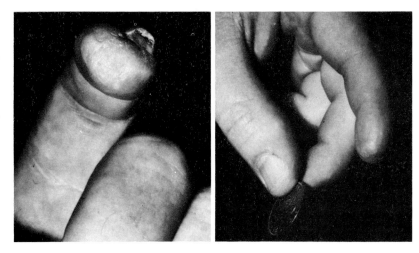

FIG. 16.4. Physiological amputation of a finger due to unsatisfactory result of graft. The owner avoids using digit with poor sensory skin cover.

abnormal mobility; the stump may be so unsatisfactory that the patient will often not use the digit, thus performing a physiological amputation (Fig. 16.4).

Elective amputations of the digital tips

The same principles apply here as to more major amputations (see Chapter 17). Much morbidity can be avoided by meticulous care. A stump should be painless, well nourished, functional and as normal in sensation and appearance as possible; scars should be well away from the contact areas when at all feasible.

Attention to the following should achieve these aims:

(1) prevention of skin adherence to underlying bone by using available subcutaneous tissue and keeping the scar, if possible, away from the pulp contact points,

(2) avoidance of neuroma formation by cutting the nerves back (p. 245), and applying heat coagulation to their cut ends,

(3) avoidance of cartilage under scar,

(4) avoidance of nail remnants,

(5) avoidance of inclusion dermoids by careful wound excision,

(6) preservation of good movement of the stump,

(7) avoidance of suturing the opposing tendons over the stump; this does not improve the function and because of the tethering can embarrass movements in the adjacent digits.

(8) avoidance of tension in the flaps; a useful manoeuvre is to cut the dorsal flap whilst holding the digit in flexion and vice versa for the palmar flap; this ensures adequate length and adequate nutrition which can be jeopardized by excessive tension. On the whole, if the tension cannot be relieved, it is probably better to shorten the phalanx to achieve adequate stump cover, with the exception of the thumb when preservation of maximal length is deemed more important.

Injuries to the nail

There has developed an unfortunate tendency to avulse the nail indiscriminately. It should always be remembered that it is a useful natural splint of the terminal phalanx if this is fractured, that it protects the sensitive nail bed and serves also as an important stimulus amplifier (p. 6).

Treatment of injuries of the nail, nail bed and nail fold

Subungual haematoma

This can be painful if under tension and should be relieved by trephining the nail usually by spinning a straight cutting needle between the forefinger and thumb.

Removal of the nail

This is recommended in troublesome small remnants or in heavy horn-like clawed nails. It can be partial by splitting the affected end longitudinally from the intact portion. Clearance of the nail from its bed is best done with sharp pointed scissors, the points being constantly directed against the undersurface of the nail; 'scoring' the nail bed or underlying bone may produce ugly distortion during nail regeneration.

Nail bed wounds which have the growth area intact can be treated by split skin grafting. Surprisingly the nail will often adhere to the grafted area in a normal fashion as it does to the original nail bed. Distortions of nail growth by scarring of the nail bed are difficult to treat but can be helped by meticulous resection of the nail bed down to periosteum. An eponychial flap may also be used.

Nail fold injuries

In cut wounds, end to end repair by suture must be accurate to avoid healing with an ugly step which is *not* self correcting. If the wound is ragged and untidy, 'even' excision is the treatment of choice followed by non-adhesive gras dressing. Scarring of the nail fold by severe infection or a burn can be managed by Barfod's technique [5]. This involves excising the nail fold and laying in two crescentric flaps taken from the sides of the fingers and based distally (Fig. 16.5).

Transplantation of a toe nail

It is possible to graft a toenail bed onto a digit, but distorted nail growth is the rule and the procedure is not reliable enough to be recommended.

Artificial nails

Often the only solution to ugly distortion of nail growth is ablation of the growth root and the use if necessary of an artificial nail.

Injuries to the terminal phalanx

The shaft and the ungual tuberosity are not infrequently the site of crushing injury when a fracture of the tuft may occur, usually comminuted. As previously mentioned, evacuation of subungual haematoma makes the patient more comfortable; preservation of the nail is advisable as a useful natural splint. No special splintage is required for fracture of the terminal phalanx in its distal two thirds except when there is an obvious distortion and immobilization is advisable. At the base of the phalanx stubbing injuries, frequently encountered in ball games such as cricket or baseball, may produce fractures into the joints; in cases of large fragments they should be reattached by suture or Kirschner wire in order to prevent irregularity of the joint surface (see Chapter 11). Avulsion of bony fragments to which the extensor or flexor tendons are attached are not infrequent, and are treated primarily as tendon injuries (vide infra). Gross damage to the joint may require arthrodesis which is carried out by excision of the articular surfaces shaping these into a cup (base of the terminal phalanx) and ball (head of the middle phalanx). The fusion is stabilized by Kirschner wires inserted in parallel (crossed wires tend to distract the surfaces) or alternatively a small size fusion peg may be used [6].

Pseudo-mallet deformity occurs in children due to a metaphyseal fracture immediately adjacent to the basal epiphysis. The nail is elevated and this is a compound

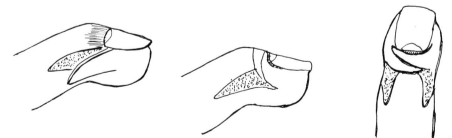

FIG. 16.5. Reconstruction of the nail fold: Barfod's technique.

injury. The nail should be preserved and after careful cleaning is repositioned under the nail fold and the fracture manipulated. The nail supports the fracture and other splintage is usually unnecessary but it can be supported by the mallet splint.

Tendon injuries

Avulsion of the extensor tendon from its insertion is a common injury, the mechanism being forced flexion of the terminal joint whilst it is being held straight; tucking in the sheets in bedmaking is a common cause. Loss of extension of the terminal phalanx is the outcome,

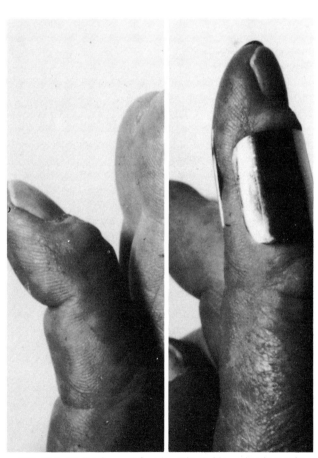

Fig. 16.6. Mallet finger deformity. The Oakley splint keeps the terminal phalanx in extension correcting the deformity whilst allowing movement at the more proximal joints.

Chapter 11). Disruption of extension may occur in one of four ways:

(1) avulsion injury with, or

(2) without a fracture (it is said that the prognosis for reattachment is better with a bony fragment since bone unites to bone more readily than tendon to bone),

(3) stubbing injury with fracture of the dorsum of the base of the terminal phalanx, and

(4) cut wound dividing the insertion of the extensor tendon.

Whatever the mechanism of injury, if it is seen soon after, there is usually a good response to splintage in extension on the Oakley splint [7] (Fig. 16.6 or similar plastic splint). The Oakley splint can be easily manufactured within the hospital or may be purchased in a ready-made series of sizes. The split ring design allows fine adjustment. Splintage does not usually hamper general use of the hand and most occupations can be continued. The patient is advised to keep the finger tip supported when the splint is temporarily removed (usually to clean and dry the skin) and at no time is the finger tip permitted to flex. The splint is removed whenever wet and in any case at least twice a day for cleansing and powdering the skin in order to prevent maceration. Six weeks of continuous wear is advised followed by temporary periods of removal for mobilizing exercises. If any extension lag develops, a further four weeks of splinting is advised. Protection during vigorous activity is recommended for a total of three months to avoid re-injuring the immature fibrous tissue of the repair. This treatment is surprisingly rewarding even when the subject presents late with a severe established mallet deformity. A period of splintage whilst awaiting surgical treatment may make this unnecessary. Failure to correct the deformity in the acute cases by this type of splintage is exceptional, provided the patient has obeyed instructions. Operative treatment may consist of tendon reattachment or simple excision of the scar and end to end suture of the tendon (see Chapter 11 for operative procedures).

Avulsion of the long flexor tendon from its insertion. The problem will vary in severity depending on the condition of the distal vinculum. If this is intact, little retraction of the tendon occurs and reattachment can be carried out through a very limited digital approach.

Retraction of the flexor tendon into the palm can be treated in one of two ways:

(1) In the recent case, re-attachment to the terminal phalanx may be tried. The bugbear of this, however, is an occasional involvement of the intact superficialis in adhesions produced by reaction to injury or surgery. The Kleinert method of elastic traction (see chapter on flexor tendon) and early movement in the post-operative management has lessened the tendency to this complication.

(2) No treatment may be required and this may be the wisest approach particularly in the injury a few days or weeks old and where terminal joint flexion is of no great importance to the patient. Caution in the approach to this problem is advised to forestall distress for both patient and surgeon alike. A complication brought to light in recent years [8] is the effect of the lumbrical action when the flexor tendon has been detached from its insertion: contraction of the flexor digitorum profundus produces instead of flexion, an extension of the proximal interphalangeal joint through the intact lumbrical. Flexion of this joint can be restored by division of the relevant lumbrical tendon.

Composite injuries

These may involve compound fracture of the phalanx, disruption of the nail bed and soft tissue. They require careful exploration and assessment and treatment along the lines described for the simpler injuries.

REFERENCES

[1] ATASOY, E., IOAKIMIDIS, E., KASDAN, M. L., KUTZ, J. AND KLEINERT, H. E. Reconstruction of the amputated finger tip with a triangular volar flap. *Journal of Bone and Joint Surgery*, 1970, **52A,** 921.

[2] MILFORD, C. Local neurovascular island flaps. In: *Campbell's Operative Orthopaedics*. Saint Louis, Mosby 1971.

[3] KUTLER, W. A new Method for finger tip amputation. *Journal of the American Medical Association*, 1947, **133,** 29.

[4] FISHER, R. H. The Kutler method of repair of finger tip amputations. *Journal of Bone and Joint Surgery*, 1967, **49A,** 317.

[5] BARFOD, B. Reconstruction of the nail fold. *The Hand*, 1972, **4,** 85.

[6] HARRISON, S. H. AND NICOLLE, F. J. A new intramedullary bone peg for digital arthrodesis. *British Journal of Plastic Surgery* 1974, **27,** 240.

[7] HELAL, B. AND MIKIC, Z. The treatment of the mallet finger by the Oakley splint. *The Hand*, 1974, **6,**76.

[8] PARKES, A. The 'Lumbrical Plus' finger. *The Hand*, 1970, **2,** –164.

CHAPTER 17

Amputations

D. W. LAMB

Amputations of the hand may result from injury, or be required following injury, or may be indicated as a planned definitive procedure.

Traumatic amputations

This is a large group which is common in injuries caused by sharp cutting implements, by a rotatory saw or when the hand is entangled in moving machinery. Examples of these injuries are described elsewhere. The general principles governing the management of such injuries has changed radically as a result of the development of microscopic surgical techniques and the ability to repair small blood vessels with a high success rate [1, 2]. Revascularization of a severed portion of the hand is much more likely to be successful where it has resulted from a clean, sharp cutting wound than in those cases associated with considerable crushing and soft tissue damage. Subject to this basic principle, replantation and revascularization should be considered when a major portion of the thumb has been severed or where several digits are involved. For its success, however, it is essential to have the necessary microscopic facilities with special surgical instruments and to pay meticulous attention to detail (see Chapter 10). The operation time may be between six and twelve hours and the optimal conditions, including a team with the required expertise, are not freely available. Thus this procedure cannot yet be considered as routine treatment, particularly for a single digit other than the thumb.

Most traumatic amputations affect the tip of the digit

and here special techniques are required (see Chapter 16). Single traumatic amputations at a more proximal level, particularly where crushing has occurred, are best treated by shortening the digit in order to provide good quality skin which has sensation and is mobile over the bone. Volar skin flaps are best in this respect (Fig. 17.1). The flap should be semicircular and long enough to provide a loose cover for the bone; it should be stitched to the shorter dorsal flap so as to form the suture line slightly dorsally. The tendons are cut at the level of amputation and allowed to retract. The nerves are cut sharply 5 mm proximal to the level of bone division and allowed to retract into good soft tissue cover and the digital arteries ligated with 5/0 catgut. Where disarticulation is carried out [3] the condyles may need to be suitably trimmed to prevent a bulbous stump. It is

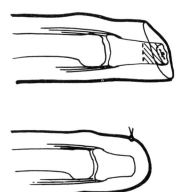

FIG. 17.1. The guillotine type amputation of finger tip treated by shortening and volar flap.

244

important that the skin closure is not carried out under tension as the skin will inevitably retract with a subsequent breakdown of the scar; it is also in these circumstances that the patient is most likely to develop problems with a neuroma of the cut digital nerve.

Where the thumb is affected or several digits involved, an attempt should be made to preserve as much length as practicable. Although the principle of preservation of maximum thumb length has been taught and practised for many years, good quality skin cover without adherence of scar or local tenderness and with good sensation present will allow much more effective use even in a shortened digit and is preferable to striving for length with a poor skin cover [4, 5].

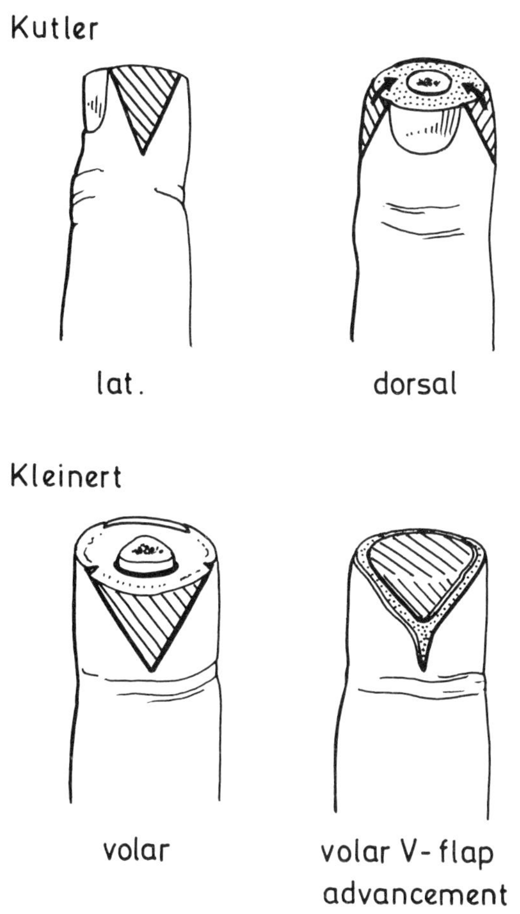

Kutler

lat.   dorsal

Kleinert

volar   volar V-flap
                advancement

FIG. 17.2. V-advancement flaps: Kutler (lateral) and Kleinert (volar).

In multiple digit amputation, particularly of the guillotine type, when further shortening would impair function, one of the methods of skin cover described in Chapters 9 and 16 will be required. The disadvantages of the adherent free skin graft with its lack of sensibility and the similar lack of sensation over the finger tip covered by distant flaps has led to an increasing use of local advancement flaps (Fig. 17.2) (see also Fig. 16.2) [6, 7].

These are very satisfactory for injuries through the more distal part of the terminal phalanx.

A single lateral V-flap advanced about 1·5 cm on the neuro-vascular pedicle to cover the tip has been used successfully [8].

In the very small child (under two years) the powers of tissue regeneration are great and only cleaning and excision of the wound is usually required.

Return to work

A return to previous employment following traumatic amputation depends on many factors including the type of work but the most important factors are the motivation of the patient and the absence of a tender stump and stiff joints [9]. The latter two factors can be influenced greatly by the surgeon [10, 11].

Definitive amputation

General principles [11]

Amputation at any site, not least in the hand, must not be delegated to an inexperienced surgeon. Any amputation stump should heal by prime intent, provide good skin cover with normal sensation and the minimum of scarring possible. To achieve these ends the surgeon must treat tissues with respect and consider the procedure as one of careful reconstruction. Delicate instruments for gentle handling are essential; dissection should be done in a bloodless field using the pneumatic tourniquet. One of the more common complications of amputation of a digit is painful neuroma of the digital nerve. There is some evidence that cauterization of the nerve by diathermy may limit neuroma formation [12]. The management of this difficult problem will be discussed later; it is much more likely to develop where there is excessive scarring with the skin being unduly

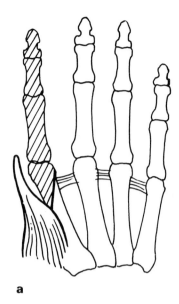

a

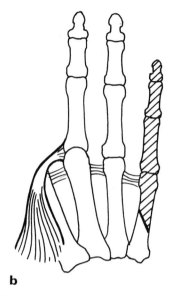

b

FIG. 17.3. (a) Index amputation through metacarpal neck with elevation of first dorsal interosseous.

(b) Closure of interosseous over bone end, and level of section of fifth metacarpal in amputation of the little finger.

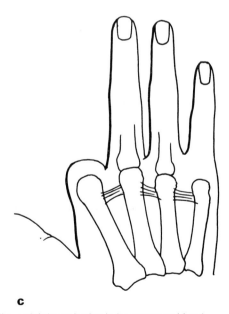

c

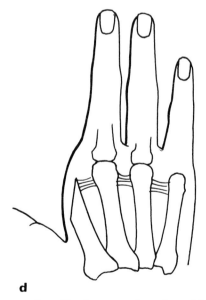

d

(c) The unsightly projecting index metacarpal head.

(d) The cosmetic outline in a properly performed index amputation through the metacarpal.

tight and adherent to the underlying structures. The management of the skin is more closely related to the development of a painful neuroma than the treatment of the digital nerve itself. This scarring may be inevitable due to the original injury but is compounded by haematoma, infection or by a careless operative technique. The best skin cover is obtained by a flap of volar skin sutured without any tension (Fig. 17.1) as provision of a trouble-free stump depends very much on mobility of the terminal tissues. Tendons and nerves should be cut cleanly and allowed to retract into soft unscarred tissue. The digital nerves should be divided distal to the bifurcation of the common digital nerve so as to avoid damage to the nerve to the adjacent digit. Before closure of the wound the tourniquet should be released and complete haemostasis obtained.

Level of amputation [13, 14]

Definitive amputation is required most frequently for the complications of trauma or infection. Severe infections of the hand and their crippling results are now fortunately seldom seen but occasionally a stiff finger may require removal. Amputation may also be needed infrequently in congenital deformity or tumour. The choice of level of amputation is of great importance [13]. Planned amputation of the thumb is very seldom required and then all possible functional length should be preserved. In other digits, amputation *distal to the insertion of the superficialis tendon* gives a useful stump provided the patient is instructed and perseveres in early active movements of the proximal interphalangeal joint in order to prevent stiffness. *Proximal to the insertion of superficialis tendon,* the stump is rarely of great functional benefit and for the index or little fingers particularly a more proximal amputation is often advised. In the index finger it is recommended that amputation should be carried out by oblique section through the metacarpal neck (Fig. 17.3a) [15]. This removes the unsightly projection of the metacarpal head (Fig. 17.3c) but preserves the attachment of the deep transverse ligament of the palm important in retaining useful breadth and power grip. In the little finger amputation is carried out obliquely through the shaft of the metacarpal (Fig. 17.3b). It is important that the first dorsal interosseous in the case of the index and abductor digiti minimi in the little finger are elevated subperiostally from the metacarpal bones

before they are sectioned. The muscle belly is then brought over the cut bone end, its tendon being sutured to the soft tissues at the base of the proximal phalanx of the adjacent digit in order to provide a good soft tissue cover and protection for the nerves (Fig. 17.3b). A skilful ablation of each of these digits can provide excellent appearance (Fig. 17.3d), so that the casual onlooker may not be aware that the digit is missing (c.f. the hand in Walt Disney cartoons). A racquet incision is used around the base of the index finger, extending along the dorsum of the second metacarpal shaft to its ulnar side, while in the little finger extension of the racquet incision is along the radial side of the dorsum of the fifth metacarpal (Fig. 17.4).

In the central two digits the best site for amputation proximal to the proximal interphalangeal joint is less well defined and may depend on the individual preference

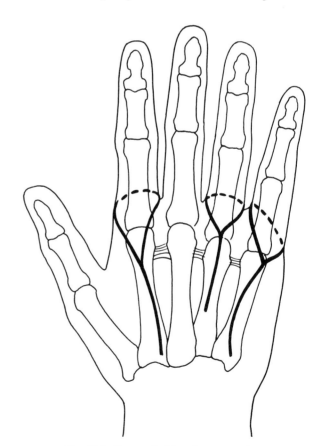

FIG. 17.4. Racquet incisions for amputation.

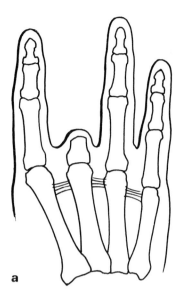

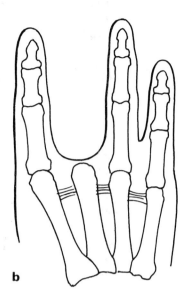

FIG. 17.5. Amputations at various levels in the middle finger.

(a) Retaining base of proximal phalanx.

(b) Disarticulation at metacarpophalangeal joint.

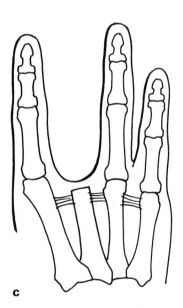

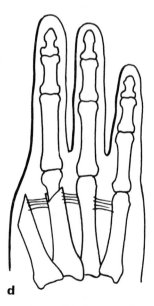

(c) Resection of metacarpal head.

(d) Transfer of the adjacent digit for cosmetic reasons following ablation of a central digit.

of the surgeon and also on the age, sex and occupation of the patient [11]. Many surgeons prefer to remove the digit through the metacarpophalangeal joint (Fig. 17.5b). This preserves the breadth of the hand and power grip but disrupts the continuity of outline of the web spaces. For this reason and also in order to prevent objects sliding out through the defect left by the missing finger, some surgeons prefer to retain a small segment of the proximal phalanx (Fig. 17.5a). In the middle ray and particularly in the female for cosmetic reasons, more proximal amputation, either through the neck of the metacarpal (Fig. 17.5c) or by complete ablation of the third ray may be considered [16]. When appearance is of particular importance and amputation of the long or ring finger is required near the metacarpophalangeal area, it is possible to transfer either the second or fifth ray to replace the parts of the missing ray with preservation of good function and with less obvious deformity

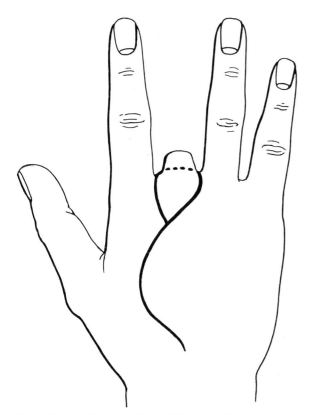

FIG. 17.6. Incision to excise middle ray and transpose index finger.

(Fig. 17.5d) [16, 17]. The incision used is shown in Fig. 17.6.

Where multiple digit amputation has occurred through the metacarpals [19] various reconstructive procedures may be considered but these are difficult and often rather disappointing (see Chapter 35).

It is seldom appreciated by others, how much mental anguish may be felt by a patient due to the lack of part of the hand. This is difficult to hide effectively from the outside world as the hand is used so much for expression and social contact (see Chapter 34). The cosmetic replacement of missing digits is of great importance to many patients and has in many ways been strangely neglected. That this is possible to the satisfaction of the patient has been shown and further mention of this topic is made in Chapter 38.

The painful stump

This is no less common in the hand than elsewhere. It is difficult to manage and is ill understood [18]. It seems that there are two main groups in which different factors may be involved.

(1) In one group, probably the majority of the patients, there is some *definite evidence of a tender neuroma* of one or both digital nerves (Fig. 17.7a). The stump frequently shows considerable scarring and adherence to the underlying tissue and bone. The mobility of the skin is impaired, and the neuroma is adherent to the scar; movement stretches the nerve and aggravates the pain. In the patient who exhibits definite evidence of neuroma and who has a poor quality stump, revision of the stump is justified (Fig. 17.7b). Following revision of the stump and resection of the neuroma the freshly cut nerve end should be diathermied and the epineurium closed carefully over the end [12]. The longer the symptoms have persisted, the less likely that the more proximal revision will give complete relief. It is possible to speculate that the pain pathways or the higher centres are affected in these cases and it is for this reason that many surgeons of great experience are reluctant to advise a proximal revision of such painful stumps. Many examples of failures of repeated more proximal amputation in giving any relief in this complication are on record.

An alternative approach is to remove the neuroma from the adverse environment. Implantation of the neuroma into adjacent bone has been tried (Fig. 17.7c), but is not reliable. A more satisfactory method is proximal dissection of the nerve and the neuroma and their implantation into a more satisfactory environment (Fig. 17.7d) well away from the scar, e.g. into the dorsum of the digit or into the interosseous muscle.

Attempts have been made to limit the neuroma formation by capping the nerve at the time of amputation with a small silicone cap (Fig. 17.7e) [20]. Sufficient evidence to prove this method is not yet available. Methods of local, nonsurgical treatment of the stump are equally unsatisfactory. The standard methods of local infiltration with an anaesthetic, with phenol or alcohol are disappointing; local percussion is not reliable in all cases, but is always worth trying [21]. Gentle tapping of

the end of the stump on a firm surface can often dull the pain; the effect is usually quite temporary.

(2) In some painful stumps *there is no obvious local abnormality* to account for the pain which is not uncommonly of a causalgic nature. The patient is often found to be of a tense, nervous and introspective disposition. Worry about the ability to return to previous employment, may aggravate a neurotic tendency in this type of individual, particularly where the amputation has resulted from industrial injury. Claims for litigation assume an undue prominence and jeopardize improvement of symptoms and recovery of function. Analgesics and antidepressants play an important part in prevention of fixation of symptoms. Time is, however, the most important factor in resolution of symptoms. Settlement

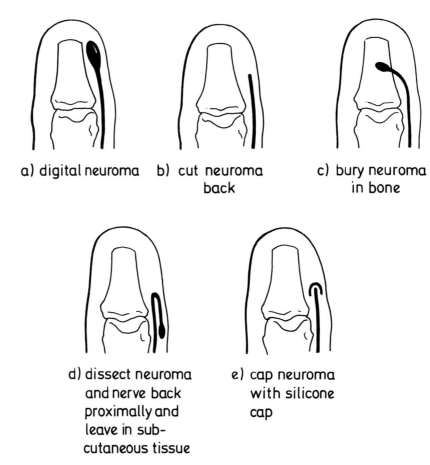

FIG. 17.7. (a) The neuroma following digital amputation. (b–e) Various methods of dealing with the neuroma.

of any litigation, when this is a prominent problem, should be expedited. No local surgery should be carried out even when symptoms persist for a long time and appear to be of considerable severity. Other methods of controlling pain such as division of the pain carrying pathways either by cordotomy or even at a higher level

may be considered. As the cordotomy would be in the cervical region, it has to be approached with great caution. The results of these procedures are not impressive and they are not recommended for routine treatment.

REFERENCES

[1] O'BRIEN, B. M. AND BAXTER, THELMA, J. Experimental digital replantation. *The Hand*, 1974, **6**, 11.

[2] O'BRIEN, B. McC. MACLEOD, A. M., HAYHURST, J. W., MORRISON, W. A. AND ISHIDA, H. (1974). Major replantation surgery in the upper limb. *The Hand*, 1974, **6**, 217.

[3] GRAHAM, W. P., KILGORE, E. S. AND WHITAKER, L. A., Trans-articular digital joint amputations. Preservation of the articular cartilage. *The Hand*, 1973, **5**, 58.

[4] PRINGLE, R. G. Amputations of the thumb. A study of the techniques of repair and residual disability. *Injury*, 1972, **3**, 211.

[5] RATLIFF, A. H. C. Amputations of the distal part of the thumb. *The Hand*, 1972, **4**, 190.

[6] ATASOY, E., IOAKIMEDIS, E, KASDAN, M. L., KUTZ, J. E., AND KLEINERT, H. E. Reconstruction of the amputated finger tip with a triangular volar flap. *Journal of Bone and Joint Surgery*, 1970, **52A**, 921.

[7] FISHER, R. H. The Kutler Method of repair of the finger-tip amputations. *Journal of Bone and Joint Surgery*, 1967, **49A**, 317.

[8] BIDDULPH, Paper read at Meeting of South African Hand Society, Durban, Sept. 1977.

[9] GRUNEBERG, R. AND SPENCE, A. J. Finger amputations and ability to work. *The Hand*, 1974, **6**, 236.

[10] HARVEY, F. J. AND HARVEY, P. M. A critical review of the results of primary finger and thumb amputation. *The Hand*, 1974, **6**, 157.

[11] SLOCUM, D. B. AND PRATT, D. R. The principles of amputations of the fingers and hand. *Journal of Bone and Joint Surgery*, 1944, **26**, 535.

[12] CONNOLLY, W. B. Paper read at Combined Meeting of British and American Hand Societies. Edinburgh. May, 1977.

[13] CHASE, R. A. Functional levels of amputation of the hand. *Surgical Clinics of North America*, 1960, **40**, 415.

[14] SWANSON, A. B. Levels of amputation of fingers and hand-considerations for treatment. *Surgical Clinics of North America*, 1964, **44**, 1115.

[15] CLAYTON, M. L. Index ray amputation. *Surgical Clinics of North America*, 1963, **43**, 367.

[16] CARROLL, R. E. Transposition of the index finger to replace the middle finger. *Clinical Orthopaedics*, 1959, **15**, 27.

[17] PEACOCK, E. E. JR. Metacarpal transfer following amputation of a central digit. *Plastic and Reconstructive Surgery*, 1962, **29**, 345.

[18] TUPPER, J. W. AND BOOTH, D. M. Treatment of painful neuromas of sensory nerves in the hand. A Comparison of traditional and newer methods. *Journal of Hand Surgery*, 1976, **1**, 144.

[19] MICHON, J. AND DORLICH, B. H. The metacarpal hand. *The Hand*, 1974, **6**, 285.

[20] SWANSON, A. B., BOEVE, N. R. AND LUMSDEN, R. M. The prevention and treatment of amputation neuromata by silicone capping. *Journal of Hand Surgery*, 1977, **2**, 70.

[21] RUSSELL, W. R. Painful amputation stumps and phanton limbs. *British Medical Journal*, 1949, **1**, 1024.

CHAPTER 18

Complicated Injuries

J. I. P. JAMES

The basic treatment of the injured hand was detailed in Chapter 8. In subsequent chapters the problems of repair of skin, tendons, nerves and bones are discussed by various contributors. The principles outlined in these chapters are of course valid in the management of the complicated injury, although complex problems arise when there are injuries to multiple tissues. These problems, both by their extent and mutual interaction, often increase the total loss of function and reduce the expected degree of recovery. The difficulties that are likely to arise in such extensive, multiple injuries and the assessment of the probable function of the hand after prolonged reconstructive surgery and rehabilitation, as is essential for such cases, does require very considerable experience and judgement.

Unless the programme can be executed by, or planned in consultation with, a surgeon skilled in hand surgery and experienced in these difficult problems, it is wise to do minimal immediate reconstruction instead of attempting unfamiliar and often difficult techniques. Inevitably such cases may be seen in remote small hospitals, or even in many bigger hospitals, without such surgeons on their staff.

In these circumstances, the essential guidelines of management must include, first of all, strict adherence to basic principles (Chapter 8): in order to remove potentially infected or ischemic tissues the wound should be excised; adequate skin cover should be provided either by closure of the wound or by grafting, care being taken to avoid thick, contracted and adherent scar. Split skin grafts are preferred at this stage to elaborate flaps but if these are unavoidable, local flaps should be

used or free transfer flaps (Chapter 9) so that the hand can be elevated. The joints should be immobilized by bandage in the correct position to prevent joint stiffness (see Chapter 8) and the limb elevated to control oedema and haemorrhage; all these measures should result in a supple hand suitable for later reconstruction in a special centre. There should be no hesitation in leaving the tendons and nerves for later surgery, if necessary expertise is lacking. It is *the stiff hand* which is often beyond the aid of even the most skilful surgeon.

In considering future reconstructive procedures in these complicated injuries it should be remembered that many months in hospital and rehabilitation may be required in contrast to a possible quick return to work if, for example, digits are reconstructed instead of amputated. There is always also a risk of undamaged or less damaged parts of the hand becoming affected by fibrosis and stiffness with significant additional loss of function although this is nearly always prevented by correct management (Chapter 8). If it is decided that reconstruction at some stage is indicated, the patient must be made aware of the likely time involved, of the number of operations needed and of the implications of a long period of rehabilitation. This is essential in order to ensure co-operation of the patient, who may even become embittered at what seems to be a lack of progress. The patient's motivation and staying power are all important; it is imperative to assess them before embarking on reconstruction which is doomed to failure if not supported by the patient's whole-hearted efforts to regain function.

This advice is cautionary to the surgeon and indicates

the solution may not be easy. However, such complicated problems can be tackled most successfully with correct planning and with the technical finesse that is now available in the surgical repair of the injured hand.

Having decided to embark upon reconstruction, and remembering the general pitfalls which have been described, consideration is given to the management of each tissue in its relationship to the other injured tissues in the hand.

Vascularity

In a recent complicated hand injury the first step is to assess the *vascularity* of the affected part of the hand or digits. If there is ischaemia, microsurgical repair of the vessels will be most clearly indicated if the affected part is vital to the function of the hand; however, the decision will be affected by the degree and complexity of the damage (Chapter 10).

Skin loss

Skin loss is in itself rarely a critical factor in deciding whether a complicated injury can be tackled or not (Chapter 9), but is a most important factor in influencing the decision and procedures in management.

As already indicated, it is often wiser for the inexperienced surgeon to use split skin grafts (p. 129) in the initial repair rather than more elaborate flaps (but see p. 139). At a later date such thin grafts can be replaced with full thickness flaps. This is particularly true in the crushed hand with severe skin loss which is rarely suitable for primary skin flaps as it is difficult to control the inevitable oedema.

Split skin grafts on the flexor surface often contract and cause flexion contractures. Such deformities at the interphalangeal joints will rapidly become irreversible and may be incorrectable, in contrast to flexion contractures at the metacarpophalangeal joint which are reversible. However, contractures of less than 30° at the interphalangeal joints are often not a serious inconvenience or loss to useful function. There is a great tendency to contracture when laceration or skin grafts have to cross flexure lines at right angles. The danger of the midline scar on the flexor aspect of a finger is well known and in judging the suitability of repair of damaged flexor skin, one has to consider how the

problems of skin contracture may be overcome by skin grafting (Chapter 9).

Tendons must glide freely under the skin. This is much more important on the dorsum where the tendons lie in areolar tissue or paratenon. On the flexor surface the tendon lies generally within specialized compartments, e.g. the fibrous flexor sheath, and therefore it is less likely here that tendons will become adherent to skin grafts and prevent tendon gliding.

Tendons with intact paratenon can glide under split skin grafts but if the tendon is bared a flap will have to be applied sooner or later.

Abrasion of all skin and tendon on the dorsum of a finger with exposure of a joint, a common buffing injury, will make a mobile, flexible finger difficult to achieve as both skin and tendon have to be replaced and the joint closed. Sometimes it is better to arthrodese the joint in a functional position and cover the area with a good skin flap rather than attempting to restore movement. A totally degloved digit is not suitable for repair and is usually better amputated.

One of the most important functions of skin on the flexor aspect is sensation for although this is also related to intact nerves the sensory organs of normal skin cannot be replaced by ordinary skin flaps. Loss of sensation particularly of the thumb and index fingers between which digits all precision work is done is therefore a critical consideration in assessing these cases. So important is sensation in these two digits that the term 'a blind hand' is used to describe its loss. In severe injuries the possibility of a neurovascular island flap graft to restore sensation and improve circulation must be remembered. A severely damaged finger with pulp skin and an intact digital nerve and artery may be worth conserving for the future as an island graft to another digit rather than being amputated as valueless.

In hands or digits with a blood supply sufficient to survive but inadequate to allow of major reconstruction the problems are difficult. There is no present method of evaluating these cases. It is however, relevant in our general considerations that a hand with impaired circulation does not stand up to hard work. There is also considerable danger when major reconstruction is undertaken in inadvertently dividing collateral vessels upon which the survival of a digit may depend. This may happen when carrying out a tendon graft for instance. Although it must be taken into consideration as a risk, since there is no accurate way of evaluation, it is not usually a factor in making a final decision to reconstruct a hand or not.

Musculotendinous injury

Direct injury to muscle is commonest in the forearm, particularly on the flexor surface. Avulsion or destruction of the flexor muscles is not uncommon in industrial injuries when the limb is pulled into moving machinery. In the hand itself, direct damage of the small muscles is much less common than irreparable damage to the motor branches of the median or ulnar nerves. In such a serious complication to an injured hand there is clearly no direct method of restoring muscle function, whether it is avulsed or denervated, although later reconstruction is possible (see Chapter 35).

Tendons can be repaired or replaced by graft (see Chapter 11). The problem in multiple injuries is usually the problem of damage to the tissue bed in which they lie and the difficulty of restoring gliding. On the extensor surface, tendons which can be sutured heal well and gliding is also easily restored when the bed is not badly damaged. Extensor tendons therefore in general repair easily in contrast to flexor tendons.

There may be extensive loss of extensor tendons over the wrist or back of the hand from avulsion. Replacing extensor tendon length even with multiple tendon loss is not difficult. However, in many of these cases there is loss of skin and possible exposure of bare bone or joints requiring a skin flap with fat to replace all scar and facilitate later reconstruction.

A particular hazard is that the distal ends of the extensor tendons become tethered and the metacarpophalangeal joints become extended and quickly stiffen. This complicates subsequent reconstruction and restoration of function considerably for in addition to damaged tendons we now have stiff joints. A common and difficult problem on the extensor surface is division or laceration of the extensor hood. Repair is followed by scarring to both superficial and deep structures in its gliding bed and may prevent full flexion even when the flexors are normal. These are particularly troublesome injuries if accompanied by a skin wound or an underlying fracture.

Multiple severe injuries to the flexor tendons present great difficulties. Although there are inherent difficulties in repairing multiple tendon injuries at the wrist these in general can be overcome if the gliding bed is undamaged or can be restored satisfactorily. Repair of all flexor tendons at the same level, however well done, is almost certain to cause adhesion between the tendons and the surrounding tissues. The amplitude of gliding on flexion is thus likely to be diminished although skilful repair may well be attended by an excellent result.

The problem of flexor tendon repair within the digits has been fully discussed (see Chapter 11). The several problems present in complicated injuries however, are most relevant to our overall discussion. In general when a digit has a damaged flexor tendon, lost skin, bone injury and digital nerve division, repair is rarely helpful even if the finger is otherwise viable.

Whilst the multiplicity of injuries to a single digit is a common reason for deciding upon amputation rather than reconstruction, the state of the other digits must also be considered. If it is the only digit left an attempt at repair should always be made. If there are other good digits much may be lost to the rest of the hand by prolonged and multiple attempts at reconstructing a single digit.

One particular problem seen in complicated injuries may present when there is damage to both extensor and flexor tendons. Though both sets of tendons may be technically well repaired adhesions may lead to extreme difficulty in regaining gliding. In the period when movement is not possible joints may also become stiff as even passive movements of the joints by a physiotherapist may not be possible with tendons stuck on both flexor and extensor surfaces. Movement in flexion or extension then becomes extremely difficult or even impossible.

It is worth reiterating that in all tendon injuries it is damage to the gliding surfaces which is likely to prove most difficult to overcome.

If there is complete destruction of the tendon bed and gliding path, repair is difficult, particularly when the fibrous flexor sheath is destroyed and it is wise to delay repair for a secondary procedure often preceded by the insertion of a silastic rod (Chapters 11 and 35).

Peripheral nerve injury

Cut nerves can be easily repaired but unfortunately the results are not accurately predictable and may be disappointing.

The factors which influence the recovery of function are discussed in Chapter 12. The decision on whether primary repair is indicated in these complicated injuries will depend on many aspects such as the state of the wound, the damage to skin, the facilities available and the technical expertise of the surgeon. It should be remembered that no harm will result from delaying the formal repair until a more appropriate occasion. If this decision is made the nerve should be lightly approximated, with correct orientation to facilitate the later repair. Some surgeons may use the technique of isolation of the nerve by Silastic sheath (p. 187).

Loss of nerve substance will usually require bridging of the defect by a nerve graft and is not a primary procedure. Avulsion of the distal end of either motor or sensory nerve prevents repair, but loss of sensation to an essential digit may be treated by a neurovascular island flap as a delayed procedure (Chapter 35).

Bone damage

Severe or complicated *bone damage* is rarely a prime reason for delaying or preventing the repair of a complex injury, although completely pulped phalanges obviously make a digit impossible to reconstruct.

Total destruction of the thumb presents a major problem. The thumb is the most important digit because by opposing to a finger, pinch and precision skills of the hand become possible and substitution is not easily accomplished. The most important requirements of the thumb are length, position and the sensation over its ulnar pulp.

Loss of the thumb is serious and when replantation and revascularisation are not possible, pollicisation of a finger or reconstruction of the thumb will make the damaged hand more useful (Chapter 35).

It does not need stressing that the more fingers that can be saved the better is function. Preservation of only one finger if it has sensation to oppose to a thumb is invaluable. A thumb which is mobile can usefully oppose to an immobile finger arthrodesed or allowed to stiffen in a functional position. Stiff fingers in a hooked position are useful even if they have no more than protective sensibility.

In conclusion, with the exception of the problems of ischaemia and total skin loss, for which there are clear cut answers, the main difficulty in deciding what to do with a complicated hand injury lies in the multiplicity of structures injured, the technical difficulties these injuries will present in reconstruction and the overall assessment of possible useful functional recovery. When skin, tendon, nerve and bone are damaged in a digit, repair is rarely useful and even when only two or three such tissues are damaged it may be an impossible task to provide a useful digit with satisfactory mobility and sensation. Although the number of structures damaged has an important bearing, the nature of the damage and feasibility of repair is at least as important. It is an obvious maxim in digital injuries of this severity to preserve all viable tissue in case they provide some function or prove useful in later reconstructive procedures. This is particularly true of the dorsal skin of fingers which can often be preserved to fill in a skin defect even if the digit itself is shattered, ischaemic and has to be amputated. A single remaining digit is almost certainly worth saving even when severely damaged whereas one or two digits similarly affected but where the other digits are intact would almost certainly be an indication for amputation.

FURTHER READING

BOYES, J. H. *Bunnell's Surgery of the Hand*, 5th edition. Philadelphia, Lippincott, 1970.

RANK, B. K., WAKEFIELD, A. R. AND HUESTON, J. T. *Surgery of Repair as Applied to Hand Injuries*, 4th edition. Edinburgh, Churchill Livingstone, 1973.

SEDDON, H. J. *Surgical Disorders of the Peripheral Nerves*, 2nd edition. Edinburgh, Churchill Livingstone, 1975.

CHAPTER 19

Burns

J. N. BARRON

The term 'burn' is somewhat of a misnomer as in its derivation it refers expressly to the effect of fire. It has been found convenient however to classify a number of different injuries under the title of 'Burns' and it is therefore necessary to consider the various sub-divisions as seen in clinical practice:

Dry heat burn   Electrical burn
Flame burn   Chemical burn
Scald   Radiation burn
Flash burn   Friction burn
Thermoelectrical burn   Frostbite (see Chapter 20)

It will be immediately apparent that with such a variety of causal agents the tissue responses to the burn injury are bound to differ.

One of the most vexing problems in this context is the assessment of burn depth, and it is here that a knowledge of the details of the injury is important. In heat burns for example it is important to know the temperature and the duration of exposure to the heat. In electrical burns the voltage and amperage are a useful guide, whereas in chemical and radiation burns the nature and strength of chemical and the type of and length of exposure to radiation should be estimated.

When we are considering burns of the hand it is important to remember that they may be only a part of the total injury, The first priority in burns management is to save life [1], and under these circumstances the hand burn may be relatively and temporarily of less importance. The great danger in the burn wound is however infection, and this is particularly important in the hand. It is therefore mandatory that in the general management of the patient, wound contamination of any kind should be avoided. For details of the general management of burns, reference should be made to the literature on the subject, as it is the purpose of this chapter to deal only with the burnt hand.

The most frequently burnt part of the human body is the hand and in up to 40 per cent of all burns treated in special burns units the hands are involved. There is of course a higher percentage of hand burns amongst those treated in casualty and accident departments. These figures are not surprising considering the nature of the injury; many hand burns occur in the act of self preservation.

The inherent structure of the hand with its relative lack of insulating subcutaneous tissue means that heat conduction to important functional mechanisms is facilitated. This is most marked on the dorsum of the hand and fingers where the skin is thin and where tendons and joints are close to the surface. The relatively large surface area of the hand and digits encourages heat absorption, thus rapid heat gain in the dermal and subdermal layers can quickly overwhelm the microcirculation causing coagulation and thrombosis. Thus progressive ischaemia is added to the original thermal insult.

From the point of view of treatment there are three types of burn [2]:

(1) *Superficial*: the epidermis (Fig. 19.1) is partly destroyed.

(2) *Dermal:* some of the dermal elements have survived.

(3) *Full thickness*: this may involve deeper structures.

In making the diagnosis of burn *depth* we have no accurate method available. Apart from the information

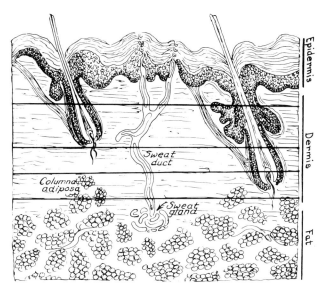

FIG. 19.1. Schematic representation of burn depth (composite diagram of the skin).

regarding the accident itself, a crude estimate can be made by *the sensitivity test*. If a pin prick can be felt it is likely to be a superficial burn, but anaesthesia generally indicates involvement of the deeper tissues. It is wise to recognise that burn depth is not static and changes such as thrombosis, oedema and infection can, in a short time, increase the gravity of the injury and a partial thickness burn today can become full thickness tomorrow. Much work has been done on the diagnosis of burn depth but has resulted in limited information of clinical value.

Aims of treatment of the burnt hand:

(1) Relief of pain.
(2) Prevention and control of oedema and thrombosis.
(3) Control of infection.
(4) Elimination of necrotic tissue as soon as possible, including early surgery and grafting when indicated.
(5) Complete healing at the earliest moment, with full range of movement in all joints.

Treatment of minor burn (superficial and not extensive)

It is usually treated at home or in the out-patient department. The pain of a small digital burn can be relieved by immersion in cold water or by pressure. Blisters should be evacuated with the displaced layer of skin left in position. Minimal dry dressings in order to protect the wound are best. Some of these minor burns, although small, may represent a dermal or subdermal injury and should remain under surgical supervision until the depth of burn is declared. There may well be an indication for surgery in some of these small injuries.

Treatment of major burns

Oedema which is so easily provoked in the hand (see p. 38 and p. 120) is one of the most potent crippling agents and every effort should be made to control it. Untreated oedema, even in a minor injury, can cause such widespread fibrosis that the hand may never recover full function. The most important factor in the control of oedema is recognition of its dangers. Unfortunately no miracle methods of treatment are available, but there are four principles of management to put into practice [3].

Elevation of the limb

Elevation of the burnt hand is urgent (see p. 120) and the patient in bed should have his arm supported in a roller towel. Control by a specially designed Polyvac arm support is also efficient.

Maintenance of the muscle pump (see p. 38)

Exercises, even if they only consist of isometric, static contractions, are valuable both in assisting venous and lymphatic return and in maintaining at the same time muscle tone. When active isotonic movements are possible without pain, joint stiffness can be largely prevented.

Avoidance of pain

Proper analgesic control and avoidance of any form of treatment which causes pain are important. Clumsy dressings, uncomfortable splints and painful movements can initiate reflex mechanisms which dilate the capillary bed with ensuing transudation. Irreversible post-traumatic sympathetic dystrophy can be a disastrous sequel to a burn injury.

Control of infection

Most burns are surface sterilised by the nature of the injury, thus those which become infected have been contaminated by the subsequent environment or by organisms in the glandular and follicular elements in the unburnt tissues. The moist necrotic pabulum arising from tissue degeneration is an excellent culture medium and it is therefore important to manage burns in such a way that the risk of infection is reduced to a minimum.

CONSERVATIVE MANAGEMENT

There are two alternatives for conservative treatment in burns less than full thickness: (1) the burnt surface is dried out immediately, or (2) isolated by dressings. Herein lies the first decision that must be made in the treatment of the burnt hand.

Drying

In general, superficial burns can be left open to dry off in elevation after blisters have been drained. Great care has to be exercised so that the dry eschar is not traumatised as this may allow the ingress of infection.

Wound isolation

Technique No. 1. The technique of isolating the burn wound in the hand by occlusive dressing is a highly skilled art. It is unwise to apply a 'pressure' dressing as it is impossible to achieve the accuracy which is necessary. After a short period of time, even with crepe bandaging, pressure in the dressing diminishes and if this occurs distally leaving a proximal tight bandage cuff, exacerbation of oedema can result. *Wound isolation with gentle support* should be aimed at. Many hours of practice are required before a good hand dressing technique can be achieved. The use of sterile polyethylene foam in its various forms is a useful adjunct to wound support. The substance most commonly employed on the burnt surface is furacin gauze, which can be tailored to fit fingers, thumb or hand and should lie comfortably without causing constriction (Fig. 19.2). This is supported by absorbent gauze and wool or polyethylene foam, the whole enclosed by a bandage of crepe or cotton. Individual finger dressing is advised in order to

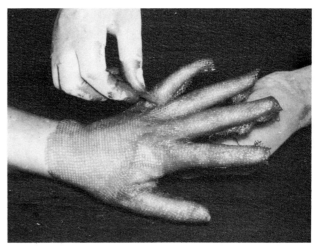

FIG. 19.2. Furacin gauze applied in strips to the hand and fingers.

prevent webbing and to allow movement (Fig. 19.3). The occlusive dressings may be left for four or five days and then changed until the wound is either healed or surgical debridement and grafting is deemed necessary. The dressing should allow as much movement as possible and any restriction should be avoided.

Technique No. 2. The hand, coated with Flamazine (silver sulphadiazine) can be *enclosed in a sterile polythene bag* secured above the wrist around a gauze wristlet and held on by a 2″ crepe bandage. Pressure should be avoided

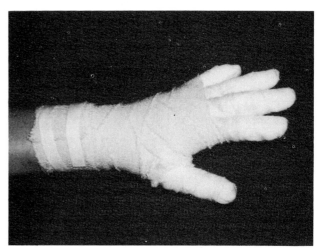

FIG. 19.3. Supporting bandage applied to allow free movement of the fingers.

at this point. The hand can be inspected through the bag. Unimpeded movements are possible. As there may be a considerable serous secretion from the wound, the bag may have to be changed several times a day.

Technique No. 3. Recently, satisfactory reports have come from the centres where *disposable polythene gloves* are being used in the management of the burnt hand. The hands are coated with silver sulphadiazine, put into the polythene gloves which are lightly attached to the wrists. It is claimed that the hand movements recover earlier and the patient is more easily able to attend to his own requirements.

The use of antibiotics

Opinions vary in this respect. Some advocate avoidance of all antibiotic cover unless there is evidence of commencing infection, others advise a routine antibiotic 'umbrella'. In essence, each case should be treated on its merits, careful observation of the patient and his wound being of paramount importance; bacteriological investigation is essential. The common invaders of the burn are pseudomonas, staphylococcus, proteus and occasionally the streptococcus.

The after-care

When the hand is healed by natural epithelialisation, dressings can be removed and full activity encouraged. Routine use of lanolin massage on the new surface is an advantage, the patient being able usually to carry this out himself twice daily. Exposure to high temperatures or to full sunlight should be avoided until the process of maturation is complete; this may take from three to six months. Most superficial burns should be healed during the third week according to circumstances. Any burn treated conservatively which is not healed at the end of the third week should be considered for surgery.

SURGERY OF THE BURNT HAND

Thermal injuries

The most important decision which must be made in the treatment of *dermal* burns is whether or not to operate,

and if so, when. In many dermal burns there is doubt whether they will develop into the full thickness variety or whether they will eventually heal without too much scarring. This will depend upon the activity of the remaining epithelial elements and upon the survival of the collagen elements in the dermis. Skill and experience are the main factors on which the decision is based.

There is however no argument about the *full thickness burn*. It should be excised and grafted.

For those who choose the surgical approach to the dermal burns the work of Janzekovic will show the excellent results which can be obtained [2]. The technique is called *'tangential' or 'laminar' excision* (Fig. 19.4). Her theory is that early removal of the coagulated epidermis and superficial dermal layers followed by immediate skin grafting preserves the deep dermal tissue with its population of hair follicles, sweat and sebaceous glands. This tissue under a conservative regimen can undergo further deterioration and expose the subcutaneous layers; it is this continuing degeneration which promotes the 'burn disease' or toxaemia.

The operation should be carried out about the third day; during this initial period the hands are isolated in dressings using flamazine on the wound surface and sufficient absorbent material to deal with any exudate. At operation under tourniquet a bloodless field is secured and with skin graft knives and scalpels the wound surfaces are tangientially excised layer by layer until the base

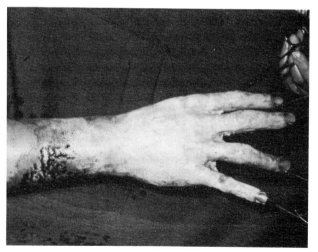

Fig. 19.4. Tangential excision of a hand burn under a tourniquet (Courtesy of Dr. Janzekovic).

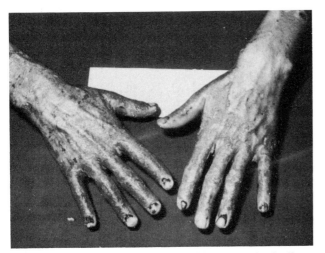

FIG. 19.5. Deep dermal burn on the tenth day showing healing with minimal scarring (Courtesy of Dr. Janzekovic).

is pale yellow or white in colour and all traces of reddish brown staining have been removed. When operating without a tourniquet, the final wound surface will contain a large number of wide bore vessels which bleed profusely. A split skin graft of equivalent thickness to the excised tissue is then cut from a suitable donor area and immobilised in position by a compressive dressing. If several pieces of graft are used they should be abutted accurately edge to edge and should fit accurately around the margins of the defect without overlapping on to the normal skin surface. In this operation it is better to remove some normal tissue rather than leave necrotic material in the wound. In other words a complete excision of necrotic tissue should be the aim of treatment (Fig. 19.5). There are many technical difficulties in the tangential excision on the fingers and in the webs it can be a time-consuming procedure. Many hand burns present with mixed partial and full thickness injuries. Both are excised and grafted in continuity. This encourages rapid primary healing and thus when necessary, reconstructive flap surgery can be commenced within a few weeks.

After-care

Postoperatively the dressings are removed in 24 hours, if necessary under sedation or anaesthesia. Any haematoma should be evacuated and the grafts adjusted in position. Subsequently they can be inspected daily or every 2 or 3 days. The earliest signs of revascularisation of the graft appear under 48 hours. Dressings can be discarded on the 8th day and a full exercise regimen commenced together with lanolin massage. Gradually the grafted skin will assume a near normal colour, the hairs from the salvaged follicles will penetrate the skin pointing eventually in their normal direction (p. 5). The glandular structures which have survived sometimes form small cysts which eventually break through to the surface. Absence of scar is a noticeable feature in all dermal burns treated this way, the full movement returning in days rather than in months. When the hand burn is part of a more widespread injury in which homografts have to be used, it is one area of the body which should have priority for any available autograft skin.

Total wound excision in the burnt hand

There is no uniformity of opinion as to when surgery is indicated in full thickness burns, some advising early or emergency excision of all diagnosable full thickness burns, others waiting for the natural sloughing process to become complete before grafting the granulating surface. In principle, the sooner the removal of the dead tissue is carried out, the better. In the electrical, thermo-electrical and chemical burns there is little difficulty as the area of full thickness loss becomes evident early. The problem is the thermal burn, because often it is a mixed dermal and full thickness lesion. It is suggested that even in these burns early excision of the necrotic tissue should be done by combining the techniques of tangential excision in the areas of dermal burn with total excision in the areas of full thickness loss. In this way early grafting becomes possible before infection has supervened, return of function is much more rapid and unnecessary scarring is avoided. Another advantage of early excision is that thicker skin grafts to cover the areas of total skin destruction can be used in the absence of infection. In some deep burns where tendons, nerves and the skeleton are exposed, a decision has to be made as to whether these structures should be sacrificed or not. It is better to leave them, unless they show evidence of charring; then they may be covered with an abdominal, groin or thoracic flap. In situations where flap surgery cannot be carried out temporary skin grafts can be used to cover these exposed structures while the patient is being prepared for more definitive surgery.

Amputations

There is a place for amputation in hand burns; the complex burns of a digit with tendon, nerve and joint destruction are best treated by this method as early as possible.

Decompression of a circumferential burn

Burns involving the whole circumference of a limb or a digit should be regarded as potentially dangerous. As the eschar dries and contracts, enormous pressures are set up inside the limb which can lead to ischaemic necrosis. Lazy 'S' shaped longitudinal incisions on the dorsum of the digits, hand and forearm will dissipate the tourniquet effect and re-establish the circulation. In very severe burns of the forearm the muscle compartments should be decompressed by dividing the deep fascia.

Thermoelectrical burns

This injury is caused by contact with an electrical heated element, usually a domestic heater or a cooker. The patient is usually a child and the burn is mainly thermal, situated on the volar surface of the palm and the digits. If an appreciable electric current has passed and found its way to earth through the dorsum of the hand or forearm and the earthed frame of the appliance, exit electrical burns may also be present. Palmar skin coagulation can be extensive in these cases and in the most severe of them the skeleton may be exposed. Wound isolation in an appropriate dressing for 3 or 4 days is advised, followed by wound excision and grafting (Fig. 19.6). Areas of dermal burns should be tangentially excised and full thickness loss burns subjected to complete debridement. All areas should be then covered with an appropriately equivalent thickness skin graft, the volar surfaces receiving the thickest skin. A successful take of a thick split skin graft gives the best result in volar burns. Exit burns should be treated similarly. In spite of early surgery some of these volar burns produce marginal scarring which contracts and requires secondary surgical correction. When healed all grafts require lanolin nourishment with simple massage for a period of months.

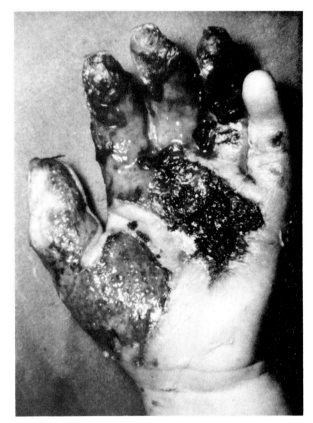

FIG. 19.6. Thermoelectrical burn of a child's hand, granulating after conservative treatment and ready for grafting.

Electrical burns

The passage of a significant amount of electricity through the body can have a devastating effect and can of course be fatal [4]. The current enters through an area of contact and, seeking the lowest resistance pathway to earth, will travel mainly along the nerves and blood vessels. More or less bizzare effects can be expected, the extent of the injury being determined by the voltage and the amperage. The three wounds which must be considered are the entrance wound, the pathway wound and the exit wound. The entrance wound may be small and covered with a dehydrated greyish slough; it can vary considerably in size. The pathway burn may include secondary entrance and exit burns if the current jumps for example between the arm and the chest wall. Such can be the cataclysmic effect on the blood vessels that a whole limb can be devascularised and require immediate amputation as an emergency procedure. In less severe cases all examples of injuries to the neuro-vascular and muscle components of the limb may be encountered. The exit wound may be at a distance, for instance, in the scalp or the foot. It can resemble an explosive wound at times and is nearly always a serious injury in itself. The main diagnostic problem is localisation of the pathway wound.

Early surgical exploration is required and is best done on the second day. Wound excision is carried out as far as possible and free skin graft cover used as the primary dressing. It is frequently necessary to carry out a staged debridement, further excisions being required as more dead tissue becomes evident. Mutilation in high voltage injuries can be severe. When eventual healing takes place the whole gamut of reconstructive surgery may be required in order to restore function. The first stage will often be a replacement of the primary skin dressing with flaps in order to provide a suitable environment for later tendon, nerve and joint surgery.

Chemical burns

These are caused by acids or alkalis. The proper antidote is seldom present at the scene of the accident and washing with copious amounts of water is usually advised. In factories where corrosive substances are in use the appropriate first aid regimen should be available. Some of these burns are full thickness and as soon as this diagnosis becomes clear excision and skin grafting is called for.

Radiation injuries

These are generally seen on the dorsum of the hand and the digits. The causal agents are considered in two groups [3].

(1) Sunburn, ultra-violet lamp and infra-red lamp. They cause irritation, pain, erythema and intradermal oedema. Severe lesions can progress to full thickness loss and must be treated according to general principles.

(2) X-rays produce two effects:

(a) firstly the *acute radiation response*, as seen in the skin which has been affected during the treatment of a malignant tumour. Evidence of this is erythema and a moist desquamation which finally heals unless the dose has been excessive. Protective treatment is all that is required.

(b) The second clinical entity which occurs as a result of exposure to X-rays is the *chronic radio-dermatitis* seen in X-ray workers. Depilation occurs and the skin glands cease to function. Changes in the basal epithelial layers lead to abnormal cell maturation, keratosis and fissuring, accompanied by loss of elasticity. These effects may not be seen for many years after exposure to X-rays has ceased. In due course ischaemic ulceration can occur and in some cases malignant change into squamous carcinoma takes place. This has a poor prognosis as node involvement and metastasis tend to be early. Osteoporosis may be found in the bones of the hand with consequent impairment of digital function. *Surgical treatment of this lesion* in its early stages is necessary to prevent inexorable degenerative processes and to protect the patient from cancer. Excision and either free graft or skin flap cover is the only method of management. When malignant change has already taken place, block dissection of axillary nodes may be necessary but generally speaking this is not a life saving procedure.

Friction burns

This injury is caused by abrasion which develops rapid heat gain in the tissues so that the insult is both mechanical and thermal. A considerable amount of foreign material may be implanted into the wound, the nature of this material varying with the injury. Road traffic accidents cause crush-friction injuries to the hand if it is dragged along the road surface. High speed belts can have a devastating effect on the hand as can fast moving pulleys. *All friction burns require debridement.* Removal of foreign material is important and on many occasions full thickness skin loss will have occurred and require flap surgery. Early skin cover is of the utmost importance.

Flash burns

These occur in the hand as the result of an explosion or electrical arcing. Most flash burns are superficial;

the outer layer of the epidermis is raised to a high temperature for a fraction of a second, the squames are charred and become dark grey or black. The only flash burn which may cause trouble is the high voltage flash or occasionally the lightning flash. These should be watched carefully in case either tangential or full thickness excision becomes necessary. *Otherwise flash burns are best left exposed and kept dry.* In due course the superficial eschar peels off leaving an unblemished skin texture.

REFERENCES

[1] MUIR, I. R. F. AND BARCLAY, T. L. *Burns and their Treatment*, London, Lloyd Luke, 1962.

[2] JANZEKOVIC, Z. *Present Clinical Aspects of Burns—a Symposium*, Ed. by M. Derganc. C. P. Mariborski Tisk, Maribor, Yugoslavia, 1968.

[3] CLARKSON, P. AND PELLY, A. *The General and Plastic Surgery of the Hand*. Oxford, Blackwell Scientific Publications, 1962.

[4] MUIR, I. R. F. The treatment of electrical burns. *British Journal of Plastic Surgery*, 1958, **10**, 292.

FURTHER READING

BURKE, J. F., BONDOC, C. C., QUINBY, W. C. AND REMENSNYDER, J. P. Primary surgical management of deeply burnt hand. *Journal of Trauma*, 1976, **16**, 593.

FLATT, A. *Proceedings of the Second Hand Club*. U.K., Westbury Press, 1962.

JANZEKOVIC, Z. A new concept in the early excision and immediate grafting of burns. *Journal of Trauma*, 1970, **10**, 1103.

POLK, H. C. AND STONE, H. H. (eds) *Contemporary Burn Management*. Baltimore, Williams and Wilkins, 1972.

SALISBURY, R. E. AND PRUITT, B. A. *Burns of the Upper Extremity*. Philadelphia, W. B. Saunders, 1976.

SALISBURY, R. E., TAYLOR, J. W. AND LEVINE, N. S. Evaluation of digital escharotomy in burned hands. *Plastic and Reconstructive Surgery*, 1976, **58**, 440.

STONE, P. A. AND LAWRENCE, J. C. Healing of tangentially excised and grafted burns in man. *British Journal of Plastic Surgery*, 1973, **26**, 20.

WEXLER, M. R., YESCHUA, R. AND NEUMAN, Z. Early treatment of burns on the dorsum of the hand by tangential excision and skin grafting. *Plastic and Reconstructive Surgery*, 1974, **54**, 268.

CHAPTER 20

Cold Injuries

J. A. BOSWICK

Cold injuries of the upper extremity usually involve the digits alone. Less then one per cent of all patients will require amputation proximal to the metacarpophalangeal joints. Total tissue loss is not great but to insure early rehabilitation and minimal loss of function, the entire extremity must be under treatment.

The mechanism of cold injury

Conditions leading to a cold injury can be divided into primary and contributory factors. Primary or basic factors are a low temperature and an adequate exposure time, without which cold injury does not occur.

A most significant contributary factor is wind velocity [6]. This combined with temperature comprises what is termed 'wind chill factor'. The basic time-temperature factor may be modified by time-wind chill factors.

A further well documented contributing factor is increased environmental humidity or local wetness. This problem is illustrated in situations where there is damage to one extremity, caused by a defective boot or glove, and the other extremity, with intact covering, shows no significant cold injury [1].

Direct contact of living tissue with cold objects will result in a much more significant cold injury than mere exposure to cold surroundings. Transfer of heat from the skin will occur more rapidly when there is direct contact with metal, glass or other cold objects. This is noticeable in patients who become comatose or unconscious and sustain a cold injury. An exposed hand will often be in contact with a snowbank, park bench, or the steering wheel of an automobile. The areas in contact with these cold objects usually will be the areas of most significant injury. This contribution of direct contact or the conduction of heat from living tissue is most pronounced when the cold object is wet, as when a wet glove is in contact with a cold metal object.

Lack of protection can contribute dramatically to a cold injury. Conversely stated, 'a minimal amount of protection may prevent a cold injury'. Minimal protection is so important in avoiding cold injury that its value must be emphasized. Experience has shown that with cold exposure of both hands, the hand protected by a thin glove had a mild or no cold injury, whereas the unprotected hand suffered injury to several digits requiring amputation of several centimeters of tissue. The amount of protection required to prevent injury is unknown, but is related to the factors of time, temperature, wind velocity, wetness and the duration and extent of contact with cold objects.

Other factors, such as age, may contribute to the severity of a cold injury. There is a strong suggestion that elderly patients exposed to cold sustain a more severe injury than younger patients. This is difficult to document since younger patients are more alert, able to move about, and more likely to detect wet clothing or contact with cold objects. The elderly patient is also more likely to have pre-existing diseases (such as arthritis, cardiac disorders, or central nervous system disease) that may prevent them from getting out of the cold.

Circulatory impairment has been considered a possible contributory factor to the significance of a cold injury.

Patients with arterial or venous disease of the lower extremity appear to have less resistance to cold than those with a normal circulatory system. However, it must be noted that the natural progress of these circulatory disorders may result in tissue loss without an added cold injury.

THE MANAGEMENT OF A PATIENT WITH COLD INJURIES

Several factors should be considered before instituting therapy:
(1) the general or systemic condition of the patient, including his response to the cold and the specific effects of the lowered temperature on other areas of the body,
(2) the condition of the injured tissue,
(3) the extent of injury.

General management

The systemic management will vary according to the extent and depth of the injury. If only the hands are involved, there is usually a mild systemic response [2]. As the extent increases, so does significant systemic changes, such as generalized hypothermia, hypovolaemia, acidosis, and hypoxaemia. In addition, alcoholic withdrawal problems and malnutrition are often present in the patient with cold injuries.

Generalized hypothermia rarely occurs in a patient with involvement of the hands only; conversely, however, severe cold injuries to the hands commonly occur in patients with generalized hypothermia. While there is some question about the best technique of re-warming a patient with systemic hypothermia, localized re-warming is generally agreed upon and will be discussed later in this chapter.

Hypovolaemia is a recognized complication of cold injury but is not usually severe, for extensive tissue damage and fluid loss is uncommon. With several extremities frozen or cold on admission to hospital, patients have presented with haematocrits as high as 60 per cent. Since most of these patients had prolonged exposure, dehydration as well as fluid loss may have played a role in the hypovolaemia. The management of this moderate hypovolaemia usually presents no problem. A balanced electrolyte solution in amounts that are twice daily fluid requirements usually corrects the hypovolaemia in 24–48 hours.

Acidosis is present in most patients with cold injuries of the hands if the tissue is cold or frozen at the time of admission. The degree of acidosis is related to the extent of injury and to the delay between injury and hospital care. Arterial pH levels as low as 7·16 have been recorded. An initial infusion of 100–300 mg of $NaHCO_3$, repeated every three to four hours, will usually restore the pH to normal in 24 hours.

Hypoxaemia with arterial oxygen levels lowered in direct relation to the duration of exposure and the decrease in metabolism is recorded. Oxygen by mask or nasal catheter restores the pO_2 to normal in eight to twelve hours.

Small vessel thrombosis and platelet aggregation have been recognized as possible factors in diminished circulation and oxygenation of cold injured tissue [7]. Low molecular weight Dextran (Dextran-40) has been used to alleviate this problem. The use of low molecular weight was compared to lactated Ringer's solution in three times the volume of the Dextran. The Dextran was infused at a rate 125/ml/hr for 4 hours utilizing 500 ml of a 6 per cent Dextran 40 solution. Lactated Ringer's solution was infused at 150/ml/hr giving 1500 ml over a 10-hour period. At the end of 3 hours the patients with cold tissue receiving Dextran 40 had an average increase in temperature at their fingertips of 5·1°F. The patients receiving the lactated Ringer's solution had less than a 1°F improvement after 4 hours.

The changes are compatible with the anti-sludging effect of Dextran 40. As platelet aggregation is diminished, circulation is improved, increasing tissue perfusion and also increasing temperature.

Alcoholic withdrawal symptoms can be a significant problem in management as over 80 per cent of these patients sustain their injury during an acute alcoholic intake [5]. If the history or evaluation suggests alcoholic addiction, early treatment is recommended to prevent the development of withdrawal symptoms. The use of sedatives (barbiturates, Sparine, chloral hydrate,

Librium) and antitremor drugs (Dilantin and MgSO$_4$), along with vitamins, is accepted therapy.

Malnourishment is not uncommon in patients who sustain cold injuries. Adequate dietary intake and supplementary vitamins should be provided as soon as possible after injury. This systemic management should not detract from the early management of the injured tissue. Patients with cold injuries are seen with tissue that is frozen, cold, blistered or cyanotic. On occasion, gangrenous tissue will be present at the time of admission due to the delay between injury and the patient's seeking medical help.

Local management of cold injured tissue

The early management of damaged tissue depends on the specific condition of the tissue when first seen. The most severe tissue condition is that of being frozen and approximately one per cent of all cold injury patients reach the hospital with frozen tissue. Some of these patients also present with generalized hypothermia, i.e. a core temperature below 32°C.

Frozen tissue requires not only local treatment, but concurrent systemic treatment, since rapid rewarming can increase or compound the problem of acidosis [8]. The most effective method of treating frozen tissue in a patient who does not have generalized hypothermia is total body warming. After drawing arterial blood for PO_2, pCO_2, and pH determinations, an intravenous catheter should· be inserted, and lactated Ringer's solution infused, with NaHCO$_3$ added if necessary. The patient should be placed in a tub or body whirlpool with the water temperature at 100°F. Water of 110°F should be added slowly. After 15–20 minutes, the water will have reached 104–105°F and skin temperature usually will have been restored to normal. If the patient has not reached a near normal temperature after 15–20 minutes, further rewarming should be done cautiously. After tissue rewarming, the management of the injured tissue should proceed according to its condition and the progress of the injury.

Lesser cold injuries require similar management but the time required for re-warming is not as great, and the temperature of the water can be maintained at 100°F, since the cold tissue will not lower the water temperature as rapidly as frozen tissue. After cold or frozen tissue is re-warmed, blistering commonly occurs.

Some patients do not seek hospital care following cold injury until blister formation has occurred, or until there is marked discolouration or cyanosis. The immediate care of damaged tissue, whether blistered or discoloured, is that it should be kept clean by frequent washings, active exercise encouraged, and the limb maintained in a functional position. Frequent washings can be accomplished in a variety of ways, depending on the general condition, other injuries, and the ability to co-operate. Patients are encouraged to wash frequently and to move their hands actively through the fullest possible range of motion. The patient sits in a body whirlpool, and, with the hands at shoulder to face level, washes and actively moves the hands thus providing an opportunity of seeing the hands move, with the hope of encouraging an increased amount of active motion each day. As motion increases, the patient is usually motivated to increase the time and enthusiasm invested in such a programme.

If a body whirlpool is not available, the same programme can be accomplished at a wash basin. In between these washings and exercises it is important to keep the tissues dry. When the feet are also involved, caution must be exercised in not allowing them to be dependent while the hands are receiving care.

The improvement in tissue perfusion by release of the sympathetic influence or sympathectomy has been frequently utilized in treating patients with cold injuries [4]. To assess the value of sympathectomy in acute cold injuries, we performed upper or lower extremity sympathectomies in one extremity in over 100 patients with bilateral cold injuries (56 lower and 49 upper). Some patients had involvement of both lower and upper extremities; in these patients only an upper or lower extremity sympathectomy was performed. The side chosen for the sympathectomy was the side with the most significant injury. An estimation of tissue loss was made at the time of injury and at 5 and 10 days after injury. There was no apparent difference in tissue survival following sympathectomy. However, the tissue on the side of the sympathectomy was drier and easier to manage. This observation prompted us to use lower extremity sympathectomy in patients with hyperhydrosis, chronic oedema and local ulcerations following cold injury. In over 60 patients treated, all but three showed an excellent response to healing of open wounds, decreased oedema and sweating [3].

Early debridement must be very conservative and limited to previously ruptured blebs or bullae. Blisters may have developed before hospital admission, or develop after the re-warming of cold or frozen tissue. They are left intact unless they interfere with movement, appear taut or the blister fluid appears purulent. Primary excision and grafting has no place in early wound care, as it is often impossible to predict accurately the extent of tissue necrosis. Hands may appear to have only partial-thickness skin loss, but, by 14 days post-injury it is obvious that there are necrotic phalanges and that amputations are required.

A programme of frequent washings and active motion should be continued until there is optimal healing of the partial-thickness wounds and definite demarcation of the full-thickness wounds. This state of care often extends to three or four months, because the amount of full-thickness injury is often over-estimated, and progressive healing requires several weeks. If only the hands are involved, most of the care, starting a few days after injury and continuing until demarcation is complete, can be rendered on an outpatient basis.

After initial care, it is important to handle the injured tissue gently. This philosophy is consistent with the earlier programme of frequent washings, gentle active motion, and minimal tissue manipulation. The injured parts should be elevated to minimize oedema, and loose crusts or dead tissue removed every two to three days. This is best accomplished after the hands have been washed, while the tissue is moist and easily separated. The loose tissue is gently trimmed to the point of firm attachment with small tissue forceps and scissors. Epithelium regenerates in areas where the wounds are partial thickness in depth, and full-thickness wounds will form granulation tissue and require grafting. In deeply injured phalanges that are non-viable the tissue will tend to contract or shrink. Only after granulation tissue develops between the healed partial thickness and obviously gangrenous tissue is amputation indicated.

During the long period of management loss of function and the development of deformities must be prevented. The role and technique for active motion have been described but correct positioning of the hands is equally important in preventing complications. The wrist should be in a dorsi-flexed position which is basic in preventing loss of function, the development of deformities, and in any programme of active hand motion. To insure that the wrist does not assume a flexed position, a wrist extension splint is worn during periods of inactivity and especially at night. This splint alone will not prevent the development of interphalangeal flexion and thumb adduction deformities and if there are signs of these developing, the splint should be modified to prevent or correct them.

Summary

The management of patients with cold injuries of the hands may be extremely simple or relatively complex. The extent of the injury and the systemic response to the cold are the major influencing factors.

In patients with extensive cold injuries, where all or a large portion of more than one extremity is cold or frozen and there has been a significant systemic response, treatment should be both systemic and local.

Treatment should be directed toward both preservation of tissue and maintenance of function of the damaged part. Minimal daily debridement and late amputation are important guidelines for care.

REFERENCES

[1] BLAIR, J. R. In: *Follow-up on Cold Injury Cases from the Korean War*. I. M. Ferrer (Editor), Fourth Conference on Cold Injury, New York, Josiah Mach, Jr. Foundation, 1955.

[2] BOSWICK, J. A., JR. 'Cold Injuries', Chapter Nine, Burns of the Upper Extremity, Salisbury and Pruitt, Vol. XIX in the Series *Major Problems in Clinical Surgery*, W. B. Saunders, Philadelphia, 1976.

[3] GOLDING, M. R. *et al.* Protection from early and late sequelae of frostbite by regional sympathectomy: Mechanism of cold sensitivity following frostbite surgery, *Surgery*, 1963, **53**, 303.

[4] GOLDING, M. R. *et al.* On settling the controversy on the benefit of sympathectomy for frostbite, *Surgery*, 1964, **56**, 221.

[5] HERMANN, G. *et al.* The problem of frostbite in civilian medical practice. *Surgical Clinics of North America*, 1963, **43**, 519.

[6] KNIZE, D. M. *et al.* Prognostic factors in the management of frostbite, *Journal of Trauma*, 1969, **9**, 749.

[7] KNIZE, D. M., WEATHERLEY-WHITE, R. C. AND PATON, B. C. Use of antisludging agents in experimental cold injuries, *Surgery, Gynecology Obstetrics*, 1969, **129**, 1019.

[8] MERYMAN, H. T. Tissue freezing and local cold injury. *Physiology Reviews*, 1957, **37**, 233.

CHAPTER 21

Drug Injection, Pressure Gun and Self-Inflicted Injuries

H. E. KLEINERT and T. W. WOLFF

DRUG INJECTION

Today's increase in the number of drug injection users in our society makes early recognition and treatment of the complications paramount.

Arterial injection can be divided into two categories: (1) accidental—by medical personnel; (2) intentional—by the drug user. In both cases, the basic pathophysiology is the same.

The most common site of injection is the antebrachial region where the brachial artery is superficial and easily entered. Variations of the presenting symptoms and signs depend upon the agent or agents injected. When the artery is accidentally injected immediate severe burning pain is felt followed by numbness of the hand. Rapid blotching of the skin and decreased temperature of the hand give it a cadaveric appearance. Late sequelae are ischaemic muscle contracture and gangrene. Exploration rarely reveals arterial thrombus at the injection site but more distal arteriolar intimal swelling and thrombosis in the wrist and hand.

Many substances given safely by vein produce catastrophies when injected intra-arterially (Fig. 21.1), and the injury is proportionate to the dilution of the injected drug. Medication injected into an artery is localized and concentrated in its field of supply whereas the same substance injected into the vein undergoes haemodilution as it circulates.

An aspect of drug injection injury in the intentional user is the 'puffy hand' syndrome secondary to chronic

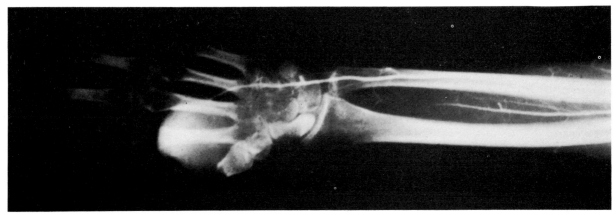

FIG. 21.1. An amputation of the thumb and index finger following accidental drug injection of the radial artery. The arteriogram depicts absent filling of the radial artery.

destruction of superficial veins and lymphatics; as peripheral veins have less adventitial support extravasation easily occurs. Intra-arterial injection may indeed be intentional after all veins have been obliterated by frequent past injections. This intra-arterial injection causes a special sensation known as a 'flash' or a 'hand trip'. 'Skin popping' is resorted to by some addicts when mainlining is no longer possible. This is a subcutaneous injection of the drug and its additive which together cause a local and severe inflammatory reaction. Abscesses are probably the most frequent complication seen in the extremity of an addict. Mycotic aneurysms can form after arterial injection. Other complications of drug injections are septic arthritis and myositis. Tissue swelling, secondary to chemical arteritis and intra-arterial thrombosis, can even produce complete ischaemia and, if left untreated, gangrene of the extremity.

Treatment

Standard management includes sympathetic nerve blocks, heparinization, and vasodilating drugs such as papaverine (100 mg injected intramuscularly). Fasciotomy of both intrinsic and extrinsic muscle groups is indicated if the extremity becomes tense. Intermittent positive pressure has been tried but rarely alleviates the need for fasciotomy.

If circulation and arterial pulsations fail to return shortly after conservative therapy is instituted arterial exploration is indicated.

Recently thrombolysin given intra-arterially has been advocated by Kartchner and Wilcox [1]. We have employed it with arterial exploration after other methods have failed to restore adequate circulation. As arteriography usually demonstrates palmar arch and digital artery thrombosis, distal thrombectomy is at best difficult and likely to be followed by recurrence of thrombosis even with heparinization. Many such extremities can and have been salvaged by early arterial exploration combined with thrombolysin given as a constant intra-arterial infusion, employing an arterial pump attached to a catheter placed in a retrograde fashion. Serial monitoring with coagulation studies is imperative. The usual dosage of thrombolysin is 100,000 units per hour until an acceptable systemic effect is achieved. Ideally the fibrinogen level is maintained at 100–200 mg/100 ml,

the euglobulin lysis time at one hour and the thrombin time at 20–30 seconds. The prothrombin time is not allowed to exceed 16 seconds. Following intra-arterial thrombolysin therapy constant intravenous infusion of heparin is started to prevent re-thrombosis. Intra-arterial thrombolysin combined with thrombectomy offers hope in cases previously thought to have inevitable gangrene from extensive thrombosis.

HIGH PRESSURE INJECTION INJURIES (PAINT AND GREASE GUN)

Since first described by Rees [2], the incidence of high pressure injection injuries of the hand has sharply increased. Previous authors pointed out that the force of injection through fine jets is as great as 6000 lb/in². Williams and Riordan stressed that the initial impact is often painless accompanied by only a stinging sensation [3]. Later the involved digit becomes very painful. Stark reported his experience with injection injuries and emphasized its seriousness and need for immediate surgery [4]. Kleinert stressed constant awareness and recognition of the severity of this injury as most important for immediate diagnosis and treatment [5].

The pathophysiology of the injection injury is a combination of chemical irritation, ischaemia and infection. (*These injuries must be treated as surgical emergencies.*) Immediate removal of the offending material lessens tissue irritation, rids the wound of contaminated material and decompresses the injured part.

Other factors influencing the severity of injury are: (1) the velocity of injection; (2) the anatomical location of the injury, and (3) the volume of material injected. If the injection is over a digital neurovascular bundle, finger pain and propagation of the material along the fascial plane is noted. Injection over a finger flexion crease enters the tendon sheath and the radial or ulnar bursa if the thumb or little finger are involved respectively. If the index, middle and ring finger tendon sheaths have been affected, thenar or mid-palmar space extravasation may be found. Injections in the finger pulp or other closed spaces have a higher incidence of gangrene.

The typical patient is male between the ages of 20 and 30 years. His occupation is commonly painter, mechanic, industrial worker, or farmer. The site of injury is probably the index finger or palm of the non-dominant hand. Immediate diagnosis is the key to a good result. A high degree of suspicion is needed when first examining these initially innocuous wounds acquired while working with or cleaning pressure guns. Individuals working on defective high pressure lines containing hydraulic fluid particularly, may present with a slightly painful, swollen finger, and with little other history. Physical examination reveals the entry wound is usually minute (Fig. 21.2). Only a few drops of the injected material can be expressed. If the patient is seen in the first few hours the involved digit may appear only minimally swollen. It may not be painful or tender; however, accompanying discoloration and/or numbness imply

serious injury. After four to six hours pain becomes intense and progressive oedema and skin changes suggest further vascular involvement (Fig. 21.3). Immediate

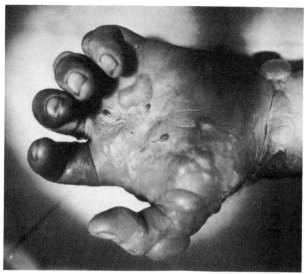

FIG. 21.3. Diffuse oedema and bleb formation illustrating the late sequelae of an overlooked high pressure paint gun injury.

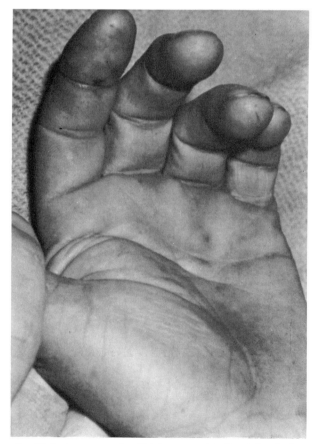

FIG. 21.2. A common site of high pressure injection injury is the index finger of the non-dominant hand. Note the innocuous appearance of entry site over distal crease.

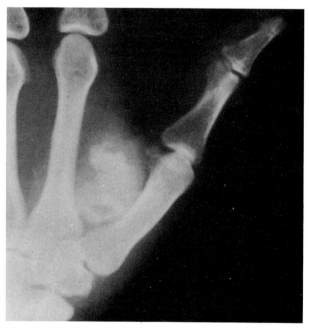

FIG. 21.4. Radiographs may be helpful in revealing the extent of the injected material.

recognition, so important since these injuries are more extensive than initial symptoms and physical findings suggest, rests on a high degree of suspicion.

Radiography is of value especially if paint, plastic, cement or other radio-opaque material has been injected (Fig. 21.4).

Treatment

Emergency management includes analgesics, antitetanus and antibiotic coverage in preparation for exploration of the wound. Axillary block is a safe, adequate emergency anaesthesia. When applying a pneumatic tourniquet the limb should be elevated but not exsanguinated with a rubber wrapper for fear of dissemination of the toxic substance. Adequate dorso-

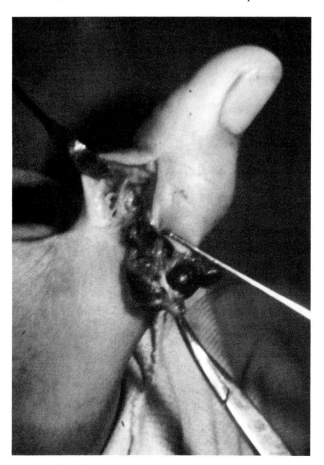

FIG. 21.5. Late excision of an oleogranuloma.

lateral longitudinal incisions are indicated in the finger with appropriate extension into the palm and forearm as needed. All foreign material should be removed as far as possible by incision proximally. Postoperatively, close observation for the need for an additional incision should be kept. If grease is the offending material and some is missed on primary debridement, excision of olegranuloma may be required weeks to months after initial treatment (Fig. 21.5).

Later symptoms and signs differ according to the material injected. With paint, paint thinner and hydraulic oil injections, the ischaemia and inflammation are severe. The patient quickly develops a fever and lymphangitis. With grease gun injuries, ischaemia is quite severe but inflammation just moderate. These patients develop decreased range of motion, late scarring and the formation of 'oleomas'.

A more recently described offending substance is the tear gas injection which causes moderate ischaemia, inflammation, and neurotoxicity.

Gangrene and subsequent amputation vary with: (1) the type of material injected, and (2) institution of adequate treatment within 24 hours. Patients injected with paint or oil did poorly even when seen within 24 hours. If treatment was delayed beyond 24 hours the amputation rate rose significantly. Reconstructive procedures are needed especially if the diagnosis is delayed. In terms of personal cost the patient has a long morbidity (an average of 6 months). Two to three operations have been noted per patient, up to ten for cases requiring extensive reconstruction. Residual disability and deformity are common particularly in cases that have been neglected.

In summary, treatment consists of immediate surgery with adequate incisions for exploration and removal of all foreign material.

SELF-INFLICTED INJURIES

Self-inflicted injuries vary in severity. The most common is the patient who indiscriminately and with slight provocation slashes the front of the wrist. Some patients in a moment of anger thrust their hand and arm intentionally through glass windows and doors under the influence of alcohol. Others with evident psychoses cause severe injury to their wrists. The psychological aspects have been alluded to by psychologists and psychiatrists [6, 7].

The typical 'self-cutter' is a 22-year-old nonpsychotic female who habitually cuts herself with a sharp object on at least two separate occasions. She is usually an intelligent, unmarried young woman unable to relate to others. She slashes her wrist indiscriminately and repeatedly at the slightest provocation but does not commit suicide. These patients have been labeled 'delicate self-cutters' to distinguish them from those who cut once, deeply and with the intent to commit suicide. A significant number of self-cutters use drugs or alcohol in excess. Most of these patients have substantial difficulty in describing their emotions and needs. Many complain of depression, emptiness and loneliness. The degree of injury ranges from the superficial wound and progresses through multiple slashes or 'hesitation marks'

to the almost complete amputation. Accordingly, the extent of the injury ranges from superficial wrist flexor tendon lacerations, partial or complete median nerve lacerations, and includes the 'spaghetti wrist' where everything is divided. One of our cases, a 24-year-old white male paranoid schizophrenic, was essentially a wrist level replantation. The patient deliberately severed his right hand through the proximal carpal row leaving only one wrist extensor intact. Following an 8 hour operation in which all structures were repaired primarily, the patient was admitted to a mental unit for psychiatric care and postoperative management. He has since been a model patient who actively uses this hand as a 'helper' for his normal extremity. Similar cases have demonstrated the value of replantation in the psychotic who purposely amputates a part of the body.

REFERENCES

[1] KARTCHNER, M. M. AND WILCOX, W. C. Thrombolysis of palmar and digital arterial thrombosis by intra-arterial thrombolysin. *Journal of Hand Surgery*, 1976, **1,** 67.

[2] REES, C. E. Penetration of tissue by fuel oil under high pressure from diesel engine. *Journal of the American Medical Association*, 1937, **109,** 866.

[3] WILLIAMS, C. S. AND RIORDAN, D. C. High velocity injection injuries of the hand. *Southern Medical Journal*, 1974, **67,** 295.

[4] STARK, H. H. Grease gun injuries of the hand. *Journal of Bone and Joint Surgery*, 1961, **43A,** 485.

[5] KLEINERT, H. E., BRONSON, J. L. AND THURSTON, J. B. The Hand: High pressure injection injuries. *Resident and Staff Physician*, 1976, **110,** 1.

[6] GARDNER, A. R. AND GARDNER, A. J. Self-mutilation, obsessionality, and narcissism. *British Journal of Psychiatry*, 1975, **127,** 127.

[7] SIMPSON, M. A. Symposium—Self injury: The phenomenology of self-mutilation in a general hospital setting. *Canadian Psychiatry Association Journal*, 1975, **20,** 429.

CHAPTER 22

Management of the Stiff Hand

R. M. CURTIS

CAUSES AND PREVENTION OF JOINT STIFFENING IN THE HAND: GENERAL REMARKS

Primary factors behind stiffening of the hand are oedema, fibrosis, collagen alteration and structural changes.

The following principles should be observed in prevention (see Chapter 8).

Elevation of the injured extremity;
Mild compression dressing;
Elimination of pain;
Prevention of haematoma; and
Prevention of infection.

An understanding of the underlying emotional factors which occur with hand injuries is important. Bunnell stated that all uninjured parts should be kept unrestrained and free to move and also that 'one should be alert to recognise early those cases that will go on to the oedematous, immobile osteoporotic hand, by recognising the signs of trophic disturbance and the disposition on the part of the patient to hold his hand completely immobile' [1]. Moberg and Stener have emphasized that contraction of the muscles pumps the tissue fluids through the limb, preventing oedema and stasis and keeping the tissues nourished [2]. A pressure point produced by the dressing or cast will lead to oedema and swelling of the injured or postoperative hand, and the dressing should be checked 12–24 hours after surgery and if necessary released at least along one border. Any point where the patient complains about abnormal pressure and pain should be checked.

Peacock stated on the basis of his clinical and experimental studies that the stiffness which follows simple immobilization is due to fixation of the joint ligaments to bone in areas normally meant to be free from such fixation and to shortening of the ligaments by new collagen synthesis [3]. It is possible that with injury we may have an imbalance between fibrin formation and lysis of fibrin.

There are a number of conservative methods of treating stiff joints or of preventing stiffening in the post-surgical stage.

Elevation is important to minimize swelling. This should be used immediately after all surgery on the hand, and when ambulatory the patient continues to keep the hand elevated.

Elastic splints and elastic traction should be used early and continuously; the amount of tension used should not produce swelling.

Molded plaster splints or casts can be applied and changed at regular intervals (daily if possible) to stretch gradually the finger joints or wrist joint into flexion or extension.

The Jobst intermittent compression unit has been very helpful in reducing the swelling in the post-traumatic and postoperative hand, and in mobilizing stiff interphalangeal joints. The hand is placed in the sleeve with the fingers in extension for 10 minutes under pressure, and then in flexion for 10 minutes. Pressure that can be easily tolerated by the patient is used increasing the time in the pneumatic sleeve gradually from 30 minutes to 1 hour, one or more times a day, and gradually increasing the millimeters of mercury pressure in the sleeve. The fact that extracellular fluid is pressed out of the hand by the intermittent pressure, and that the tight capsular ligaments are stretched first into extension and then into flexion, makes it possible to mobilize some joints where splinting and other methods of treatment have failed.

Local heat therapy by warm water soaks or whirlpool baths is helpful, as is hot wax therapy. Occasionally a patient may be helped with alternating warm and cold baths. This seems to be particularly helpful in the sympathetic dystrophies.

Stellate ganglion blocks and local nerve blocks, or blocks with local anesthesia of the painful trigger areas, may be helpful. In sympathetic dystrophy, the stellate ganglion block or sympathectomy can relieve pain and decrease oedema.

Exercise. The need for active use of the hand in mobilizing stiff joints cannot be overemphasised and also the use of passive exercises to improve the range of motion. The force applied must not increase the swelling or pain in the joints which are stiff.

Medical treatment. Various drugs are available for systemic use which may be helpful. Two of the most effective are butazolidin and prednisone. The local use of 10 mg of triamcinolone following extensive dissections, such as tendolysis or fasciectomy, is of definite help in reducing postoperative swelling. This may also be used in an amount of 2 mg injected intra-articularly in the small finger joints. Sympathetic blocking agents (Etamon or Priscoline) may be of value, and some of the tranquilizers seem to aid in the patient's recovery.

In the following section specific causes and treatment options for stiffness of the metacarpophalangeal and proximal interphalangeal joints are discussed with particular attention to ankylosis and operative procedures. Subsequently a range of surgical procedures for relief of thumb contracture are discussed.

METACARPOPHALANGEAL JOINTS

Anatomy (see p. 17)

Ankylosis

The following limit metacarpophalangeal joint flexion:
(1) adhesions of the extensor tendons over the dorsum of the hand or adhesions of the extensor hood mechanism over the metacarpophalangeal joints;
(2) thickening of the dorsal synovium of the joints;
(3) contracture of the collateral ligament (cordlike portion);
(4) insufficient skin coverage or scar of the skin over the dorsum of the hand, as in a burn; and
(5) bony block within the joint.

Immobility of the metacarpophalangeal joints, for whatever reason, and particularly if there is swelling with the deposit of oedema fluid about the ligamentous tissue and extensor tendons, leads to adhesions of the extensor mechanism, to contracture and adhesions of the collateral ligaments, or thickening of the entire capsular ligamentous structure.

This is seen in hands in which there has been infection, trauma of all types, burns with scar contracture over the dorsum of the hand, congenital aplasia of the metacarpophalangeal joints, and in certain systemic diseases such as rheumatoid arthritis and dermatomyositis.

Conservative treatment

The prevention of this very disabling abnormality is of primary importance. It can be best achieved by following the general principles discussed above, i.e. (1) early motion of the metacarpophalangeal joints, (2) elevation of the injured extremity to prevent oedema, (3) elimination of plaster casts or splints which immobilize the joints, and (4) early elastic band traction in patients who are developing this clinical entity [4].

Early after injury, rubber band traction should be used along with the use of a small volar plaster splint, worn 12 to 24 hours a day, or the Bunnell knuckle bender splint, to improve flexion and extension. This dynamic splinting can be coupled with various forms of physiotherapy (see Chapter 36). Alternating positive pressure with a compression unit can be of great help in reducing oedema of the hand and in mobilizing the joints.

If progress is being made with conservative treatment, operative release should be delayed. However, if after several months there is no progress in the range of active or passive motion in the metacarpophalangeal joints, surgical release of these joints is indicated. Capsulectomies on metacarpophalangeal joints which can be actively flexed as much as 65° are not indicated. Where joints are fixed in full extension or have a range of motion less than 65° of flexion, one can expect to improve the range of motion by operation.

Bunnell stated that the essentials for the success of capsulectomy are good surrounding tissue, good nerve supply and nutrition, redundant dorsal skin and good extensor and flexor tendons and intrinsic muscles [5].

Operative procedures

Where there is a stiff metacarpophalangeal joint the choice lies between capsulectomy and arthroplasty. The decision will depend on the appearance of the metacarpal head and the base of the phalanx in the radiograph. A good range of motion in the metacarpophalangeal joint may be salvaged by capsulectomy even when the radiograph shows considerable joint damage. When there is advanced destruction arthroplasty is usually required.

Capsulectomy of the metacarpophalangeal joint

The extensor tendons are exposed by four straight longitudinal incisions over the metacarpals and the tendon split longitudinally for a distance of approximately 2·5 cm on either side of the joint [5]. The aponeurotic or extensor hood is then retracted to either side and the attachments of the extensor tendon to the base of the proximal phalanx are severed when these are present. The synovium which forms the dorsal part of the capsule of the joint between the base of the phalanx and the head of the metacarpal is excised, for this may be greatly thickened in severe cases. This dorsal capsule is excised from one collateral ligament across to the opposite collateral ligament over the dorsum of the joint (Fig. 22.1a).

Since it is the cordlike portion of the collateral ligament that limits flexion, it can be released from its attachment just beneath the tubercle on either side of the head of the metacarpal (Fig. 22.1b), leaving it attached to

the accessory collateral ligament but freeing any adhesions which may have formed between the cord portion of the collateral ligament and the head of the metacarpal (Fig. 22.1c). Pressure against the base of the proximal phalanx will then carry the proximal phalanx into flexion beneath the head of the metacarpal.

If there is much thickening in the ligament, a section of the cordlike portion of the ligament should be removed near its metacarpal attachment and the remainder of the ligament left attached to the accessory collateral ligament. This will prevent ulnar deviation of the finger which is seen when too much of the ligament is removed and is particularly apt to occur in the patient with ulnar nerve palsy. Care must be taken not to sever the attachment of the interosseous tendon into the base of the

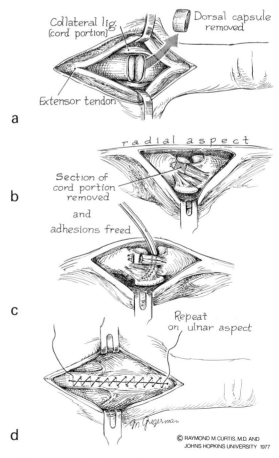

FIG. 22.1. Capsulectomy of the metacarpophalangeal joint.

phalanx for this may also lead to ulnar deviation of the fingers.

If the phalanx does not drop into flexion beneath the head of the metacarpal, then a curved periosteal elevator should be inserted around the head of the metacarpal to recreate the volar pouch beneath the head of the metacarpal; in long-standing cases, this pouch becomes obliterated when the volar plate becomes adherent to the metacarpal head.

The excursion of the extensor tendons over the dorsum of the hand should be checked. If these are not gliding freely, they should be tenolyzed over the dorsum of the hand, and if necessary, over the dorsum of the wrist and into the forearm. In addition, one may need to free the extensor hood well onto either side of the metacarpophalangeal joint. Before closure of the extensor tendon, 2 mg of triamcinolone should be placed into each joint, and another 10 mg distributed beneath the extensor tendons on the dorsum of the hand if they have been tenolyzed. The extensor tendon is closed with a running suture of 4–0 stainless steel wire (Fig. 22.1d). A pressure dressing is applied with the metacarpophalangeal joints in moderate flexion, care being taken to avoid such a severe degree of flexion as to cause the extensor tendons to open over the joint. This is left in place for 72 hours, and then a volar plaster splint applied to allow rubber band traction into flexion by leather loops around the proximal phalanges.

This elastic splinting must be continued as long as necessary, both day and night. After four to six weeks, a Bunnell knuckle bender splint may be used. During the period of elastic splinting, active extension is allowed and there is rarely any difficulty achieving complete active extension. If there is a problem with finger extension, a dynamic splint for extension is alternated with one for flexion.

Arthroplasty

This is indicated for severe destruction of the metacarpal head and/or base of phalanx where release of the capsular ligament may not provide a satisfactory range of motion [6]. It is indicated in the rheumatoid hand (see Chapter 25), in osteoarthritis with marked deformity of the joint, and in destruction of the joint after trauma. The best arthroplasty result is obtained by the use of a joint prosthesis interposed between the metacarpal and the proximal phalanx [7].

PROXIMAL INTERPHALANGEAL JOINTS

A surgeon treating a crippled hand is confronted frequently with a hand that fails to function properly because of limitation of flexion or extension in the interphalangeal joints. Bunnell noted that it is the narrow joint space present in the interphalangeal joints which results in limitation of motion where there is even the slightest shortening of the capsular ligaments, as might be produced by lack of use or by oedema of the ligaments and subsequent fibrosis [5].

This shortening with limitation in motion may occur despite the most rigid attention to proper splinting and to physical and occupational therapy, and to proper reduction of fractures or dislocations. However, more often it follows the improper use of these methods of treatment [8].

Anatomy (see p. 19)

Conservative treatment of injuries to the proximal interphalangeal joint by means of physiotherapy and splinting should follow the principles stated previously. However, for a severely ankylosed joint in extension or flexion, a capsulectomy may be needed to restore function.

Ankylosis of the proximal interphalangeal joint in extension

The surgeon who intends to correct a limitation of flexion of the proximal interphalangeal joint must have in mind the various mechanical factors that may limit this motion. These are:

(1) scar contracture of the skin over the dorsum of the finger;

(2) contracted long extensor muscle or adherent extensor tendon;

(3) contracted interosseous muscle or adherent interosseous tendon;

(4) contracted capsular ligament, particularly the accessory collateral ligament;

(5) retinacular ligament adherent to capsular ligament;

(6) bone block or exostosis;

(7) adherence of the flexor tendons within the finger.

Before surgical correction of the lack of flexion of the interphalangeal joint, it is important to determine by clinical and radiographic examination which anatomical structures are limiting flexion, and to exclude a true ankylosis by bony fusion or block.

Bunnell, Doherty, and Curtis described various test positions of the hand and fingers to determine which structures are to blame [9].

Capsulectomy of the proximal interphalangeal joint in extension (Fig. 22.2)

The interphalangeal joint is approached by a dorsal curvilinear incision on either side of the joint (Fig. 22.2a). The incision is deepened through the skin and subcutaneous tissue to expose the transverse retinacular ligament (see p. 30).

By approaching the joint from the distal edge of this ligament it can be lifted and retracted proximally (Fig.

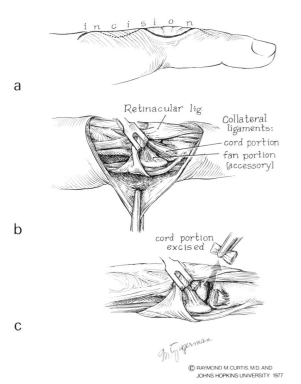

FIG. 22.2. Capsulectomy of the proximal interphalangeal joint stiff in extension.

22.2b) from the collateral ligament of the proximal interphalangeal joint, the middle portion of which can be removed on either side (Fig. 22.2c) [10].

In some longstanding cases the volar synovial pouch becomes obliterated, and must be re-formed with a small curved elevator or by forcing the base of the middle phalanx into flexion. Where there is an associated contracture of the interosseous muscle, the tendon is lengthened by tenotomy at the junction of the longitudinal fibres with the middle slip of the extensor tendon, allowed to slide proximally where it is sutured to the extensor aponeurosis. Excision of a triangle including the longitudinal fibres from the interosseous and lumbrical muscles, as recommended by Littler [11] is also effective.

If there is severe contracture of the interosseous muscle with flexion deformity at the metacarpophalangeal joint as well, it may be necessary to tenotomize this tendon proximal to the metacarpophalangeal joint and divide the volar capsular ligament of the metacarpophalangeal joint.

If necessary, the extensor tendon mechanism should be freed over the dorsum of the finger. The dissection and freeing of contracted tissues must continue until there is a free range of motion of the middle phalanx about the distal end of the proximal phalanx. This necessitates freeing the extensor tendon from the phalanx, opening the dorsal synovium of the joint, resection of the collateral ligaments, and a release of the contracted interosseous tendon mechanism.

One may elect to place 2 mg of triamcinolone acetonide (Kenalog) into the interphalangeal joint after this procedure. The hand is then placed in a dorsal plaster splint, using mechanics' waste and mild compression, with the fingers in moderate flexion at the proximal interphalangeal joints. Within 48–72 hours rubber band traction is begun either by leather loops over the finger tips or by traction through the nail gradually pulling the fingers into the flexed position. It may be necessary to alternate between rubber band traction for flexion at the interphalangeal joints and rubber band traction for extension of the fingers, together with active exercise. Elastic splinting is continued until the patient can maintain, by active and passive exercise, the range of motion obtained at surgery. In some cases this requires part-time splinting for three or four months.

Indications and results

When the proximal interphalangeal joint can be flexed actively to 75° or more, it is better to rely on conservative measures of physiotherapy and splinting to achieve additional flexion. In those who have a lesser degree of flexion and even in those whose fingers are held in rigid extension but without bony ankylosis, one can expect to improve flexion by operation. The more anatomical structures there are involved in the limitation of motion, the poorer the end result [12]. If the only limiting factor is the capsular ligament, then capsulectomy of the collateral ligaments gives a good result both for flexion and extension. If it is necessary to free the extensor tendon over the proximal phalanx or cut the interosseous tendons in addition to a capsulectomy of the collateral ligaments the result is not as successful. This is particularly true of the severely scarred finger where the increase in motion may be only 20–30°; in most cases as much as 80° is gained which usually means the difference between a hand that could be used for work and one that could not. Full function should not be expected by this procedure, but one can expect to improve it.

This approach is applicable to a joint stiff in extension, of whatever etiology, if the joint surfaces are not too badly destroyed. In the latter instance, an arthroplasty with a joint prosthesis is the procedure of choice (see Chapter 25).

Sprague, and Harrison reported their results of the surgical treatment of the stiff proximal interphalangeal joint [13, 14]. The latter author recommends division only of the main collateral ligament and the dorsal capsule for the joint stiff in extension.

Ankylosis of the proximal interphalangeal joint in flexion

Causes

The mechanical factors that may limit extension of a finger at the proximal interphalangeal joint are:

(1) Scar of the skin on the volar surface of the finger.

(2) Contraction of the fascia in the finger, as in Dupuytren's contracture.

(3) Contracture of the flexor tendon sheath within the finger.

(4) Contracted flexor muscle or adherent flexor tendon.

(5) Contraction or adherence of the volar plate of the capsular ligament.

(6) Adherence of the retinacular ligament to the collateral ligaments.

(7) Adherence of the collateral ligaments with the finger in the flexed position.

(8) Bony block or exostosis.

Frequently, more than one structure is involved in flexion contracture. e.g. In congenital flexion contracture of the finger, where all tissues from the skin to the joint capsule, and even the joint itself, may be involved (see Chapter 24) or in long standing Dupuytren's contracture where the skin will be short; there will be a thick strand of contracted fascia; the flexor superficialis tendon may be contracted and the volar capsule and the accessory collateral ligaments may contract or adhere in such a way as to prevent extension.

Capsulectomy of the proximal interphalangeal joint in flexion (Fig. 22.3)

Operative release of the finger in an acutely flexed position is usually through a midlateral incision which is deepened to expose the flexor tendon sheath and the joint itself (Fig. 22.3a). (A Z-plasty on the flexor surface of the finger may be preferable in Dupuytren's contracture.) A good approach is to excise a portion of the flexor tendon sheath over the proximal interphalangeal joint and see whether or not this simple excision will allow any extension. In some instances, it may be the only structure which is contracted.

The flexor tendons are then checked to see whether they are adherent over the proximal phalanx or whether they are contracted. If severely contracted, it may be necessary to tenotomize and lengthen them in the forearm.

The retinacular ligament is freed from the lateral capsule and the volar capsule is then excised. The accessory collateral ligament is resected on either side through separate mid-lateral incisions (Fig. 22.3b). Subluxation of the middle phalanx may occur if the cord portion of the lateral ligament is completely severed. In some instances, it will be necessary to divide the retinacular ligament. This release of all contracted structures will allow extension of the joint which is fixed in moderate

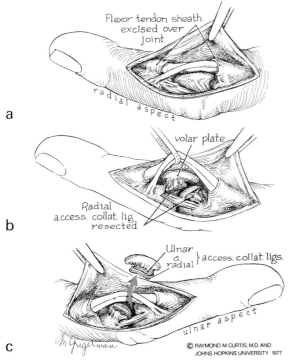

FIG. 22.3. Capsulectomy of the proximal interphalangeal joint stiff in flexion.

extension by a Kirschner wire. The wire is removed in one week and active motion of flexion and extension begun with rubber band traction.

In a Dupuytren's contracture, a partial volar capsulectomy is used with excision of the accessory collateral ligaments (Fig. 22.3c) when excision of the thickened fascial band does not allow full extension of the joint [15].

THUMB CONTRACTURE

To achieve grasp, power and precision pinch, that is, the most useful hand functions, there must be no limitation in motion of the thumb. To improve the function of the stiff and contracted thumb, we must achieve as nearly as possible these normal ranges of motion. If this is not possible, then the thumb must be brought into its most functional position, taking into consideration the needs of each individual patient and the functional loss of use as demonstrated on careful examination.

Anatomy (pp. 35–51)

Causes of thumb contracture and its prevention

Trauma to the hand or upper extremity, from whatever cause, which leads to swelling of the hand with the deposition of fibrin, followed by the laying down of fibroblasts of a dense scar in and about the thumb with the subsequent shortening of muscles, fascia, joint capsules, and tendons is the most common cause of thumb contracture.

Burns, avulsion injuries, and infection produce contracture by both fibrosis and muscle shortening, as well as by the actual loss of skin in the thumb web and palm of the hand. There is need for all the skin of the hand for perfect function, for there is no excess skin present.

Fractures by malunion can narrow the thumb web. Ischaemia of the hand leads to fibrosis and contracture of the first interosseous and the short adductor muscles, as well as of the deep and superficial heads of the flexor pollicis brevis. In cerebral palsy, spasticity of the short adductor and the flexor pollicis brevis, causes thumb contracture.

It also occurs in congenital anomalies, e.g. in arthrogryposis, and with anomalies of the extensor tendons in the 'clutched thumb' [16] and an abnormal swelling of the flexor pollicis longus in the congenital stenosing tenovaginitis. Dupuytren's contracture and rheumatoid arthritis are other frequent causes.

To prevent thumb contracture oedema must be controlled by compression bandaging and elevation, together with early motion when possible. The thumb must be maintained in palmar abduction by orthoplast or plaster splints to prevent thumb web contracture, both in the closed injury and the open wound, as well as in burns. Prompt cover of open wounds with adequate partial thickness skin grafts or pedicle flaps prevents scar contracture.

Conservative treatment

If the contracture is mild and there is no skin loss and muscles function normally, physiotherapy including careful passive stretching of the thumb into its normal ranges of motion, can be beneficial. These measures are supplemented by elastic traction or moulded plaster splints which are changed every other day, gradually stretching the contracture.

Surgical correction of thumb contracture

This is indicated in severe contractures or those cases where progress is no longer being obtained by conservative treatment.

To correct surgically the contractures of the thumb all of the anatomical structures which may be responsible must be considered [17, 18]. These are the skin, fascia overlying the first interosseous muscle, muscles including the first interosseous, the adductor, the flexor pollicis brevis, extensor pollicis longus and brevis, the long abductor and flexor pollicis longus, and the capsular ligaments of the thumb joints.

Careful clinical examination of the thumb will disclose which anatomical structures are primarily responsible for the contracture.

Operative procedures

The surgeon must plan for skin cover, release of the deep contractures and maintenance of the release, and the following procedures are available.

Skin release

This may be dealt with by:
  (1) Z-plasty.
  (2) Z-plasty with partial thickness skin graft.
  (3) Partial thickness skin graft only.
  (4) Dorsal rotation skin flap with skin graft.
  (5) Skin flap from distant region with pedicle.
  (6) Microvascular free flap.

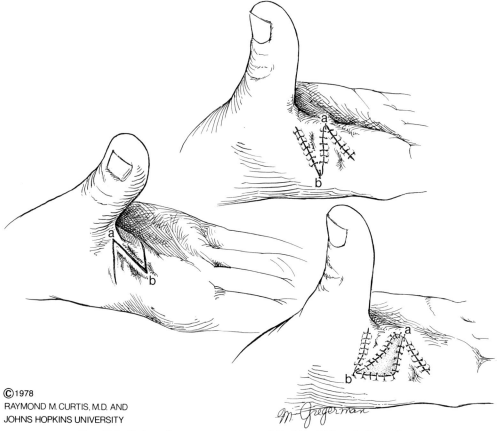

©1978
RAYMOND M. CURTIS, M.D. AND
JOHNS HOPKINS UNIVERSITY

Fig. 22.4. Z-plasty for scar contracture and Z with addition of skin graft.

Z-plasty is the most simple method when there is only a linear scar in the web. The central incision parallels the web, the palmar limb is parallel to the thenar crease and the dorsal limb parallel to the extensor pollicis longus tendon. (See Chapter 9, pp. 135, 136, Fig. 9.14.) A Z-plasty with skin graft (Fig. 22.4) or a large partial thickness graft is the procedure of choice when there is an actual deficiency of skin in the web; however, there must be a good bed in the form of good muscle to which the graft can be applied.

The dorsal rotation skin flap (Fig. 22.6a) is used when there is good dorsal skin and additional skin is needed in the web. This gives excellent coverage when it is necessary to release or excise the ischaemic and contracted first dorsal interosseous and adductor muscles.

A skin flap from the abdomen (Fig. 22.5), groin or cross-arm is reserved for those cases where a flap rotation is not possible. This technique is of particular value when there has been extensive contracture with loss of skin, and in those instances where the fibrotic muscles have to be excised in order to release the contracture.

The cross-arm flap is excellent both cosmetically and functionally [19]. It is raised as a diamond-shaped area over the front of opposite biceps.

The microvascular free flap offers another method of providing excellent skin cover for the contracted web, and is likely to be used increasingly in the future.

Technique of muscle release

In severe thumb contracture, the operator proceeds step by step to correct the deformity [20, 21]. All dissection

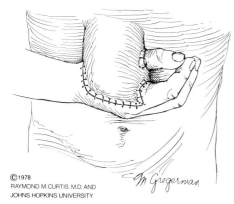

FIG. 22.5. Skin flap from abdomen.

is done under tourniquet. Where there is good dorsal skin for the rotation flap, this is elevated in such a fashion (Fig. 22.6a) as to expose the first interosseous muscle and its origin from the thumb metacarpal. Using sharp dissection, the muscle is removed from the metacarpal from distal to proximal (Fig. 22.5b), using great care as one reaches the base of the thumb metacarpal in order to visualize but not damage the radial artery (Fig. 22.6a) which may be the sole source of blood supply to the thumb (see p. 50). After complete release of the first interosseous muscle, the next structure visualized and found to be tight will be the adductor muscle. The tendon of the adductor is divided near its insertion so that it may be lengthened by a free tendon graft (Fig. 22.6d) if the muscle is functional or alternatively may be released at its origin. The first interosseous and adductor may be so affected by fibrosis that they will have to be excised. The volar ulnar neurovascular bundle to the thumb lies immediately palmar to the adductor and must be avoided.

Following muscle release, the thumb may be stretched away from the palm but if this is not possible, the next step is to release the dorsal capsular ligament of the trapezio metacarpal joint (Fig. 22.6c), leaving the strong volar ligament attached. This capsular release will usually allow the thumb metacarpal to be abducted and rotated into a position of opposition. Where there has been extensive injury to the wrist or carpal area, it may be necessary to excise the trapezium to mobilize the thumb. Replacement with a prosthesis is rarely necessary since there is so much scarring about this area that even while mobility is achieved, no instability results.

If the thumb metacarpal is still held in a flexed position toward the palm, the short flexor will have to be released (Fig. 22.6c). This can be done through dorsal exposure, but the operator must expose the volar digital arteries and nerves as they course along on either side of the flexor pollicis longus tendon and carefully retract them before releasing the muscle.

If the volar skin overlying these muscles is contracted, an incision releasing this tight tissue will expose the flexor pollicis brevis for the tenotomy. Where skin is contracted volarly as well as dorsally. and in the web, the skin incision may extend volarly from the base of the thumb to the dorsal base of the thumb, that is, completely encircling the thumb. It is this type of contracture which usually requires excision or release of all the small

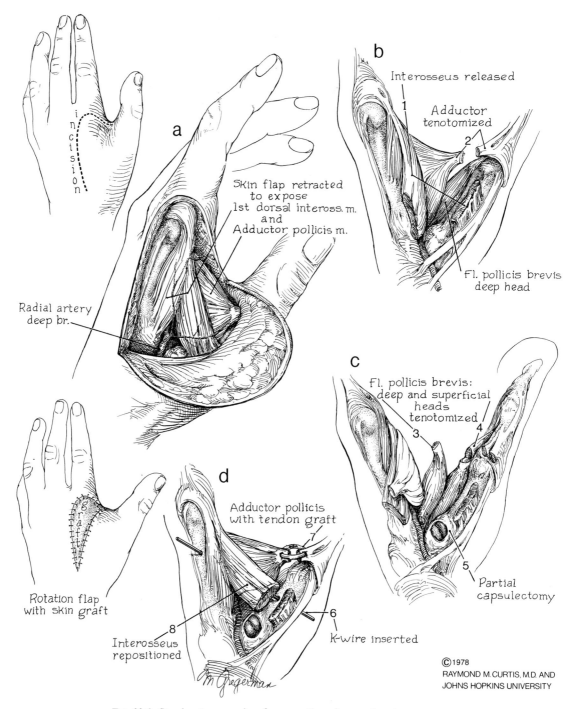

FIG. 22.6. Step-by-step procedure for correction of severe thumb contracture.

Within the image:

a — Skin flap retracted to expose 1st dorsal inteross. m. and Adductor pollicis m.; Radial artery deep br.; incision

b — Interosseus released; 1; Adductor tenotomized; 2; Fl. pollicis brevis deep head

c — Fl. pollicis brevis: deep and superficial heads tenotomized; 3; 4; 5; Partial capsulectomy

d — Adductor pollicis with tendon graft; 7; 6 K-wire inserted; 8 Interosseus repositioned; Rotation flap with skin graft

©1978 RAYMOND M. CURTIS, M.D. AND JOHNS HOPKINS UNIVERSITY

muscles of the thumb and a pedicle flap for skin coverage of the defect. The web should be released until there is an angle of approximately 40° between 1st and 2nd metacarpals.

Maintenance of released web space

Once the thumb has been released, it is held in the corrected position by Kirschner wires passing from the thumb metacarpal to the index metacarpal (Fig. 22.6d). These are maintained until there is soft tissue healing and any skin grafts are stable enough to allow dynamic splinting to maintain the operative correction.

A corrective osteotomy of the metacarpal may be needed to position the thumb, especially where there has been a malunion of a fracture.

With proper early treatment of the injured thumb and thumb web, hand function can be preserved. The positioning of the thumb in abduction and slight opposition by proper splinting from the day of injury, in conjunction with early skin coverage of open wounds, can prevent thumb contracture in most instances. When thumb contracture does occur, however, it is possible to correct poor functional position by the correct preoperative assessment of the anatomical causes and their correction by surgical means.

REFERENCES

[1] BUNNELL, S. *Surgery of the Hand*, 3rd ed., pp. 313–314. Philadelphia, Lippincott, 1956.

[2] MOBERG, E. AND STENER, B. Injuries to the ligaments of the thumb and fingers. Diagnosis, treatment and prognosis. *Acta Chirurgica Scandinavica*, 1953, **106,** 166.

[3] PEACOCK, E. E., Jr. Some biochemical and biophysical aspects of joint stiffness: Role of collagen synthesis as opposed to altered molecular bonding. *Annals of Surgery*, 1966, **164,** 1.

[4] PRATT, D. R. Joints of the hand and fingers—their stiffness, splinting and surgery. *California Medicine*, 1947, **66,** 22.

[5] BUNNELL, S. *Surgery of the Hand*, 2nd ed., p. 301. Philadelphia, Lippincott, 1948.

[6] FOWLER, S. B. Mobilization of metacarpophalangeal joint, arthroplasty and capsulotomy. *Journal of Bone and Joint Surgery*, 1947, **29,** 193.

[7] SWANSON, A. F. Flexible implant arthroplasty for arthritic finger joints. Rationale, technique, and results of treatment. *Journal of Bone and Joint Surgery*, 1972, **54A,** 435.

[8] PEACOCK, E. E. Preservation of interphalangeal joint function: a basis for the early care of injured hands. *Southern Medical Journal*, 1963, **56,** 56.

[9] BUNNELL, S., DOHERTY, E. W. AND CURTIS, R. M. Ischemic contracture, local, in the hand. *Plastic and Reconstruction Surgery*, 1948, **3,** 424.

[10] CURTIS, R. M. (1975) Joints of the hand. In: *Hand Surgery*, 2nd ed., Flynn, J. E., ed. pp. 222–239. Baltimore, Williams and Wilkins, 1975.

[11] HARRIS, C., Jr. AND RIORDAN, D. C. Intrinsic contracture in the hand and its surgical treatment. *Journal of Bone and Joint Surgery*, 1954, **36A,** 10.

[12] CURTIS, R. M. Capsulectomy of the interphalangeal joints of the fingers. *Journal of Bone and Joint Surgery*, 1954, **36A,** 1219.

[13] SPRAGUE, B. L. The proximal interphalangeal joint contractures and their treatment. *Journal of Trauma*, 1976, **16,** 259.

[14] HARRISON, D. H. The stiff interphalangeal joint. *The Hand*, 1977, **9,** 102.

[15] CURTIS, R. M. Volar capsulectomy in Dupuytren's contracture. Les Monographies Du Groupe D'Etude de la Main, Tubiana, R. and Hueston, J. T. eds. pp. 165–167. Paris: Expansion Scientifique Française, 1972.

[16] WECKESSER, E. C. Congenital flexion—adduction deformity of the thumb (congenital 'clasped thumb'). *Journal of Bone and Joint Surgery*, 1955, **37A,** 944.

[17] BROWN, P. W. Adduction—flexion contracture of the thumb. *Clinical Orthopaedics*, 1972, **88,** 161.

[18] LITTLER, J. W. The prevention and correction of adduction contractures of the thumb. *Clinical Orthopaedics*, 1959, **13,** 182.

[19] MUTZ, STERLING B. Thumb web contracture. *The Hand*, 1972, **4,** 236.

[20] HOWARD, L. D. Contracture of the thumb web. *Journal of Bone and Joint Surgery*, 1950, **32A,** 267.

[21] BOYES, J. H. Bunnell's *Surgery of the Hand*, 5th ed. p. 254. Philadelphia, Lippincott, 1970.

CHAPTER 23

Volkmann's Contracture

K. TSUGE

This condition first described by Richard von Volkmann [1] nearly a century ago is generally considered to result from spasm of the main arteries of the forearm as a consequence of trauma to the elbow or forearm. The severe and prolonged but incomplete interruption of arterial blood supply, together with venostasis, produces acute ischaemic necrosis of the flexor muscles.

During the early phase, there is marked swelling of the forearm and hand with vesicle formation of the skin. The marked increase in internal pressure caused by the swelling contributes greatly to the muscle ischaemia. The most marked ischaemia occurs in the deeply situated muscles such as the flexor pollicis longus and flexor digitorum profundus, but severe ischaemia is evident in the pronator teres and flexor digitorum sublimis muscles, and comparatively mild ischamia occurs in the superficially located muscles such as the wrist flexors. The muscle degeneration which follows is most marked in the middle of the forearm with the severity decreasing peripherally, forming a so-called 'ellipsoid shaped infarct' as described by Seddon [2].

The acute symptoms of this condition are known as the five 'Ps', that is *pain*, *pallor*, *puffiness*, *pulselessness* and *paralysis*. Naturally, these changes are not necessarily all present at the same time. The most diagnostic findings will be the palpable induration in the flexor muscles. Another sign of ischaemia of the flexor muscles is exacerbation of pain with passive finger extension. The weakness or absence of a radial pulse is an indication of the onset of impending ischaemia. The cause of sensory deficit is ischaemia and mechanical compression due to oedema. The median nerve which lies near the centre of the necrotic muscles is usually more severely involved than the ulnar nerve which lies on the periphery. Early recognition of these signs is very important because progression of such findings demands surgical decompression before the muscles develop the irreversible changes.

Emergency treatment

When aggravation of ischaemia is suspected, any constrictive cast or bandage should be removed and if displacement of a fracture is found, gentle reduction or correction of the alignment should be attempted so as to improve circulation. The course of the patient is observed for an hour or two, and if the circulatory disturbance fails to improve, a zig-zag incision is made from the anterior aspect of the elbow down the proximal half of the forearm and the fascias of the flexor muscles are incised so as to release muscle compression and examine the major vessels. If there is arterial spasm, papaverine is applied to bring about relaxation, and if there is vascular damage or thrombosis, appropriate measures instituted which may require resection of the damaged segment of vessel. Any fracture should be reduced and immobilized with Kirschner wires at the same time so as to give skeletal stability. A minimum of dissection is advised and where possible percutaneous insertion of the wires.

After surgery the arm is elevated and maintained in the corrected position by a bivalved cast avoiding any tightness and compression, and the state of circulatory recovery is observed.

Late treatment

When more than 24 or 48 hours have elapsed since the onset of symptoms and irreversible changes have oc-cured in the muscle, all subsequent measures adminis-tered should be considered late therapy. If severe swelling is present, decompression by fasciotomy may be con-sidered, but as there will probably be blistering of the skin there is an increased risk of infection, and at this stage it is not considered a strong indication. The sub-sequent procedure would be to wait for bone union and improvement of the skin condition before attempting further surgery. The optimal time would be 3–6 months later.

The extent of muscular degeneration varies con-siderably, and with the passage of time, some of the necrotic muscles become regenerated. However, some become absorbed and undergo fibrosis, which with cicatrization gradually causes contracture. Contracture due to scarring, in addition to paralysis of the intrinsic muscles resulting from nerve ischaemia, causes deformity of varying degree.

The cases can be classified into three types, mild, moderate and severe, and their respective symptoms, characteristics and treatment will be discussed.

Mild type

This type may also be called the localized type. Muscle degeneration is limited to part of the flexor digitorum profundus and flexion contracture involves only two or three fingers. Generally, contracture develops in the ring finger followed by the long, and then extends to the little and index fingers with the thumb the last digit to be affected. This is an interesting finding in that it indicates that muscle degeneration caused by ischaemia spreads from the mid-section of the flexor digitorum profundus. Sensory disturbance is either absent or slight, and even when present immediately after injury, it gradually im-proves.

Although it is sometimes caused by supracondylar fracture, in most cases it is due to non-fracture injury such as crushing of the forearm. The largest number of cases is found in young people in their twenties, which is different from findings of the moderate type to be dis-cussed next and may be considered characteristic of this

type. Further, it is noteworthy that cases of this type are on the increase recently.

Treatment, when the interval after development is short, gives good results by the combination of a dynamic splint, physical therapy and functional training. In longer standing cases, surgery is indicated, but the extent of muscle contracture is usually limited, and thus dissection or excision of the affected area will suffice. However, if degeneration is more extensive and three or four fingers are affected, flexor muscle sliding is indicated.

A zig-zag incision from above elbow to lower forearm is used and the flexor muscles are released from the medial epicondyle, from the ulna subperiosteally and from the interosseous membrane using the ulnar periosteal incision (Fig. 23.1). These procedures are performed while extending the fingers from time to time to determine the degree of improvement. Particular attention must be paid to avoid traumatizing the com-mon interosseous artery and the anterior interosseous artery, vein and nerve (Fig. 23.1). If the median and ulnar nerves pass through the scarred portion of the muscles, neurolysis is indicated and the ulnar nerve is usually transposed to the antero-medial side of the elbow joint. After surgery, the forearm is kept in supination, the wrist in dorsiflexion and the metacarpo-phalangeal joints in slight flexion with the fingers ex-tended for 2–3 weeks, after which exercise is begun. The patient is instructed in the use of a dynamic splint.

Moderate type

In this, which, may also be called the typical type, muscle degeneration involves flexor digitorum profundus and flexor pollicis longus with varying degree of de-generation of the superficial muscles [3]. The classic signs include flexion contracture of all digits, a flexed wrist, sensory disturbance in the median and ulnar nerve dis-tribution and claw deformity of the hand due to intrinsic muscle paralysis. Most cases are due to supracondylar fracture occurring between five and ten years.

Treatment consists of muscle sliding operation and tendon transfer after excision of necrotic muscles [4].

Muscle degeneration is more extensive than the mild type, and the area requiring muscle release is more ex-tensive. In addition to the extent of muscle release re-quired for the mild type, it is necessary to detach the

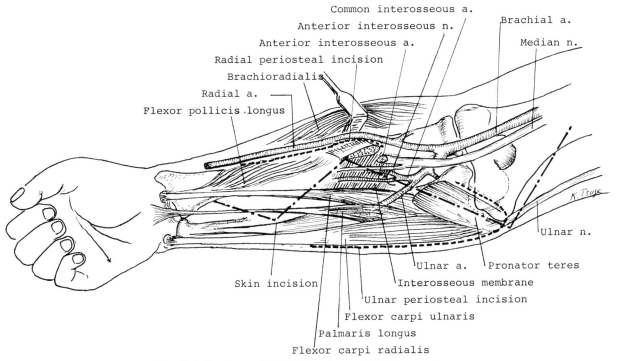

FIG. 23.1. Anatomy and incision lines for muscle sliding operation.

flexor pollicis longus and the pronator teres from the radius using the radial periosteal incision (Fig. 23.1) and advance all flexor muscles distally. Thus, flexion contracture of the digits and wrist can be removed, and restoration of some supination be expected. Neurolysis of the median and ulnar nerves is performed. The nerves located in the area which corresponds to the necrotic site are reduced to about two-thirds or one-half of their normal size due to pressure and strangulation. The normal gloss and elasticity are missing and the impairment is more severe in the median nerve than in the ulnar nerve. After surgery, the same procedures as those for the mild type are used.

If muscle release has been adequate and the postoperative care carried out correctly, recurrence is infrequent and it is possible to obtain satisfactory results (Fig. 23.2a–d).

However, when degeneration is extensive and severe, although the deformity can be corrected by a radical sliding operation, flexion of the digits will be disturbed. In such a case, tendon transfer should be considered either simultaneously or as a secondary procedure.

A similar zig-zag incision is used. Protecting the nerves and vessels, the necrotic portion of the muscles is excised after checking the color and determining the degree of muscle degeneration by palpation. The superficial muscles where degeneration is comparatively mild and those with considerable excursion are selected as the power source, while the deep flexors with severe degeneration are excised.

The decision of whether to perform tendon transfer together with the excision of necrotic muscles or as a secondary procedure, should be made on the basis of whether or not a power source is available and also the presence or absence of joint contracture. For further discussion of this, refer to the section on the severe type.

Severe type

The severe type includes cases with degeneration of all flexor muscles and also varying degree of degeneration of the extensor muscles, and where the degree of neurological disturbance and extent of contracture are severe.

The age distribution is most frequent in the five to ten years group as in the moderate type, but occurs also in young people with barbiturate or carbon monoxide poisoning.

Early excision of the degenerated muscles and neurolysis should be performed to restore sensation and function of the intrinsic and extensor muscles. Reconstruction should be carried out by tendon transfer as a secondary procedure, usually about six months or more after the primary operation. The brachioradialis or wrist extensor may be used as the power sources. Following the release of flexor tendons, the sublimis tendons are removed, and after smooth movement of each profundus tendon has been achieved, tendon transfer is performed. In a child seen relatively soon after injury and with little joint contracture, the results are generally satisfactory.

Where a sufficient power source for tendon transfer is not available, free muscle transplantation can now be performed by the recently developed microsurgical techniques [5]. The pectoralis major or gracilis muscle are used as the transplant muscle. There are some problems such as the former being rather excessive in volume while the latter is slightly inadequate, but the choice of use depends upon the individual case. The nerves, arteries and veins serving the muscle are separated and with the aid of a microscope the arteries and veins are anastomosed with their counterparts of the forearm and the nerves are sutured to the anterior interosseous nerve. After about three months, muscle contraction occurs

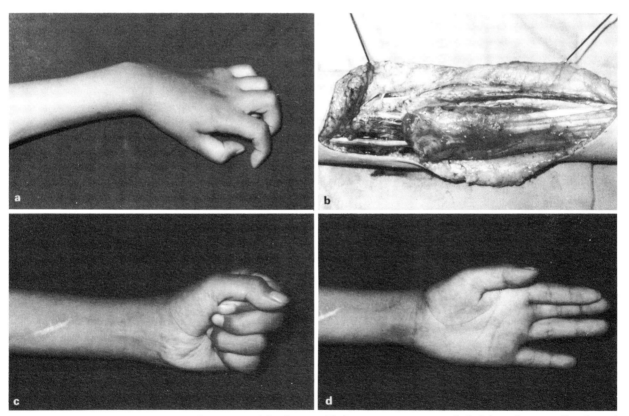

FIG. 23.2. Nine-year-old boy, 11 months after supracondylar fracture. Moderate type contracture of all digits and sensory disturbance in the median and ulnar nerves were noted.
(a) Pre-operative findings.
(b) Flexor muscles were advanced about 3 cm.
(c) and (d) Finger-extension and flexion four years after surgery.

followed by gradual increase in strength and a useful amount of muscular function can be obtained.

However, in old cases with severe joint contracture, treatment is very difficult. Most patients will have to be satisfied with procedures such as pedicle skin graft, tenodesis, arthrodesis and osteotomy for correction of the deformity alone.

REFERENCES

[1] VOLKMANN, R. Die ischämischen Muskellämungen und Kontrakturen, *Zentralblatt für Chirurgie*, 1881, **8**, 801.

[2] SEDDON, H. J. Volkmann's Contracture: Treatment by Excision of the Infarct. *Journal of Bone and Joint Surgery*, 1956, **38B**, 152.

[3] SEDDON, H. J. Volkmann's Ischaemia. *British Medical Journal*, 1964, **1**, 1587.

[4] TSUGE, K. Treatment of Established Volkmann's Contracture. *Journal of Bone and Joint Surgery*, 1975, **57A**, 925.

[5] IKUTA, Y., KUBO, T. & TSUGE, K. Free Muscle Transplantation by Microsurgical Technique to treat severe Volkmann's Contracture. *Plastic and Reconstructive Surgery*, 1976, **58**, 407.

CHAPTER 24

Congenital Abnormalities of the Hand

Malformations of the hand are amongst the most common of congenital abnormalities. Birch-Jensen in a study in Denmark, estimated that 1 in 6000 births would have a congenital abnormality of the hand [1]. Conway and Bowe described one malformation of the upper limb in every 626 live births [2]. The most accurate figures which we have available have been assessed on the Edinburgh Register of the Newborn [3]. The anomalies range from those of great severity and complexity to relatively minor deformities which are of little or no clinical significance. The deformity may be unilateral or bilateral and strictly localized to the hand or involve other parts of the upper limb. This involvement may be an isolated feature or part of a complicated series of abnormalities and perhaps of a designated syndrome (Table 24.2).

Congenital anomalies of the hand present a difficult problem in both classification and treatment. Treatment may vary from country to country, from centre to centre in the same country and amongst individual surgeons. A major difficulty in evaluating the effectiveness of treatment arises from the differing methods of assessment and classification of the deformity. In order to further knowledge and provide a sound basis for treatment, it is essential that there should be a classification that can be followed universally. The classification commissioned by the American Society for Surgery of the Hand and prepared by Entin *et al* [4] has been accepted by the International Federation of Hand Societies and is recognized as the most simple and useful classification available. This chapter will be based on this type of classification (Table 24.1).

TABLE 24.1. Classification for congenital abnormalities of upper limb

(1) **Failure of formation of parts**
(2) **Failure of differentiation (separation) of parts**
(3) **Duplication**
(4) **Overgrowth (gigantism)**
(5) **Congenital constriction band syndrome**
(6) **Miscellaneous**
(7) **Generalized skeletal abnormalities**

GENETICS

RUTH WYNNE-DAVIES

It is fortunate that the many complex and varied anatomical types of hand deformity can, from the point of view of aetiology, be classified fairly simply [6]. They can be grouped as: (1) the isolated deformities, (2) those forming part of the malformation syndromes, or (3) part of the generalized skeletal dysplasias (discussed later in this chapter). The 'isolated' hand deformities may be accompanied by similar changes in the feet, but they form a clearly defined group. The malformation syndromes consist of multiple congenital defects, not only of limbs but also of other systems in the body such as the cardiovascular, genitourinary or the branchial arch region.

It is of obvious importance to establish whether an individual belongs to the 'isolated' or to the 'syndrome' group and to be aware that the hand deformity, present at birth, may be an early warning that other problems may develop at a later age. Table 24.2 lists the commoner

TABLE 24.2. Some syndromes and skeletal dysplasias associated with congenital hand defects

Hand defect	Syndrome or dysplasia	Onset age of other signs	Clinical description	Inheritance
Transverse absence	none			
Longitudinal absence Radial	Fanconi's anaemia	Childhood or later	Pancytopenia, sometimes leukaemia	Autosomal recessive
	Thrombocytopenia—absent radius	Infancy	Thrombocytopenia, may be transient	Autosomal recessive
	Holt Oram	Infancy	Congenital heart, usually septal defect	Autosomal dominant
	Chromosome anomalies (Trisomy 13 and 18)	Birth	Mental deficiency and multiple congenital defects	Sporadic
Ulnar	de Lange	Birth-infancy	Mental deficiency, dwarfism, eyebrows meet in the middle	Sporadic
Ring constrictions	none			
Short thumb	Diastrophic dwarf	Early infancy	Short-limbed dwarfism with contractures and clubfoot	Autosomal recessive
	Fibrodysplasia ossificans progressiva	Childhood	Ossification of muscle aponeuroses	Autosomal dominant
	Rubinstein–Taybi	Infancy	Mental deficiency, beaked nose with nasal septum below alae	Sporadic
Short 4th/5th metacarpals	Turner's (XO)	Infancy and later	Webbed neck, barrel chest, amenorrhoea, may be multiple congenital defects	Sporadic
	Pseudohypoparathyroidism	Adult	Hypocalcaemia with mental deficiency, tetany and metastatic calcification Parathormone resistant	X-linked dominant
Short, dysplastic or absent terminal phalanges	Craniocleidodysostosis	Infancy or later	Absent clavicles, bulging forehead wide symphisis pubis	Autosomal dominant
	Pycnodysostosis	Infancy or later	Short stature, open fontanelles, micrognathia, increased bone density, absent clavicles	Autosomal recessive
Syndactyly massive	Apert group	Birth	Craniostenosis, mental deficiency, some forms with polydactyly	Autosomal dominant and recessive forms
limited	(innumerable syndromes, often involving the heart, face or palate)			

TABLE 24.2—*continued*

Hand defect	Syndrome or dysplasia	Onset age of other signs	Clinical description	Inheritance
Polydactyly pre-axial post-axial	Rarely Several lethal forms of short-limbed dwarfism	Birth	Often very short ribs and respiratory failure	Autosomal recessive and sporadic forms
	Chromosome anomalies (Trisomy 13 and 18)	Birth	Mental deficiency and multiple congenital defects	Sporadic
	Chondroectodermal dysplasia	Birth or later	Dysplastic nails and teeth, short-limbed dwarfism, congenital heart defect	Autosomal recessive
Symphalangism	Diastrophic dwarf (rarely)		(see short thumb above)	
Camptodactyly	Marfan's	Childhood or later	Long limbs, ectopia lentis, joint laxity, aortic aneurism	Autosomal dominant
	Congenital contractural arachnodactyly	Birth	Long limbs, multiple contractures	Autosomal dominant
	Homocystinuria	Childhood or later	Long limbs, mental deficiency, ectopia lentis, osteoporosis and thrombotic tendency	Autosomal recessive
	Freeman–Sheldon	Infancy	'Whistling face', feeding difficulties, club foot	Autosomal dominant
	Diastrophic dwarf		(see short thumb, above)	
Macrodactyly	Neurofibromatosis	Childhood or later	Café-au-lait patches, scoliosis, cutaneous and other neuro-fibromata, sometimes congenital pseudarthrosis of the tibia	Autosomal dominant
Dysplastic nails	Chondroectodermal dysplasia		(see post-axial polydactyly, above)	
	Pycnodysostosis		(see absent terminal phalanx, above)	
	Nail-patella syndrome	Childhood or later	Small or absent patellae, iliac horns, dislocated head of radius, sometimes later kidney failure	Autosomal dominant
	Metaphyseal chondrodysplasia type McKusick	Infancy	Short stature, irregular metaphyses	Autosomal recessive

congenital hand defects with the age at which the associated malformation syndrome develops.

Any disorder with a genetic basis must be either a chromosome defect, a single-gene disorder (dominant or recessive, either autosomal or X-linked) or multifactorial, (that is, the influence of multiple genes together with the influence of environmental factors). The malformation syndromes may have any pattern of inheritance, but the isolated hand deformities, if genetic at all, are usually of autosomal dominant inheritance. This means that an affected individual married to a normal individual has a 50 per cent risk of passing the deformity on to his children or, on average, half of them will be affected. Unaffected individuals do not usually carry the gene and there is no risk to their children, though a word of caution is needed in that 'skipped' generations can occur, and, particularly with post-axial polydactyly, genetic advice should be rather more cautious. Since precisely the same anatomical defect can be produced by the action of completely different genes, or indeed be non-genetic, one must have an informed picture of the family background as well as taking every care to ensure whether the hand deformity is the only defect in the child; even then, meaningful genetic advice cannot always be given.

Isolated deformities of autosomal dominant inheritance

The *lobster claw* deformity of the hands and feet is characterized by a missing middle ray. It is a rare deformity but appears to be regularly dominant. *Symphalangism*, often accompanied by massive fusion of the tarsal bones, is also very uncommon and regularly dominant. *Brachydactyly* occurs in several different forms, all having this same pattern of inheritance. Shortening of the middle phalanges may be accompanied by absence of the terminal phalanges, and, rarely, shortening of the proximal phalanges may be accompanied by an 'absence' defect distal to this. In *stub thumb* only the first digit is involved.

A simple bifid thumb is non-genetic but a *triphalangeal thumb* is of dominant inheritance, as may be other forms of pre-axial polydactyly. *Post-axial polydactyly* is rather more common and often accompanied by an extra fifth toe. It is uncertain whether it is of dominant or multifactorial inheritance. The proportion of affected near

relatives is only 12–15 per cent [3], not the typical 50 per cent shown in the other conditions described here. *Camptodactyly* is often of dominant inheritance. The flexion contracture of the little finger (and sometimes of the ring finger as well) is rarely present at birth, developing usually during the early years of childhood.

Syndactyly and polysyndactyly are sometimes dominant, though they also occur as sporadic events. Syndactyly is a very frequent finding in the malformation syndromes.

Isolated non-genetic deformities

The isolated defects which are characteristically sporadic include the transverse 'absence' defects and ring constrictions, nearly always the longitudinal 'absence' defects such as the rare condition of absent ulna, or the commoner, radial club hand, and also isolated shortening of metacarpals, macrodactyly and pre-axial polydactyly (not triphalangeal).

DEVELOPMENT OF THE UPPER LIMB AND HAND

K. KUCZYNSKI

The upper limb bud appears at the twenty-sixth day after fertilization. The ectoderm overlying the developing bud undergoes some thickening along the margin of the bud, forming a longitudinal apical ectodermal ridge (AER) (Fig. 24.1). This ridge is present during the fifth week of the development and then regresses. It plays an important role in the growth and differentiation of the limb.

The development proceeds with a proximodistal gradient. The bud grows rapidly and becomes subdivided into the hand plate with lateral and medial surfaces, like the remainder of the limb bud, and becomes separated by a slight constriction from the proximal segment. The pre-axial and post-axial borders can be identified also. At first the hand plate looks like a paddle, but soon its flange-like margin acquires a scalloped appearance as the digital thickenings are formed. The digital rays become well marked and the thumb diverges from the rest of the digits. About 48 days after fertilization the digits are well formed and separated.

The developing limb bud has considerable self-differentiating capacity. However, the above broad plan of development is subject to further control which is associated with interaction between the apical ectodermal ridge and the underlying mesoderm. It is thought that the formation of the limb begins with the mesoderm which influences the overlying ectoderm to acquire metabolic properties leading to formation of the AER which is necessary for further limb elaboration. The distal part of the limb outgrowth is influenced by the ridge to a great extent.

The limb development may also depend on the cell death process applied quite early to the proliferating cell masses. This process is known to occur in many organs, e.g. in formation of joint cavities there is necrosis of cells,

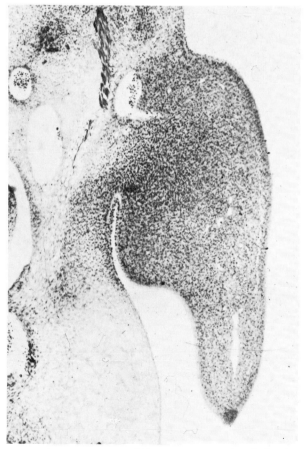

FIG. 24.1 Human embryo of 12 mm crown-rump length showing nipple-like appearance of apical ectodermal ridge in cross-section.

and it is thought that it sweeps along the pre-axial and post-axial borders of the limb to appear finally in the web spaces leading to the separation of the digits [7]. Unless the normal cell death process is under control, abnormalities may occur due either to insufficiency or excess of cell destruction. The lysosomes play an important role in the digestive processes inside the cell and act on the cell itself and on the extracellular material if released. Thus any modification in the activities of lysosomes and release of the hydrolytic enzymes affects the development of the limb.

Skin and appendages

The specialized skin of the palmar aspect of the hand is probably derived from the AER. As early as the commencement of the fetal period, the flexure lines of the digits are present, but those on the palm appear later. The precise pattern of the palmar ridges and grooves, which form the basis of the fingerprints, is established during the fourth month and remains constant. The sweat glands begin to form in the fifth month, the ducts reaching the surface in the seventh month. Differentiation in the dorsal skin lags behind that on the palmar aspect. The hair follicles become apparent at the end of the fourth month and the future nail areas can be demonstrated microscopically during the fourth month, but the growth of the definitive nail itself does not begin until the fifth month. By full term the tips of the nails just reach the ends of the digits.

Chondrification

The cartilaginous skeleton of the hand appears in the embryos of about 12 mm crown–rump length at the end of the seventh week (Fig. 24.2). By the early fetal stage all elements are chondrified. The rudiments of the ossa centralia are usually present and may remain separate.

Ossification

Figure 24.3 shows the general pattern. The ossification in the metacarpal bones and phalanges is usually completed between 17 and 19 years but in the carpus not until

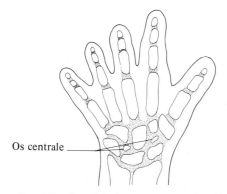

FIG. 24.2 Chondrification of the hand. Diagram of cartilaginous skeleton of the hand at the end of the second month. Note there are no joint cavities.

20–25 years. Variations include: (1) radial os centrale which may fail to fuse with the scaphoid, (2) the hook of hamate may remain separate, (3) the secondary ossification centre of the first metacarpal may be in the head of the bone, (4) the styloid process of the third metacarpal may be separate, (5) the distal phalanges may be occasionally bifurcate, (6) the thumb may have three phalanges. The sesamoid bones are cartilaginous in the child and begin to ossify about the thirteenth year of life. They may show variations in number and site.

Joints

As mentioned above, the joint cavity arises by necrosis of the central part of the interzone between the cartilaginous rudiments of the hand skeleton. This occurs in the wrist joint and the digital joints in the late embryonic stage (25–30 mm crown–rump length) and in other joints of the hand somewhat later.

Muscles

The pre-muscle mass in the limb bud mesenchyme can be seen during the fifth week, the more distant hand musculature lagging behind. The nerve trunks are seen entering these masses, but it is generally agreed that the muscles, like most tissues of the hand, develop *in situ* and not by migration. There are wide variations in the arrangement of the muscles of the hand [8].

Innervation

With the appearance of the limb bud the nerves of the segments opposite to it grow into the mesenchyme of the bud to be distributed to the dermis and the muscle masses differentiating *in situ*. Therefore both are supplied segmentally. The intrinsic muscles of the hand are considered to be supplied by the first thoracic nerve; the eighth cervical may contribute. The distribution of both cutaneous and motor branches show considerable variation. The specialized sensory endings related to the epidermodermal junction and associated with fine touch localization and discrimination develop relatively late. Their differentiation begins at fourth month and is not well established until one year of life and goes on throughout life.

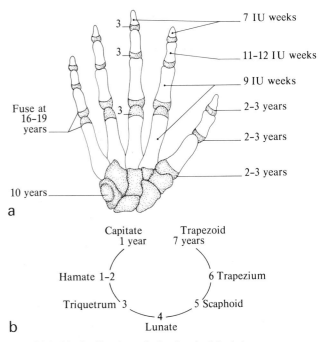

FIG. 24.3 (a) Ossification of the hand. Stippled areas are cartilaginous at birth. Numbers at stippled areas indicate in years, time of appearance of ossification centres. (b) Ossification of the carpus. Numbers indicate in years the appearance of primary centres.

Arteries

At first the vascular plexus of the limb bud is supplied by several consecutive intersegmental branches of the dorsal aorta opposite the bud. Soon however one of them (lateral branch of the seventh cervical) enlarges and becomes the axial artery. The terminal axial segment, the interosseous artery, breaks up into a distal capillary plexus, from which later the digital branches arise. When the median artery is formed, it joins the hand plexus but later is replaced by radial and ulnar arteries. Therefore it is not surprising that the arrangement of the arterial supply of the hand is subject to wide variations [9 & 10].

GENERAL PRINCIPLES OF MANAGEMENT [11–18]

D. W. LAMB

Surgery is seldom an urgent consideration but it is of great value for the surgeon to see the child as soon after birth as possible. This allows an early assessment of the situation, getting to know the parents and to advise on a likely programme of management. A simple explanation of any possible effects on function and whether improvement of the appearance is possible will allay parental anxiety.

The types of deformity can be divided into those which are amenable to surgery and those where surgery is of little or no value. Parental concern is often extreme and there is, not unnaturally, an underlying sense of guilt in that they may have been responsible for the deformity in some way which they do not understand. The early concern of the parents is about the appearance and the surgeon will be under considerable pressure to do something about this, but it should be explained that function is more important than appearance. Surgery to improve the appearance is only justified if it will be accompanied by a definite improvement, or at least no detriment, in function. The young child has a quite extraordinary facility to compensate for anatomical abnormalities and to develop a very useful functional pattern of activities. The decision by the surgeon whether surgery is justified can be extremely difficult and very careful and sometimes prolonged assessment of the functional pattern is required. Supervision under an experienced occupational therapist to assess what functions, particularly those of self care, can or cannot be done is an important prelude to any surgical treatment.

In some types of congenital abnormality such as the simple types of syndactyly, polydactyly and ring constriction (p. 327) [19], there is well documented evidence that skilful surgery can improve function. The correct timing of operation, the likely number of operations and the type of postoperative rehabilitation required is well known. Accordingly, a planned programme of reconstructive surgery can be carried out at the optimal time. This may vary, and be influenced by the physical and mental development of the child. Surgery might be delayed in a puny or undersized child or in a child with other more serious congenital abnormalities, and would be avoided in a child with defective mental development or impaired sensation in the hand.

The aim of surgical treatment is to provide a hand that has active control for pinch and grasp with good sensory appreciation both for tactile sensation and for proprioception and stereognosis. This implies good sensory skin cover without scarring and an appearance as near normal as can be provided.

Certain general principles will govern the decision regarding the type of operation. Soft tissue procedures can usually be carried out at an early age, particularly where operation is likely to change a prehension pattern [20]. Any bone or joint procedure, or where tendon transfers are required to improve function, are best delayed as long as possible, provided this does not lead to any serious impairment of function.

It is very seldom that parents are not deeply appreciative of the efforts being made and they will give full co-operation provided a clear programme is explained even though this may involve multiple operative procedures. Where the deformities are complex and of an unusual type, it is often difficult for the surgeon to provide such a planned programme and there is a tendency to delay treatment as there is no clear cut knowledge of what benefit will be obtained. However, it is always wise for operation to be carried out early where the prehension pattern is likely to be changed by surgery. It is usually a mistake to change a prehension pattern which has been developed over many years. In the bilateral case a decision is particularly difficult, and where one upper limb is normal it is more justifiable to carry out procedures for cosmetic reasons rather than for function. In the more bizarre and complicated deformities, each individual case has to be assessed on its own merits.

The children have to be under review for a prolonged time as recurrence of deformity is likely during growth, particularly if there is unequal muscle balance. Close co-operation with the parents, the paediatrician and the family doctor are necessary during this period. Many patients come from considerable distances and the facilities provided by an inpatient self-care centre in which mother and child can be accommodated, has proved to be invaluable. The occupational therapist is a leading member of the team looking after these children and much of the success of any programme depends upon her ability to gain the confidence of parent and child (p. 297).

The *management* of each group shown in Table 24.1 is now considered in detail.

FAILURE OF FORMATION

D. W. LAMB

Failure of formation or arrest of development forms a large group of the congenital abnormalities of the upper limb and hand. It is seldom that these are genetically patterned or inherited [3, 21], with the exception of the central defect known as 'lobster claw hand' which not infrequently runs through families as a dominant mutation.

Terms such as ectromelia and hemimelia have been used to describe these sometimes bizarre deformities. These terms are seldom accurate, are meaningless to most people and apt to lead to confusion about the exact clinical deformity.

Kay *et al.* recommend two distinct categories in this group (Table 24.3) [5].

Transverse, in which there is a complete absence of structures distal to a certain point in the upper limb (terminal transverse deficiencies; 'congenital amputations').

Longitudinal, which can be grouped into proximal (humeral), and distal (radial, ulnar and central) and a combination of these (Table 24.4). They are described according to a clinical and radiological assessment of the bony structures which are deficient.

TABLE 24.3.

Failure of formation
  (1) Transverse
  (2) Longitudinal
      Pre-axial
      Central
      Post-axial

TABLE 24.4 Longitudinal absence

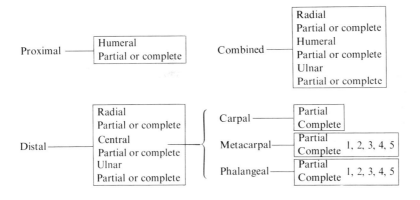

Transverse terminal deficiencies

These may occur at any level from the shoulder downwards (Table 24.5). As a general rule, the management is by prosthetic replacement similar to that utilized for acquired amputation at the same level. There are, however, some details in general management which may differ, and these are illustrated by a description of the management at the three most common levels.

TABLE 24.5 Transverse absence

Level of absence		
Arm	Complete Upper $\frac{1}{3}$ Middle $\frac{1}{3}$ Lower $\frac{1}{3}$	
Forearm	Complete Upper $\frac{1}{3}$ Middle $\frac{1}{3}$ Lower $\frac{1}{3}$	
Carpal	Complete Partial	
Metacarpal	Complete Partial	
Phalangeal	Complete Partial	

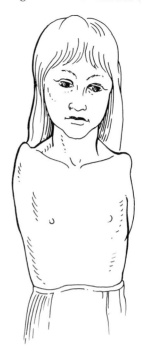

FIG. 24.4. Bilateral amelia (complete absence of arm).

Arm, complete

This is fortunately rare, except when resulting from Thalidomide where bilateral absence of the upper limbs was common (Fig. 24.4) [22]. Conventional body-powered prostheses are of no functional value and a prosthesis powered by some external source of energy is required. Much of the pioneering work was done by Marquhardt in Heidelburg, using carbon dioxide gas, and this has proved to be the cheapest, safest and least heavy power source. Simpson developed a sophisticated prosthesis providing five degrees of freedom of movement including elevation at the shoulder, side to side movement across the body, flexion of the elbow, forearm rotation and prehension [23]. Active pronation and supination, not easily obtained in a body-powered prosthesis, has led to a significant improvement in the functional capacity of the externally-powered prosthesis and,

combined with the position awareness of the terminal device by the introduction of the Servo system, has led to very precise positioning of the artificial hand or powered split hook (see Chapter 34).

Forearm upper third

This is the commonest site of terminal transverse absence in the upper limb. The appearance is characteristic (Fig. 24.5a), and radiography usually shows presence of the upper portions of both forearm bones and a normal elbow. The forearm length is usually 6–7 cm at birth and by the time the child is fully grown is seldom more than 10 cm in length.

Early prosthetic fitting is indicated [24]. This requires easy access to provision and repairs of the prosthesis and close co-operation with an occupational therapist, skilled in the training of the young child in prosthetic use [25, 26]. During the first 5 or 6 months no prosthetic replacement is indicated, but the time is well spent in acquainting the parents with the intended programme and, if possible, demonstrating the successful prosthetic management of such a deformity. At 6 months, when bi-manual upper limb function is developing a simple, light, plastic one piece prosthesis is introduced (Fig. 24.5b). The child finds this of some value in bi-manual grasp, soon becomes adapted to the feel of the prosthesis and accepts it as part of the body image.

At the crawling stage, this prosthesis is often a help and of value when pulling up on chairs or tables in attempting to stand. Prehension function is not introduced in the first year. The best prehension in a unilateral below elbow amputee remains the active opening split hook, moti-

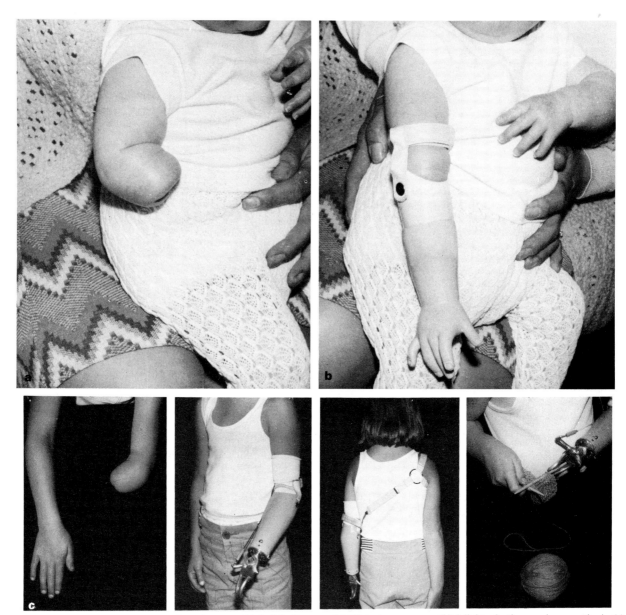

FIG. 24.5. Terminal transverse absence from the upper third of the forearm. (a) Clinical appearance. (b) A light, plastic one-piece prosthesis. (c) To aid prehension a split hook mechanism is added to the prosthesis between 12 and 15 months shown in a child with left below elbow terminal absence.

vated by body power, despite any new developments in artificial hands (see Chapter 34). Between 12 and 15 months of age, a quick release mechanism and split hook is introduced into the prosthesis. Therapist and mother show the child how the split hook can hold objects to be manipulated with the normal hand. Between 15 and 18 months a motivating cord operated by loop from the opposite shoulder is incorporated to give active prehension (Fig. 24.5c). At this stage, the occupational therapist trains the child in the use of the prosthesis and encourages a similar programme at home. If there has been a close link between the parents, surgeon, prosthetist and occupational therapist, the programme is usually smooth and most parents can see that the split hook, despite its ugly appearance, has definite functional value (Fig. 24.5c).

A check is made at 3-monthly intervals to ensure that the prosthesis is being worn and is functional. With good parental guidance, continuous use of the prosthesis is common. Before the child attends school, the therapist visits the school and explains the situation to the teacher. In this way most children merge into the school atmosphere without more than temporary embarrassment. A major problem occurs at adolescence and again guidance and help from a therapist is important at this stage. At this age, the appearance of the split hook is particularly conspicuous and the alternative of a satisfactory cosmetic glove or cosmetic glove and hand replacement is important (see Chapter 34). Many adolescents will abandon the prosthesis but, after 2 or 3 years of limited use, return to a full use of the prosthesis is again usual, particularly if well trained from an early age.

In summary, while a prosthesis provides only an assistance for the normal hand, the resulting function is infinitely superior to that without a prosthesis in a world full of gadgets and equipment designed for the two-handed [27].

Recent experience with the myoelectric prosthesis, developed for use in young children about the age of three years by Dr. Sorbye of Sweden, has been very encouraging and may be the method of future management.

Transverse carpal—partial (Fig. 24.7a)

This is the next most common level of terminal transverse absence. The appearance is characteristic and sometimes there are vestigal remnants of the digits (Fig. 24.6). It can

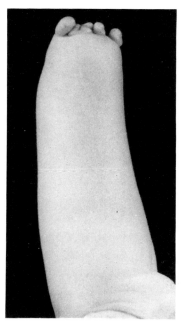

FIG. 24.6. Partial transverse carpal absence showing remnants of digits.

be assumed that these will neither grow nor be of any functional benefit. The absence is at the intercarpal level and it is usual for a good range of radiocarpal movement to be present. Both bones of the forearm appear normal but may not grow as much as on the normal side. Management at this level is difficult and controversial. There is no useful surgical reconstructive procedure. The length of the forearm segment is so useful for holding objects down on a flat surface for manipulation with the other hand that there is seldom any functional benefit from prosthetic replacement. It is particularly important to remember that the valuable sensation is lost by enclosing the stump in a prosthesis. There are, however, various ways of providing improved prehension, without the loss of sensation.

(1) A volar plate is attached to the front of the forearm (Fig. 24.7b), and utilizing stump movement against the surface of the volar plate allows objects of varying sizes to be gripped (Fig. 24.7c and d).

(2) A socket can be constructed around the forearm leaving the end open for sensation and providing prehension by a split hook attached to the dorsum of this socket.

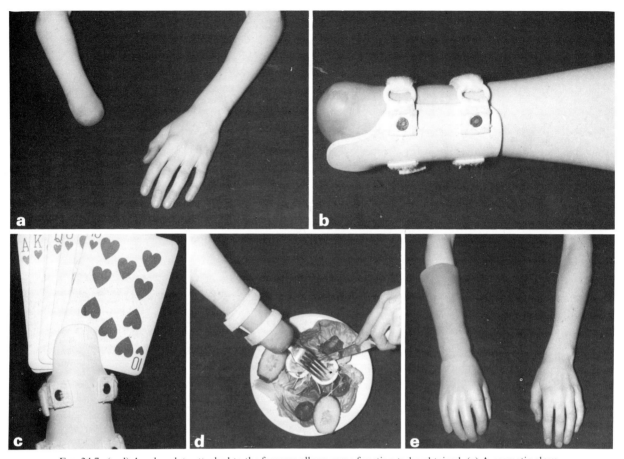

FIG. 24.7. (a–d) A volar plate attached to the forearm allows some function to be obtained. (e) A cosmetic glove.

(3) It is possible to harness the movement of the radio-carpal joint (Fig. 24.8a, b) to drive an artificial hand and provide pinch between the thumb and the side of the index finger (Fig. 24.8c, d). This is a relatively new design and while it provides good cosmetic replacement and some function, it has the disadvantage of the loss of sensation. It is particularly of value in the adolescent sensitive about the appearance who may also benefit simply from a cosmetic glove (Fig. 24.7e).

Longitudinal absence

Humeral

Absence of the humerus may be partial or complete. Partial absence of the humerus is rare but usually occurs at the proximal end and is seen in the deficiencies resulting from Thalidomide, and is commonly associated with radial distal absence. There is weakness of muscle control at the shoulder so that normal elevation is limited and shoulder movement is restricted and of little functional benefit.

In complete absence the forearm and hand project from shoulder level. The forearm and hand may be normal, but it is more usual for the forearm bones to be short or deficient in radial or ulnar components and with abnormality of the hand, often resulting in only three digits (Fig. 24.9). The common term used in this abnormality is phocomelia because the limb resembles that of a seal. This term is of little use in clinical description or management, and it is better to indicate the bone structures which are defective on clinical and radiological

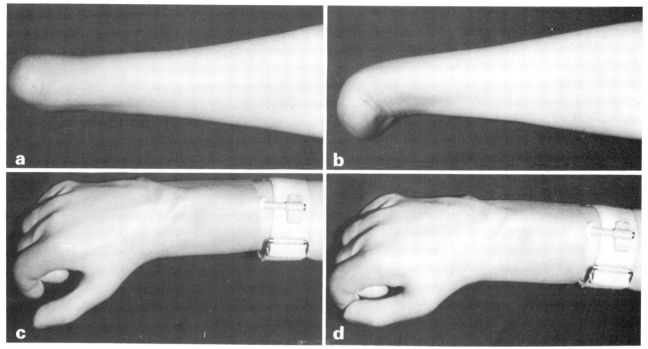

FIG. 24.8. An artificial hand powered by wrist movement (a) and (b) give pinch between the thumb and the side of the finger (c) and (d).

examination. The main problem is the functional loss resulting from the shortness of the limbs particularly if bilateral [28]. At an early age, the hands, which frequently have some useful function, are able to meet the mouth and face and join each other across the front of the body. As the body increases in size, the limb does not grow proportionately and the ability to reach the face or to clasp with the other hand in front of the body is lost.

Treatment

An operation to stabilize the shoulder by turning the clavicle downwards and implanting it into the deficient humerus has been described. The functional benefits do not justify this procedure.

Surgery may be indicated to improve digital function, particularly if there are only two digits of good function but unable to get a satisfactory grip. Rotational osteotomy of one of the digits to bring it into a position for opposition to the other digit, is sometimes justified. As a general rule, the management is conservative [29]. The child is trained in self-care activities to enable as

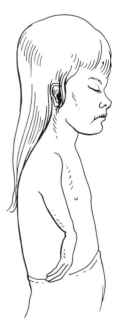

FIG. 24.9. Humeral longitudinal absence showing the flipper-like appearance, showing a three-digit hand.

much independence as possible. The shortness of the limbs makes toilet function increasingly difficult, particularly as the child gets older. Various aids and clothing adjustments carried out by the occupational therapist can play a very important part in management.

Conventional prostheses may give some apparent lengthening of the limb and help to fill the sleeves of clothes, but are often rejected. However, the range of activities can often be enhanced by the provision of external powered prostheses, as used in the amelic child. The problem of fitting is more difficult as the appliance has to be constructed around the shortened limbs and leads to rather an unsightly appearance; the benefits obtained from the powered prostheses rarely justify their use.

Distal radial deficiency (Radial club hand)

Distal radial deficiency is rare [1, 3]. Its rarity means that any one surgeon is unlikely to have much personal experience. Most series consist of an accumulation of cases from other sources [30–32]. Absence of the radial component was a most common deformity resulting from Thalidomide, and there have been several reports of its management [33–36].

Causation

Any factor which adversely influences the development of the upper limb bud between the twenty-eighth to the forty-second day may result in this deformity due to damage to the apical ectoderm [37]. In recent years, the most common cause has been Thalidomide. The clinical and radiological features in those cases known to be due to Thalidomide and those of unknown aetiology show very little difference apart from the increased incidence of proximal humeral deficiencies in Thalidomide.

Effects of the causative factor on the development of other important systems during the same period lead to a frequent association with abnormalities of the cardiovascular, the gastrointestinal, the genitourinary systems and many others, the potential combination being almost unlimited, and it is important to exclude these before considering surgery.

Heredity

Absence of the radius is found in three conditions which

are of varying degrees of inheritance (see Table 24.2): (1) the Holt–Oram syndrome, (2) Fanconi syndrome, and (3) trisomy 17.

None of these conditions was noted in the series described by Lamb [37]. In thirty-three cases of this series Wynne-Davies found no evidence of an inherited pattern in 337 third-degree relatives. Thrombocytopaenia may be associated with absence of the radius. It may be evident at an early stage, although uncommon in the small child, but may develop as the child grows older and should be kept in mind before embarking on surgery.

Anatomy

There are many excellent descriptions which stress that it is important to realise that there is an abnormality of all the tissues on the radial side of the forearm and hand [30, 37–40].

There is often a striking limitation of the range of elbow movement, particularly of active flexion. This appears to be related partly to the bony structure of the joint and partly due to failure of development of the biceps and brachialis muscles. The triceps muscle is often better developed and may favour the extended elbow position.

Muscles arising from the lower lateral aspect of the humerus and from the radius itself are usually absent. The most important functional loss results from absence of the radial carpal extensors and the profundus of the index.

The radial vessels and nerve are usually deficient and the territory of the nerve is taken over by the median nerve. It lies well over to the radial side of the wrist and in about 25 per cent of cases divides into two main terminal branches at the junction of the middle and lower third of the forearm [37]. The more radial division takes over the distribution of the radial nerve and the other passes through the carpal tunnel in the usual way. The deformity may be unilateral or bilateral, and in a recent survey 72 per cent were bilateral [37]. The radius may be completely absent (total aplasia) (Fig. 24.10a), partially absent (partial aplasia) (Fig. 24.10b), when the upper part of the bone is present, or the bone may be apparently complete but short (hypoplasia) (Fig. 24.10c). Absence of the trapezium is usual and of the scaphoid in over 90 per cent [39]. The other carpal bones are usually present but may have undergone varying degrees of fusion. In the

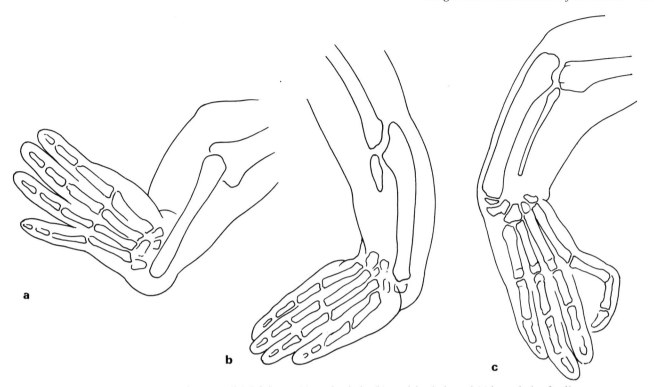

FIG. 24.10. Anatomy of distal radial deficiency: (a) total aplasia, (b) partial aplasia, and (c) hypoplasia of radius.

vast majority the thumb is absent but may be present in very deficient form, the so-called 'floating thumb' (*pouce flottant*) or 'dangle thumb' (Fig. 24.11). It is very rare indeed for the thumb to approach normality.

Function of the upper limb and hand

This varies considerably and is dependent on the structure of the joints, particularly of the elbow and of the hand, and on the muscles which are functioning. The most striking feature is the tendency to stiffness of the elbow in extension. The stiffness limits function considerably, although in the early years, because of the shortness of the arm and the radially deviated position of the hand, the hand can reach the mouth and face without the necessity for elbow flexion. In many cases flexion of the elbow may slowly return until active flexion to at least 90° is obtained, and this can be speeded by corrective splinting of the wrist and physiotherapy to encourage elbow movement. The continuing presence of a stiff ex-

tended elbow is an absolute contraindication to any surgical correction of the wrist deformity.

The range and diversity of movement of the joints of the hand is considerable, varying from those where there

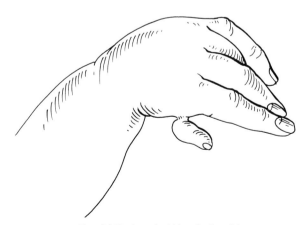

FIG. 24.11. A typical 'dangle thumb'.

is no movement and the condition resembles an arthro-grypotic hand to those where there is relatively normal movement. As a general rule it can be stated that the function and range of movement increases from radial to ulnar side. The thumb when present is rarely of functional value. The metacarpophalangeal joints of the other digits usually have a restricted range of flexion but have excessive hyperextension. The proximal interphalangeal joints have flexion contractures, usually between 30° and 40° in the radial two digits and less than 10° in the little finger. In a review of representative cases the active range of movement in this joint averaged 24° in the index, 35° in the long, 57° in the ring and 70° in the little finger. The movement of the terminal joint is usually less restricted but in about a quarter of the cases there is absence of the index profundus.

In a review of the activities of daily living in a group of children, it was found that in the unilateral deformity function was little affected [37]. In the more severe bilateral cases the function was found to be about two-thirds of the normal for the same age (based on a points system). No children with bilateral deformity were completely independent in self-care activities due to a combination of shortness of the limb, stiffness of the elbow and poor hand function.

Management

As the deformity is usually mobile and correctable at birth, splintage in the corrected position is indicated. A light splint is applied along the radial side of forearm which can be removed to allow cleaning and washing but otherwise should be worn continuously (Fig. 24.12). Once the child has started to make use of the hands the splint can be removed during the day but should be worn regularly at night. Normal activity is allowed during the day, and in the radially deviated position it is usual for the ulnar digits to be used for prehension (Fig. 24.13).

Attempts are made to mobilize the stiff elbow by physiotherapy, and active use is encouraged while corrective splintage on the wrist is maintained (Fig. 24.14).

It is usually possible to control the deformity during the first 2 or 3 years, but gradually the ulna grows away from the carpus deviating it radially and volarwards. At this stage, provided there is elbow flexion to at least 90°, consideration should be given to operative correction of the wrist deformity [37, 38, 41, 42]. This is always indicated in the unilateral problem where the improvement in appearance is an important consideration. Where it is bilateral, and provided there is good elbow flexion and mobile hand joints, operative correction should be considered on both sides. In a series reported there has been no adverse affect on function [37].

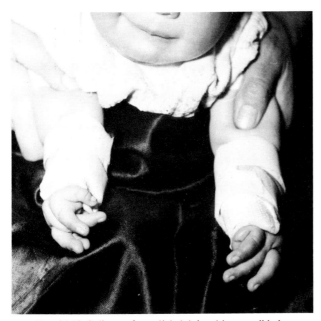

Fig. 24.12. Splintage for radial club hand in a small baby.

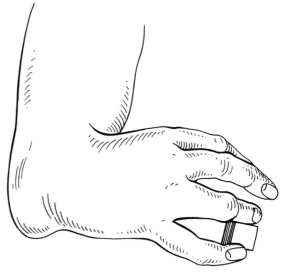

Fig. 24.13. Ulnar prehension in the uncorrected deformity.

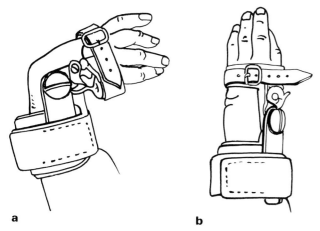

a   b

FIG. 24.14. A small 'ratchet' type splint (a) before and (b) after treatment. This can correct a soft tissue contracture, and also be used to control the corrected deformity.

Many previous operative procedures have been described, but the only operation now considered to be applicable and successful is that of centralization of the carpus on the ulna (Fig. 24.15) [43].

Technique of centralization

The soft tissues are exposed through a curved incision on the dorsum of the hand from the head of the second metacarpal to the head of the ulna and then deviating across the carpal crease from ulnar to radial side and then extending up the volar aspect of the forearm (Fig. 24.16). The radial nerve and vessels are usually absent and the median nerve is lying on the radial side of the wrist immediately subjacent to the deep fascia. The nerve is identified before freeing the many tight soft tissue structures on the radial side of the carpus. The cartilaginous carpus is lying on the radial side of the lower ulna and has to be dissected free in order to remove sufficient part of the centre of the carpus to enable placement of the lower ulna into the resulting notch. This usually means removal of the lunate and capitate. The lower end of the ulna is dissected extra-periosteally and inserted into the carpus to a depth equal to its transverse diameter (see A, Fig. 24.15) and fitted snugly to obtain stability. The radial carpal extensors are usually absent and as there is the deforming influence of the flexor carpi radialis it is transferred to the dorsum of the hand. When the hand has been corrected and placed over the ulna there may be a flexion contracture of the fingers due to tightness of the superficialis muscle. If the fingers cannot be passively extended in the new position, the muscle is lengthened at the musculotendinous junction.

The wrist is stabilized in position by a Kirschner wire passed along the third or fourth metacarpal shaft across the carpus. the centre of the epiphyseal line of the ulna and up the ulnar medullary cavity (Fig. 24.17).

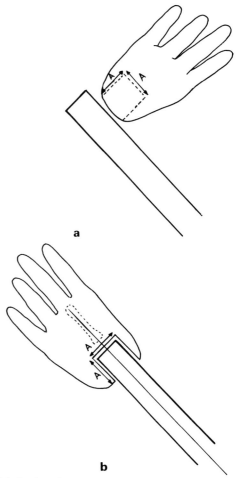

a

b

FIG. 24.15. The principles of centralization.

(a) Sufficient of the central carpus is removed to accommodate the lower ulna.

(b) The position is maintained by a Kirschner wire across the centre of the lower ulnar epiphysis and the third metacarpal.

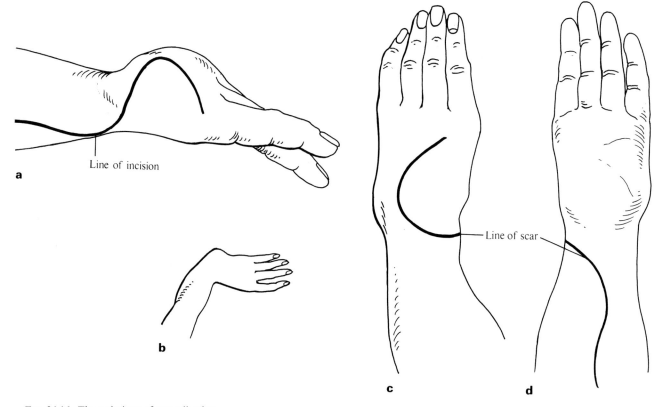

Line of incision

a

b

Line of scar

c   d

Fig. 24.16. The technique of centralization.

(a) A curved incision on the dorsum extends from the head of the second metacarpal across the head of the ulna, deviates across the carpal crease to the radial side of the wrist and extends up the volar aspect of the forearm. A Z-plasty can be used if the skin is tight on the radial aspect of the wrist.

(b) The preoperative deformity.

(c) Dorsal and (d) volar views of the postoperative correction.

It is a feature of absence of the radius that the forearm remains short and is seldom more than two-thirds of the normal length of the ulna and usually between half and two-thirds [30, 32]. Provided there is care in freeing the lower end of the ulna with a minimum of soft tissue dissection and the wire is passed across the centre of the lower ulna epiphysis, there is no evidence that there is any premature cessation of growth.

Considerable swelling of the hand occurs after operation and postoperative elevation should be continued until all swelling has settled. A plaster cast is then applied from the metacarpal heads to above the elbow which is immobilized at 90°. External support should be maintained for 6 months.

The Kirschner wire may be left for several years without detriment to growth. Usually the wire is extruded at one or other end within a few weeks and the external splintage becomes even more important.

Following correction of the wrist deformity a further assessment of function is made and where the index finger has good joint movement and tendon control, consideration should be given to its pollicization by which significant improvement in prehension function of the hand can be obtained.

To compensate for the short forearm, lengthening of the ulna by about 3 cms has been described [44]. While this may improve the appearance it is unlikely to improve any hand function which is present.

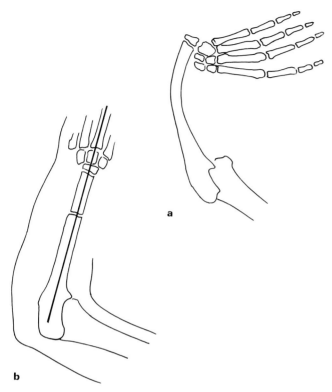

FIG. 24.17. (a) Preoperative, and (b) postoperative positions after centralization. Note Kirschner wire and corrective osteotomy required due to the bowing of the ulna.

Pollicization

Absence of the thumb is a significant functional disability. Remarkable adaptation occurs in the young child born without a thumb, but there is no doubt that there is impairment of overall function and self-care activities, particularly when bilateral.

Pollicization is well described [45–50]. The general opinion is that pollicization should be considered where the joints and muscle control of the radial digit are sufficiently good to allow some function of the transposed digit in the thumb position. There are reservations whether this is justified in unilateral absence, and it might be considered by some only on one side in bilateral cases. As a general principle the operation is best done at an early age so that the new pattern of prehension is easily acquired and does not require alteration of a previous pattern.

Technique

The technique described by Buck–Gramcko will give reliable results [49, 50]. The skin incision described by Barsky is used (Fig. 24.18). To facilitate exposure of the extensor mechanism in the region of the proximal interphalangeal joint of the index a straight dorsal extension from the incision is used along the proximal phalanx. The incision is deepened from the dorsum through the intermetacarpal space and the deep transverse ligament divided. This allows separation of the interossei and metacarpals in order to expose the neurovascular bundle. The vessel bifurcation is identified distal to the nerve division and the vessels to the radial side of the long finger are isolated and divided (Fig. 24.19). The common digital nerve to the second interspace is gently separated into its radial and ulnar components as far proximally as possible. The skin flap is reflected and dissected round the palmar aspect where the neurovascular bundle is again identified and if there is a radial digital vessel to the index finger it is identified and protected. This vessel is not infrequently absent. With the neurovascular supply to the index digit now protected the metacarpal is again exposed from the dorsal aspect. The first dorsal and palmar interosseous muscles are identified, dissected from the second metacarpal and the tendons are detached from their insertions. The metacarpal is stripped subperiostally and the proximal three quarters of the shaft is removed, leaving the head of the metacarpal. The digit can now be rotated through 150° into the position of the thumb and the metacarpal head stitched into its new position where it becomes the new trapezium (Fig. 24.20). The length of the new thumb should be such that its tip is approximately at the level of the proximal interphalangeal joint of the extended long finger (Fig. 24.21).

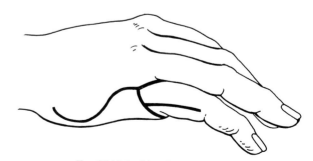

FIG. 24.18. Incision for pollicization.

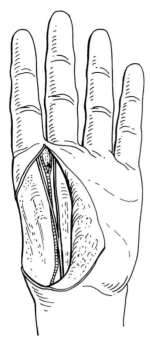

FIG. 24.19. Technique of pollicization showing the neurovascular bundle to the interspace between the index and middle fingers. The flap has been elevated to expose the nerve and vessels on the volar aspect. The artery to the middle finger has been divided and the nerve is being separated into two components.

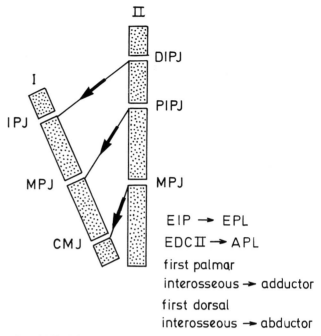

FIG. 24.20. Diagram showing how the components of the index digit are transposed into the thumb. The head of the second metacarpal becomes the new trapezium. The interossei are inserted in the extensor at the level of the old proximal interphalangeal joint and what is now the metacarpophalangeal joint of the new thumb.

The first dorsal and palmar interosseous tendons are attached to the extensor tendon at the level of the original proximal interphalangeal joint which will now become the metacarpophalangeal joint of thumb. This boosts the extensor power of the digit and the first dorsal interosseous becomes the new short abductor of the thumb and the palmar interosseous the adductor (Fig. 24.20).

It is seldom that any adjustment is needed for the long tendons. In the young person the flexor invariably tightens up and provides adequate flexion. It is occasionally necessary to shorten and tighten the extensor tendon, seldom at the original procedure, but rather at a later date if the extensor power of the new thumb is unsatisfactory.

Distal ulnar deficiency

Absence of the ulnar side of the forearm is very rare being approximately ten times less common than distal radial absence. Birch–Jensen reported an absent ulna in

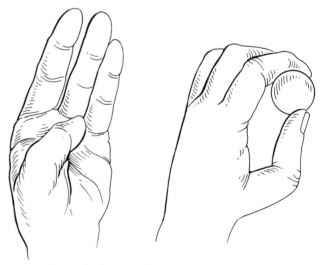

FIG. 24.21. Following pollicization the tip of the thumb should be at the level of the proximal interphalangeal joint of the extended long finger, for a good cosmetic and functional result.

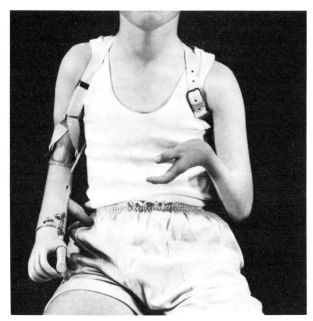

FIG. 24.22. Bilateral total absence of ulna and ulnar digits with fixed contraction of the elbows in flexion. The contracture has been corrected partially on the right side to allow use of a prosthesis.

1/100 000 live births [1]. The deformity consists both of the bone and soft tissue components; the bone deficiency may be complete or partial. There is usually absence of the ulnar side of the carpus and the ulnar digits (Fig. 24.22), but occasionally there is a lesser degree of absence of the ulnar component of the forearm with a normal hand.

Abnormalities of the elbow joint are common and vary in degree from an almost normal articulation to fixed flexion contractures (Fig. 24.22).

The deficiency is commonly unilateral. Carroll in a study of twenty-three patients over a 20 year period found no examples of bilateral involvement [51].

The condition is seldom associated with other congenital abnormalities with the exception of the Cornelia de Lange syndrome.

Treatment

Splintage is indicated to prevent progressive deformity during the first 6–12 months. The deformity is rarely as severe as that due to absent radius, but if there is a progressive ulnar club hand deformity the fibro-cartilaginous band which often replaces the absent bone should be resected [51–53].

When growth has ceased arthrodesis of the carpus to the lower radius may be indicated to correct any deformity.

In partial ulnar absence the upper third of the ulna is usually present. As the forearm grows there is a tendency for the upper end of radius to dislocate proximally and to displace on to the radial side of the lower humerus.

The cosmetic appearance can be improved by an operation in which the upper third of the radius is excised and the lower two-thirds implanted into the upper ulna (Fig. 24.23) [54]. This improves the appearance, gives some stability to the forearm and the function, particularly at the elbow, may be improved.

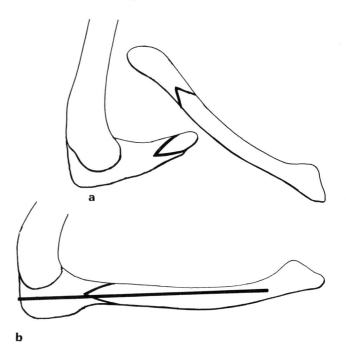

FIG. 24.23. Treatment of distal ulnar deficiency.

(a) Preoperative view showing displacement of upper end of radius. This is resected to create a wedge that is inserted into a corresponding groove in the remaining upper third of the ulna.

(b) Postoperative appearance showing the creation of a one bone forearm. The position is maintained by an intramedullary Kirschner wire.

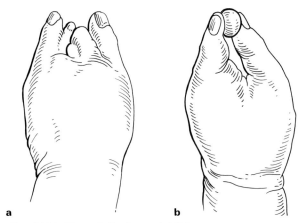

FIG. 24.24. Group 1 distal central deficiency.
(a) Partial absence of central digits.
(b) Prehension between thumb and little finger is provided after resection of central metacarpals and vestigial digits.

Distal central deficiencies [14, 15, 55]

There are two main types of distal central deficiency:

(1) The central part of the hand, including a variable part of the metacarpals, is present but the digits are missing partially or completely (Fig. 24.24a). This is the more common type and is a sporadic non-genetic deformity which is usually unilateral.

(2) The central part of the hand as far proximally as the carpus is absent resulting in a classical lobster claw hand (Fig. 24.25). This may involve only the middle metacarpal ray or sometimes all three central meta-

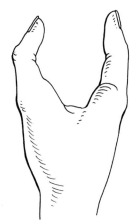

FIG. 24.25 Group 2 distal central deficiency showing the lobster claw effect.

carpals. The deformity is often bilateral, is hereditary with a dominant gene and may be associated with a similar deformity of the feet.

In both types the thumb and little finger are of a varying degree of normality, being sometimes entirely normal, with the potential to provide useful functional prehension between the two components.

Treatment [55]

This depends on whether functional improvement can be obtained. Surgery purely to improve the appearance is only justified if it can be associated with functional improvement.

Group 1. Surgery is indicated when the central metacarpals obstruct the apposition of the radial and ulnar components and prevent useful prehension. The mobility of the thumb can be improved appreciably by deepening the thumb web with resection of the second metacarpal to enable opposition to the little finger. Sometimes removal of all the central metacarpals is required (Fig. 24.24b). If this does not provide satisfactory pinch and grasp a corrective osteotomy through the fifth metacarpal shaft is carried out to rotate the ulnar component into a functional position. Cosmetic replacement of the missing component of the hand can be provided for social occasions (see Chapter 36).

Group 2. The function of the lobster claw deformity often is very good. Where the whole of the central part of the hand is missing the remnants usually provide good opposition between thumb and little finger and no surgery is indicated.

Where only the third metacarpal ray is missing then the skin cleft can be excised to bring the remaining metacarpals into close apposition, thus improving the appearance of the hand but at the same time retaining its function [55].

FAILURE OF DIFFERENTIATION
R. J. SMITH

Congenital radioulnar synostosis [56, 57]

Radioulnar synostosis occurs most commonly at the proximal end of the forearm. When the distal radioulnar joint is synostotic, it is rarely affected alone. Occasionally synostosis is associated with pre-axial abnormalities, including hypoplasia of the thumb and radial side carpal coalescence. It is bilateral in 60–70 per cent of cases; males are affected more frequently than females.

Often there is a family history of other defects of the upper limbs. The abnormality appears to be inherited as a dominant phenotype with variable expression. If severe and diffuse abnormalities are associated with synostosis, the patient may have a chromosome abnormality such as is found in Klinefelter's syndrome with XXY, XXXY or XXXXY phenotype. In these patients, the defect appears to be carried by the Y chromosome.

During the seventh and eighth week of embryonic development, the radioulnar anlage separates from distally to proximally forming the radius and ulna. It is at this time that failure of differentiation leads to synostosis and persistence of the embryonic position of forearm pronation.

Two main types of congenital radioulnar synostosis have been described:

(1) *Primary.* The proximal ends of both the radius and ulna are fused for a distance of about 2–6 cm (Fig. 24.26). The radial head is absent and the synostotic area consists of cancellous bone without a central cortical layer.

(2) *Secondary.* There is a shorter and less intimate area of bony fusion with cortical bone visible radiographically in the fusion mass. The radial head is present and may be dislocated anteriorly or posteriorly.

The primary type of synostosis occurs three times as frequently as the secondary type. There is a spectrum of bony abnormalities which lies between these two extremes. Many patients will have a primary type of synostosis in one forearm and the secondary type in the other.

With proximal radioulnar synostosis, the radius distal to the fusion is typically stout and somewhat arched, the ulna is slender and atrophied, the interosseous space is widened and the hand is often ulnarly deviated at the wrist. Bony deformities are frequently accompanied by absence of the brachioradialis, pronator teres, pronator quadratus and supinator muscles. Whether muscle atrophy is primary, or secondary to the synostosis, is unclear.

The principal physical finding is a fixed pronation deformity which, in nearly half, will exceed 60°. The forearm may be shortened, and the bowed radius is apparent clinically. There is frequently a mild fixed flexion contracture of the elbow, decrease in the carrying angle and prominence of the dislocated radial head. With increased wrist mobility, apparently due to lax ligaments, many patients are able to achieve up to 45° of rotation of the hand at the radiocarpal joint.

Function will depend upon the severity of the deformity and whether or not it is bilateral. With severe fixed pronation contractures of the forearm, the patient

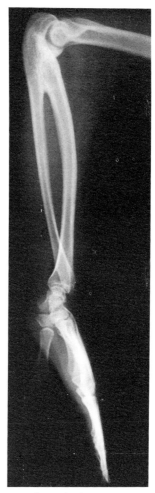

FIG. 24.26. Lateral radiograph of proximal radioulnar synostosis with a 90° pronation deformity of the forearm. It shows the more frequent primary type synostosis with fusion of proximal radius and ulna for several centimetres.

cannot compensate by shoulder rotation and will find it awkward to write, eat or hold small objects.

Treatment

If the deformity is mild and unilateral, no treatment is needed. If, however, there is awkwardness and difficulty in using the hands due to severe deformity, surgical treatment should be considered.

In an attempt to provide active motion, many surgical methods have been used. These have included radial osteotomy distal to the synostosis site with interposition of muscle, metal or a plastic cap. Others have divided the synostosis longitudinally and interposed local tissues or metallic or plastic sheets. Most of these procedures have been unsuccessful. Postoperative problems have included severe angulation of the distal radial fragment, pseudoarthrosis, poor active motion due to the absence of the pronator and supinator muscles or, frequently, reformation of bone about the interpositional material with recurrence of a rigid synostosis. A 'swivel' operation has also been recommended to restore active motion to the rigid forearm [57]. A metallic dowel is placed in the medullary cavity of the radius at the osteotomy site just distal to the synostosis. The distal ulna is resected and the extensor carpi ulnaris tendon is divided. Its distal end is threaded through the ulna to reconstruct the ulnar collateral ligament of the wrist. The proximal end is transferred dorsally either to the tendon of the brachioradialis or to the radial styloid in order to achieve active supination of the forearm. Unfortunately, this imaginative procedure has not met with consistent success.

A more conservative plan is to decrease severe deformity by osteotomy and derotation of the pronated forearm into a more functional position. Any angulatory deformity can be corrected by appropriate wedge resection at the osteotomy site. Recommendations as to how and when the osteotomy should be performed have varied. The most frequent complications following derotational osteotomy have included postoperative angulation at the osteotomy site and vascular disturbance due to torsion of the brachial, radial or ulnar vessels.

As the results of operations to obtain active rotation of the forearm have been disappointing, we make no attempt to achieve and maintain active supination of the forearm. If there is pronation of more than 45° either unilaterally or bilaterally, rotational osteotomy is recommended.

Osteotomy is performed between 5 and 7 years of age in order to decrease the risk of vascular complications and to enable a normal prehensile pattern to develop during childhood. If unilateral, the forearm is placed in 20° of pronation and if bilateral, the dominant side is placed in about 30° of pronation and the assistive limb in neutral. Shoulder rotation will permit the child to bring both hands parallel to a table top for such activities as writing, typing and playing keyboard instruments. Neutral rotation or mild pronation will look best when the patient is walking and the limbs are at the side.

Good bone-to-bone apposition is achieved by rotational osteotomy through the synostosis site. Any angulation deformity is corrected by wedge resection. If the operation is performed distal to the synostosis, the displacement of the tubular bones by rotation will create a gap with a delay in bone healing.

Operative technique

Under tourniquet control, a longitudinal incision is made over the dorsal subcutaneous surface of the ulna from its olecranon to the junction of the proximal and middle thirds of the forearm. The synostosis is exposed subperiostally and divided transversely by a sagittal power saw. A Kirschner wire is driven through the olecranon from the osteotomy. The forearm is rotated into the desired position. If angulatory correction is desired, an appropriate wedge is then removed from the distal osteotomy site. Bone surfaces are opposed and the Kirschner wire is driven distally into the radius. One or two oblique Kirschner wires are then drilled through the osteotomy site to maintain the position. If there is evidence of vascular impairment on release of tourniquet, the oblique wires are removed and the rotational correction is reduced slightly. Periosteum is closed with absorbable sutures. The skin is closed about a small drain. An above-elbow long arm cast is applied for about 2 months, by which time the osteotomy is usually healed.

Derotation may be difficult in an older patient due to a taut radioulnar interosseous membrane and the dorsal incision must be extended distally to elevate the interosseous membrane from the radius. Particular care must be taken to protect the anterior and posterior interosseous nerves.

Symphalangism (rigid digits) [58–61]

John Talbot, first Earl of Shrewsbury, had stiff ring and little fingers of both hands; fourteen generations of his descendants have had a similar condition. William Brown, a possible descendant, emigrated from Scotland to Virginia in 1740. Of Brown's 684 descendants in ten generations, 350 have had symphalangism and many have had talonavicular fusion. Cushing called the abnormality symphalangism, or 'hereditary anchylosis (sic) of the proximal phalangeal joints' [58].

The condition is transmitted as an autosomal dominant trait, and half the members of a family are likely to be affected. In over 20 per cent of patients there is also symphalangism of the distal joints of the toes. Concurrent synostosis between the stapes and the petrous portion of the temporal bone, causing hearing loss, may occur, but rarely have other stigmata been associated. Non-hereditary symphalangism is frequently found in patients with diastrophic dwarfism, Hurler's syndrome, dysplasia epiphysealis multiplex and Apert's syndrome.

Hereditary symphalangism affects the ulnar digits more frequently than the radial and the thumb is rarely involved. There is no sex predilection. It is bilateral in 50 per cent of cases. The proximal interphalangeal joint is affected three times as frequently as the distal, and the metacarpophalangeal joints are affected in only 3 per cent of patients with symphalangism.

Affected fingers are short and slender, the skin appears tight and shiny, lacking normal flexion and extension creases. Although the distal interphalangeal joint may compensate for more proximal rigidity by flexing up to 90° with attempts at grasp, the patient cannot make a fist. Radiographs taken during infancy or early childhood may be misleading as a wide epiphyseal radiolucency may be mistaken for a joint space (Fig. 24.27).

Treatment

Children with symphalangism are accustomed to other members of the family with straight fingers and think 'there is nothing wrong with it'. Indeed, such families usually talk of those members who have 'straight fingers' (symphalangism) and those who have 'crooked fingers' (normal interphalangeal joints). Surely no treatment would be indicated in these cases unless there is a moderately severe functional disability.

Stretching exercises are useless. If use of the hands is awkward and difficult because of inability to grasp objects, one might consider arthroplasty or arthrodesis. Replacement arthroplasty in a growing child is contraindicated as the small fingers would be shortened still further by damage to the epiphyses. Arthroplasty in adults would be of little value as any tendon apparatus which may be reconstructed would scarcely be able to impart strong stable motion to the newly constructed joint. Thus, osteotomy and arthrodesis of the conjoined phalanges is often the only reasonable procedure by which the affected fingers may be flexed to a position which would permit grasp. If osteotomy is to be performed, it is usually best delayed until late in adolescence when the epiphyseal plates are closed.

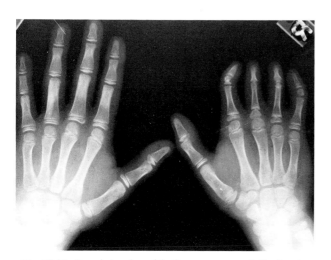

FIG. 24.27. Symphalangism of the fingers accompanied by brachydactyly and incomplete simple syndactyly. The syndactyly has been released. This radiograph shows total absence of the middle phalanges of the middle and ring fingers with abortive middle phalanges of the index and little fingers. As there is no proximal interphalangeal joint motion of the index and little fingers, all four fingers have symphalangism. Note the abnormal epiphyseal plate of the proximal phalanx of the middle finger.

Syndactyly [63, 65]

Incomplete separation of adjacent digits is among the more common congenital deformities of the hand. It occurs approximately once in every two to three thousand births.

In the sixth week of intrauterine life, digital buds appear and grow rapidly from the palm. By 7–8 weeks, the fingers become well developed and well formed. If, during the seventh or eighth week, the finger buds are slowed in their growth, the subsequent growth of fingers and webs will take place at a uniform rate resulting in syndactyly.

'Complete syndactyly' refers to webbing of the fingers to the fingertips. Digits with 'incomplete syndactyly' have a web extending more distally than the middle of the proximal phalanx but not to the end of the terminal phalanx. The syndactyly is 'simple' if skin alone is joined, and 'complex' if the bones of adjacent digits are fused. Acrosyndactyly is the lateral fusion of digits at their distal ends, usually with a proximal fenestration or space between the digits distal to the normal web. Brachy-syndactyly refers to shortened fingers which are joined laterally. The treatment of each of these deformities varies.

Syndactyly may be associated with other deformities such as absent or multiple digits, diffuse musculoskeletal abnormalities, craniofacial dysostosis or other visceral anomalies.

The cause of syndactyly varies as well. Acrosyndactyly is usually due to exogenous factors (see section on annular grooves, p. 327). Endogenous syndactyly is due to a genetic interference with early fetal development.

Syndactyly—endogenous, unassociated with remote abnormalities

There is a family history of similar abnormalities in about 20 per cent of patients with syndactyly. White races have a higher prevalence than black races, and males are affected twice as frequently as females.

It affects the third web in over 50 per cent, the fourth web in 30 per cent, the second web in 15 per cent and rarely involves the thumb web. Syndactyly is more frequently unilateral than bilateral.

Finger deformities depend upon the extent of the syndactyly, whether or not it is complex, and the comparative size of the adjacent fingers.

Partial, simple syndactyly

This produces little, if any, functional impairment. The child is able to flex and extend the fingers without difficulty and inability to abduct the syndactylous digits causes no serious handicap. The fingers may grow normally with little deformity or limitation of motion, and treatment is directed at improving appearance and permitting a wider grasp.

Complete, simple syndactyly

Fingers approximately the same size (Fig. 24.28). The deformity is likely to be mild and consist mainly of a mild rotation of each of the syndactylous digits towards each other. Motion may be virtually normal and there is little angulatory deformity.

Fingers of different sizes. The fingers rotate towards each other and the larger of the two angulates towards the lesser finger which tethers it into flexion. Angulation, flexion and rotation deformities progress as growth continues.

Complex syndactyly between fingers of different sizes

The deformity is still more severe than in the previous two groups and it is best to free the fingers early in an attempt to prevent further deformity and to correct contractures. As the difference in size of the adjacent fingers of the second and fourth webs is greater than the difference between those of the third, they usually require an earlier release. Although surgery may be delayed for several years in order to minimize scarring and distal web migration, with increasing deformity it is often best to release the syndactyly well before the age of 1 year. Even with non-deforming, simple syndactyly, if surgery can be completed before the age of 18 months, the child will not be exposed to the social stigma which is often associated with 'webbed fingers'.

Treatment [66, 70, 71]

Partial simple syndactyly. Many methods have been described to treat partial simple syndactyly. In the first web, a four-flap z-plasty can deepen the cleft between the thumb and index finger without the need of a skin graft. Incomplete webbing between two fingers can be deepened with a butterfly flap. However, if the web extends past the distal third of the proximal phalanx, we prefer to use interdigitating triangular flaps to create the new commissure, zig-zag incisions to separate the sides of the fingers (Fig. 24.28), and skin grafts to cover the fingers adjacent to the commissure.

An inverted, V-shaped incision is made on the dorsum of the fingers with its base at the metacarpal heads of the syndactylous digits. The apex of the flap is placed at the neck of the proximal phalanx of the longer of the digits. The entire dorsal flap is centred radial to the midline of the webbed fingers (Fig. 24.28a).

The palmar web flap is made with its base just proximal to the proximal digital flexion crease and is offset ulnarly. The apex lies just proximal to the middle digital crease (Fig. 24.28b).

The dorsal incision is then continued in a zig-zag fashion first radially, then ulnarly, finally back to the midline between the nails and then straight distally. The apices of each of the zig-zags lie at the level of the interphalangeal joints (Fig. 24.28a). On the volar side, the incision complements that of the dorsum, continuing first ulnarly, then radially and finally straight between the pulps to join the dorsal incision (Fig. 24.28b).

The triangular flaps are elevated with a thin layer of subcutaneous fat. By blunt dissection, the areolar tissue is separated between the proximal phalanges of the syndactylous digits and the neurovascular bundles are identified. If there is distal bifurcation of the vessels, one branch must be ligated and sectioned. The vessels should be left with the border digits in cases of a single web so that the more important finger gets the vessels. If three fingers are webbed, the finger requiring web release on either side is given the benefit of two vascular bundles. If the digital nerve bifurcates distally, its fascicles may be gently dissected apart as far as the distal palm.

The zig-zag incisions are developed deeply and the multiple triangular flaps dissected with a thin layer of subcutaneous tissue. The longitudinal grooved portion of the conjoined fingernail is excised. Sutured side to side, the triangular flaps at the sides of the fingers are interdigitated. These flaps must not be pulled tightly or sutured under tension. Open areas will invariably remain at the opposing sides of the bases of each of the freed fingers. Additional open areas may also remain at the tips of the fingers in the region of the pulp. The surgeon must avoid the temptation to close the defects at the bases of the fingers without a skin graft. If the web skin is sutured to the finger skin, contracture and secondary angulation results. A skin graft is *always* necessary after releasing syndactyly by this method. A

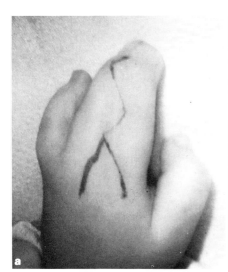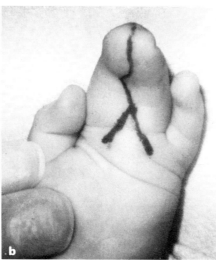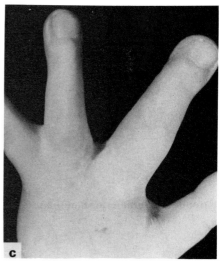

FIG. 24.28. Complete simple syndactyly showing (a & b) well formed thumb and little finger. There is a complete skin bridge between the remaining two fingers, but no bony fusion. The web is reconstructed with interdigitating triangular flaps. Complementary zig-zag incisions are used to separate the digits.

(c) 2 years postoperatively there is excellent separation of the fingers. Both the appearance and function of the hand are improved. The interdigitating triangular flaps with full thickness skin grafts at adjacent bases of the separated fingers give a good web.

full thickness skin graft is taken from the groin crease, defatted and sutured into the defects. The donor site is closed with absorbable suture material and collodion. The tourniquet is released and haemostasis obtained. If there is any area of blanching, the tight sutures are removed.

The skin grafts are covered by a petrolatum wide mesh gauze which is sutured to the skin with fine absorbable catgut. The fingers are widely separated and wet cotton is placed over the gauze. Layer upon layer of soft cotton is then placed in the newly created web space until the fingers are held firmly in extension and abduction. Cotton wadding is also placed in the webs of the adjacent fingers. The dressings are held in place with stretch gauze and an above-elbow plaster protects the entire wound.

Unless there is a change in the colour of the fingertips, the dressings are not removed for 3 weeks, at which time the wound is inspected through the wide mesh gauze. The hand is immobilized for an additional 3 weeks. Six weeks after surgery, all dressings are removed. It is rarely necessary to apply a splint after that time. Figure 24.28c shows the result 2 years after separation.

Complex syndactyly. A similar technique is used for complex syndactyly. The conjoined distal phalanx and nail are sharply transsected longitudinally with a scalpel blade. An osteotome or saw is rarely necessary. A full thickness skin graft may be applied directly over the bone and will usually 'take'. If osteotomy causes instability at the distal interphalangeal joints, longitudinal Kirschner wires are inserted through these joints for 6 weeks. Figure 24.29a shows preoperative example of complex syndactyly and 24.29b the result of separation after 1 year. If there are two webs affected, only one should be released at a time. If three are affected, the second and fourth webs are released simultaneously and the third web is released some months later. Simultaneously releasing the webs on both sides of a finger unnecessarily jeopardizes its circulation.

A small, hypoplastic digit may lie between two well formed syndactylous fingers. Although it may be technically feasible to construct three digits from this conglomerate, usually neither the functional nor the aesthetic result is satisfactory. It is far better to create three fingers of normal length than four fingers, one of which is small, misshapen and lacks active motion.

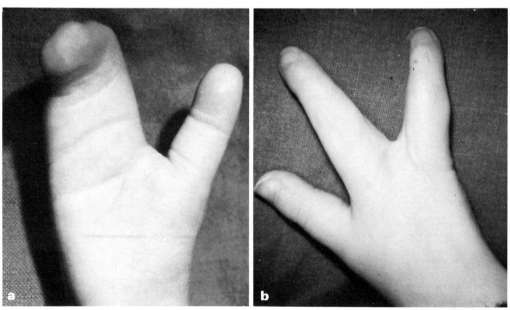

FIG. 24.29. Compound syndactyly showing (a) complete, compound ectrosyndactyly. The ulnar two fingers are absent, the index and middle fingers are webbed to the tips and the distal phalanx of each of the fingers is fused laterally.

(b) One year postoperatively, the full thickness skin grafts at adjacent surfaces of the bases of the fingers are barely noticeable. A good web and good alignment of the fingers are maintained.

Brachysyndactyly (Poland's syndactyly)

Simple, incomplete syndactyly may be associated with shortening of all digits to between 35 and 50 per cent of their normal length. This anomaly is rare, is usually unilateral and the middle and distal phalanges are principally involved (Fig. 24.30a).

Brachysyndactyly may be associated with ipsilateral pectoral hypoplasia with absence of the sternal and costal heads of the pectoralis major, pectoralis minor, and serratus anterior. There is often deficient pectoral and axillary hair, scanty subcutaneous tissue over the pectoral muscles, asymmetry of the nipples or breasts and, in some cases, hypoplasia of the entire upper extremity. A tight web in the anterior axillary fold may limit abduction of the shoulder. Although the eponym 'Poland's syndrome' has been used, the relationship between pectoral hypoplasia and brachysyndactyly was apparently not appreciated by Poland [67–69]. His report merely described the two sets of anomalies in the same dissection but he drew no inferences about their association with each other.

The condition is best treated by syndactyly release with reconstruction of a new web at the level of the MP joints. There is apparent lengthening of the fingers if the web is made proximal to its proper anatomical location. This will improve both the function and the appearance of the hand (Fig. 24.30b). Shoulder abduction may be increased by excising the fibrous band in the anterior axillary fold (often a fibrous remnant of pectoralis major) and lengthening the skin with multiple Z-plasties. Large local flaps should be avoided in order to prevent the transfer of axillary hair to the front of the shoulder.

Syndactyly with craniofacial dysostosis (Apert's syndrome) [62, 64]

Acrocephaly associated with abnormalities about the hands and feet is called Apert's syndrome (Fig. 24.31a & b).

The deformities are most severe. There is usually complex, complete syndactyly of all the fingers and the thumb. The hand is spoon-shaped with the thumb short and radially deviated at its tip. The little finger may be relatively spared and may share only a skin

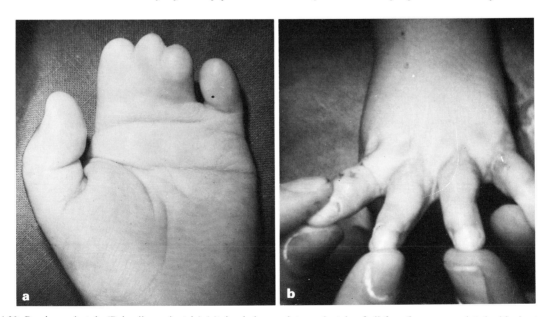

FIG. 24.30. Brachysyndactyly (Poland's syndactyly) (a) simple incomplete syndactyly of all four fingers, associated with shortening of the digits (brachysyndactyly) which usually spares the thumb.

(b) The border digits are first released. Later the central digits are released. Full thickness skin grafts cover denuded opposing areas of the fingers. The fingers appear relatively longer when they are separated than preoperatively.

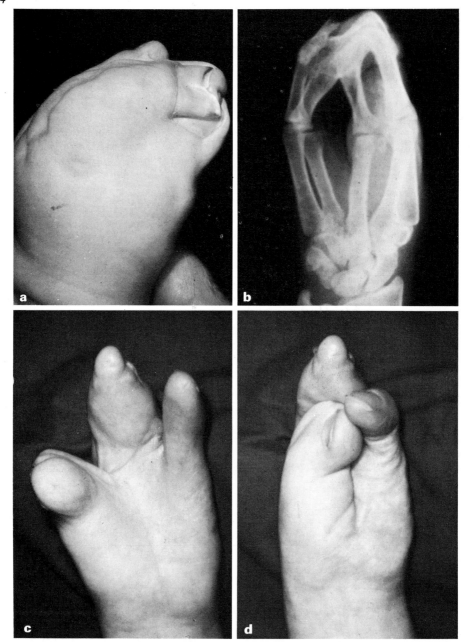

Fɪɢ. 24.31. Complex syndactyly with craniofacial dysostosis.

(a)   Typical severe bilateral, complete complex syndactyly with webbing of all interdigital clefts, ulnar deviation of the fingers, radial deviation of the distal joint of the thumb, one conjoined fingernail.

(b) With longstanding complex syndactyly there are changes at the metacarpophalangeal and interphalangeal joints. Note the flattening of the metacarpal heads.

(c & d) A functional trident hand is formed, enabling partial independence in carrying out activities of daily living and in the workshop. Separation of the middle and ring fingers appeared unnecessary for either functional or aesthetic purposes.

web (simple syndactyly) with the ring finger. Typically, the fingers are stiff and exhibit symphalangism; the metacarpals are short; the proximal phalanx of the thumb may be delta shaped. As both hands are involved, function is poor: food is scooped to the mouth and cups and toys must be held between the two paddle-shaped hands.

Fortunately, Apert's syndrome is rare, occurring once in every 200 000 births and results from a single gene in heterozygous form or by mutation. There are few opportunities to study inheritance patterns.

The severe cerebral problems may contraindicate any reconstructive surgery to the hands. Yet, with advances in neurosurgical procedures, and newer techniques of plastic surgery to the facial bones, many of these patients can now expect to live a relatively normal life. The hand surgeon may expect to be challenged more frequently to do what he can to sort out the jumble of bones, tendons and skin of the two deformed hands.

It is probably best to separate out the border digits (thumb and little finger) first. Later, the other digits may be separated. The magnitude of the syndactyly is so extensive that a better functioning hand usually can be reconstructed by amputating one of the fingers. Frequently, resection of the ring or middle finger may provide enough skin to permit the separation of three independently functioning fingers and a good opposable thumb. Tendon remnants of an amputated finger often can be transferred to an adjacent digit. Frequently, osteotomy of the base of the thumb or of one of the fingers may be necessary to align the digits properly after syndactyly release.

Although operation never can create a normal or 'good-looking' hand, the multiple operative procedures are usually well worth the effort (Fig. 24.31c & d). Even for the institutionalized patient, the restoration of prehension may allow self-caring, helping others, and engaging in various play and work activities. As there is a great deal which has to be done to rehabilitate these hands, it is usually wise to begin surgery early so that proper prehensile habit patterns can be formed.

Acrosyndactyly

This will be discussed in the section on 'ring constriction syndromes'.

DUPLICATION

R. J. SMITH

Polydactyly [72, 73, 75–77]

Accurate statistics of the incidence of polydactyly are difficult to obtain, since an extra finger is often tied-off or removed in the delivery room shortly after the birth of the child. Only a small nubbin of skin may remain and the parents and child are unaware of its origin.

Polydactyly is usually transmitted as an autosomal dominant with variable expression. Over 100 family pedigrees have been traced throughout the Middle East, Eastern Europe and Africa with several generations possessing six or seven fingers on either hand. It is believed that polydactyly is more common in the black than the white races. Review of statistics at the University of Iowa, where the population is almost exclusively white, has revealed 14 per cent of all hand deformities to be polydactyly.

Other associated abnormalities of the limbs including syndactyly of the hands and polydactyly and syndactyly of the toes may be found. Supernumerary digits are a frequent stigma of trisomy 13–15. In patients with chondro-ectodermal dysplasia, the Ellis–van Creveld syndrome, there is autosomal recessive inheritance of short limbs, defective teeth, rudimentary nails and polydactyly. The Laurence–Moon–Biedl–Bordet syndrome [77] consists of polydactyly, obesity of the Fröhlich's type, retinitis pigmentosa, genital hypoplasia and mental retardation. This syndrome is thought to be caused by a hypothalamic disturbance. As retinitis pigmentosa in these patients frequently may be manifest first by night blindness and only gradually result in decreasing visual fields, the physician should be alert to the possibility of more serious abnormalities elsewhere if polydactyly is asymmetrical and associated with obesity.

If polydactyly is unassociated with chromosomal abnormalities or with visceral dysplasia, hand abnormalities are bilateral in approximately two-thirds of the patients. The supernumerary digit is found most frequently at the borders of the hand [79]. Approximately 50 per cent of the cases show a reduplication of the thumb and, in 30 per cent, the little finger (Fig. 24.32). The central fingers are involved in perhaps 15 per cent of cases and the index finger is reduplicated rarely. The digit adjacent to the supernumerary finger or thumb is usually shorter and more slender than normal and may lack a full complement of normal musculotendinous structures.

Supernumerary digits may take one of several forms. Most frequently, the extra digit is short, has neither bone nor cartilage and appears as a flaccid soft tissue appendage lacking any motion or stability. This has been designated Type I by Stelling [80]. Type II has been classified as digit duplication which contains relatively normal components of bone and tendon and which articulates with a bifid metacarpal or phalanx. Type III is most infrequent and consists of a complete digit possessing its own metacarpal and all normal soft tissue elements. Frequently, the reduplicated digit may be incompletely separated throughout its length from the adjacent thumb or finger. The proximal end of the supernumerary digit may form a trapezoidal or delta phalanx or metacarpal with an abnormal or J-shaped epiphyseal plate (p. 330). Often with complex syndactyly-polydactyly, it may appear that there is but one broadened digit with a longitudinal furrow at the finger nail. Roentgenographic examination will permit accurate diagnosis in these cases. With central polydactyly, an extra metacarpal may lie obliquely or transversely in the centre of the palm causing deviation of the adjacent metacarpals and angulation of the fingers.

Treatment

With Type I polydactyly, the supernumerary digit is often tied off in the delivery room and allowed to slough. This is not advisable as there are risks of bleeding from necrosed vessels. Frequently an unsightly bump remains from a bifid metacarpal head. It is preferable to excise the supernumerary digit and any protuberant portion of the metacarpal head through an oval incision when the child is about 1 year old.

Duplication of the thumb may occur in several forms. Wassel [81] described seven types depending upon whether there is incomplete duplication of the distal phalanx, the proximal phalanx or the metacarpal (Types I, III and V), or total duplication of the distal phalanx, proximal phalanx, or metacarpal (Types II, IV and VI). He also classified triphalangeal thumbs as a type of polydactyly (Type VII).

A bifid distal phalanx usually appears as a widened tip

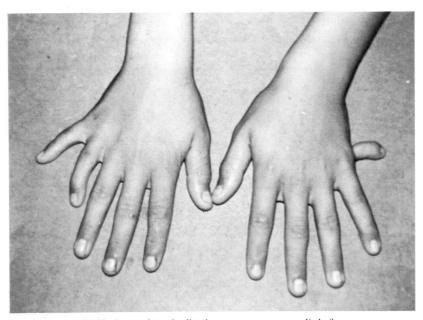

Fig. 24.32. Post-axial reduplication or supernumerary little fingers.

of thumb with a ridged or furrowed thumb nail. Resection of the bifurcated portion of the distal phalanx is often unsatisfactory as the narrowed thumbtip is angulated and protrudes from a broad base. For this reason, Bilhaut recommended central wedge resection of opposing surfaces of the bifid distal phalanx so as to narrow the thumbtip by approximation of the osteotomized surfaces [74]. A similar procedure was recommended by Bilhaut and Cloquet for total duplication of the distal phalanx. These procedures risk damaging the epiphyseal plate and are not suitable for cases with mild widening. With more severe widening or with total duplication of the distal phalanx, the radial supernumerary digit should be excised with the portion of the head of the proximal phalanx with which it articulates (Fig. 24.33). The collateral ligament is preserved and allowed to remain attached to the neck of the proximal phalanx. It is then sutured into the remaining phalanx at the thumbtip so as to maintain stability at the interphalangeal joint. Surgery is advised at 18 months of age.

In severe angulation at the interphalangeal joint (Fig. 24.34), arthrodesis may be required at the age of 8–10 years, with care to avoid damage to the epiphyseal plate.

A similar procedure is performed with duplication more proximally. If there is duplication of the proximal and distal phalanges (Type IV) (Fig. 24.35), a racquet-shaped incision is made about the metacarpophalangeal joint of the supernumerary thumb. Usually, the radial thumb is the smaller and has less function. If the ulnar thumb is the more affected, it is removed. If the radial digit is to be removed, the insertion of the abductor pollicis brevis is identified and preserved, if the ulnar thumb, the adductor pollicis tendon is preserved. The collateral ligament is detached distally and, if possible, stripped with the periosteum to the metacarpal neck. The supernumerary digit is excised with the articular surface of the metacarpal with which it articulates. The metacarpal is appropriately shaped so that it forms a smooth surface with the remaining proximal phalanx. Collateral ligament and appropriate tendon are sutured to the base

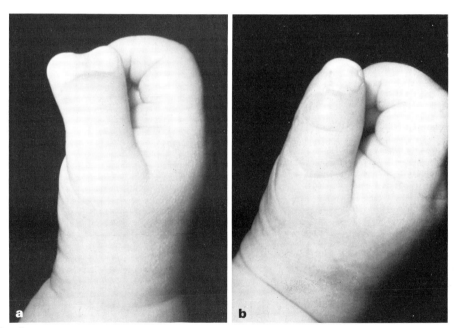

Fɪɢ. 24.33. Bifid thumb.

(a) A bifid proximal phalanx with duplication of the distal phalanx (Wassel Type III) is treated by excision of the supernumerary distal phalanx and the radial half of the proximal phalanx. Stability to the distal phalanx is preserved by suturing the dorsal apparatus of the duplicated radial thumb to the base of the distal phalanx of the remaining thumb to create a collateral ligament. The thumbtip is immobilized with a longitudinal Kirschner wire for about four weeks postoperatively.

(b) Postoperative condition.

of the proximal phalanx and, if necessary, a thin Kirschner wire is placed through the metacarpophalangeal joint for four weeks to hold the thumb in its correct position.

Careful attention must be paid to the tendons of the preserved digit which may be off-centre, tending to deviate the tip, and partial resection or transfer of the tendon to balance the thumb may be necessary. If the remaining thumb is deficient in its flexor or extensor apparatus, a tendon from the sacrificed thumb may be used for transfer. If skin on the concave side of the thumb is tight, Z-plasty or a local rotation flap may prevent recurrence of the angulatory deformity. Post-operatively, the thumb is immobilized for a period of

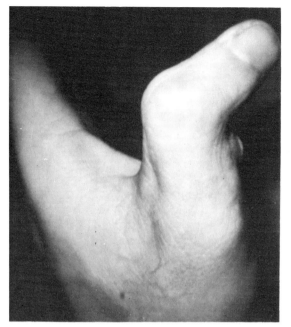

Fig. 24.34. Seventeen years previously, a supernumerary distal phalanx was excised and apparently no attempt was made to reconstruct the soft tissues on the ulnar side of the interphalangeal joint. Gradually, the distal phalanx deviated radially and the head of the proximal phalanx became progressively more deformed.

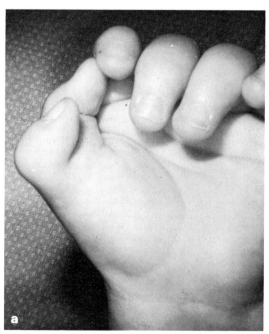

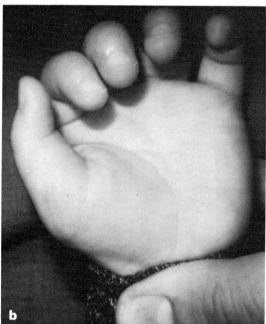

Fig. 24.35. Duplication of the thumb.

(a) The proximal and distal phalanges of the thumb are duplicated (Wassel Type IV). As the appearance and motion of the more ulnar thumb is virtually normal, there is no question but that the radial digit is to be removed.

(b) The radial digit has been excised. The radial condyle of the first metacarpal was removed and the abductor pollicis brevis sutured to the radial base of the proximal phalanx to preserve metocarpophalangeal joint stability. The appearance of the hand is much improved.

about 4 weeks. If deviation develops at the site of duplication, tendon transfer or arthrodesis must be considered when the child is older.

Polydactyly of the little finger is treated similarly by removing the ulnar supernumerary digit, preserving or reconstructing the muscular and ligamentous structures on the ulnar side of the remaining little finger. At the metacarpophalangeal joint, the abductor digiti quinti is preserved and sutured to the ulnar side of the proximal phalanx and with duplication more distally, a part of the dorsal apparatus of the excised finger may be preserved to reconstruct the collateral ligament at the proximal or distal interphalangeal joint.

With duplication of index [82], middle and ring fingers the supernumerary digit usually is hypoplastic and may be joined to its neighbour in a complex syndactyly. With a jumble of extra metacarpals and phalanges in the centre of the hand, one should plan reconstruction to achieve the best function and appearance by preserving those parts of the removable digits which may be required for the remaining fingers [83]. If the super-

numerary digits are hidden and cause no functional harm, they should be left untreated.

Is it justifiable to excise a supernumerary digit which causes no functional harm? In most societies, any deviation from the normal is considered a deformity. To subject a child to the taunts of his playmates, the reflected guilt of his parents and the often horrified glances of strangers because of a correctable congenital deformity of the hand is unwise and unnecessary. Although function should be our first priority in planning reconstructive surgery of the hand, aesthetics cannot be ignored.

Ulnar dimelia and mirror hands [84, 86] (Fig. 24.36a)

Ulnar dimelia with mirror hand is rare but sporadic cases are reported [87, 88].

Despite its rarity, there is a clinical pattern of associated deformities. The thumb and thenar muscles are absent. There are usually two, three or four hypoplastic

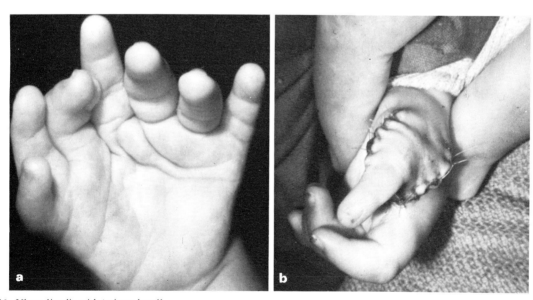

FIG. 24.36. Ulnar dimelia with 'mirror hand'.

(a) The four ulnar digits of this left hand appear relatively normal. The four radial digits are based upon two metacarpals. R1 is biphalangeal and appears more like a thumb than a finger. R3 and R4 are syndactylous. Intrinsic muscles of the palm insert onto the radial side of R1. Both forearm bones are similar and at the elbow have the configuration of two ulnae. At the wrist, they flare and give the appearance of two radii. There was good elbow motion but the wrist tended to fall into palmarflexion.

(b) The R3 digit was selected to remain as a thumb as it appeared to have the best motion and position. The R1, R2 and R4 rays were excised.

digits, each with three phalanges, flexion deformity at the interphalangeal joints and varying degrees of simple syndactyly. The carpal bones are difficult to identify. Typically there is a central lunate from which a series of carpal bones radiates, representing symmetrical pairs of triquetrum, hamate and capitate. Because of the natural arch of the palm, the radial supernumerary digits are pronated relative to the more 'ulnar' fingers. The wrist is deviated radially. Of the two ulnae, the radial one is more slender but each will articulate with the humerus, the articular surface of which is abnormal, possessing two trochleae. The proximal end of the humerus, the scapula and the clavicle often show less extensive abnormalities.

The anomaly may be unilateral or bilateral. In at least one case [85], bilateral duplication of the ulna and absence of the radius was associated with bilateral duplication of the fibulae and absence of the tibiae.

The deformity is frightening and grotesque to the layman. A string of fingers dangles from the infant's hand and it will be covered with oversized mittens by the embarrassed parents. Early surgical correction is indicated to avoid prolonged psychological trauma to the family which is inevitably sensed by the child. The infant is observed carefully to determine which of the radial digits is best suited functionally to serve as a thumb (Fig. 24.36b). The selection of the expendable fingers is more difficult when there are three or four from which to choose. After the choice is made, the extra digits are removed with their metacarpals and the carpal bones more proximally. The variability in carpal configuration is such that each case must be planned separately. The stability of the remaining fingers must be achieved by reconstructing the collateral ligaments. Often, tendons of the adjacent sacrificed fingers can be used to stabilise the remaining digits.

OVERGROWTH (GIGANTISM, MACRODACTYLY)

R. J. SMITH

Macrodactyly, or gigantism of a digit, may be primary, or secondary to tumour or exogenous factors. In the primary or true macrodactyly, there is enlargement of all tissues of the involved finger giving it an elongated, broadened and swollen appearance. In over 80 per cent

of patients, macrodactyly is unilateral; in 70 per cent of cases there is multiple finger involvement, the fingers being always adjacent. Of 132 macrodactylous digits reviewed by Barsky [89], 26 involved the thumb, 46 the index finger, 41 the middle finger, 16 the ring finger and in only 3 were the little fingers involved. In none of these cases was there a family history of similar abnormality.

In primary macrodactyly, finger enlargements may be seen at birth or develop within the first 2 years. Disproportionate enlargement of the involved fingers may continue with swelling of the contiguous areas of the palm but growth usually ceases after puberty. Of 16 patients with macrodactyly reported by Khanna *et al*, none had syndactyly or polydactyly [94]. Eight were static and 8 progressive. Of the static type, all had enlargements of only one finger without involvement of the contiguous palm (Fig. 24.37). Of the progressive type, all had involvement of two or more digits as well as thickening of the palm. The phalanges of the macrodactylous digit are increased in length and breadth. Typically, the growth centres show advanced maturation so that the skeletal age of the involved phalanges may be as much as one or two years greater than the chronological age of the patient or the skeletal age of the uninvolved fingers. Asymmetric growth of the phalanges usually causes deviation of the fingers towards the less involved side. The finger nail is broad and unfurrowed. The skin is relatively normal in colour and texture but may be somewhat bulbous in areas of fat hypertrophy. Occasionally, there may be diminution of sensibility, but trophic changes are uncommon.

In the affected digits, the blood vessels are elongated and angiography has revealed hypertrophy usually affecting the vessels of only one side. The subcutaneous fat is markedly hypertrophic and has the appearance of adult abdominal fat. Large fat globules are found throughout the volar aspect of the finger intimately associated with the nerves. The most consistent and distinctive pathological changes are in the digital nerves, which are broad, tortuous and covered by a rather thick epineurium lacking the lustre and sheen normally seen in a child. Nerve branches are intimately adherent to the fat globules which appear to envelop them. On histological section, there is a proliferation of the fibrous endoneurium and perineurium which causes coarseness of the axon cylinders, narrowing of the myelin and compression of the axons. The fatty and bony enlargement of the finger is restricted to the area in which these nerve changes are found. Basset *et al* have found a proliferation of fibroblastic tissue between the bone cortex and the periosteum in the region of peripheral nerve fibrosis about which there was increased osteoid in one phalanx and bone destruction in another [90]. The close association between peripheral nerve abnormality and macrodactyly [95], as well as the occasional association of neurofibromatosis with enlarged digits, inevitably has led many to question whether primary macrodactyly is a *forme fruste* of neurofibromatosis [92]. However, this association appears unlikely. Neurofibromatosis is usually an inherited disorder and many members of a family show various stigmata of the disease including café-au-lait spots, scoliosis, pseudarthrosis of the tibia

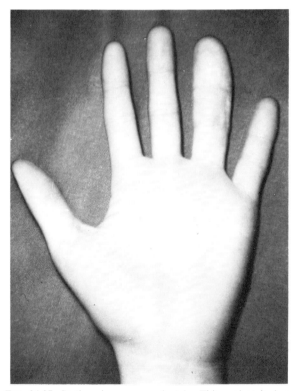

FIG. 24.37. Static primary macrodactyly. This patient had no stigmata of neurofibromatosis, no abnormalities elsewhere and no family history of gigantism. The soft tissues of the ring finger were grossly enlarged but there was no involvement of the palm. Typical of static macrodactyly, only one finger was involved. Excision of excessive soft tissues provided the finger with reasonable function and appearance.

and diffuse peripheral nerve changes. Such is not the case with primary macrodactyly. In addition, the fibro-lipomatous changes found about the branches of the median nerve with primary macrodactyly are quite different from the neuropathology of neurofibromatosis.

Nonetheless, the possibility of a neurogenic cause of macrodactyly remains. Inglis has suggested a neuro-intrinsic factor which may be the cause of the finger hypertrophy [92]. Others have suggested a disturbance in growth limiting factors as the cause of the deformities. To date, no mutation, chromosomal abnormality, nor genetically determined factor has been associated with macrodactyly. Although macrodactyly of the fingers may rarely be associated with macrodactyly of the toes (the abnormality is three times more frequent in the hands than in the feet), it is rare that there are any other associated skeletal or visceral changes. There have been reports of radio-capitellar dysplasia with radial head dislocation in patients with macrodactyly. Whether this abnormality is related to the finger deformity or is coincidental is unclear.

Secondary macrodactyly may be due to neurofibromatosis (with the stigmata of neurofibromatosis found elsewhere), haemangioma and other vascular abnormalities, lymphoedema—which may occasionally be secondary to proximal annular bands, or to skeletal abnormalities with bone tumours or endocrine dysfunction. Even acromegaly may be considered a type of secondary macrodactyly of all digits. In each of these conditions, the treatment of macrodactyly is usually secondary to the treatment of the underlying disorder.

Treatment of primary macrodactyly

A macrodactylous digit is unsightly, stiff and usually functions poorly. The goals of surgery are to decrease its size, prevent its continued growth, correct its angulatory deformity and, if possible, increase motion at its stiffened joints.

If macrodactyly involves only one finger which is unsightly, deformed and stiff, serious consideration should be given to its amputation. A three-fingered hand with a normal thumb is usually more functional and more aesthetic than one with a reconstructed macrodactylous digit. If the family does not wish amputation, or if multiple fingers are involved, reconstructive surgery is indicated.

Various means have been used in the past to prevent increased growth of the finger. These have included epiphyseal stapling, epiphyseodesis [91, 93], arterial ligation and nerve transection. With epiphyseal arrest, the longitudinal growth of the finger can be halted but the phalanges remain broad and continue to increase in diameter and the soft tissue enlargement proceeds unchecked. Ultimately, the finger may be of normal length but will look bulbous and unattractive. Arterial ligation is not successful and nerve division, to prevent the formation of 'neural intrinsic factor', interferes with the sensibility of the finger and gives disappointing results in control of finger growth.

If the finger is too large (Fig. 24.38a), it may be reduced in size by resection of the distal end of the middle phalanx and the proximal end of the distal phalanx [96]. An arthrodesis of the distal interphalangeal joint is then performed and the digit shortened (Fig. 24.38b). Angulatory deformity (Fig. 24.38a) may be corrected by wedge resection (Fig. 24.38b). The resulting bulge of excessive soft tissue at the volar aspect of the finger

should be resected three months after osteotomy. Excessive fatty tissue at the pulp and volar side of the finger and at the branches of the digital nerve may be removed at this time. Excess skin is resected with care taken to preserve the circulation to the fingertip. Frequently, soft tissue resection must be performed in two separate stages subsequent to osteotomy and bone shortening. If the nail is excessively broad, both the nail and its matrix may be partially removed and the eponychial fold resutured about the new nail margins.

Some surgeons have advocated narrowing of the phalanges in a macrodactylous digit by longitudinal osteotomy through the joint surfaces. This procedure appears to jeopardize the stability and motion of the joints postoperatively. Limited motion may be caused by osteophytes which form about asymmetrical joint surfaces. Arthroplasty might be considered in such fingers. To date, there have been no reports of arthroplasty of the stiffened joints of a reconstructed macrodactylous digit.

When considering surgical reconstruction for macro-

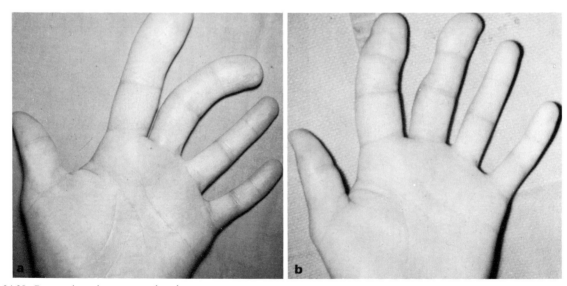

FIG. 24.38. Progressive primary macrodactyly.

(a) Marked enlargement of bone and soft tissue of the index and middle fingers and the contiguous area of the palm causes unsightly deformities and awkward, inefficient grip in this patient with progressive macrodactyly. There were no other abnormalities. Ulnar deviation of the middle finger is due to asymetrical involvement of the digit with maximum enlargement to its radial side. Thus, like a thermocouple, the finger angulates ulnarly.

(b) The fingers have been shortened and straightened by resection/angulation osteotomies accompanied by excision of excessive soft tissue. Although function was improved, the aesthetic result is somewhat indifferent. (Smith, R. J. and Lipke, R. W. In *Management of Peripheral Nerve Problems*, G. E. Omer and M. Spinner. Fig. 42.8, 705. Philadelphia, Saunders, 1980.)

dactyly, one must be aware of the possibility of the deformities worsening in patients with progressive poly-dactylous involvement. In these patients, the results of surgery are usually less satisfactory than in those with static macrodactyly.

CONGENITAL CONSTRICTION BAND SYNDROME

R. J. SMITH

Annular grooves and acrosyndactyly (constriction band syndrome)

Congenital transverse grooves may appear anywhere about the limbs. They are most frequent in the distal portion and in the hands. Index, middle and ring fingers are affected with approximately equal frequency, the little finger less often and the thumb rarely. Annular grooves are twice as frequent in the upper limb than the lower and only occasionally is the lower limb involved alone.

Annular grooves occur sporadically and are not genetically transmitted. Associated abnormalities occur in the involved limb at or distal to the pathological grooves. Cleft palate and cleft lip have been described in association but may well be coincidental.

The cause is still unresolved although Streeter, McKusick and others favour an endogenous aetiology. Streeter refers to focal necrosis of mesenchymal elements predetermined by germ cell abnormality and leading to a primary circumscribed tissue deficiency [108]. McKusick believes the grooves may be due to focal necrosis on a vascular basis [103]. In the first half of the 19th century, Montgomery and Simpson suggested an exogenous cause and that the grooves were the result of compression by the amnion or umbilical cord [104, 107]. Browne described an amnion with several perforations associated with amputated fetal parts in an infant with annular bands [97]. Field and Krag reported histological studies of the placentas of two infants with congenital amputation of the fingers and toes and constricting bands about the fingers and ankles, both of whom had abnormality of the amnion [98].

Annular grooves lie at right angles to the longitudinal axis of the limb. They may vary in severity from a superficial depression in the skin one-third of the way around a finger to a deep, circumferential band which causes amputation of all parts distal to it. These amputated and gangrenous portions of the limbs on occasion have been delivered at birth. More frequently, they appear to resorb during gestation. The severity of soft tissue and bony changes depends upon the location and the depth of the band. If it extends through skin and subcutaneous tissue, the distal portion is enlarged and oedematous, often giving the hand a balloon-like appearance of congenital elephantiasis. With deeper grooves, tendons may be damaged, nerves and vessels compressed, and bone indented, causing loss of sensibility and motion at the fingertips. With more severe involvement, vascular embarrassment at the time of birth may be so extensive that gangrene will supervene unless treatment is rendered promptly (Fig. 24.39a).

Congenital annular grooves are associated with syndactyly in over 50 per cent of cases. Typically, this is an *acrosyndactyly* which involves the more distal portions of the fingers and a sinus is usually present at the level of the proximal phalanges (Fig. 24.39b). The web proximal to the sinus is rarely normal and usually extends well distal to the web of the adjacent digit. The fingernails in the area of acrosyndactyly are usually abnormal and may be absent. Although acrosyndactyly rarely involves lateral fusion of adjacent fingers incomplete interphalangeal joint motion is common.

Bilateral asymmetric involvement of the upper limbs is common and the same patient may have a mild incomplete annular band in one digit, a deeper one in another and acrosyndactyly or amputation of other fingers (Fig. 24.40). The limb proximal to the annular bands is usually normal and ossification centres and limb growth usually proceed normally. Exogenous amputations often show scarring at the stump. Amputations are often multiple and variable in different limbs and can only be considered exogenous if the remaining skeleton shows no developmental abnormality except for those which are caused by the grooves. Anomalies can be considered endogenous if there is more proximal bone or soft tissue abnormality or if the defects are bilaterally symmetrical. Only endogenous deformities will have an hereditary history.

Treatment

This is twofold:

(1) Release of the circumferential band to re-estab-

lymphatic and venous drainage from the distal portions and to prevent the groove from deepening and causing further soft tissue damage;

(2) Release of any syndactyly.

Release of bands. If, at birth, a circumferential annular groove jeopardizes the distal circulation, early surgery is indicated to prevent gangrene. With less severe bands, surgery may be delayed for several months.

Excision of the grooves and Z-plasty are usually sufficient to release constriction and to re-establish the lymphatic drainage. The groove and soft tissue involvement are usually more severe dorsally than volarly. Dissection of the dorsal tissues is less hazardous than dissection volarly in the neighbourhood of small nerves and arteries.

Surgery is thus performed first at the dorsum of the finger or hand, the groove being excised rather than incised in order to remove the granulation tissue at its depth. One or two Z's with 60° angles are fashioned, the flaps transposed, and held in place by 5–0 absorbable sutures. The limb is appropriately splinted and protected until healed. The volar side of the groove may be re-leased 3–6 months later. Although several fingers may be released simultaneously, it is both unwise and unnecessary to excise a band circumferentially in one stage. When dissecting and transposing the Z-plasty flaps on the volar side of the finger, one should be particularly alert to protect the soft tissue structures which lie just deep to the groove to be excised.

With deep involvement of the annular groove, tendons, nerves, and even bone may be affected. Secondary reconstructive procedures such as tendon transfers or grafts, nerve grafts and skeletal reconstruction should be postponed until Z-plasty flaps are healed and oedema has subsided. It has been reported that with deep grooves on the volar aspect of the fingers, skin replacement may be achieved by means of a cross-finger flap. We have not found this necessary.

Release of acrosyndactyly. The extent of acrosyndactyly may vary from a simple, distal skin bridge to a mass of several digits joined at their distal phalanges as though they had been tied together with a string. Attention must also be directed towards the webs proximal to the interdigital sinus. The sinus is usually small and its proximal

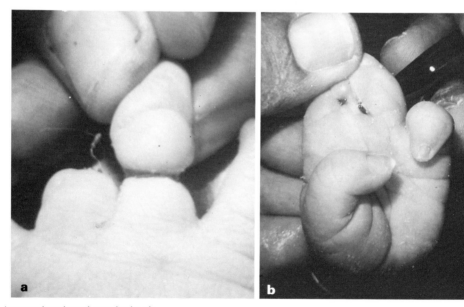

FIG. 24.39. Acrosyndactyly and annular bands.

(a) This newborn with a tight annular band around the middle finger required immediate release in order to save the fingertip. The dorsum of the band was excised and the skin transposed by means of Z-plasties.

(b) The typical sinus of acrosyndactyly on the volar aspect.

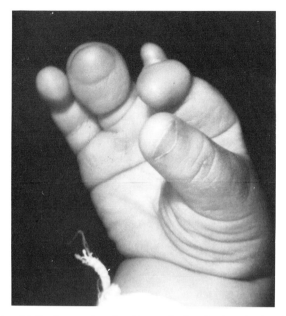

FIG. 24.40. Acrosyndactyly with annular bands. Annular bands involving all four fingers of the right hand with partial amputations of the index and middle fingers. Simple syndactyly of the second web released previously and the first stage of circumferential Z-plasty of the ring finger was performed. Further reconstructive surgery includes release of the annular band around the little finger, volar release of the annular band of the ring finger and release of the annular band around the index finger both volarly and dorsally.

border may be tilted distally or volarly, radially or ulnarly. It is best to deepen the web at the same time as the syndactyly release. Shallow, incomplete annular grooves may be freed at the same time. If there is oedema and a tight constricting band, however, the band should be released at least six months to a year prior to freeing the syndactyly.

The techniques of syndactyly release are similar to those used for other types of syndactyly (Fig. 24.28). Interdigitating volar and dorsal V-incisions create the web. Zig-zag incisions at the volar and dorsal sides of the fingers create complementary flaps. Full thickness skin grafts are placed at denuded areas. Due to the hypertrophy of the subcutaneous tissues which is so often present, defatting the flaps will usually permit the sides of the fingers to be closed without difficulty. Residual limitation of motion of the interphalangeal joints should

be expected in these patients, even with excellent release of the syndactyly.

In some cases, absence of a central digit leaves an unsightly space in the middle of the hand and small coins, beads and other playthings will fall from the grasp. Holding screws and bolts, hair grips and buttons will be awkward with a fenestrated grasp. For these reasons, ray transfer may be useful as a late reconstructive procedure.

MISCELLANEOUS

R. J. SMITH

A group of minor deformities, difficult to classify.

Triphalangeal thumb [109–112]

Triphalangeal thumbs occur once in every 25 000 births. The extra phalanx appears usually between a relatively normal proximal and distal phalanx and may be wedge-shaped, giving an ulnar tilt to the thumbtip. There may also be duplication of the thumb either on the same or on the opposite hand. Triphalangism may represent an arrest in development of a supernumerary or bifid thumb, or the extra phalanx may represent a phylogenetic throwback with restoration of a lost or missing middle phalanx of the thumb.

It often appears as a dominant inherited trait which has been followed in up to five generations in one family and is frequently associated with other congenital anomalies of the hand, including polydactyly, syndactyly and partial aplasia or hypoplasia of the radius of the same or opposite limb. In some patients, there is absence of the thumb in one hand and a triphalangeal thumb in the other.

A radial-most digit which is triphalangeal may be an extra finger rather than a triphalangeal thumb and in such a five-fingered hand, the radial digit lies parallel to the adjacent digit (Fig. 24.41), and is attached by a deep transverse metacarpal ligament. Its muscular and tendinous structures are similar to those of the fingers and on its ulnar side is a typical interdigital web unlike that between a thumb and index finger.

The treatment of the triphalangeal thumb depends upon its size, stability and the nature of any angulatory

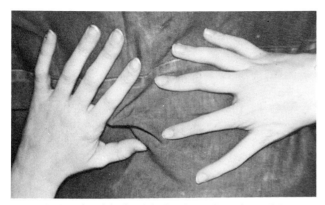

FIG. 24.41. The right hand is five-fingered as the radial-most digit has the length, circumference and general configuration of a finger rather than a thumb. In these cases the epiphyses will usually be in the finger position rather than the thumb position.

deformity. It will also depend upon whether there is duplication of the thumb adjacent to the site of triphalangism. With a small, wedge-shaped extra phalanx, excision of the excessive bone and arthrodesis of the proximal to the distal phalanx will usually correct angulatory deformity and appropriately diminish the size of the thumb. If the extra phalanx is rectangular and the deformity is mainly one of excessive length, both stability and appearance are improved by segmental resection of the distal end of the proximal phalanx and the proximal end of the middle phalanx. The neck of the middle phalanx is then held to the shaft of the proximal phalanx with oblique Kirschner wires. By this procedure, the thumb is shortened and the normal number of joints and phalanges is restored.

Simple resection of the extra phalanx in cases of triphalangeal thumb will be unsuccessful in restoring normal alignment to a deviated thumb if the opposing articular surfaces of the distal and proximal phalanges are not parallel and stability of the newly created joint often will be poor. In a five-fingered hand, pollicization of the radial-most digit to create a broad first web and to shorten and rotate the radial finger is usually rewarded by improved function and appearance.

Delta-phalanx deformity [113–116]

The delta-phalanx refers to a triangular or delta-shaped phalanx with an abnormally shaped epiphyseal plate

[113]. A similar abnormality may occur in the metacarpals. Occasionally, triangular remnants of phalanges may be present in hands with polydactyly or in triphalangeal thumbs. In these cases, the epiphyseal plate is horizontal but the development of the phalanx is abnormal. The abnormal shape of the phalanx causes lateral or medial deviation. If a phalanx or metacarpal has a proximal and distal articular surface which are not parallel, corrective osteotomy may be performed after the age of four or five in order to improve the function and the appearance of the affected digit. With an abnormal central phalanx in the triphalangeal thumb, partial excision of the central phalanx and its arthrodesis with the proximal phalanx is recommended as discussed in the section on *Triphalangeal thumb*.

The classical delta-phalanx with a J-shaped epiphyseal plate is of particular interest both because of its etiology and treatment. This abnormality is most frequent in the proximal phalanx of the thumb and in the little finger. The epiphyseal plate lies in the normal transverse plane in the portion of the digit closest to the centre of the hand (ulnar side of thumb and radial side of little finger). At the outer border of the affected digit (radial side of thumb and ulnar side of little finger), the epiphyseal plate curves distally and longitudinally. The distal articular surface of the involved phalanx slopes proximally at the side of the phalanx with the abnormal epiphyseal plate. Thus, with the thumb, the epiphyseal plate is transverse at its ulnar half and longitudinal at its radial half. The distal end of the affected phalanx slopes proximally at its radial side causing the distal phalanx to be radially deviated (Fig. 24.42a). The opposite deformity occurs in the little finger. The distal phalanges of the involved finger or thumb are also abnormal and Watson and Boyes [115] have suggested that the abnormality represents an abortive formation of a supernumerary digit. We have found that this type of delta-phalanx is not always associated with supernumerary digits. It does, however, appear to represent a complex syndactyly. The portions of the digit distal to the abnormal phalanx are either completely or incompletely duplicated. The nail is broad and often furrowed longitudinally. There is usually a bony fenestration in the wide, distal phalanx.

The deformity caused by the delta-phalanx is unsightly and the digit is awkward. If possible, surgical correction should narrow the digit, lengthen and straighten the phalanx and destroy the abnormal portion of the

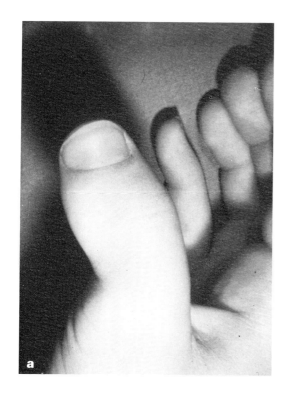

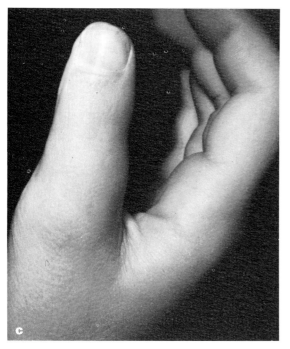

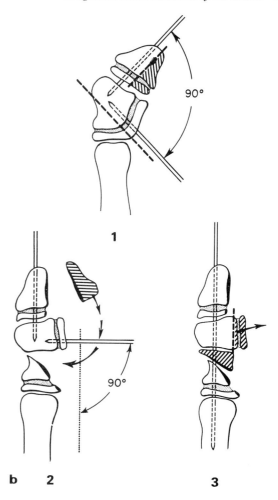

FIG. 24.42. Delta-phalanx.

(a) Frequently, the delta-phalanx, which is often trapezoidal in shape, has a J-shaped epiphysis, transverse to the convex side and longitudinal to its concave side. The phalanx represents a complex syndactyly with an abortive digit to its radial side. Note the broadened distal phalanx with a perforation towards its distal end as well as the broadened thumbnail. The deformity is quite unsightly.

(b) The thumb is narrowed, the abnormal epiphyseal plate excised and the deformity corrected by removing supernumerary portions of the distal phalanx and the longitudinal portion of the epiphyseal plate and performing an open wedge osteotomy at the base of the delta-phalanx. Excised portions of the distal phalanx are used as a free graft to fill the open wedge osteotomy.

(c) The thumb is narrowed and alignment improved by this procedure.

epiphyseal plate. We have found that these goals can frequently be obtained by the following method [114] (Fig. 24.42b):

A Kirschner wire is passed longitudinally through the tip of the digit distal to the delta-phalanx. The supernumerary bone is excised. A second Kirschner wire is placed in the delta-phalanx in the coronal plane perpendicular to the first wire and distal to the transverse portion of the epiphyseal plate (Fig. 24.42b1). The delta-phalanx is divided just proximal to the second Kirschner wire. The second wire is then swung in the coronal plane until it is perpendicular to the longitudinal axis of the proximal segment of the involved digit (Fig. 24.42b2). The bone chips of the excised supernumerary phalanx are placed in the open wedge created by the movement of the second wire. The first Kirschner wire is then passed longitudinally through the osteotomy site and into the more proximal portion of the digit (Fig. 24.42b3). The second wire is removed. Occasionally, the skin to the concave side of the digit requires lengthening by means of Z-plasty or skin graft (Fig. 9.14). By this procedure, the digit is straightened (Fig. 24.42c), the

abnormal articular surface of the delta-phalanx is made parallel to the transverse axis of the digit and continued epiphyseal growth can be expected.

Camptodactyly [118, 119, 121, 122]

By definition, camptodactyly refers to a bent finger. By common usage, however, the term is applied to a congenital or developmental flexion contracture of the proximal interphalangeal joint of a finger unrelated to trauma, systemic disease or neurological abnormality (Fig. 24.43a). Neither the metacarpophalangeal nor the distal interphalangeal joints are usually affected and there is neither joint swelling nor thickening of the palmar aponeurosis. The little finger is the one characteristically affected.

There is a strong hereditary predisposition and the deformity has been traced through as many as five generations of a family showing an autosomal Mendelian dominant trait. Up to two per cent of the population may be affected and in just over two out of three, the

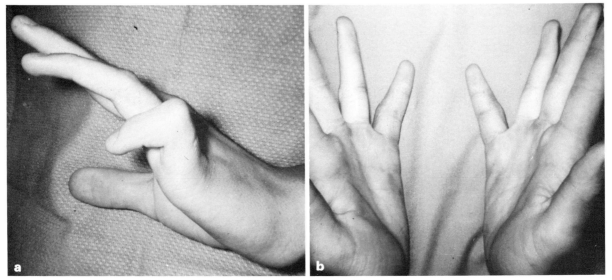

FIG. 24.43. (a) Camptodactyly with flexion of the proximal interphalangeal joint of the little finger. If the deformity can be completely corrected by wrist and metacarpophalangeal joint flexion, transsection of the flexor superficialis is advised. If there is weak proximal interphalangeal joint extension, this tendon may be withdrawn from the palm and then transferred to the dorsal apparatus in the manner of the Bunnell intrinsic transfer.

(b) This patient required only superficialis tenotomy and was able to achieve improved (although not complete) proximal interphalangeal joint extension even with his wrist dorsiflexed.

abnormality is bilateral, the right hand being usually more severely involved. Sixty-two per cent of the patients are females. Occasionally, contracture of the little finger is associated with similar contractures of the ring finger and, less frequently, of the middle and index fingers. Flexion contractures associated with brachydactyly, supernumerary digits, syndactyly or arthrogryposis are not considered as cases of typical camptodactyly.

Although the deformity may be present at birth, it usually is not noted until later in childhood. Up to the age of ten, the contracture is usually mild, unassociated with changes in the skin or fascia and may be diminished by holding the wrist or metacarpophalangeal joint in flexion. The contracture may remain unchanged for several years and then, during the growth spurt, may suddenly become more severe. The deformity does not increase past the age of 20 years. Although flexion deformity of the proximal interphalangeal joints may be as great as 90°, the finger retains ability to flex completely. After several years, a fold of volar skin may bowstring across the proximal segment of the finger and secondary changes of the proximal interphalangeal joint will appear as the finger rotates into supination.

Treatment

For mild deformity, treatment is neither sought nor indicated as function is usually normal. When the de-formity is more severe, treatment may be indicated to improve function and appearance.

Corrective splinting is frustrating and rarely succeeds in improving the attitude of the flexed finger. Virtually every structure about the base of the finger has been implicated as a deforming factor in camptodactyly. If proximal interphalangeal joint extension is improved by palmar flexing the wrist or proximal phalanx, the flexor digitorum superficialis is probably one of the deforming forces. If there is full active interphalangeal joint extension with wrist palmar flexion, the superficialis is divided close to its insertion and the finger splinted in extension for 4 weeks (Fig. 24.43b). If there is full passive but weak active extension of the proximal interphalangeal joint, the detached superficialis is transferred to the lateral band of the dorsal apparatus similar to the Stiles–Bunnell transfer for ulnar nerve palsy.

Where the flexion contracture is unaffected by flexion of the wrist or metacarpophalangeal joints, a radiograph often reveals bone changes about the proximal interphalangeal joint with a sulcus at the proximal articular surface of the middle phalanx and soft tissue surgery will almost certainly be unsuccessful. If flexion contracture remains after release of flexor superficialis but X-ray is normal, the proximal insertion of the volar plate and the attachment of the accessory collateral ligaments to the plate are divided. Tight volar skin may be released by Z-plasty or skin graft but where extensive soft tissue

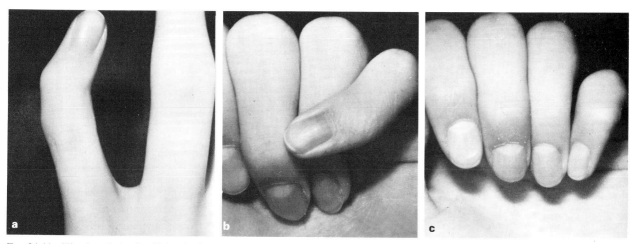

FIG. 24.44. Clinodactyly is a familial trait of unequal growth of both sides of the middle phalanges of the little finger (a), causing difficulty in typing, playing musical instruments, and grasping due to the overlapping little finger (b). Closed wedge osteotomy of the middle phalanx improved the alignment of the little finger (c).

release is required at the time of flexor superficialis tenotomy, the results of surgery are often disappointing. Surgery should thus be restricted to deformities which can be corrected preoperatively by wrist and meta-carpophalangeal flexion as capsular and skin contractures are likely to be relatively mild and superficialis tenotomy more successful. It has been recommended that in severe cases, the neck of the proximal phalanx may be divided and the distal fragment angulated dorsally to increase the apparent extension at the proximal interphalangeal joint. This procedure should be avoided as it may rob the finger of its excellent flexion.

Clinodactyly [120]

Angular deformity of the little finger, may occur (Fig. 24.44a), usually due to unequal growth of the sides of the middle phalanx. There is a familial tendency and it may be associated with chromosomal or genetic abnormalities.

The deformity may obstruct finger flexion (Fig. 24.44b) and is corrected by wedge osteotomy of the middle phalanx (Fig. 24.44c).

Kirner's deformity [117, 123, 124]

An infrequent but unsightly deformity of the fingertip may be caused by dysplasia of the epiphysis of the distal phalanx of the little finger (Fig. 24.45a). Occasionally, the deformity may affect several of the fingers. It appears more frequently in girls than boys, there is often a family history of similar abnormalities and the onset of the deformity usually does not occur until the child is 8–10 years of age. The distal segment of the finger gradually

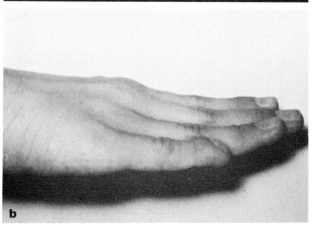

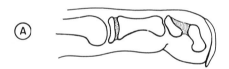

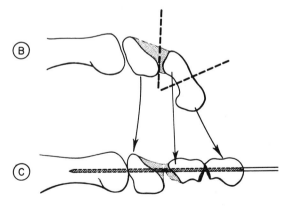

Fig. 24.45. Kirner's deformity is a flexion at the epiphysis of the distal phalanx of the little finger (a). It is due to an epiphyseal abnormality and may be corrected by appropriate osteotomies. Most patients find the deformity neither disabling nor particularly unsightly (b). It is important to differentiate this deformity from a mallet finger as neither splinting nor tendon exploration would be of any benefit. (c) Stages in operative correction of Kirner's deformity by osteotomy and Kirschner wire fixation.

enlarges, there is increasing convexity of the fingernail and the fingertip curves volarly and radially (Fig. 24.45b). The deformity may continue to increase for several years but is not painful. There are no associated abnormalities of the neurovascular structures or tendons about the affected finger. Radiographs reveal a broadened epiphyseal plate, often with irregularity of the metaphysis. The distal phalanx is curved volarly and radially with the apex of the concavity about the middle third of the phalanx (Fig. 24.45b).

For mild deformity, no treatment is indicated. If the deformity becomes severe and causes functional problems, as with typing or playing musical instruments, or if the patient finds its appearance objectionable, transverse correctional osteotomy would be justified. Occasionally, two osteotomies must be performed in the distal phalanx and the bone segments realigned and held with a Kirschner wire (Fig. 24.45c). No effective treatment has been described for correction of the nail deformity.

GENERALISED ABNORMALITIES OF THE SKELETON

RUTH WYNNE-DAVIES

Individually the skeletal dysplasias are rare, but collectively they form a large group of diseases characterized by a generalized disorder of bone and cartilage growth. Many patients are of short stature and there may in addition be some structural defect, such as the post-axial polydactyly in chondroectodermal dysplasia, cleft palate in spondyloepiphyseal dysplasia congenita, or congenital cataract in Conradi disease. In contrast to the malformation syndromes, the skeletal dysplasias often cannot be diagnosed clinically at birth, and when they do become apparent, the hand is unlikely to be the first point drawing the clinician's attention to the disease. However, examination of the hand is of interest in that it reflects the generalized disease and it is also of some importance in the differential diagnosis within this group of bone dysplasias.

The diagnosis of skeletal dysplasias from hand radiographs is made simpler by noting whether the changes are predominantly epiphyseal or metaphyseal, or whether both regions are affected; whether there is increased bone density, anarchic development of bone or any special structural defects such as absent terminal

phalanges or a short first metacarpal; these latter are noted in Table 24.2.

Predominantly epiphyseal changes

The commonest disorder in this group is *multiple epiphyseal dysplasia*. The disease develops at about 2 years of age and is of autosomal dominant inheritance. The fingers are short and stubby. Modelling of the shafts and the metaphyseal areas is relatively normal, but the epiphyses of all digits and the carpal bones are small, irregular and late in appearing (Fig. 24.46). In the severe

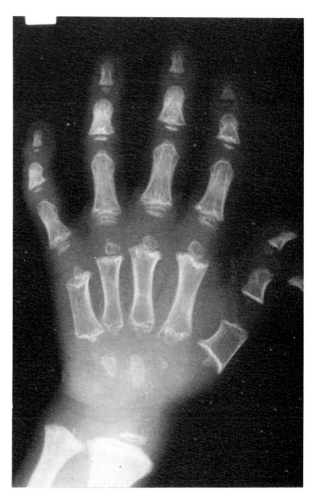

FIG. 24.46. Boy aged 8 years with multiple epiphyseal dysplasia. There is a little irregularity of the metaphyseal areas but it is predominantly epiphyses which are small and late in appearing.

form of multiple epiphyseal dysplasia the patient is likely to be stunted and most joints in the body are affected. Premature osteoarthritis is inevitable. The severe form of multiple epiphyseal dysplasia must be differentiated from the milder Ribbing type, which is of later onset and *without* changes in the wrist and hand.

Predominantly metaphyseal changes

Here the metaphyses tend to be broadened and irregular but the epiphyses are relatively normal and secondary osteoarthritis is not a feature. *Classical achondroplasia*, a short-limbed form of dwarfism has characteristic (though mild) changes in the hand. The trident appearance is well known, with stubby fingers, particularly short metacarpals and some flaring of the metaphyseal areas. This is one of the skeletal dysplasias that can be diagnosed clinically at birth and it is of autosomal dominant inheritance.

There are many different *metaphyseal chondrodysplasias*, of varying severity and patterns of inheritance. The *Jansen type* is the rarest, but has the most striking appearance in the hand, with almost normal epiphyses and expanded, cyst-like and fragmented metaphyseal

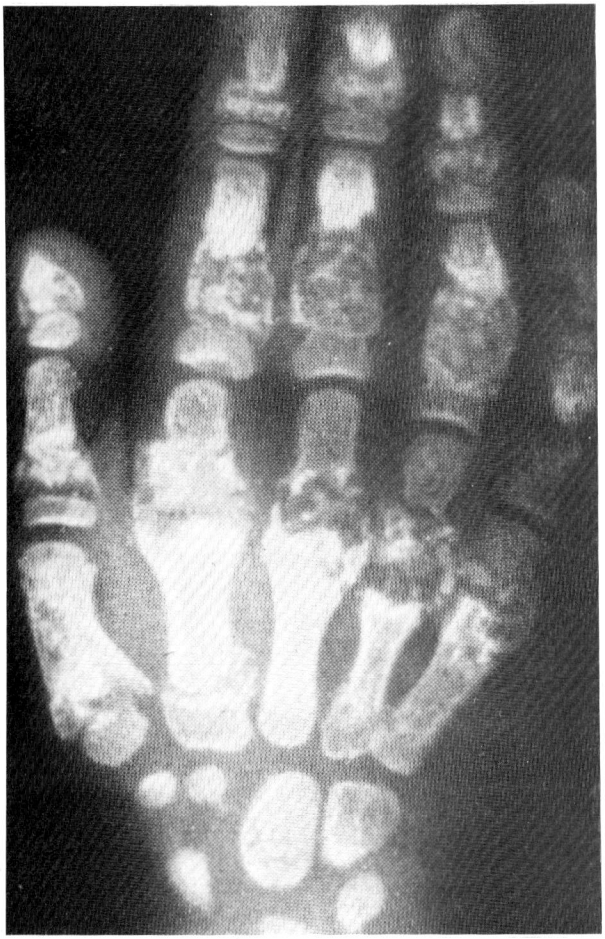

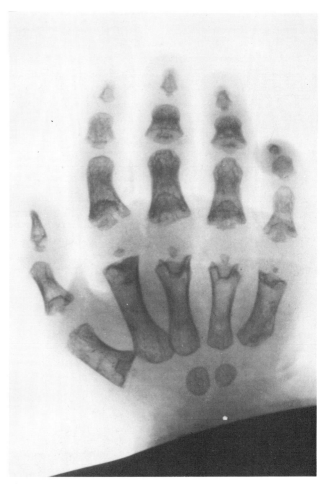

FIG. 24.47. Boy aged 7 years with metaphyseal chondrodysplasia type Jansen. The epiphyses are almost normal but the metaphyses are much expanded and cyst like.

FIG. 24.48. Boy aged 15 months with metaphyseal chondrodysplasia type McKusick. Epiphyses are normal but the metaphyses are wide and irregular.

areas (Fig. 24.47). The patients are dwarfed, all long bones in the body being similarly affected. *Type McKusick* is rather more common and considerably less severe. It may be apparent at birth or becomes so during early infancy. It is of autosomal recessive inheritance, thus there is a one in four chance that the parents will have a second affected child. The hands have short, wide phalanges and irregular metaphyseal areas with scalloping (Fig. 24.48). The rather similar *type Schmid* does not become apparent until about 2 years of age, and in contrast to type McKusick the hands are little affected, though there may be some metaphyseal

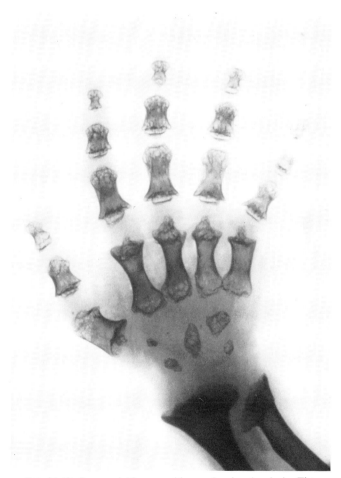

FIG. 24.49. Boy aged 10 years with pseudoachondroplasia. The epiphyses are small and late in appearing and metaphyses are very irregular.

sclerosis and irregularity at the lower end of the radius and ulna.

It is important to differentiate the metaphyseal chondrodysplasias from other diseases of bone affecting the metaphyses, in particular rickets (both nutritional and metabolic) and the hypophosphatasias, (congenita and tarda), diagnosis being made from abnormalities of blood chemistry in these latter diseases.

Both epiphyseal and metaphyseal changes

The commonest in this group of diseases is *pseudoachondroplasia*, a short-limbed form of dwarfism with irregular vertebrae as well as affected epiphyses and metaphyses of long bones. The hands are short and stubby with expanded metaphyses, and the epiphyses are small, late appearing and very irregular (Fig. 24.49). Unlike classical achondroplasia the disease is not apparent until about 2 years of age and premature osteoarthritis is inevitable and severe. There is more than one form of pseudoachondroplasia since both autosomal dominant and recessive forms have been described.

The storage diseases, in particular the *mucopolysaccharidoses* and *mucolipidoses* also have epiphyseal, metaphyseal and vertebral changes. It is typical of the group that the radiographic signs are similar in all of them, though the degree of involvement of the skeleton varies considerably. None of the mucopolysaccharidoses can be diagnosed at birth (except by biochemical means), and all are of recessive inheritance. Figure 24.50 is an example of Hurler's disease, which becomes clinically apparent around 6 months of age. The hand is characteristic, with generalized coarse trabeculation of bone, a pointed base to the second to fifth metacarpals, bullet-shaped phalanges and late appearance of the epiphyses. In Morquio's disease (Fig. 24.51) the pointed metacarpal bases are similar, as are the irregular and late appearing epiphyses, but there is here the distinguishing feature of constriction of the metacarpal shafts.

Increased density of bone

The best known of this group is *osteopetrosis* in which the congenital form is of great severity and of recessive inheritance, while the tarda form is milder, and of dominant inheritance. On radiography (Fig. 24.52) there is overall increase of bone density, some failure of modelling and sometimes an appearance of a 'bone-within-a-bone'.

Other members of the 'increased density' group are pycnodysostosis, sclerosteosis (with accompanying syndactyly), Engelmann's disease and other even rarer forms. All have some failure of long bone modelling in addition.

Anarchic development of bone

These disorders with their irregular asymmetrical bony changes are perhaps more allied to tumours than to skeletal dysplasias. The best known is *diaphyseal aclasis*,

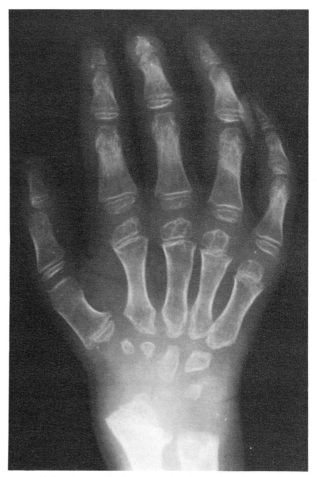

FIG. 24.51. Boy aged 12 years with Morquio's disease. Both metaphyses and epiphyses are involved, there is the same pointed base of the second to fifth metacarpals as in Hurler's disease but here the metacarpals are 'waisted'.

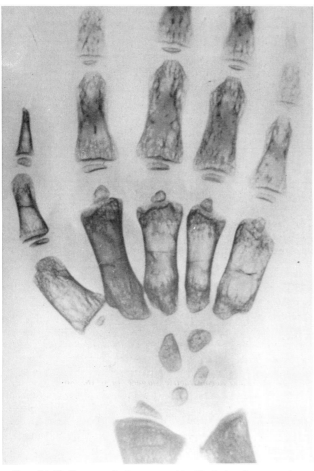

FIG. 24.50. Boy aged 3 years with Hurler's disease. The trabeculae are coarse, the second to fifth metacarpal bases are pointed and phalanges bullet shaped.

which may present with small exostoses of the digits. These rarely attain large dimensions and may even disappear, though the usual outcome is that growth of the exostosis stops with growth of the child. The condition is of autosomal dominant inheritance and usually becomes apparent around the age of 5 years.

Other members of this 'anarchic' group are sporadic, not inherited, and although lesions may be bilateral, they are rarely symmetrical. *Ollier's disease* (multiple enchondromatosis) not infrequently involves the bones of the hand (Fig. 24.53), with metacarpal and phalangeal lesions expanding over the whole length of the bone.

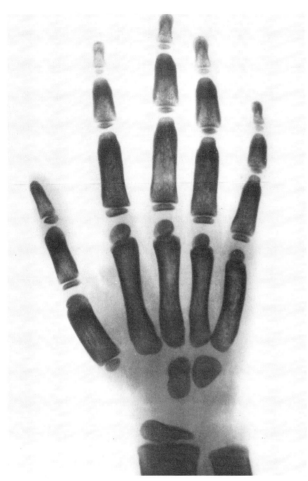

FIG. 24.52. Girl aged 4 years with osteopetrosis tarda. Bone density is increased and there is failure of modelling.

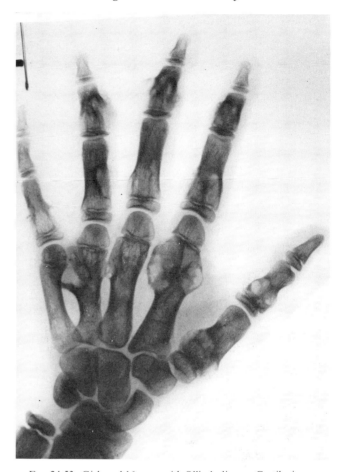

FIG. 24.53. Girl aged 16 years with Ollier's disease. Cartilaginous masses have developed asymmetrically in the metaphyseal regions expanding down the shafts.

Huge cartilaginous masses may develop giving rise to very considerable deformity which may require amputation. The lesions do not usually progress after puberty. The rather similar *Maffucci's syndrome* is accompanied by multiple haemangiomata or lymphangiomata of the soft tissues. Malignant change is reported only rarely in Ollier's disease, but is a characteristic feature of Maffucci's. *Melorheostosis* is characterized by sclerotic linear streaks along the length of a bone. Soft tissue contractures are present and deposits of bone around the joints add to the stiffness and limitation of movement. It is one of the few general affections of the skeleton in which pain is a feature.

REFERENCES

[1] BIRCH-JENSEN, A. *Congenital Deformities of the Upper Extremities.* Odense, Andelsbogtrykkeriet, 1949.

[2] CONWAY, H. AND BOWE, J. Congenital deformities of the hands. *Plastic and Reconstructive Surgery*, 1956, **18**, 286.

[3] ROGALA, E. J., WYNNE-DAVIES, R., LITTLEJOHN, A. AND GORMLEY, J. Congenital limb anomalies. Frequency and etiological factors. *Journal of Medical Genetics*, 1974, **11**, 221.

[4] ENTIN, M., BARSKY, A. AND SWANSON, A. Classification of congenital anomalies. *The Hand*, 1972, **4**, 215.

[5] KAY, H. W. International classification. *Inter-Clinic Information Bulletin*, 1975, **14**, No. 3.

[6] TEMTAMY, S. AND McKUSICK, V. A. Synopsis of hand malformations, with particular emphasis on genetic factors. In

Birth Defects: Original article Series 5, Part 3, pp. 125–184. New York, National Foundation. March of Dimes, 1969.

[7] SAUNDERS, J. W., Jr., GASSELING, M. T. AND SAUNDERS, L. C. Cellular death in morphogenesis of the avian wing. *Developmental Biology*, 1962, **5,** 147.

[8] Le DOUBLE, A. F. *Traité des Variations du Système Musculaire de l'homme*. Paris, Schleicher Frères, 1897.

[9] EDWARDS, E. A. Organisation of the small arteries in the hand and digits. *American Journal of Surgery*, 1960, **99,** 837.

[10] COLEMAN, S. S. AND ANSON, B. J. Arterial patterns in the hand. *Surgery, Gynecology and Obstetrics*, 1961, **113,** 409.

[11] LAMB, D. W. The reconstruction of congenital deformities of the hand. *British Journal of Hospital Medicine*, 1974, **12,** 627.

[12] JAMES, J. I. P. AND LAMB, D. W. Congenital abnormalities of the limbs. *Practitioner*, 1963, **191,** 159.

[13] ENTIN, M. A. Reconstruction of congenital abnormalities of the upper extremities. *Journal of Bone and Joint Surgery*, 1959, **41A,** 681.

[14] BARSKY, A. J. Congenital anomalies of the hand. *Journal of Bone and Joint Surgery*, 1951, **33A,** 35.

[15] BARSKY, A. J. *Congenital Anomalies of the Hand and their Surgical Treatment*. Springfield, C. C. Thomas, 1958.

[16] BARSKY, A. J. Reconstructive surgery in congenital anomalies of the hand. *Surgical Clinics North America*, 1959, **39,** 449.

[17] TACHDJIAN, M. D. *Paediatric Orthopaedics*. Philadelphia, Saunders, 1972.

[18] KELIKIAN, H. AND DOUMANIAN, A. R. A. Congenital abnormalities of the hand. *Journal of Bone and Joint Surgery*, 1957, **39A,** 1002.

[19] PATTERSON, T. J. S. Congenital deformities of the hand. *Annals of the Royal College of Surgeons of England*, 1959, **25,** 306.

[20] LITTLER, J. W. Principles of reconstructive surgery of the hand. In *Reconstructive Plastic Surgery*, J. M. Converse, Vol. 4, 1648. Philadelphia, Saunders, 1964.

[21] WYNNE-DAVIES, R. *Heritable Disorders in Orthopaedic Practice*. Blackwell Scientific Publications, Oxford, 1973.

[22] LAMB, D. W., SIMPSON, D. C., SCHUTT, W. H., SPEIRS, N. T., SUTHERLAND, G. AND BAKER, G. The management of upper limb deficiencies in the thalidamide type syndrome. *Journal of the Royal College of Surgeons of Edinburgh*, 1965, **10,** 102.

[23] SIMPSON, D. C. AND SUNDERLAND, G. D. The development and control of a powered prosthesis for children. *Health Bulletin*, 1964, **22,** 67.

[24] MACDONNELL, J. A. Age of fitting upper extremity prostheses in children. *Journal of Bone and Joint Surgery*, 1958, **40A,** 655.

[25] LAMB, D. W. *et al.* Congenital absence of the upper limb and hand. *The Hand*, 1971, **3,** 193.

[26] SWANSON, A. B. Restoration of hand function by the use of partial or total prosthetic replacement. *Journal of Bone and Joint Surgery*, 1963, **45A,** 276.

[27] BLAKESLEE, B., ed. *The Limb Deficient Child*. Los Angeles, University of California Press, 1963.

[28] LAMB, D. W. *et al.* Phocomelia of the upper limb. *The Hand*, 1971, **3,** 200.

[29] JENTSCHURA, G., MARQUARDT, E. AND RUDEL, E. M. *Behandlung und Versorgung bei Fehlbildunger und Amputationen der Oberen Extremitat*. Stuttgart. George Thumer Verlag, 1963.

[30] HEINKEL, H. V. A. Aplasia and hypoplasia of the radius. Studies on 64 cases and on epiphyseal transplantation in rabbits with the imitated defect. *Acta Orthopaedica Scandinavica*, 1959, Supplement 39.

[31] KATO, K. Congenital absence of radius. *Journal of Bone and Joint Surgery*, 1924, **6,** 589.

[32] McCON, M. B. *Radial Club Hand*. A review of 106 cases. Thesis for Ch.M. (Orth.) Liverpool, 1974.

[33] LLOYD ROBERTS, G. C. *Orthopaedics in Infancy and Childhood*, London, Butterworth, 1971.

[34] PULVERTAFT, R. G. Aplasia and hypoplasia of the radius. *The Hand*, 1969, **1,** 60.

[35] PULVERTAFT, R. G. Twenty-five years of hand surgery. *Journal of Bone and Joint Surgery*, 1973, **55B,** 32.

[36] LAMB, D. W. The treatment of radial club hand. *The Hand*, 1972, **4,** 22.

[37] LAMB, D. W. Radial club hand. *Journal of Bone and Joint Surgery*, 1977, **59A,** 1.

[38] BORA, F. W., Jr., NICHOLSON, J. T. AND CHEEMA, H. M. Radial meromelia. The deformity and its treatment. *Journal of Bone and Joint Surgery*, 1970, **52A,** 966.

[39] O'RAHILLY, R. Radial hemimelia and functional anatomy of the carpus. *Journal of Anatomy*, 1946, **80,** 179.

[40] SKERIK, S. K. AND FLATT, A. E. The anatomy of congenital radial dysplasia. Its surgical and functional implications. *Clinical Orthopaedics*, 1969, **66,** 125.

[41] ENTIN, M. A. Reconstruction of congenital aplasia of radial component. *Surgical Clinics of North America*, 1964, **44,** 1091.

[42] RIORDAN, D. C. Congenital absence of the radius. *Journal of Bone and Joint Surgery*, 1955, **37A,** 1129.

[43] LIDGE, R. T. Congenital radial deficient club hand. *Journal of Bone and Joint Surgery*, 1969, **51A,** 1041.

[44] DICK, H. M., PETZOLOT, R. L., BOWERS, L. R. AND RENNIE, W. R. Lengthening of the ulna in radial agenesis—a preliminary report. *Journal of Hand Surgery*, 1977, **2,** 175.

[45] BARSKY, A. J. Congenital anomalies of the thumb. *Clinical Orthopaedics*, 1959, **15,** 96.

[46] EDGERTON, M. T., SNYDER, B. AND WEBB, W. L. Surgical treatment of congenital thumb deformities. *Journal of Bone and Joint Surgery*, 1965, **47A,** 1453.

[47] LITTLER, J. W. The neurovascular pedicle method of digital transposition for reconstruction of the thumb. *Plastic and Reconstructive Surgery*, 1953, **12,** 303.

[48] WHITE, W. E. Fundamental priorities in pollicisation. *Journal of Bone and Joint Surgery*, 1970, **52B,** 438.

[49] BUCK-GRAMCKO, D. Operative treatment of congenital malformations of the hand. *The Hand*, 1972, **4,** 33.

[50] BUCK-GRAMCKO, D. Pollicisation of the index finger. Methods

and results in aplasia and hypoplasia of the thumb. *Journal of Bone and Joint Surgery*, 1971, **53A,** 1605.

[51] CARROLL, R. E. AND BOWERS, H. Congenital deficiency of the ulna. *Journal of Hand Surgery*, 1977, **2,** 169.

[52] RIORDAN, D. C., MILLS, E. H. AND ALLREDGE, R. H. Congenital absence of ulna. *Journal of Bone and Joint Surgery*, 1961, **43A,** 614.

[53] WATSON, H. K. AND BOHNE, W. H. The role of fibrous bone in ulnar deficient extremities. *Journal of Bone and Joint Surgery*, 1971, **53A,** 816.

[54] STRAUD, L. R. Congenital absence of the ulna. *American Journal of Surgery*, 1965, **109,** 300.

[55] BARSKY, A. J. Cleft hand: classification, incidence and treatment. Review of the literature and report of 19 cases. *Journal of Bone and Joint Surgery*, 1964, **46A,** 1707.

[56] HANSEN, O. H. AND ANDERSON, N. O. Congenital radio-ulnar synostosis. Report of 37 cases. *Acta Orthopaedica Scandinavica,* 1970, **41,** 225.

[57] KELIKIAN, H. *Congenital Deformities of the Hand and Forearm*, pp. 939–967. Saunders, Philadelphia, 1974.

[58] CUSHING, H. Hereditary anchylosis of the proximal phalangeal joints (symphalangism). *Genetics*, 1961, **1,** 90.

[59] ELKINGTON, S. G. AND HUNTSMAN, R. G. The Talbot fingers: a study in symphalangism. *British Medical Journal*, 1967, **1,** 407.

[60] FLATT, A. E. AND WOOD, V. E. Rigid digits or symphalangism. *The Hand*, 1975, **7,** 197.

[61] SMITH, R. J. AND LIPKE, R. W. Treatment of congenital deformities of the hand and forearm. *New England Journal of Medicine*, 1979, **30,** 344.

[62] APERT, E. De l'acrocephalosyndactylie. *Bulletins et mémoires de la Société médicale des hôpitaux de Paris*, 1906, **23,** 1310.

[63] BARSKY, A. J. *Congenital Anomalies of the Hand and their Surgical Treatment*, pp. 26–47, Springfield, C. C. Thomas, 1958.

[64] HOOVER, G. H., FLATT, A. E. AND WEISS, M. A. The hand and Apert's syndrome. *Journal of Bone and Joint Surgery*, 1970, **52A,** 878.

[65] KELIKIAN, H. *Congenital Deformities of the Hand and Forearm*, pp. 331–407, Philadelphia, Saunders, 1974.

[66] KETTLEKAMP, D. B. AND FLATT, A. E. An evaluation of syndactyly repair. *Surgery, Gynecology and Obstetrics*, 1961, 133, 471.

[67] MCDOWELL, F. On the propagation, perpetuation and parroting of erroneous eponyms such as "Poland's syndrome". *Plastic and Reconstructive Surgery*, 1977, **59,** 561.

[68] POLAND, A. Deficiency of the pectoral muscles. *Guy's Hospital Reports*, 1841, **6,** 191.

[69] RAVITCH, M. M. Poland's syndrome—a study of an eponym. *Plastic and Reconstructive Surgery*, 1977, **59,** 508.

[70] SKOOG, T. Syndactyly. A clinical report on repair. *Acta chirurgica Scandinavica*, 1965, **130,** 537.

[71] ZACHARIAE, L. Syndactyly. *Journal of Bone and Joint Surgery*, 1955, **37B,** 356.

[72] BARSKY, A. J. Congenital anomalies of the hand. *Journal of Bone and Joint Surgery*, 1951, **33A,** 35.

[73] BARSKY, A. J. *Congenital anomalies of the Hand and their Surgical Treatment*, Springfield, C. C. Thomas, 1958.

[74] BILHAUT, A. Guerison d'un Pouce Bifide par un Nouveau Procede Operatoire. *Congress Française de Chirurgie*, 1890, **4,** 576.

[75] BOYES, J. H. *Bunnell's Surgery of the Hand*, 4th ed., pp. 80–81. Philadelphia, 1964.

[76] KANAVEL, A. B. Congenital malformations of the hands. *Archives of Surgery*, 1932, **25,** 282.

[77] KELIKIAN, H. AND DOUNANIAN, A. Congenital anomalies of the hand. *Journal of Bone and Joint Surgery*, 1957, **39A,** 1002.

[78] LEVY, M., LOTEM, M., FRIED, A. AND PETAH-TIQUVAH. The Laurence–Moon–Biedel–Bardet syndrome. *Journal of Bone and Joint Surgery*, 1970, **52B,** 318.

[79] O'RAHILLY, R. Morphological patterns in limb deficiencies and publications. *American Journal of Anatomy*, 1951, **89,** 135.

[80] STELLING, F. The upper extremity. In *Orthopaedic Surgery in Infancy and Childhood*, 2nd ed., pp. 282–402, ed. A. B. Ferguson. Baltimore, Williams & Wilkins, 1963.

[81] WASSEL, H. D. The results of surgery for polydactyly of the thumb. *Clinical Orthopedics*, 1969, **64,** 175.

[82] WOOD, V. E. Duplication of the index finger. *Journal of Bone and Joint Surgery*, 1970, **52A,** 469.

[83] WOOD, V. E. Treatment of central polydactyly. *Clinical Orthopedics*, 1971, **74,** 196.

[84] HARRISON, R. G., PIERCESON, M. A. AND ROAF, R. Ulnar dimelia. *Journal of Bone and Joint Surgery*, 1960, **42B,** 549.

[85] LAURIN, C. A., FAVREAU, J. C. AND LaBELLE, P. Bilateral absence of the radius and tibia with bilateral reduplication of the ulna and fibula. A case report. *Journal of Bone and Joint Surgery*, 1964, **46A,** 137.

[86] MUKERJI, M. Congenital anomaly of the hand. Mirror hand. *British Journal of Plastic Surgery*, 1957, **9,** 222.

[87] PINTILIE, D., HATMANU, D., AOLARU, I. AND PANOZA, G. Double ulna with symmetrical polydactyly. Case report. *Journal of Bone and Joint Surgery*, 1964, **46B,** 89.

[88] SANDROW, R. E., SULLIVAN, P. D. AND STEELE, H. H. Hereditary ulnar and fibular dimelia with peculiar facies. A case report. *Journal of Bone and Joint Surgery*, 1970, **52A,** 367.

[89] BARSKY, A. J. Macrodactyly. *Journal of Bone and Joint Surgery*, 1967, **49A,** 1255.

[90] BEN BASSET, M., CASPER, J., KAPLAN, I. AND LARAN, Z. Congenital macrodactyly. A case report with three years follow-up. *Journal of Bone and Joint Surgery*, 1966, **48B,** 359.

[91] BOYES, G. Macrodactylism—A review and proposed management. *The Hand*, 1977, **9,** 172.

[92] INGLIS, K. Local gigantism (a manifestation of neuro-fibromatosis). Its relation to general gigantism and to acromegaly illustrating the influence of intrinsic factors in disease when development of the body is abnormal. *American Journal of Pathology*, 1950, **26,** 1059.

[93] JONES, K. G. Megalodactylism. A case report treated by

epiphyseal resection. *Journal of Bone and Joint Surgery*, 1963, **45A**, 1704.

[94] KHANNA, N., GUPTA, S., KHANNA, S. AND TRIPATHI, F. Macrodactyly. *The Hand*, 1975, **7**, 215.

[95] SMITH, R. J. AND LIPKE, R. W. Surgical treatment of peripheral nerve tumours of the upper limb. In: *Management of Peripheral Nerve Problems*, eds. G. E. Omer and M. Spinner, 701–708. Philadelphia, Saunders, 1980.

[96] TSUGE, K. Treatment of macrodactyly. *Plastic and Reconstructive Surgery*, 1967, **39**, 590.

[97] BROWNE, D. The pathology of congenital ring constriction. *Archives of Diseases of Childhood*, 1957, **32**, 517.

[98] FIELD, J. H. AND KRAG, D. O. Placental studies on the development of congenital constricting bands and congenital amputation of the fingers. *Journal of Bone and Joint Surgery*, 1973, **55A**, 874.

[99] FISCHL, R. A. Ring constriction syndrome. *Transactions of the International Society of Plastic and Reconstructive Surgeons*. Fifth Congress, Australia, pp. 657–670. Butterworth, 1971.

[100] FLATT, A. E. *The Care of Congenital Hand Anomalies*, pp. 213–277. C. V. Mosby, St. Louis, 1977.

[101] KINO, Y. Clinical and experimental studies of the congenital constriction band syndrome, with an emphasis on its etiology. *Journal of Bone and Joint Surgery*, 1975, **57A**, 636.

[102] KOHLER, H. G. Congenital transverse defects of the limbs and digits (intrauterine amputation), *Archives of the Diseases of Children*, 1962, **37**, 263.

[103] MCKUSICK, V. A. *Mendelian Inheritance in Man*, 2nd ed., 248. Baltimore, Johns Hopkins Press, 1968.

[104] MONTGOMERY, W. F. Further observation on spontaneous amputation of the limb of the foetus in utero (as cited in Kalekian). *Dublin Medical Chemical and Scientific Journal*, 1833, **2**, 49.

[105] PATTERSON, T. J. S. Congenital ring constrictions. *British Journal of Plastic Surgery*, 1961, **14**, 1.

[106] PATTERSON, T. J. S. Ring constrictions. *The Hand*, 1969, **1**, 57.

[107] SIMPSON, J. Y. Cases illustrative of the spontaneous amputation of the limbs of the foetus in utero with remarks (as cited in Kalekian). *Dublin Journal of Medical Science*, 1836, **10**, 220.

[108] STREETER, G. L. Focal deficiencies in foetal tissues and their relation to intra-uterine amputation. *Contrib. Embryology*, 1930, **22**, 1.

[109] ABRAMOWITZ, I. Triphalangeal thumb in a Bantu family. *Journal of Bone and Joint Surgery*, 1959, **41B**, 766.

[110] LAPIDUS, P. W., GUIDOTTI, F. P. AND COLETTI, C. J. Triphalangeal thumb—report of six cases. *Surgery, Gynecology and Obstetrics*, 1943, **77**, 178.

[111] PHILLIPS, R. S. Congenital split foot (lobster claw) and triphalangeal thumb. *Journal of Bone and Joint Surgery*, 1971, **53B**, 247–257.

[112] CARSTAM, N. AND THEANDER, G. Surgical treatment of clinodactyly caused by longitudinally bracketed diaphysis. *Scandinavian Journal of Plastic and Reconstructive Surgery*, 1975, **9**, 199.

[113] JONES, G. B. Delta-phalanx. *Journal of Bone and Joint Surgery*, 1964, **46B**, 226.

[114] SMITH, R. J. Osteotomy for 'delta-phalanx' deformity. *Clinical Orthopedics*, 1977, **123**, 91.

[115] WATSON, H. K. AND BOYES, J. H. Congenital angular deformities of the digits. Delta phalanx. *Journal of Bone and Joint Surgery*, 1967, **49A**, 33.

[116] WOOD, V. E. AND FLATT, A. E. Congenital triangular bones of the hand. *Journal of Hand Surgery*, 1977, **2**, 179.

[117] BLANK, E. AND GIRDANY, B. R. Symmetric bowing of the terminal phalanges of the fifth fingers in a family (Kirner's deformity). *American Journal of Roentgenology, Radium Therapy and Nuclear Medicine*, 1965, **93**, 367.

[118] MOORE, W. G. AND MESSINA, PATRINA. Camptodactylism and its variable expressions. *Journal of Heredity*, 1936, **27**, 27.

[119] OLDFIELD, M. C. Camptodactyly: flexion contracture of the fingers in young girls. *British Journal of Plastic Surgery*, 1956, **8**, 312.

[120] POZNANSKI, A. K., PRATT, G. B., MANSON, G. AND WEISS, L. Clinodactyly, camptodactyly, Kirner's deformity and other crooked fingers. *Radiology*, 1969, **93**, 573.

[121] SMITH, R. J. AND KAPLAN, E. B. Camptodactyly and similar atraumatic flexion deformities of the proximal interphalangeal joints of the fingers. *Journal of Bone and Joint Surgery*, 1968, **50A**, 1187.

[122] WELCH, J. P. AND TEMTAMY, S. A. Hereditary contractures of the fingers (camptodactyly). *Journal of Medical Genetics*, 1966, **3**, 104.

[123] CARSTAM, N. AND EIKEN, O. Kirner's deformity of the little finger. *Journal of Bone and Joint Surgery*, 1974, **52A**, 1653.

[124] KIRNER, J. Doppelseitige Verkrummung des Kleinfingergliedes als Seldstandiges Krankenheitsbild. *Fortschitte auf dem Gebiete der Rontgenstrahlen und der Nuklearmedizin*, 1927, **36**, 804.

FURTHER READING

FLATT, A. E. *The Care of Congenital Hand Abnormalities*. St. Louis, Mosby, 1977.

WYNNE-DAVIES, R. *Heritable Disorders in Orthopaedic Practice*. Oxford, Blackwell Scientific Publications, 1973.

CHAPTER 25

The Hand in Rheumatoid Disease

MEDICAL ASPECTS OF MANAGEMENT

T. M. CHALMERS

The benefits which may accrue to patients with rheumatoid arthritis from co-operation between the physicians and orthopaedic surgeons responsible for their care are now generally recognized. The importance of this combined medical–orthopaedic approach is nowhere more apparent than in the management of the problems presented by the involvement of the structures in the hand in the disease process. It has also become clear that the experience gained from such co-operation over the years and the information obtained from prospective studies of the natural history of the disease have resulted in a more discriminating selection of patients for operative treatment.

The medical management of rheumatoid arthritis in the hands rests on the same basic principles as apply in the management of the disease in other joints.

First, the physician is concerned with the relief of pain, stiffness and disability which are the rather non-specific and subjective cardinal features of diseases of the locomotor system. Next, it is important to prevent deformity or to correct it when already established. Thirdly the physician is concerned with measures which may assist in inducing and maintaining the remissions which are a characteristic feature of the natural course of this disease. Finally, there is the responsibility of ensuring that function is restored to the highest possible level for the individual patient.

Clearly, to achieve these aims, the rheumatologist cannot function in isolation but must form part of a team whose members include—the patient, the family doctor, surgeons and anaesthetists, nursing staff, physiotherapists, occupational therapists, social workers and by no means last, the secretarial staff essential for maintaining communication between the various members. The physician in the team has several roles. He is not infrequently the person responsible for the initial selection of patients for consideration for operation. His decision must depend on several factors but obviously a prerequisite is an awareness on his part of the indication for and the feasibility of surgery in individual cases. The physician must, therefore, be familiar with current developments and opinion in orthopaedic surgery. He should also be familiar with the repertoire of the surgeons with whom he works and with the various factors which may influence the results of operation. Occasionally, enthusiasm must be tempered with discretion according to the circumstances of the individual patient.

Perhaps the prime concern of the physician, once a problem potentially amenable to surgical intervention has been identified, is to undertake an assessment of the patient's general physical state. In particular, he must ascertain what evidence there is of rheumatoid disease affecting systems other than the locomotor. Is there evidence, for example, of severe anaemia, or involvement of the respiratory system (pleurisy or parenchymal lung disease), the cardiovascular system (valvular disease, pericarditis or especially peripheral vasculitis which might affect healing by introducing the hazard of ischaemia)?

The physician is also concerned with the supervision of the patient's medication. He should be familiar with and draw attention to any known allergies. Undesirable drug interactions should be avoided and in this regard the hazards of the simultaneous exhibition of various non-steroidal anti-inflammatory drugs and anticoagulants of the coumarin group should be recognized and avoided. If the patient has been taking oral synthetic corticosteroids, the anaesthetist should be informed and in this regard the hazard should be recognized of proprietary preparations, e.g. Delta butazolidin and Elestol whose names do not immediately indicate clearly their steroid content. It should be remembered that the chelating agent, D-penicillamine, currently popular in some centres for long-term treatment, may introduce problems of delayed wound healing and difficulties with elective arthrodesis.

Two particular facets of pre-operative management which fall within the province of the physician and merit mention are the correction of obesity and correction of the anaemia which is a common feature of inflammatory joint disease; both these features may influence post-operative progress.

Finally, certain routine preoperative precautions are advisable. These include the estimation of current haemoglobin, leucocyte and platelet counts, and the estimation of prothrombin activity. Next, in view of the hazard of luxation in the cervical spine in rheumatoid arthritis, lateral radiographs of the cervical spine on flexion and extension are indicated, in view of the manipulation of the neck inherent in intratracheal intubation for purposes of anaesthesia.

It will be clear that in different centres, there may be considerable overlap in the various members of staff immediately responsible for these details of preoperative and postoperative care. There can be no argument, however, that the success or failure, of operative treatment in patients with rheumatoid disease depends as much on attention to these details as on the niceties of surgical technique. Many undertakings, though technically beyond criticism, have failed to achieve the potentially optimum result as a result of the neglect of these simple, fundamental measures.

GENERAL PRINCIPLES OF SURGICAL MANAGEMENT
W. A. SOUTER

In the early 1960s, during the general upsurge of interest in the surgical management of rheumatoid arthritis, most of the pioneer efforts were concentrated on the knee and hand. More recently, surgery of the lower limb has become even more important because of new arthroplasty techniques which are often dramatically successful. In contrast, although surgery can play an important role in management of the rheumatoid hand, there has been perhaps some tempering of the early enthusiasm with the realization that, in the presence of severe disease, only a limited degree of surgical success can be achieved in such a complex and finely balanced structure. This chapter attempts to define the state of progress in this surgical field and to provide some idea of the measure of success of the various techniques in vogue at the present time.

Role of surgery

Surgery is merely a local intervention in a systemic disease and should only be undertaken in conjunction with skilled medical treatment supervised, if possible, by a specialist rheumatologist. In ideal circumstances, the physician and surgeon should see the patient together in a combined medicosurgical clinic when a programme based on both disciplines can be planned. The extent of joint involvement and the severity of the general illness initially may present such a picture that any surgery may appear to be totally impracticable, yet after a spell of hospitalization and modern medical treatment, the condition may be improved dramatically so that in the end a relatively small number of residual problems fully capable of surgical solution remain.

As a general working rule, surgery should probably not be undertaken until after at least 6 months of adequate medical treatment. Thereafter, however, if significant synovial hyperplasia persists, especially with attendant pain, serious consideration should be given to synovectomy either of joint or tendon.

In the late stages of the disease with destruction of joints or disruption of tendons, surgery may have a major role to play in the reconstruction and restoration of function.

The aims of surgery

The relief of pain is first and foremost, but restoration of function runs a very close second. Thirdly, early intervention aims at prevention of further joint damage but the prophylactic value of synovectomy remains unproven and is still a matter of controversy. Indeed, the relative failure of synovectomy to halt the inexorable progress of disease in the digital joints [1–3] is one of the main disappointments in this field. The fourth goal, cosmetic improvement, can frequently be fairly easily achieved but usually commands a relatively low priority. Nevertheless for some patients it may be of prime importance [4], and this applies to both sexes.

Guiding principles

These have been discussed elsewhere by the author in considerable detail [4] and may be summarized as follows:

Deformity should, in most patients, be only regarded as an indication for surgery if accompanied by pain or serious loss of function. For example, even in the presence of quite severe volar subluxation and ulnar drift at the metacarpophalangeal joints, the hand may retain remarkably good power grasp and if three point pinch is not impaired, radical reconstruction of these joints may not be necessary.

The surgical programme should be tailored to the individual patient. A very careful clinical assessment should be made of the patient as a whole; the surgeon should be in possession of a complete picture, not only of physical disabilities but also of the patient's personality, intelligence, motivation, occupational requirements and hobbies. The hand cannot be treated successfully in isolation. It is important that the surgeon should define clearly in his own mind what he wishes to achieve for that particular patient, and these objectives should be carefully explained to the patient.

It is essential that a good surgeon–patient relationship be established early. This demands the highest exercise of the traditional art of our profession. Once trust between surgeon and patient has been securely established, it will survive even in the face of an inexorable advance of the disease or a surgical failure. In the absence of such rapport, however, a progressive deterioration is liable to arouse intense resentment and to be attributed to the incompetence of the surgeon. It is helpful if the latter can identify himself with the patient and thus gain some insight into his often unspoken fears of the progress of the disease. An attempt should also be made to dispel as far as possible the natural dread of surgical procedures.

The surgical programme should proceed from simple, high success operations to the more complex procedures requiring considerable co-operation, perseverance and determination from the patient. The sequence of procedures must, of course, vary quite widely according to the pattern of involvement in any given patient. However, the following sequence is useful where an extensive surgical programme is required.

(1) Dorsal wrist surgery; extensor tendon synovectomy and excision of head of ulna with wrist stabilization where necessary;

(2) Flexor tendon surgery;

(3) Metacarpophalangeal joint surgery;

(4) Proximal interphalangeal joint surgery and correction of finger deformities;

(5) Realignment of the thumb in the most useful position relative to the reconstructed fingers.

Dorsal wrist surgery is usually highly successful in relieving pain and improving function and being first in a surgical programme helps to gain the patient's confidence and also ensures a painless, stable wrist as a base on which to build the later surgical reconstruction. Placing flexor synovectomy next in sequence ensures that optimum function is restored to both the extrinsic muscle groups prior to reconstruction of the joints. The metacarpophalangeal joints should probably be dealt with first since the functional recovery achieved here will determine the optimal treatment and alignment of the proximal interphalangeal joints and the thumb, especially in cases where arthrodesis is contemplated at the latter sites.

The surgical programme should be staged in such a way as to inflict at any one sitting the minimal insult to the hand compatible with a reasonably rapid completion of the programme. It is preferable to perform a series of carefully staged and relatively small operations rather than carry out a single major onslaught likely to result in considerable oedema and serious problems of remobilization. In particular, major extensor and flexor tendon surgery should not be undertaken at the same sitting, nor should extensive tenosynovectomy be coupled with major joint reconstruction. Moreover, it is desirable that the postoperative induration should be allowed to resolve as fully as possible with concomitant recovery of function before the next stage of surgery. Finally, it is probably best not to operate on both hands at one sitting, since this is likely to entail a distressing loss of independence for the patient, at least until the bulky dressings have been reduced [5].

THE DORSUM OF THE WRIST
W. A. SOUTER

This is one of the sites most frequently involved by rheumatoid arthritis. Not only the synovial sheaths of the extensor tendons, but also the radioulnar, radiocarpal and intercarpal joints may be affected. The tendon and joint lesions are closely interrelated both with regard to the mutual pathogenesis and to the overall severity of the clinical picture.

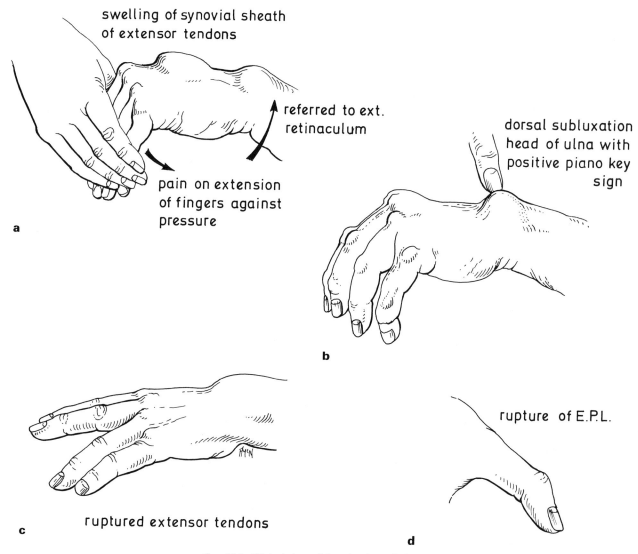

FIG. 25.1. Clinical signs of dorsal wrist pathology.

Clinical presentation

Tendon disease is characterized by pain, tenderness, swelling, loss of power and impairment of muscle function, triggering and, in some cases, actual tendon rupture.

Hyperplasia of the tendon synovium presents as mild to gross boggy swelling on the dorsum of the wrist in the line of the affected tendons (Fig. 25.1a). Ability to extend the fingers and thumb should be carefully checked. Pain at the distal edge of the extensor retinaculum during extension of the fingers against resistance may indicate serious tendon involvement and impending rupture and is an indication for decompression.

The examiner must guard against making a false diagnosis of extensor rupture. This is most likely in severe metacarpophalangeal joint subluxation and ulnar drift where the extensor tendons have slipped into the hollows between the metacarpal heads with impairment of finger extension. If the alignment of the tendons is first corrected by passive extension of the fingers, this position can often subsequently be maintained actively by the patient with the outline of the intact tendons clearly seen.

Involvement of the distal radioulnar joint presents as soft tissue swelling, dorsal subluxation of the end of the ulna, painful reduction in the range of supination and pronation, and a positive 'piano-key' sign (acute pain produced by sharply depressing the dorsally subluxated distal end of the ulna) [6] (Fig. 25.1b).

In involvement of the intercarpal and radiocarpal joints, marked restriction of movement, especially extension, is commonly encountered. However, severe pain arising in these joints is comparatively uncommon unless there is also marked instability of the wrist. Where volar subluxation with instability of the radiocarpal joint is suspected clinically, it is important to obtain radiological corroboration. Swelling of the extensor synovium can give an illusion of volar subluxation and the wrist with incipient volar subluxation may yet remain quite stable because of the development of a prominent bony buttress on the anterior edge of the radius, so that in the absence of significant pain surgery may not be required.

Where definite subluxation is present, the posterior edge of the distal radius should be palpated since if this has been eroded into a sharp ridge of bone realignment of the joint is urgently required to avoid attrition rupture of the extensor tendons.

Pathology

Extensor tendons

The severity and extent of involvement may vary very widely in different patients, or indeed, in the same patient at different times. The swelling may be minimal or may amount to quite a bizarre tumour on the dorsum of the wrist. The disease, moreover, may be present across the back of the whole wrist (Fig. 25.2), or confined to the radial wrist extensors and the extensor pollicis longus, or the extensor carpi ulnaris, or, less commonly, the extensor digitorum communis. Significant involvement of the abductor pollicis longus and extensor pollicis brevis is uncommon.

The diseased synovium is thick and has a felted and highly vascular appearance, or alternatively may present markedly villous hyperplasia. In the presence of gross swelling, it is usual to find in addition to synovial hypertrophy that the sheath contains fibrinoid debris or a large number of melon seed bodies (Fig. 25.3). In the early phase the visceral synovial layer is easily stripped from the tendons which appear healthy. Later, the synovium becomes adherent and some minor fraying of the surface of the tendons may be seen. Later still, the synovium penetrates between the collagenous bundles of the tendon with disruption of its substance. Nodules of hyperplastic synovium or rheumatoid granulomas may occur on the surface of, or within, the tendons (Fig. 25.3). Intratendinous nodules are frequently the site of fibrinoid necrosis [7] and may have a frankly necrotic, caseous appearance and indicate impending rupture. The progressive nature of the lesions has been well described and classified [8].

Although rupture may indeed occur, a gradual thinning and tendon attenuation is more usual, continuity being maintained by slender strands of fibrous tissue lying within the synovial sheath. This elongation is frequently of such an extent that for all practical purposes normal function is lost. Tendons most frequently involved are extensor digiti minimi, extensor digitorum communis to the ring and little fingers (Fig. 25.1c), and extensor pollicis longus (Fig. 25.1d), in decreasing frequency [9].

The tendons are not necessarily most at risk when the pathology is florid [10]; rupture can, in fact, occur in rather inconspicuous disease and it is important that the surgeon is not lulled into a false sense of security.

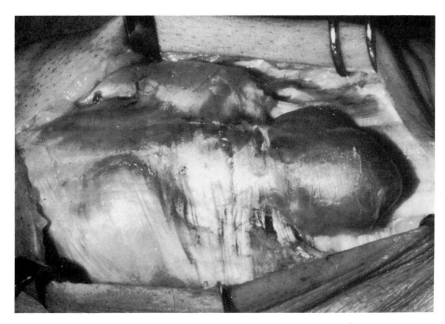

FIG. 25.2. Severe tenosynovitis on dorsum of wrist. Note the bulging synovial sheath with the stretched and attenuated extensor retinaculum. The bulging area seen on the lower left is due to dorsal subluxation of the head of the ulna and synovial hyperplasia within the inferior radioulnar joint.

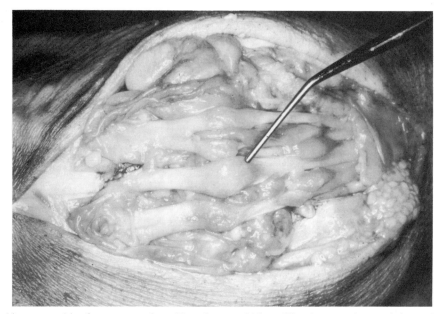

FIG. 25.3. Rheumatoid tenosynovitis of extensor tendons. Note the very thick proliferative synovium and the tendon nodules arranged linearly across the dorsum of the wrist just distal to the original site of the extensor retinaculum. Some melon seed bodies are seen on the lower right.

Considerable argument exists as to the actual cause of tendon rupture. Vaughan Jackson believes that the main cause is the protrusion of a small spicule of the eroded and dorsally subluxated head of the ulna through the dorsal capsule of the radioulnar joint [11–13]. Others, while accepting the occurrence of such attrition rupture, have advanced a multifactorial aetiology for most ruptures [5] and have tended to lay considerable emphasis on synovial hyperplasia in conjunction with tight compression under the extensor retinaculum [6, 9, 14–16]. In support of this view, there is no doubt that tendon nodules and the sites of tendon rupture are most commonly to be found at the distal edge of the extensor retinaculum (Fig. 25.3), or in flexor tendons under the flexor retinaculum or just proximal to the edge of the palmar digital fibrous sheaths [8]. Moreover, experience shows that following decompression of the extensor tendons, spontaneous regression of the synovial hyper-

plasia will frequently occur and tendon rupture is rare [10, 14, 16].

Even where bony attrition has clearly contributed to tendon damage, it should be remembered that the tendon itself was probably already the seat of quite advanced rheumatoid changes including inflammatory cellular infiltration, separation, disintegration and fragmentation of collagen bundles, fibrinoid degeneration and necrosis [6, 7, 17].

Radioulnar joint

Tendon disease on the dorsum of the wrist seldom exists in isolation. Very frequently there is major involvement of the distal radioulnar joint with marked synovial hyperplasia, destruction of the articular disc, stretching or disruption of the capsule or ligaments and dorsal subluxation of the head of the ulna [6] (Fig. 25.4).

Radiocarpal and intercarpal joints

Erosion of these joints is common. Notching of the carpus and joint narrowing lead to gross bone erosion, sometimes with virtual disappearance of the proximal carpal row and major destruction of the anterior margin and surface of the radius so that the carpus and hand subluxate volarward and proximally (Fig. 25.5a).

Intercarpal bony ankylosis may occur and also take place between the medial edge of the distal radius and the lunate [18]. Where this occurs, the scaphoid settles into a deep notch between the newly formed bar of bone and the radial styloid so that a remarkable degree of stability may be present. In some cases a prominent volar shelf or osteophyte may persist or develop along the anterior margin of the radius so that the carpus sinks into a deep cavity in the distal end of the radius, thus conferring a stability reminiscent of the egg and cup deformity observed at the metacarpophalangeal joint [19].

Arthrography shows that early in the disease, abnormal communications develop between the radioulnar, radiocarpal, intercarpal and carpometacarpal joints, and in some cases with the extensor and flexor synovial sheaths [20]. Exuberant synovium in some wrists disrupts and penetrates the dorsal radiocarpal ligaments as pouching herniations seen not infrequently during surgery.

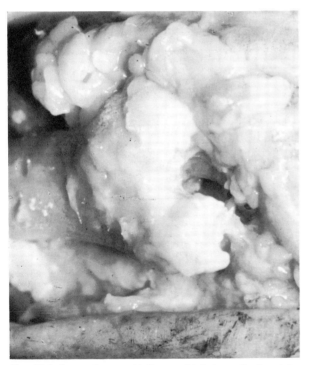

Fig. 25.4. Severe rheumatoid disease of inferior radioulnar joint with hyperplastic synovium and marked erosion of ulnar head. The drill holes seen on the distal ulnar shaft mark the ideal level for bone section.

The alignment of the wrist and its interrelationship with the extensor force and radioulnar lesions on the one hand and the development of ulnar drift of the fingers on the other has attracted considerable attention.

Backdahl in his classic description of the 'Caput ulnae syndrome' [6], first stressed the unique role of extensor carpi ulnaris as a stabilizer of the wrist. Electromyographic studies showed that this muscle alone among the extensors is active during palmar flexion of the wrist. When the muscle slips anteriorly, in cases of dorsal subluxation of the ulnar head, the activity is lost, and the whole balance of the wrist is upset so that the medial side of the carpus is rotated forwards and the carpus as a whole falls into radial deviation. The importance of this in the pathogenesis of ulnar drift of the fingers (p. 361) was first stressed by Shapiro [21] and discussed in greater

depth by Stack and Vaughan-Jackson [22]. In a review of arthrodesed wrists it appeared that ulnar drift was more likely where the arthrodesis was in radial deviation [23]. Further evidence of the important influence of wrist alignment on the development of finger deformity was shown by the fact that where the wrists had been fused in more than 5° of ulnar deviation the relatively unusual deformity of radial drift of the fingers was liable to occur. The biomechanical reason for these developments is explained by Landsmeer in his description of bi-muscular, bi-articular [24], three-bone systems with their tendency to collapse into a zig-zag pattern if a third stabilizing force is absent. Linscheid and Dobyns point out that the impaired stabilizing force is the foreshortened, eroded proximal carpal row, the eventual posture of the wrist being dependent on whether the strut falls into an ex-

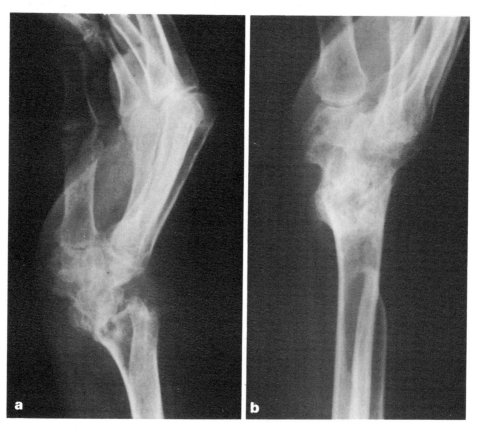

FIG. 25.5. Unstable rheumatoid wrist. (a) The marked preoperative volar subluxation is clearly seen. Following dorsal stabilization and excision of head of ulna a sound fibrous ankylosis has been achieved. (b) 8 years after original surgery shows good maintenance of alignment.

tesded or flexed position relative to the radius [25]. The whole subject is excellently reviewed and summarized by Flatt [5].

Operative technique

Surgical management of dorsal tenosynovitis

Rheumatoid patients often have extremely atrophic subcutaneous tissues on the dorsum of the hand. The curvilinear or lazy-S type of incision traditionally recommended for a dorsal approach to the wrist often necessitates the division of several of the main longitudinally running veins. Primary healing may be slow with some degree of ischaemic necrosis along the wound margins, sometimes with dehiscence [6, 14, 15, 26, 27]. Because of this, a straight midline longitudinal approach (Fig. 25.6), which can be deepened between the basilic and cephalic venous systems to the plane of the extensor retinaculum is recommended. As the wound flaps are elevated the

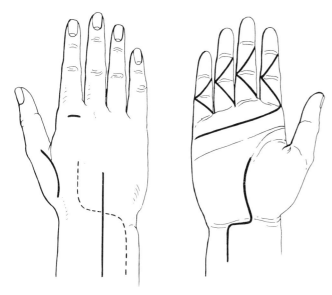

Fig. 25.6. Commonly used incisions in tenosynovectomy. The mid-line longitudinal dorsal incision has been found to give superior healing to the dotted curvi-linear. The accessory incisions shown over the thumb and over the head of the 2nd metacarpal are utilized during repair of extensor pollicis longus by transfer of extensor indicis proprius.

Note the Bruner type incisions which give excellent access for clearance of the digital theca during flexor synovectomy.

radial nerve and the dorsal branch of the ulnar nerve can both be easily identified on the deep surface of the superficial fascia and preserved. It might be thought that the scar would be subject to longitudinal contracture but this has not presented a problem.

The extensor retinaculum is divided along its ulnar margin in the line of the extensor carpi ulnaris and reflected towards the radial side of the wrist, the septa between the tendon compartments being carefully sectioned until exposure of the radial wrist extensors. It is not usually necessary to carry the dissection further radialward to include the abductor pollicis longus and extensor pollicis brevis compartment. The elevated retinaculum should either be slipped under the radial skin margin or covered with a moist swab to prevent its drying out.

The tendons should next be systematically stripped of their synovial sheaths. The visceral layer should be incised longitudinally over each tendon; it will usually be found relatively easy to unroll the sheath from around the tendon merely by a few light strokes of the knife on the areolar tissue binding the synovium to the face of the tendons. Any nodules on or within the tendon are removed with fine dissecting scissors while the tendon is stretched over the pulp of the surgeon's finger [28] (Fig. 25.7). Following synovectomy, the extensor retinaculum is replaced deep to the tendons and sutured into position, where it may provide strengthening to the dorsal capsule of the wrist. The wound is then closed in two further layers with or without suction drainage according to the preference of the surgeon. A fluffed gauze supporting bandage, incorporating a volar plaster slab to maintain the wrist in neutral position [15] and the metacarpophalangeal joints in extension, is then applied. It may be retained for 10–14 days, by which time sound healing should have occurred and full mobilization of the wrist and extensor tendons may be commenced. Active interphalangeal joint exercises are encouraged from the outset. If there has been any attenuation and elongation of the tendons, a period of dynamic splintage may be helpful in reducing the extension lag (Fig. 25.8a). The Rancho long opponens splint with metacarpophalangeal extensor assist [29] is very useful [16]. A rest splint to maintain the metacarpophalangeal joints in extension at night is used.

The results of extensor synovectomy are usually good. Straub and Ranawat in fifty-six wrists found good to excellent results in no less than forty-six cases, while four cases were rated as poor [9]. Kessler and Vainio in reviewing a result of sixty-six wrists, reported good to excellent results in forty-four, but stressed that the result was dependent on the degree of involvement of the underlying joints and advocated excision of the ulnar head where there was radioulnar disease [30].

Some believe that radical extensor tendon synovectomy is unnecessary and that it is the decompression of the synovium which is fundamental. These surgeons confine the operative procedure to transposition of the retinaculum deep to the hyperplastic synovial sheath and await spontaneous resolution of the hyperplastic synovial tissues. The simplicity of this technique [10] with its avoidance of any danger of postoperative tenodesis, has recently been re-examined in a series of fifty-seven wrists [14] with spontaneous resolution of the synovial hyperplasia in 82 per cent of cases within approximately 8 weeks.

Distal radioulnar joint

In most patients undergoing dorsal tenosynovectomy, the radioulnar joint is itself the seat of fairly advanced disease. Thus, excision of the ulnar head and synovectomy of the distal radioulnar joint tends to be an integral part of the routine surgery of the dorsal wrist. Conversely, in not a few patients, disease of the distal radioulnar joint may exist without any significant involvement of the extensor tendons and in these circumstances the ulnar head is excised through a short direct longitudinal incision developed between the extensor digiti minimi and extensor carpi ulnaris. About one inch of bone is removed subperiosteally (Fig. 25.4), and the periosteal sleeve plicated with several transverse purse string sutures so as to reduce it to a fibrous cord stabilizing the distal cut end of bone.

Ulnar head resection is for the most part dramatically successful [27, 31, 32] in the relief of pain and improvement in function.

Neither ulnar subluxation of the carpus nor painful instability or clicking of the lower end of the ulna is any great problem postoperatively. Jackson *et al*, in a series of 111 cases, recorded eight cases in which postoperative ulnar deviation of 20–30° developed [32]; in only one of these was corrective surgery necessary and all had bony erosions. Rana and Taylor reported ulnar subluxation in nine of their eighty-six cases, but in none was function adversely affected [27]. For those concerned by the potential risk of ulnar subluxation, an osteotomy

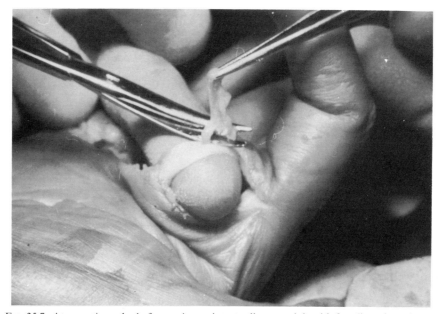

Fig. 25.7. Atraumatic method of removing an intratendinous nodule with fine dissecting scissors.

of the distal third of the ulna coupled with a screw fusion of the distal radioulnar joint [33, 33a] or the use of a silastic ulnar head implant [34] may offer useful alternatives, and are perhaps to be recommended where the preoperative radiological findings suggest that ulnar subluxation is a very definite risk. Where the head of the ulna and the triangular articular disc are still reasonably well preserved, Linscheid and Dobyns merely advocate synovectomy of the joint followed by reconstruction of the ligaments using remnants of the original dorsal radioulnar ligaments and portions of the extensor carpi ulnaris or flexor carpi ulnaris tendons [25]. Rana and Taylor noted painful instability of the distal stump of the ulna in twenty-two of their eighty-six cases of ulnar head resection. This is particularly liable to occur if too much bone has been resected [27]. Backdahl suggested that re-positioning of the extensor carpi ulnaris over the distal

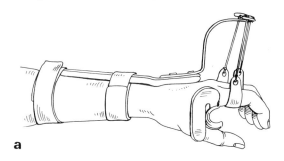

a

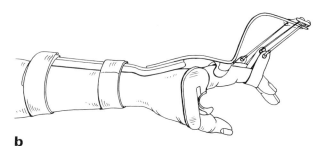

b

FIG. 25.8 Dynamic brace for use in postoperative mobilization after tenosynovectomy.

(a) The Rancho long opponens splint with metacarpo-phalangeal joint extensor assist which can be useful after extensor tendon synovectomy, especially in the presence of attenuation or excessive laxity of the tendons.

(b) The same basic splint with a proximal interphalangeal joint extensor assist and lumbrical bar which can be helpful in pro-moting recovery of finger extension after flexor synovectomy.

ulnar stump by a small fascial sling might increase the stability of the ulna and that it also appeared to restore the normal physiological activity of this muscle during active wrist flexion [6]. Jackson *et al* similarly advocated the suture of the extensor retinaculum both deep and superficial to the extensor carpi ulnaris so as to fashion a retaining sling [32]. If painful clicking and instability of the distal end of the ulna occurs postoperatively, stability may be restored by securing the stump of the bone to the radius or to the tendon of the flexor carpi ulnaris with a sling of fascia lata or palmaris longus [35].

Wrist joint

The radiocarpal and intercarpal joints are frequently involved by rheumatoid disease and some advocate early synovectomy in the management [5, 20, 36–38]. Radical synovectomy of these joints, however, is difficult without further destruction of the already impaired interosseous ligaments or indeed without damaging further the articular surfaces. Moreover, it is compara-tively uncommon for these joints to be painful even in the presence of quite marked erosive disease [27, 39].

It is advisable to limit surgery of these joints to those relatively few patients with either significant pain or disabling instability. Where these criteria exist, treatment should be dorsal stabilization [9] or arthrodesis. As a temporary measure in those awaiting surgery or as a palliative procedure in those unfit for surgery, splintage of the unstable, painful wrist may be very worthwhile [15, 40].

Dorsal stabilization is usually undertaken in conjunc-tion with extensor synovectomy and excision of the ulnar head. Following these procedures, the dorsal radio-carpal ligaments are reflected and a thorough clearance of all synovium, remnants of cartilage and fibrinoid debris from the radiocarpal and intercarpal joints carried out. The distal radius is trimmed to provide a fairly stable surface against which to position the remnant of carpus. The wrist should be secured in a neutral or 5–10° palmar flexion position by the insertion of three Kirschner wires, two usually being passed obliquely from the ulnar border of the carpus or 5th metacarpal and one from the radial border of the second metacarpal into the opposite cortex of the radius. The dorsal ligaments are sutured back and reinforced with the transposed extensor retin-aculum. If the tourniquet is not released before closure, suction drainage should be mandatory as marked swelling and haematoma formation can follow. The forearm and hand should be supported postoperatively in a fluffed gauze bandage with supporting plaster slab. At 10 days, this is changed to a closely fitting forearm plaster cast which is retained for a further 10 days. Thereafter, external splintage can be abandoned, but the Kirschner wires should be left *in situ* for a total of 6 weeks. This procedure is very valuable in relieving pain, confers remarkable stability (Fig. 25.5b), and it usually has the advantage of leaving approximately 20–30° of movement, which may be of considerable help in positioning the wrist for different activities. By leaving the carpal surface intact and fashioning an anterior shelf buttress on the radius the postoperative range of movement and stability may be further increased [41].

Where wrist instability is very marked and equally where there is a definite tendency for the wrist to collapse into ulnar deviation, *arthrodesis* is to be preferred. Sound bony fusion can usually be achieved fairly readily without resorting to multiple cancellous grafts or a cortico-cancellous strut. However, in the presence of very severe erosion, the addition of a bone graft [5, 9, 15, 42] may be advisable, plaster immobilization being maintained for 8–12 weeks. Securing the wrist with an intramedullary Steinman pin driven through the third metacarpal, carpus and radius has been found highly effective. It may be advisable to reinforce this temporarily with an obliquely placed Kirschner wire to control rotation (Fig. 25.9). Postoperatively the forearm and hand are immobilized with a short arm cast for 6 weeks.

Millender and Nalebuff advocate a somewhat similar technique using the retrograde insertion of a Steinman pin to emerge between the second and third or third and

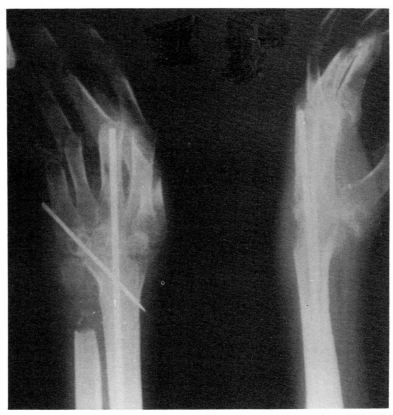

FIG. 25.9. Internal fixation for fusion of the rheumatoid wrist by a Steinmann pin driven through the third metacarpal across the carpus and into the radius supplemented by an oblique Kirschner wire to control rotation.

fourth metacarpals [43]. The pin is then driven up into the radius and the fixation is reinforced by the insertion of two staples, as originally recommended by Mannerfelt and Malmsten [26] who obtained fixation with a Rush pin inserted from the ulnar side of the base of the third metacarpal and driven deeply into the medullary cavity of the radius. With this technique, they advise that plaster immobilization can be dispensed with.

Arthrodesis of the wrist can be an immense boon as it creates a stable base on which the weakened forearm musculature can more effectively activate the digits. In bilateral arthrodesis one wrist should be fused in 10° palmar flexion so as to leave the patient independent as regards toilet function.

Efforts are being made in the direction of replacement arthroplasty notably those of Swanson using a stemmed silastic spacer with a dacron core [44], Meuli using a ball and socket, metal on high density polythene bearing [45], and Gschwend using a linked type of implant [46]. Such procedures at present are experimental but may come to fill a definite place in the management of bilateral wrist problems. A fairly conservative arthroplasty using silastic sheeting between the distal radius and carpus is at present being explored in less severely involved wrists [47]. This work is yielding some interesting results with regard to the re-appearance of what seems to be a significant joint space on either side of the interposed membrane.

Management of extensor tendon rupture

Where tendon ruptures have occurred it is usually impossible to achieve continuity by direct suture because of the length of tendon which is involved and the degree of retraction. Various methods of repair may be used [48], i.e. suture to adjacent tendons, insertion of tendon grafts or transposition of intact tendons of sufficient length and excursion. Bridge grafts have not proved particularly successful due to a marked tendency for adhesion with resultant tenodesis. Suture to intact adjacent tendons is also not without problems. Although suturing the distal stump of say the tendons to the ring and little fingers into the side of the intact tendon to the middle finger, may appear a simple solution, in practice the result often leaves a great deal to be desired. It can be very difficult to achieve the correct tension and if the distal stumps are sutured too tightly, tenodesis in extension will result

with marked loss of flexion [16]. Function may be restored but its excursion is limited and full flexion and extension of the ulnar digits are seldom regained [48]. It may be preferable to use the extensor indicis proprius for the reconstruction of ruptured tendons to the ring and/or little finger. Whatever technique is used, the results may prove disappointing, and in a recent series of twenty-five such cases treated by a variety of techniques, only fifteen patients were satisfied [49].

For the extensor pollicis longus tendon rupture (Fig. 25.1d), the standard treatment is transposition of the extensor indicis proprius. Alternative motors are extensor pollicis brevis [49a] or extensor carpi radialis longus [48]. Riddell considered that the limited excursion of the latter tendon and its more radial alignment tended to yield a less than ideal result [50], but Shannon and Barton found that the recovery of extension after the use of extensor carpi radialis longus was just as acceptable as with extensor indicis proprius [49], while the more restricted flexion was not considered to be a significant handicap by any of their patients. Where multiple ruptures have occurred (Fig. 25.1c), Nalebuff recommends the transposition of extensor indicis proprius [48], usually to the thumb, while the finger extensors may be repaired by the transposition of one or two tendons of the flexor digitorum sublimis, each of which can be subdivided into two strips as recommended by Boyes for the management of radial nerve palsy [51].

Savill advocated an extension of his conservative approach to the surgery of dorsal tenosynovitis to embrace the management of tendon rupture [16, 52]. He believed that simple decompression of the tendons and of the hyperplastic synovium followed by 2–3 months of dynamic splintage while awaiting spontaneous regeneration of the attenuated and elongated extensors was all that was required. Although less certain than formal tendon transfer it may be preferable in its final result to side-to-end suture of adjacent tendons and may be an extremely useful technique in gross disruption of many tendons where the availability of motors is limited. However, it should be clearly realized that the advocacy of this technique was always allied to a policy of not carrying out a formal synovectomy but merely relying on release of the extensor retinaculum. Given the continued presence of synovium around the elongated strands of the disrupted tendons, spontaneous recovery would frequently seem to be possible. If, however, a radical synovectomy is performed and the attenuated tendon strands are left exposed to the bare surface of the retinaculum, the formation of dense adhesions is inevitable and active extension will never be achieved. Postoperative adhesions may also vitiate the results of formal tendon repair and Vaughan-Jackson has suggested that synovium, even in its diseased condition, may be useful for covering the suture line and has emphasized that in such cases one must spring-clean the area with discretion [12, 13].

FLEXOR TENDONS
W. A. SOUTER

Flexor tenosynovitis may be much less obvious than disease on the extensor aspect, and thus in mild cases may frequently go unrecognized. Fully developed it can be extremely disabling and painful. It is by no means uncommon; Brewerton found evidence of flexor tendon involvement in 42 per cent of an unselected series of 300 rheumatoid patients [53].

In florid cases at wrist level, loss of the normal

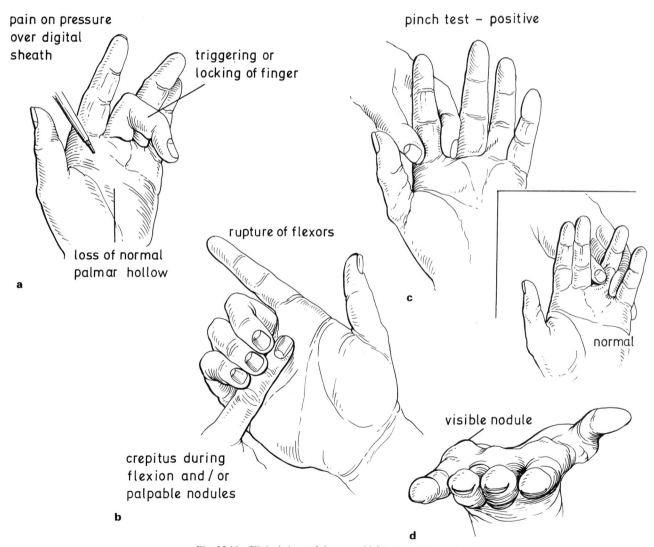

Fig. 25.10. Clinical signs of rheumatoid flexor tenosynovitis.

hollowing of the palm may be apparent (Fig. 25.10a) with marked swelling both above and below the flexor retinaculum. Signs of median nerve compression are not infrequent and should be carefully looked for [54]. Barnes and Currey in a carefully controlled series of forty-five patients found that 69 per cent had clinical or electrical evidence of nerve compression [55]. In the author's own review of eighty cases, forty-seven had evidence of median nerve involvement as presenting symptoms [56].

Marked limitation of finger flexion due to the sheer bulk of volar hyperplastic synovium is commonly present. A considerable discrepancy may exist between the active and passive flexion of the fingers, referred to by Wissinger as 'flexor lag' [57]. Tenderness may be elicited over the front of the wrist and over the line of the flexor sheaths at the base of the fingers. Palpation of the palm during active flexion of the fingers may reveal marked crepitus (Fig. 25.10b). The lateral pinch test (p. 7) (Fig. 25.10c) may reveal boggy swelling in front of the proximal phalanx of one or more digits [52]. Triggering is a frequent accompaniment of such pathology due to the presence of nodules [58] (Fig. 25.10a and d). These are commonly situated on one or both tendons at the proximal end of the fibrous flexor sheath or on the profundus tendon just distal to the sublimis tunnel [59]. In assessing the presence of nodules at this latter site, the absence of active flexion in the terminal interphalangeal joint when the proximal interphalangeal joint is held in maximal passive flexion may be of value [60]. As with the extensor tendons, uncontrolled disease may eventually result in marked fraying and attenuation of the tendons or frank rupture (Fig. 25.10b).

Treatment is by release of fibrous retinacula and synovectomy of the tendons. Whereas extensor tendon synovectomy can be embarked on with a fair guarantee of a worthwhile result, this is not so with flexor synovectomy, where great care must be exercised in the handling of the tendons. A detailed rehabilitation programme may be required to achieve a worthwhile result and this type of surgery should only be undertaken in units with considerable experience of hand and rheumatoid surgery and with excellent physiotherapy facilities [10, 52, 56].

Surgical procedure

Exploration at wrist level is done through a curvilinear incision in the thenar and wrist creases with an extension along the ulnar side of the forearm (Fig. 25.6), the transverse carpal ligament being divided. Usually the synovial reaction at wrist level is comparatively mild, mainly taking the form of a thick, adhesive felting around the tendons, especially the profundus, rather than a profuse, proliferative hyperplasia, although this latter pathology does occur and can be very florid indeed. In these hyperplastic cases, the synovial sheath may be full of fibrinoid debris or melon seed bodies. In the usual adhesive reaction the surgery can be confined to a simple division of the transverse carpal ligament. With more florid pathology radical synovectomy should be performed. Paradoxically, however, if there is evidence of gross fraying of tendons, there may be a place for simple decompression. Too radical surgery may cause marked adhesions in the carpal tunnel, precipitate frank rupture, or, where rupture has already occurred, jeopardize the possibility of spontaneous tendon healing with restoration of at least some function, even if only through mass action of the flexor group [10].

Mannerfelt and Norman have stressed the importance of looking for any sharp spicules of bone within the carpal tunnel which may have been responsible for attrition rupture [61]. In their own series of twenty-five cases of flexor tendon ruptures, attrition by a bony spur was found in eleven. Such spicules are most likely to be found in relation to an eroded scaphoid or trapezium with resultant rupture of the flexor pollicis longus, and less frequently the index flexors. Disruption of the scapholunate articulation may similarly result in exposure of roughened areas of either bone in the floor of the carpal tunnel [25].

The distal part of the palm and the proximal ends of the fibrous flexor sheaths are explored through a transverse incision in the distal palmar crease. Here a much more proliferative or villous type of synovial hyperplasia is likely to be seen (Fig. 25.11). There is often marked attenuation of the overlying fibrous flexor sheath due to herniation of the synovium between its transverse fibres, so that in late cases the only areas of the sheath remaining intact may be the definitive pulleys. These should be carefully preserved, particularly the proximal pulley, otherwise a disastrous degree of bow-stringing with subluxation and flexion contracture of the metacarpophalangeal joints may result [56]. This type of gross deformity may also follow flexor synovectomy if the

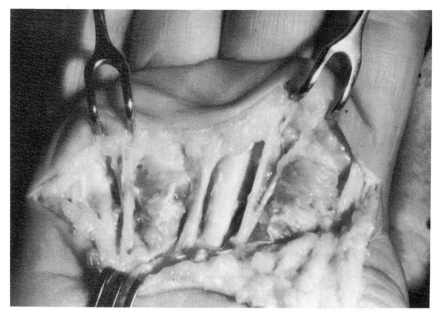

FIG. 25.11. Flexor tenosynovitis. The synovium surrounding the tendons to the right index and ring fingers is markedly hyperplastic. The proximal part of the fibrous flexor sheath appears very attenuated. The synovium and fibrous flexor sheaths around the little and middle finger tendons are essentially normal.

latter is carried out prior to the correction of volar subluxation of the metacarpophalangeal joints [62].

In clearing digital tendons, the fibrous flexor sheath should be incised along its radial margin for about an inch and carefully elevated from the underlying hyperplastic synovium. The latter is stripped from around the tendons and any nodules of synovium on the surface of or within the tendons removed by a similar technique to that described for the extensors (Fig. 25.7). Sairanen reported satisfactory results following the removal of such nodules in sixty-five out of seventy-five patients followed for 1–2 years [58]. However, in the ten remaining cases the beneficial effects only lasted for a few months, after which triggering recurred.

When the synovectomy of the proximal digital theca has been completed, the excursion of the tendons should be tested to see whether or not it approaches normal. If there is still marked restriction of finger flexion on passive traction, it must be assumed that there is pathology distal to the sublimis tunnel and exploration of the individual digits over the proximal phalanx may be required. If extensive dissection has already been undertaken in the palm, especially in the presence of significant

fraying of the tendon surfaces, it may be better to leave the digital exploration until satisfactory movement of the tendons within the wrist and palm has been regained.

Where the index finger has to be explored, the palmar wound can be extended as a mid-lateral radial incision. For the other digits, the Bruner zig-zag incision is extremely useful, as this gives excellent direct exposure of the sheath (Figs. 25.6 and 25.12). Clayton has recently condemned this incision as predisposing to postoperative stiffness, and advocates a return to the use of a mid-lateral incision [63]. In those cases requiring digital exploration, the cause of obstruction to the free movement of the tendons will usually be found to be an aggregation of hyperplastic synovium and/or a nodule on the profundus tendon just distal to the sublimis tunnel. This should be very carefully removed with as little surface damage to the tendon as possible. Very occasionally, florid pathology may be found to exist within the sheath right down to the terminal interphalangeal joint and radical clearance of the entire sheath may then be necessary. In such cases, a pulley over the middle phalanx, in addition to the usual proximal pulley, should be carefully preserved.

The recovery of movement after flexor synovectomy can present many difficulties. The patient may not only experience considerable loss of flexion, but also loss of extension. The use of static splints (Fig. 25.13) are of great value in providing counter pressure at the different joint levels while the patient is actively exercising [16, 40]. A dynamic brace, such as the Rancho long opponens splint with lumbrical bar and proximal interphalangeal joint extensor assist (Fig. 25.8), or the Swanson brace is of great help in improving the range of extension [40, 64]. An intensive physiotherapy programme for 2 or even 3 months may be required before a satisfactory return of function is obtained. The eventual functional result following flexor synovectomy at the wrist and palmar levels should be highly satisfactory, but where the fingers have had to be explored distally, especially in the presence of even a minor degree of tendon damage, the results may be poor. Flatt [5] and Clayton [63] claim that the results can be improved by excision of half of the sublimis tendon so as to increase the space in which the remaining tendons have to glide.

Where gross fraying of both tendons is found, it may be worthwhile excising the sublimis and leaving only the profundus in the hope that this will facilitate the recovery of a better range of movement in the postoperative period [57, 65, 66].

Apart from persistent restriction of movement, the other main long-term complication of flexor synovec-

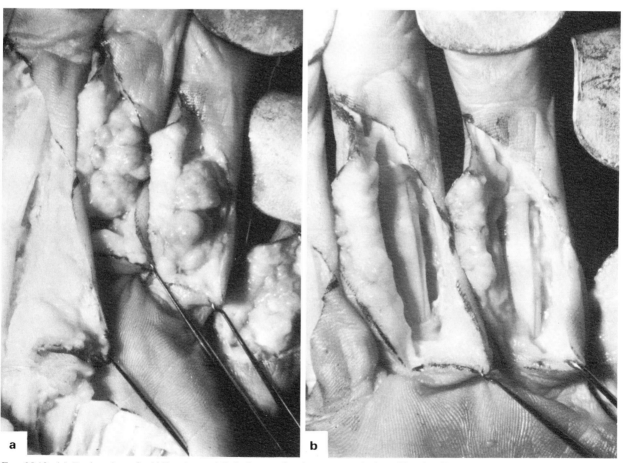

FIG. 25.12. (a) Exploration of middle, ring and little fingers showing very marked proliferative disease within the digital theca. (b) The tendons fully stripped of diseased synovium. Note the excellent exposure achieved through the Bruner incisions.

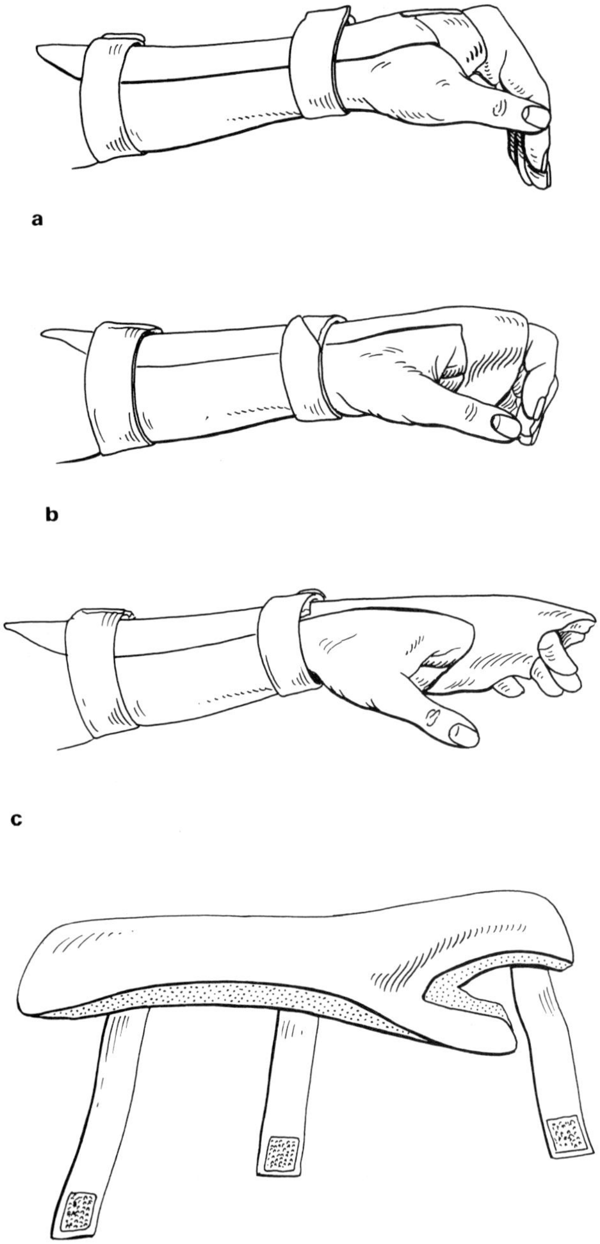

FIG. 25.13. Functional static braces. (a–c) For helping with post-operative programme following flexor tendon synovectomy. (d) Rest splint for use after both extensor and flexor tenosynovectomy.

tomy is recurrence of synovial hyperplasia. Jackson and Paton in their series of thirty-six cases followed for 6–37 months did not find recurrence a problem [66]. However, Dahl, Mikkelsen and Sorensen, in a series of twenty flexor synovectomies followed for 1–6½ years found evidence of recurrence in 37 per cent, though in very few to such an extent that re-operation had been necessary [67]. In the author's own series of eighty cases with a follow-up ranging from 2–16 years (mean 7 years), twenty-three showed some degree of recurrence and in thirteen of these this contributed materially to a poor result [56].

Rupture of flexor tendons presents an extremely difficult problem. In the case of rupture of a profundus tendon in the presence of an intact sublimis, there is certainly no place for attempting any tendon graft. If the patient should subsequently be troubled by instability of the terminal joint, this can be dealt with by tenodesis or arthrodesis.

Where both tendons have ruptured but at a slightly different level, it may be possible to restore single tendon activity by anastomosing the longer proximal motor to one of the distal stumps, if possible the profundus. Where rupture has occurred at wrist or palm, restoration of function may be achieved by the insertion of a short bridge graft. Again in the palm a sublimis from an adjacent intact finger might be transposed to the profundus at the site of the rupture [13]. Where immediate reconstitution by any of the above methods seems inappropriate, it is inadvisable to carry out a tendon graft at the time of the original synovectomy; rather, perhaps, silastic rods should be left *in situ*, in the hope of carrying out a definitive tendon graft at a later date. It is possible that with further development of artificial tendons, this might be an ideal situation for their use.

INTRINSIC CONTRACTURE

D. W. LAMB

One of the postures which the hand may adopt in rheumatoid disease is that of the 'intrinsic plus' position (Figs. 25.14 and 15). While this position may be largely due to joint disease there may be a contributing component of tightness of the intrinsic muscles and the deformity appears occasionally to be due almost entirely to the latter. In the routine examination of the rheumatoid hand an attempt should always be made to determine if there is an element of intrinsic muscle tightness. The classical test of trying to flex the proximal interphalangeal joint while the metacarpophalangeal joint is held in full extension (Fig. 5.14) [68–70] is difficult to perform in the rheumatoid hand because of pain and the destructive changes in the joints. However, an attempt should be made and the metacarpophalangeal joint held in maximal extension while the passive range of flexion of the proximal interphalangeal joint is tested in radial deviation, in neutral position and in ulnar deviation. As deviating the finger towards the radial side during the test tightens the ulnar intrinsic, it will often be found that the degree of flexion at the proximal interphalangeal joint will increase from radial to ulnar test position. The intrinsic tightness prevents satisfactory flexion of the proximal interphalangeal joint and produces the pattern of prehension known as 'the long pinch' (Fig. 25.14).

If intrinsic tightness is a factor a release of the hood [71] should be carried out (p. 366; Fig. 25.20); if joint damage is minimal the result can be very satisfactory.

Intrinsic tightness may be a cause of progressive hyperextension (swan necking) at the proximal interphalangeal joint (p. 364) (Figs. 25.15 and 25.19). Release of the tight intrinsics will probably not correct by itself this deformity or prevent its deterioration. The ulnar slip of the intrinsic tendon should in addition be transposed volar to the proximal interphalangeal joint along the line of the retinacular ligament [72, 73].

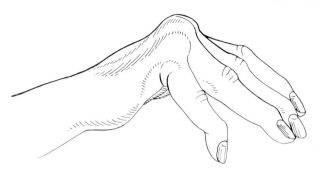

FIG. 25.15. Intrinsic tightness showing a marked flexion of the metacarpophalangeal joints with volar subluxation and swan neck deformity of little and ring fingers.

ULNAR DRIFT
D. W. LAMB

The term ulnar drift is used to describe the deviation of the fingers at the metacarpophalangeal joints so common in the rheumatoid hand and which may develop slowly and imperceptibly but tends to progress relentlessly [74–78] (Fig. 25.32). A variety of complex factors may play an interwoven part in development of this deformity:

(1) A normal tendency to slight ulnar deviation at the metacarpophalangeal joint of the index is aggravated when this joint is swollen and the capsule stretched and this tendency may be a factor leading to early displacement of the other fingers [79, 80].

(2) Ulnar deviation tends to be more marked in the dominant hand suggesting that activity of the hand, particularly the pull of the flexor and extensor tendons, may be a factor.

(3) Radial deviation at the wrist, a common deformity, tends to increase the ulnar deviating force of the long flexor and extensor tendons [81, 82].

(4) The grip of the thumb against the other digits during prehension tends to push the fingers ulnarwards and the use of a stick may be an augmenting factor in this respect.

(5) Tightness of the intrinsic muscles which may result from spasm or contracture has a greater tendency to affect the ulnar intrinsics [74], and may influence the development of ulnar drift. The little finger (where the ulnar intrinsic is the abductor digiti minimi) tends eventually to be more displaced than any of the others.

(6) Joint erosion and destruction of articular cartilage

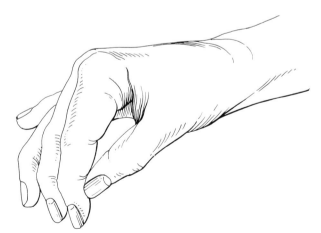

FIG. 25.14. The long pinch which is necessary in this deformity because of the inability to flex the interphalangeal joints. The fingers are in the intrinsic plus position due to intrinsic tightness.

of the metacarpal head, usually in the area deep to the attachments of the collateral ligaments, produces collateral instability and allows ulnar displacement as the radial collateral ligament is longer than the ulnar, and is probably one of the most significant factors resulting in ulnar drift [83].

Treatment

In the management of ulnar drift consideration is given to three stages in its development [84]:

(1) when the deformity can be corrected actively by the patient,

(2) when the deformity can be corrected passively, and

(3) when it cannot be corrected.

In the first two stages soft tissue procedures may realign the structures around the joint, balance them and prevent deterioration.

Stage 1. All that is required is adjusting the play of the tendons around the metacarpophalangeal joint. If the extensor tendon is displaced to the ulnar side, it should be realigned in the centre and held in place by loops made from the intertendinous bands. At the same time the insertion of the ulnar intrinsic is transferred to the radial side of the adjacent digit [85], and the extensor indicis proprius tendon may be moved to a more radial attachment near the base of the proximal phalanx of the index. Harrison [86] has stressed the importance of re-alignment of the middle finger in early ulnar drift.

Stage 2. When passive correction alone is possible, there is often also volar displacement of the base of the phalanx. Deterioration in volar displacement may be prevented by the extensor loop operation [85, 86]. A strip of the central portion of the main extensor tendon is divided proximal to the metacarpal head. A hole is drilled in the base of the proximal phalanx through which the strip of the tendon is passed, brought out and sutured back to the parent tendon which controls the volar displacement. To control the associated ulnar drift, the strip is brought back deep to the radial collateral ligament before it is rejoined to the main extensor tendon.

Stage 3. When the deformity is not correctable, soft tissue procedures alone are not likely to help; the only satisfactory procedure is a joint replacement (p. 377).

This is used when impairment of the overall function of the hand and/or degree of pain from the metacarpophalangeal joint destruction are sufficient to justify surgery. See p. 378 for indications for joint replacement.

THE THUMB
D. W. LAMB

Grip is severely affected in the rheumatoid hand by a combination of factors which have already been described. Between one-half and two-thirds of rheumatoid hands show a significant degree of involvement of the thumb [87]. As power grip in these patients is severely reduced, they are very dependent on precision grip for their limited hand activity and any involvement of the thumb affects this seriously. During the early stages of synovial hyperplasia, considerable relief of pain and possible prevention or delay of future deformity may be obtained by *synovectomy* of the metacarpophalangeal joint, usually the earliest joint involved. If the synovitis is allowed to progress, a tendency for

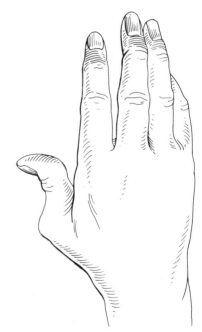

Fig. 25.16. The classical thumb deformity with flexion at the metacarpophalangeal joint and hyperextension at the distal joint.

forward subluxation of the base of the proximal phalanx gradually leads to a flexion deformity of the metacarpophalangeal joint (Fig. 25.16). In the early stage of this deformity, before it becomes fixed, *transfer of the extensor pollicis longus tendon into the base of the proximal phalanx* may be indicated to control the displacement [88]. Progressive destruction of the metacarpophalangeal joint and volar subluxation of the proximal phalanx will gradually lead to a fixed deformity. Contracture of the short flexor and also sometimes of the adductor muscle develops and the extensor pollicis longus tendon is displaced ulnarwards leading to secondary hyperextension of the interphalangeal joint (Fig. 25.16). This deformity can be corrected initially, but if allowed to progress, fixed contractures of the metacarpophalangeal joint in flexion and of the interphalangeal joint in extension develop, commonly associated with a tight adduction web contracture [89]. The metacarpophalangeal joint is the key to the situation and where the damage is too great to be rectified by synovectomy and the transfer of the extensor pollicis longus tendon, the joint should be arthrodesed [90]. In some cases the deformity of the interphalangeal joint is reversible and active flexion may be regained once the metacarpophalangeal joint is stabilized. Where the intrinsic contracture is marked, it is necessary to treat it before the arthrodesis of the metacarpophalangeal joint, by releasing the flexor and adductor muscles either at their origin or insertion. It is most easily done at the insertion, but this may weaken the power of the thumb subsequently and the earlier stages are best treated by a release and slide of the muscle origins. While this is the most typical deformity of the thumb, with the key to its development in the metacarpophalangeal joint, it must be appreciated that other deformities may occur.

Severe and progressive disease of the carpometacarpal joint of the thumb is by no means unusual in rheumatoid disease and may be the main joint or, indeed, the only one involved in the digit. A tendency to progressive lateral subluxation of the base of the metacarpal may be associated with contracture of the adductor. It is sometimes difficult to determine whether the joint displacement is the prime factor followed by secondary muscle contracture or whether the muscle contracture is responsible for the subluxation of the base of the metacarpal. In this type of deformity, excision of the trapezium and replacement with a silastic prosthesis as described by

Swanson (p. 381) can give a very satisfactory result [91]. Where there is adduction contracture, it is essential to release it during operation or subluxation will recur. When subluxation at the carpometacarpal joint occurs as part of the classical deformity affecting all three joints a combined treatment of all the affected joints is required.

A third type of deformity of the thumb is subluxation or dislocation of the carpometacarpal joint, associated with a reverse type of deformity at the metacarpophalangeal joint which becomes hyperextended (Fig. 25.17). A secondary flexion deformity of the interphalangeal joint occurs due to muscle imbalance. This disabling and unsightly deformity requires correction both at the carpometacarpal joint by excision of the trapezium and joint replacement and also usually by arthrodesis of the metacarpophalangeal joint.

When the interphalangeal joint is severely damaged a radial deviation deformity may occur due to the prolonged effect of pinch between thumb and index (Fig. 25.18). Where this occurs in association with a contracted thumb web this deformity increases the span of grip and its correction by fusion may be unwise.

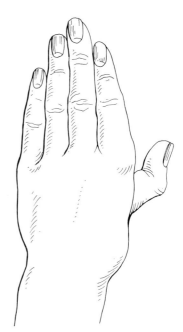

Fig. 25.17. Classical deformity of the thumb in rheumatoid disease showing the adducted metacarpal with hyperextension at metacarpophalangeal joint and flexion at interphalangeal joint.

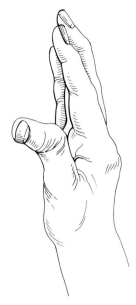

FIG. 25.18. Typical thumb deformity in rheumatoid disease showing the destructive changes in the interphalangeal joint with a valgus deformity occurring at that level to compensate for the fixed adduction contracture of the first metacarpal.

Deformity of the thumb may occur in rheumatoid arthritis as a result of tendon rupture where the joints themselves are not severely involved. In the classical rupture of the extensor pollicis longus tendon, the standard procedure is the transfer of the extensor indicis proprius tendon; results as good as those obtained for the common rupture after Colles fracture can be achieved. Spontaneous rupture of the flexor pollicis longus tendon may also occur and has been shown to be due usually to an attrition rupture at the base of the thumb in the floor of the carpal tunnel. Provided that the bed can be made smooth, a free tendon graft may have a better chance than is usual in other digits treated by flexor tendon grafting in rheumatoid disease.

SWAN NECK DEFORMITY

E. A. NALEBUFF

One of the most common finger deformities encountered in rheumatoid disease is the swan neck deformity [92], which is characterized by hyperextension of the proximal interphalangeal joint with distal joint flexion (Fig. 25.19a). It may be associated with and is usually accen-

tuated by metacarpophalangeal joint flexion deformity. Many factors can lead to the swan neck deformity. It is the end result of imbalance, the origin of which can be either at the metacarpophalangeal, proximal or distal interphalangeal joint. With the metacarpophalangeal joint fixed in flexion, the major extensor force leads to proximal interphalangeal joint hyperextension. Alternatively, rupture of the flexor digitorum superficialis or proximal interphalangeal joint synovitis with stretching of the volar plate has the same effect. Just as proximal interphalangeal joint hyperextension leads to distal joint flexion, the reverse is true. Thus, attenuation of the distal extensor attachment with its mallet deformity can

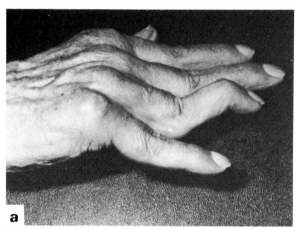

a

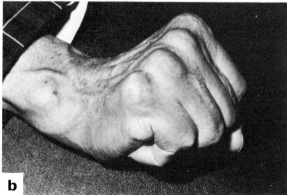

b

FIG. 25.19. Type 1 swan neck deformity.

(a) Typical swan neck deformity of ring finger with hyperextension of the proximal interphalangeal joint and flexion of the distal interphalangeal joint.

(b) Demonstration of full flexibility of the interphalangeal joints, showing no functional loss in spite of severity of deformity.

be the precursor to the hyperextended proximal interphalangeal joint.

As both of these are influenced by the mobility of the proximal interphalangeal joint, we must determine both the passive and active motion of the finger in all positions. Using this approach, we can assess readily which swan neck deformity is of functional significance and understand precisely the objective of any surgical procedure [93]. We must ask whether the patient has any functional loss? If not, what deformity (metacarpophalangeal, proximal or distal interphalangeal) needs to be corrected? If there is functional loss, how is this to be corrected? The choices may be obvious and simple, but in many cases this is not so. Therefore, a variety of surgical procedures have been devised, most of which are effective if applied at the right time. Swan neck deformities can be classified into four types based upon the proximal interphalangeal joint's mobility and condition [94]. In Type 1 there is full mobility of the digit in all positions (Fig. 25.19b). In Type 2 the joint is limited in only certain positions related to intrinsic tightness. In Type 3 there is limited joint motion in all positions. In Type 4 the joint surfaces are damaged and either cause the limitation of motion or would be painful if motion could be re-established. The surgical management of each Type differs.

Type 1

The deformity presents more as a cosmetic postural alteration than any functional loss. If surgery is contemplated, it is carried out either to improve the appearance or possibly to prevent progression of deformity. The surgical choice is made depending upon where the abnormality is greatest. The most deformed joint is probably the site of origin. A primary mallet deformity usually exceeds in degree the secondary proximal interphalangeal joint hyperextension. With the proximal interphalangeal joint as the site of origin, its hyperextension will overshadow the distal joint flexion. In both of these examples, a metacarpophalangeal joint flexion deformity may or may not be present. Treatment is directed at correcting the alignment rather than improving motion and surgical procedures include *distal joint fusion, proximal interphalangeal joint volar dermadesis, tenodesis* or *retinacular relocation* [95]. At the metacarpophalangeal joint, *arthro-*

plasty is the method used to eliminate any fixed flexion deformity.

Distal joint fusion

The distal joint flexion deformity is corrected and controlled by fusion (p. 494). Attempts to restore active extension are doomed to failure.

Control of the proximal interphalangeal joint hyperextension itself can be accomplished by several methods, all of which attempt to provide a volar restraint using soft tissues to limit the joint extension just short of the neutral position.

Dermadesis

This simple method involves removal of an elliptical wedge of skin from the volar aspect of the joint. The resultant skin tightening restricts the joint's extension. The skin is removed carefully by sharp dissection to avoid injury to the venous plexus underneath. The tips of the wedge usually extend to the limits of the volar skin creases, and its width varies according to the degree of hyperextension, but usually measures 1.5 cm at its mid-portion. Dermadesis is an easy, quick procedure which can be added to the other more extensive operations. The major fault with this procedure is that in time the volar skin may stretch. In Type 1 deformity originating in the distal joint dermadesis is sufficient to correct the swan neck. When the origin of the deformity is at the proximal interphalangeal joint, a more substantial checkrein, less apt to stretch out, is needed.

For this *tenodesis* of one slip of the flexor digitorum superficialis is used as the restraint against full joint extension [96]. No loss of active flexion or strength should occur, and the procedure can be done in conjunction with distal joint fusion, proximal interphalangeal joint or metacarpophalangeal joint surgery. A volar zig-zag incision centred over the proximal interphalangeal joint flexion crease is used to expose the flexor tendon sheath which is then opened. The flexor tendons are identified and one of the two superficial flexor tendon slips is divided 2 cm proximal to the joint. This slip is dissected carefully to its terminal attachment avoiding injury to the vincula. It is then woven into the thick margin of the flexor tendon sheath and sutured under tension to limit extension of the joint by 15°. Postoperatively, the joint is held in slight flexion with a curved dorsal splint. The proximal interphalangeal joint is usually protected against hyperextension for 6 weeks.

Retinacular reconstruction

An alternative method to provide a check hyperextension utilizes the ulnar-lateral band [97], which is divided proximally and separated from the extensor mechanism distally. It is then passed retrograde volar to the proximal half of Cleland's ligament (p. 472) before being sutured to the flexor tendon sheath. This reconstitutes an oblique retinacular ligament which, under appropriate tension, will prevent proximal interphalangeal joint hyperextension. In theory, this technique also restores distal joint hyperextension, if the terminal extensor tendon attachment is intact. In most digits with rheumatoid swan neck deformity, traction on the displaced lateral band does not extend the distal joint. For this reason, its main achievement (like flexor tenodesis) is to limit proximal interphalangeal joint hyperextension.

Type 2

This is characterized by limited mobility of the proximal interphalangeal joint directly related to intrinsic tightness (p. 360). The surgical procedures used at the proximal and distal interphalangeal joints in Type 1 can also be used to correct the digital deformity in Type 2 but, by themselves, will not improve the active mobility of the proximal interphalangeal joint. In order to achieve this, *intrinsic release* is required [98].

This may be carried out in conjunction with arthroplasty of the metacarpophalangeal joints (p. 377), or as a separate procedure (Fig. 25.20). In those patients without associated metacarpophalangeal joint deformity, a longitudinal incision 2 cm in length is made along the dorsoulnar border of the extensor apparatus at the base of the proximal phalanx (Fig. 25.20a). The oblique fibres of the ulnar intrinsics are resected as a triangle of tissue (Fig. 25.20b) which can be done under local anaesthesia as an outpatient. The radial intrinsics are usually left as they are not a significant deforming force and are helpful in maintaining improved digital alignment following correction of the more common ulnar deviation.

It should be emphasized that Type 1 and Type 2 swan

neck deformities do not usually present difficult problems. More complex decisions and treatment are required in Types 3 and 4, where limitations of proximal interphalangeal joint motion is present in all positions of the digits.

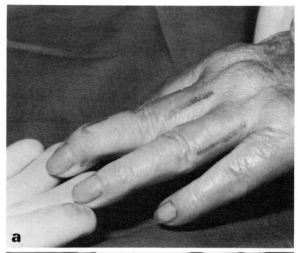

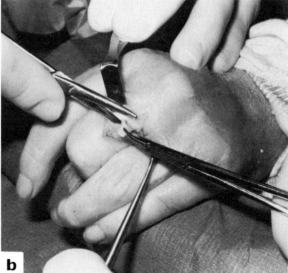

FIG. 25.20. Type 2 swan neck deformity, treated with intrinsic release.

(a) Incisions used for intrinsic release carried out over the proximal phalanx.

(b) Excision of the ulnar-oblique fibres of the extensor mechanism. Note full flexibility of the proximal interphalangeal joint.

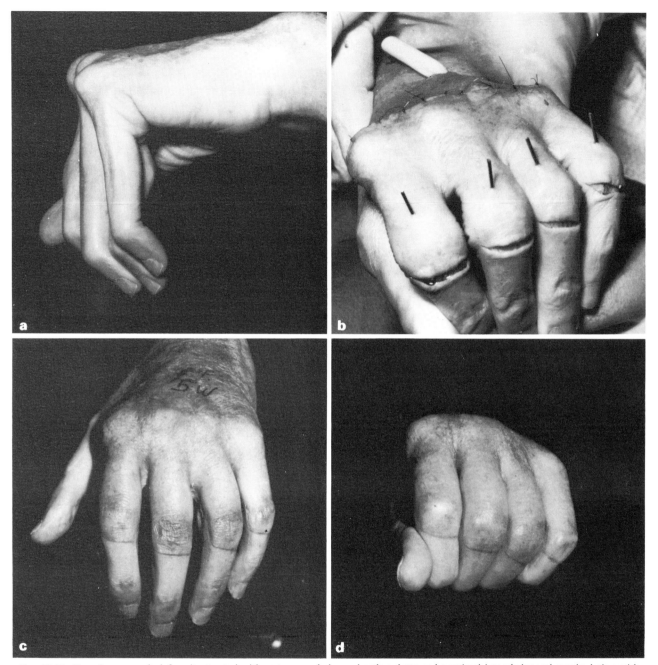

FIG. 25.21. Type 3 swan neck deformity, treated with metacarpophalangeal arthroplasty and proximal interphalangeal manipulation with skin release.

(a) Severe swan neck deformity with complete inability to flex the proximal interphalangeal joints with metacarpophalangeal joints flexed.

(b) Appearance of hand following metacarpophalangeal arthroplasties, proximal interphalangeal manipulation with Kirschner wire fixation. Note skin relaxing incisions distal to the proximal interphalangeal joint.

(c) The improved posture of the hand 5 weeks following surgery. Note the spontaneous closure of the skin release incisions.

(d) Postoperative active flexion.

Type 3

Patients have significant functional loss and are particularly inept at grasping small objects. They make a poor fist and often cannot bring the fingertips to within several inches of the palm (Fig. 25.21a and Fig. 25.14). The surgical goal is to improve motion and although the operative procedures previously described can be utilized a meaningful improvement in the proximal interphalangeal joint mobility must be obtained.

Although the deformities are severe and motion is often non-existent, the proximal interphalangeal joint surfaces are intact, and it is the soft tissue problems alone that have to be overcome. What factors must be considered? First, the tissues that limit passive flexion of the proximal interphalangeal joint. Secondly, those structures which can limit active motion, once passive motion has been restored. This allows an orderly approach to these complicated matters, and, if followed to conclusion, can be quite successful in restoring significant mobility to the seemingly hopeless finger. To restore passive flexion to the stiff proximal interphalangeal joint, the techniques utilized include proximal interphalangeal joint manipulation, skin release and lateral band mobilization.

Proximal interphalangeal joint manipulation

In many patients the joint can be gently manipulated under anaesthesia into a flexed position. If the finger is then maintained in 80° of flexion by either Kirschner wire fixation or taping, the tight extensor mechanism and collateral ligaments will gradually stretch. Discomfort associated with joint manipulation is minimal and reactive swelling does not occur. When the fingers are allowed to resume the extended position after 7–10 days the hard fought for flexion is easily reproduced without pain. This technique may be combined with

metacarpophalangeal arthroplasties [99–101] in those patients with stiff swan neck deformities and severe metacarpophalangeal joint involvement (Fig. 25.21b). It is important to maintain the proximal interphalangeal joints in flexion with tape support during the many hours the patient is not actively exercising. Proximal interphalangeal joint manipulation is an effective method to gain 80–90° of proximal interphalangeal joint motion, but two additional factors need to be considered. The first deals with the overlying skin and the second deals with the status of the flexor tendons providing active power to the joint. If the patient has loose dorsal skin over the proximal interphalangeal joint associated with hyperextension, then 80–90° of flexion is possible without undue skin tension. However, in many the skin is tight when held in moderate flexion and blanching, followed by skin necrosis may occur. To prevent this an associated skin release can be combined with proximal interphalangeal joint manipulation.

Skin release

An oblique incision (Fig. 25.22d) is made across the dorsal aspect of the middle phalanx just distal to the proximal interphalangeal joint with care to avoid injury to the underlying veins. The open wound reduces the tension over the joint (Fig. 25.21b) and any blanching noted prior to the incision is eliminated. It is not necessary to cover the defect with a skin graft, although this could be done with any skin removed by dermadesis. Because there has been no actual 'skin loss' the defect will gradually close spontaneously leaving an inconspicuous scar (Fig. 25.21c and d). By leaving the wound open, drainage is unobstructed and swelling, thereby, minimized. It is emphasized that the relaxing tissue should not be directly over the proximal interphalangeal joint in order to keep the delicate extensor mechanism well covered by intact skin. The placement of this incision

---

Opposite

FIG. 25.22. Type 4 swan neck deformity.

  (a) Preoperative extension demonstrates swan neck deformities of the ring and small fingers.

  (b) Restricted active flexion of the ring and small digits.

  (c) Lateral band release of the ring digit and preparation for arthroplasty of the proximal interphalangeal joint of the little finger.

  (d) Passive flexion achieved of the proximal interphalangeal joints of the ring and little fingers following surgery. Note the distal portion of the incision left open to facilitate drainage.

  (e) Volar view demonstrates incision used to check excursion of flexor tendons at the time of surgery.

  (f) Postoperative active flexion.

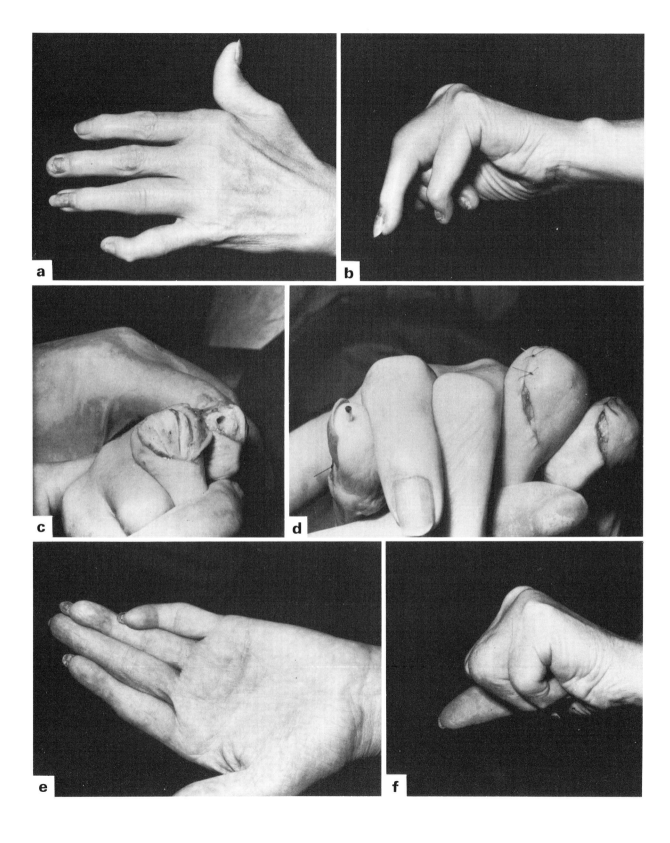

over the middle phalanx leaves a less important part of the extensor mechanism exposed. If a dorsal incision is required to expose the proximal interphalangeal joint itself, it can be curved to create an intact flap over the proximal interphalangeal joint with an extension obliquely across the middle phalanx which is left open. This is particularly helpful when performing a lateral band release to achieve increased passive flexion in those patients for whom closed manipulation seems unsuitable.

Lateral band mobilization

Dorsal displacement of the lateral bands is common and these may become somewhat adherent. The normal volar shift which usually occurs in flexion is absent and releasing the lateral bands from the central slip allows them to glide volarly as the joint is manipulated into flexion. Two parallel incisions (3 cm in length) are made in the expansion on each side of the central slip. The lateral bands with their intact transverse retinacular ligaments along the volar borders are separated from the underlying joint capsule. It is then usually possible to manipulate the joint into flexion (Fig. 25.22c). The central slip is preserved but Z lengthening may occasionally be needed. The collateral ligaments usually stretch without difficulty but may require a proximal release. The dorsal skin will not close and it is advisable to suture only the proximal portion of the incision, leaving the distal oblique lip open to minimize tension as described in skin release.

Restoration of active flexion

Although passive flexion of the proximal interphalangeal joint can be restored by joint manipulation and/or lateral band release, there is no guarantee that the patient will be able to utilize the motion actively unless the flexors are functioning. The only sure way to check the flexors is to have the patient flex the digit during operation under local anaesthesia, wrist block or intravenous regional anaesthesia. A less certain, but effective, method to check the flexors is by applying traction to them in the palm. When flexor tendon problems are suspected a transverse palmar incision is made, the flexor tendon sheath is opened and the tendons inspected (Fig. 25.22e). Traction is applied to both superficial and deep flexors to axcertain whether or not the proximal interphalangeal joint flexes.

If full flexion of the proximal interphalangeal joint is not obtained it indicates that the tendons are adherent either to each other or to the flexor tendon sheath. The digital sheath is then exposed and opened through a volar zig-zag incision and a tenolysis carried out. There may be isolated flexor tendon nodules which need to be removed. A major portion of the flexor tendon sheath should be preserved to prevent bowstringing. However, it is essential that free gliding of the flexor tendons be achieved before closing the wound. Where the superficial flexor tendon is badly scarred, it may be excised leaving the intact profundus tendon to flex actively the interphalangeal joints.

Postoperative management

To achieve significant motion, one must not only perform the correct surgical procedure but also carry out specific postoperative care. The proximal interphalangeal joints will gradually lose motion unless the passive mobility is maintained by splinting and the active motion is continued by exercises. During the immediate postoperative period, the proximal interphalangeal joints are fixed in flexion with either Kirschner wires or tape support. If the flexor apparatus has not been exposed, Kirschner wire fixation is very effective in eliminating pain and provides a constant stretch to the contracted soft tissues. On the other hand, taping the fingers in flexion allows intermittent extension and active exercises. This is advisable if the flexors have been surgically released. The fingers are taped in flexion following removal of the Kirschner wire fixation and continued until the proximal interphalangeal joint tightness has been eliminated. It is not uncommon for the fingers to be taped in flexion at night for several months following surgery.

Although significant improvement in mobility can be achieved by the procedures outlined (Fig. 25.21d), occasionally gradual loss of motion occurs or increase in pain is noted, as the proximal interphalangeal joint surfaces deteriorate. In some of our patients deterioration of this type has led to recurrent stiffness and what would then be classified as a Type 4 swan neck deformity.

Type 4

None of the previous surgical procedures at the proximal interphalangeal joint can be relied upon to eliminate pain or restore movement. Either fusion or arthroplasty can correct the hyperextension deformity, but only the latter can restore mobility. The choice between these two procedures depends upon several factors including the digit involved, the state of the metacarpophalangeal joint, the lateral supporting structures and the flexor apparatus.

Currently the flexible implant arthroplasty is favoured particularly for the ulnar digits. The ability to flex the proximal interphalangeal joints of the ring and small fingers enhances grasp. In contrast, fusion of the index proximal interphalangeal joint in approximately 25° of flexion provides lateral stability in pinch. However, the digit involved is only one factor to consider. The size of the intramedullary canals must be evaluated, particularly if metacarpophalangeal deformities co-exist. There is a limit regarding the capacity of the intramedullary canals of the proximal phalanx to accept a prosthetic stem from each end. When faced with a patient with a Type 4 swan neck deformity in whom proximal interphalangeal arthroplasty is considered (Fig. 25.22a and b) one must take into account the timing of surgery at the proximal interphalangeal joint in relationship to the metacarpophalangeal joint. Although it is possible to carry out simultaneous arthroplasties at both levels, it is usually advisable to stage the procedures. Metacarpophalangeal surgery should be done initially as stiff proximal interphalangeal joints actually enhance the proximal result, the flexor power being concentrated at moving the metacarpophalangeal joints. Initially the stiff proximal interphalangeal joints are manipulated into flexion and held temporarily with Kirschner wire fixation. At a second stage (usually several months later), proximal interphalangeal arthroplasty using the Swanson technique is performed (p. 379) [99–101] (Fig. 25.22c and d). Lessons learned from restoring motion to the stiff Type 3 swan neck deformities may be utilized, including dorsal skin release (Fig. 25.22d), and exploration and testing of the flexors (Fig. 25.22e). Again, the importance of postoperative exercises and splinting cannot be over emphasized.

With good soft tissues and intact tendons, one can anticipate 60° or 70° of active proximal interphalangeal joint motion with arthroplasty (Fig. 25.22f).

Proximal interphalangeal joint fusion

This is an accepted salvage procedure in Type 4. The deformity is corrected and the proximal interphalangeal joint placed in a functional position. The index finger should be fused in approximately 20–25° of flexion with increasing flexion for the other digits, proceeding ulnarward. The maximum flexion for the small finger should not exceed 40°. The technique utilizes a curvilinear dorsal skin incision with splitting of the extensor apparatus in a longitudinal fashion. The finger is then manipulated into flexion, and the articular surfaces removed with a small rongeur. Crossed Kirschner wires are used to obtain stabilization of the joint in the appropriate degree of flexion. External splints are used to supplement the internal fixation for the initial 4–6 weeks. Tightness of the dorsal skin may be a limiting factor, and occasionally the distal portion of the incision is left open, as described under skin release (p. 368). It is important to check the rotation of the fingers which are being brought into a flexed position. This is particularly important when multiple digits are fused in flexion.

Summary

The rheumatoid swan neck deformity represents an imbalance of the flexor and extensor forces acting upon the various digital joints. In the mild Type 1 and Type 2 active motion is still present, and, therefore efforts are directed toward correcting the deformity, and, perhaps minimizing the risk of further progression. In the Type 3 passive motion must be restored initially, and then active motion. In the Type 4 the choice is between arthroplasty and arthrodesis based upon a number of factors including the digit involved, the status of the adjacent joints and associated soft tissues. With the use of an orderly approach to the swan neck deformity, it is possible to restore significant function.

RHEUMATOID BOUTONNIÈRE DEFORMITY

A. W. B. HEYWOOD

Approximately 15 per cent of rheumatoid patients develop boutonnière deformity in one or more fingers. Caused by erosion and stretching of the middle extensor slip at its insertion, it consists of flexion of the proximal interphalangeal joint and extension of the metacarpophalangeal and distal interphalangeal joints (Fig. 25.23).

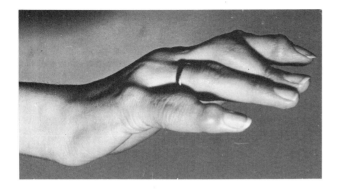

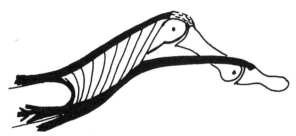

FIG. 25.23. Established boutonnière deformity in the middle finger. Pre-boutonnière synovial blow-outs in the little finger. Mechanism of deformity is shown in the sketch.

The deformity must be distinguished from other causes of flexion of the proximal interphalangeal joint, notably flexor tenosynovitis and volar capsular contracture which are not associated with hyperextension of the neighbouring joints of the digit.

Pathogenesis

The first lesion is synovial invasion and attenuation of the attachment of the middle slip to the base of the middle phalanx. As the slip retracts the joint flexes, and stretching of the transverse retinacular fibres allows volar migration of the lateral bands which finally cross the axis of rotation of the joint and become flexors instead of extensors. The deformity is now self-perpetuating: attempts to extend the finger result in ever more flexion of the proximal interphalangeal joint with extension of the neighbouring metacarpophalangeal and distal interphalangeal joints (Fig. 25.24).

Three clear stages in the evolution of the deformity must be recognized clinically.

Stage 1 (pre-boutonnière). Synovitis of the proximal interphalangeal joint. When the swelling demarcates itself into two soft pouting ridges on either side of the middle slip on the midline dorsally, erosion and stretching are under way and boutonnière deformity is threatened (Fig. 25.23).

Stage 2 (Mobile boutonnière). The tendon lesion is established and active extension is lost, while passive motion is still possible (Fig. 25.25).

Stage 3 (Fixed boutonnière). Articular destruction and tendon adhesion fix the joint in flexion deformity which slowly increases until fibrous ankylosis takes place (Fig. 25.26).

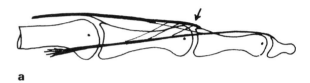

a

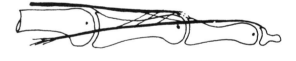

b

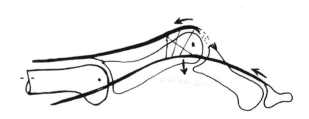

c

FIG. 25.24. Pathogenesis of the deformity.
(a) Normal anatomy. Arrow shows the site of the lesion.
(b) Yielding of middle extensor slip insertion with proximal migration. Volar drift of lateral bands which thus become flexors.
(c) Inevitable flexion of proximal interphalangeal joint and extension of metacarpophalangeal and distal interphalangeal joints.

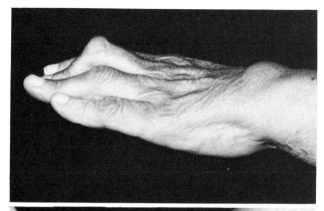

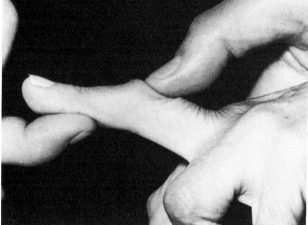

Fig. 25.25. Testing for passive extensibility of the joint before undertaking tendon reconstruction. This finger is in stage 2, advancing towards stage 3.

Management

The deformity is usually compatible with fair function so most do not come to surgery. Each case must be assessed on its own merits in the light of the stage of local pathology, the function of the hand and the general state of the disease.

Stage 1 (Pre-boutonnière)

Full medical treatment is mandatory. Intra-articular injection therapy may still be of benefit. Physiotherapy has no place at this stage: the accent should be on rest, so manual exertion should be reduced to a minimum.

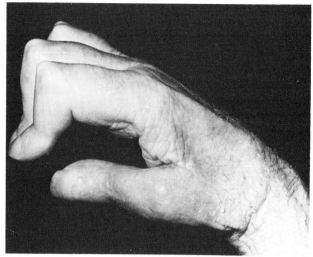

Fig. 25.26. Late fixed boutonnière deformity. Tendons and joints are all fibrosed.

Surgical synovectomy should be strongly considered as a prophylactic measure in selected cases. Factors favouring a decision to perform synovectomy include:

(1) Reasonable control of the systemic disease on a medical regime.

(2) Persistent severe pain.

(3) Good preservation of articular surfaces.

(4) Other fingers which have already developed boutonnière deformities should act as prognostic pointers to those already in Stage 1 but not yet deformed.

Surgical synovectomy. The joint is approached by two parallel incisions on either side of the middle slip. At closure, the stretched transverse retinacular fibres are double breasted to draw the lateral bands dorsally. Mobilization started on first or second day ensures that motion is not lost.

Stage 2 (Mobile boutonnière)

Surgical repair is indicated when other joints are relatively undamaged but multiple boutonnières are impairing function. Results of late salvage surgery are less satisfactory than early tendon repair at this stage. It is more important to repair the index and middle fingers than the little finger. The younger the patient, the more she may need the repair. Cosmetic considerations may also be important.

Repair of extension mechanism. Any attempt at repair must achieve two objects: the middle slip must be re-inserted, and the lateral bands must be replaced on the dorsum. Many techniques have been described [102–106]. Figure 25.27 shows a selection of three of these.

In Heywood's technique (Fig. 25.28), a flap of skin, its fat and dorsal veins carefully preserved, is elevated through a curved dorsolateral incision (Fig. 35.1). Two longitudinal incisions in the extensor expansion, 6–7 mm apart extend on either side of the middle slip from the middle of the proximal phalanx to the base of the middle phalanx, and a transverse cut joins these two limbs 6–7 mm proximal to the insertion. The middle slip is then dissected proximally and the capsule reflected distally to afford easy access for synovectomy if required. The lateral bands are now freed anteriorly to bring them and the rest of the extensor expansion dorsally, leaving the oblique retinacular ligament *in situ*. The ulnar lateral band is cut through at its distal junction with its fellow.

It and the middle slip are grasped with a moist swab and drawn distally while flexing the distal joint simultaneously. The whole extensor apparatus is thus pulled distally to its normal position. The middle slip now overlaps the thickened dorsal capsule where it must be fixed with two mattress sutures, the most distal of which

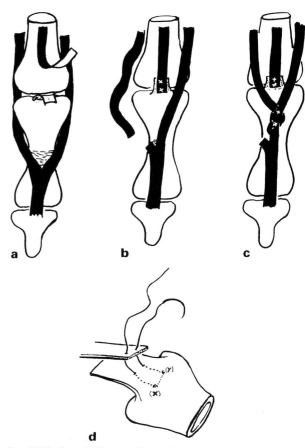

FIG. 25.28. Steps in Heywood's repair of the extensor mechanism.
(a) Elevation of the middle slip and drawing it distally.
(b) Mobilization of the lateral bands and transection of the ulnar lateral band which is also pulled distally. Suture of the middle slip onto the dorsal capsule and periosteum.
(c) End-to-side suture of the ulnar lateral band into its fellow on the dorsum of the middle phalanx to afford maximum cohesion.
(d) Detail of the key suture of middle slip into dorsal capsule and the base of the middle phalanx. The needle must exit at (X) and pass under the periosteum to exit again at (Y) before returning through joint capsule. When the purchase on periosteum is insufficient, a fine drill hole should be made through bone for the suture.

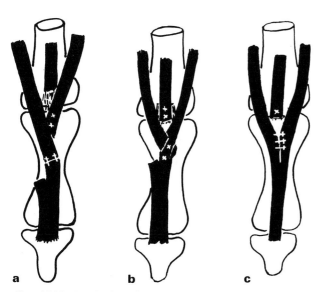

FIG. 25.27. A selection of methods for repair of the mobile rheumatoid boutonnière deformity.
(a) Matev [105]. The lateral bands are mobilized. One slip is transferred to the base of the middle phalanx, the other being lengthened.
(b) Heywood [103]. The middle slip is advanced onto the dorsal capsule and one lateral band is sutured end-to-side to its fellow on the dorsum of the middle phalanx.
(c) Nalebuff and Millender [109]. The middle slip is advanced and the lateral bands are sutured side-to-side on the dorsum.

goes down distally through the dorsal capsule to pick up a transverse bit of periosteum on the base of the middle phalanx (Fig. 25.28d). The end of the ulnar lateral band is now laced twice through the radial lateral band just distal to the proximal interphalangeal joint at such a tension that the end-to-side anastomosis comes to lie centrally (Fig. 25.28c). The site of junction is 6–7 mm distal to the joint, distal enough to allow free flexion but proximal enough to prevent button-holing of the joint in flexion. Finally, the thin transverse retinacular fibres preserved medial to the lateral bands are folded over the middle slip repair, and held there with one suture. A diagonal Kirschner wire holds the joint nearly straight for 14 days and a light plaster slab holds the distal joint flexed at 45°. A removable straight splint is worn for 6 weeks. Gentle mobilization may start on the 14th day, increasing gradually from the 21st day.

In this technique it is important to preserve the regenerated dorsal capsule of the joint as described. The tissue has always been found to be thick enough to hold sutures. Moreover, preservation of its synovial lining enhances the recovery of joint motion once the Kirschner wire has been removed. Twenty-seven out of 29 patients were satisfied with the results at review one to thirteen years after operation (Fig. 25.29). As indicated in Table 25.1, the improvement seen in the first five years tends to diminish in the second five-year period as it does with all arthritis surgery, due to stiffness caused by the slowly advancing disease.

TABLE 25.1. Summary of results of extensor mechanism repairs on rheumatoid boutonnière fingers over a period of 1–13 years. Twenty-nine patients with repairs to forty-five fingers: four index, sixteen middle, twenty-one ring and four little fingers.

	Preoperative	Postoperative	
		1 year	5 years +
PROXIMAL INTERPHALANGEAL JOINT			
Average extensor lag	61°	8°	8°
Average range of active motion	20°	72°	45°
Average range of passive motion	80°	75°	45°
DISTAL INTERPHALANGEAL JOINT			
Average posture when finger held straight	Hyperextended 8°	Flexed 5°	5°
Average range of active motion	15°	42°	35°

Extensor tenotomy

When extensor lag of the proximal interphalangeal joint is less than 30° and hyperextension of the distal interphalangeal joint is the main disability, Fowler's [102] extensor tenotomy as elaborated by Dolphin [107] and

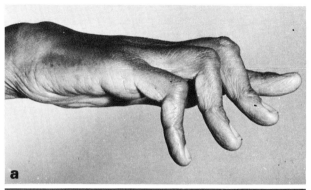
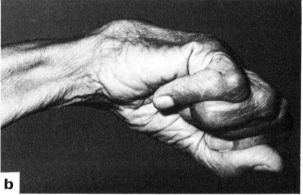
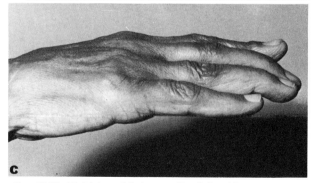

FIG. 25.29. Multiple mobile boutonnière deformities.
 (a) Before tendon reconstruction.
 (b) Fingers flexed.
 (c) Several years after reconstruction: fingers extended.

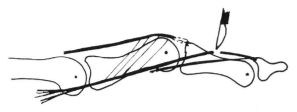

FIG. 25.30. Open extensor tenotomy (Fowler [102]). It is essential to leave intact the oblique retinacular ligament of Landsmeer volar to the extensor mechanism.

Nalebuff [106] may be sufficient (Fig. 25.30). To avoid postoperative mallet deformity, the oblique retinacular ligaments must be preserved. Therefore an open operation is required; and splinting of the distal interphalangeal joint may be needed for some weeks.

Stage 3 (Rigid boutonnière)

An early fixed flexion deformity with intact articular surface may occasionally be mobilized by physiotherapy and a dynamic splint, to enable tendon repair to be carried out successfully.

In most cases, the approach has been to accept the deformity or at most offer arthrodesis of the proximal interphalangeal joint at from 20° flexion (index) to 40° flexion (little finger). However, Swanson reports good results after replacement arthroplasty [108], and this is supported by Nalebuff [109] and others. Arthroplasty is likely to gain more acceptance in future, though results can never match those of reconstructive surgery done at an earlier stage.

ARTHROPLASTY IN THE RHEUMATOID HAND

A. B. SWANSON

The improvement following arthroplasty of the digital joints, particularly of the metacarpophalangeal, is predictable and rewarding if appropriate indications and careful technique are applied.

There has been in the past few years a great progress in the development of arthroplasty methods for the small joints. It is now possible to achieve predictable results in reconstruction of the destroyed arthritic joints and the surgeon has a great responsibility in understanding and selecting the most appropriate treatment;

he has also an important role in the rehabilitation of these patients.

In recent years a large number of recognized varieties of arthroplasty, based on different mechanical and biological concepts, have been developed and in many cases have given satisfactory results. This account, however, will deal only with those devised by the author which in general have given the patients prolonged periods of pain relief and a considerable degree of useful function.

Arthroplasty should approach as near as possible the ideal of a pain-free, mobile, stable, durable and salvageable joint. Three different concepts of arthroplasty for finger reconstruction have emerged: resection arthroplasty, mechanical joint replacement and resection arthroplasty combined with a flexible implant insertion.

Resection of bone in a stiffened joint can improve movement by shortening skeletal structures and by relative lengthening of the soft parts and by providing new gliding surfaces; it also allows nature to develop a new supporting fibrous articular capsule, but the results of this procedure are unpredictable.

In *mechanical joint replacement* the function is completely substituted by a mechanical model; this approach has certain attractive engineering possibilities but has

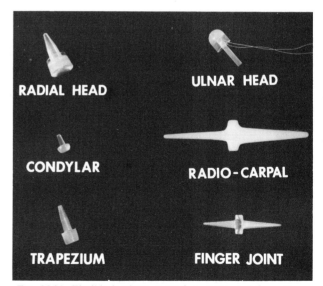

FIG. 25.31. Flexible implants most frequently used for arthroplasty of destroyed joints in the upper extremity; they are made of high performance silicone elastomer.

met with mixed success because of bone absorption and implant lossening.

In order to obtain a simple and reproducible arthroplasty flexible implants have been designed and developed as an adjunct to resection arthroplasty [110–116] (Fig. 25.31). *The flexible implant resection arthroplasty* could be expressed simply in: BONE RESECTION + IMPLANT + ENCAPSULATION = NEW JOINT.

The flexible implant acts as a dynamic spacer maintaining the internal alignment of the reconstructed joint and provides support for the capsule and ligaments developing around it. The latter has been named 'the encapsulation process'. The useful adaptability of the new capsule and ligaments is flexible to such an extent that when increased mobility is desired, e.g. in the finger arthroplasty, motion can be started early; on the other hand when greater stability is required such as in the carpal, radiocarpal and metacarpophalangeal joint of the thumb reconstruction, the period of the postoperative immobilization can be extended.

It is important that an arthroplasty procedure should be amenable to further use when required; this implies preservation of bone and soft tissues so that a further procedure can be performed. Provision of this requirement by the flexible implant arthroplasty is of particular importance [115]. If an implant fractures and instability necessitates its removal, a functioning resection arthroplasty remains. Modern implants have very much greater resistance to tear propagation than the original material. The bone removal in this method is minimal and as its absorption practically never occurs an arthrodesis using a bone graft can be easily done.

The metacarpophalangeal and interphalangeal joints of the fingers

Metacarpophalangeal deformities are especially noticeable and at the same time are most amenable to treatment by arthroplasty. Precise anatomical dissection, soft tissue release, prevention of oedema and early supervised movement in functional planes are essential for good results.

With involvement of both metacarpophalangeal and proximal interphalangeal joints, the former should have first priority in the reconstructive and rehabilitation programme. Tendon imbalance or bone and joint malalignment should be corrected if the long-term result is to be satisfactory.

Metacarpophalangeal joint implant arthroplasty

General considerations. The ideal motion following this procedure should provide adequate flexion of the ulnar fingers for grasp while flexion of the index and long fingers should be enough for pinch activities. Abduction of the fingers, especially of the index, and their full extension are also important. A meticulous postoperative rehabilitation programme, including positioning and control of movement by dynamic bracing and physical therapy during the first 6–8 weeks, is as important as surgery. Alternating flexion–extension exercises should be started within the first week to obtain the required range of movement; lateral movements should be prevented. Passive and active exercises along with splinting are carried out under supervision until the patient understands the instructions and is able to carry them out independently.

A frequent disabling deformity is the pronated index, when the finger presents its relatively less useful lateral surface for opposition. This deformity originates mainly in the metacarpophalangeal joint and thus its arthroplasty should include the following measures of correction of pronation tendency by using soft tissue constraint across the joint and by provision of active supinating forces as well:

(1) the long extensor tendon should not be reefed too far radially as this would aggravate the deformity;

(2) as the first dorsal interosseous, when palmarly subluxated, contributes to pronation, it should be replaced to the normal position in order to stabilize the index;

(3) the ulnar intrinsic should be released only if severely tight;

(4) the finger can be rotated out of pronation by reattaching the radial collateral ligament dorsally on the metacarpal;

(5) the implant should be inserted with the finger in slight supination.

Stabilization of the implant stem against rotational forces is also dependent on the reaming of the medullary canals in a correct rectangular and axial alignment. Postoperative control of rotation with dressing and dynamic bracing is also important. The patient should be instructed to avoid a pure lateral pinch; three point pulp pinch or supported lateral pinch should be always recommended instead.

Indications for arthroplasty include the following, either singly or in combination:

(1) stiff metacarpophalangeal joint;

(2) evidence of joint destruction or subluxation;

(3) ulnar drift considered not correctable by surgery of soft tissues alone;

(4) contracted intrinsic and extrinsic musculature and ligaments.

(5) severe pain.

A typical radiograph showing joint destruction, subluxation and severe ulnar drift is seen in Figure 25.32a. Figure 25.32b shows the postoperative correction.

Surgical procedure. A transverse dorsal incision is made over the metacarpal necks. The intercapitular veins (p. 37) are preserved. The extensor hood is incised on the ulnar side and parallel to the extensor tendon. The neck of the metacarpal is transected without splintering the bone and leaving part of the metacarpal flare with the shaft. The collateral ligaments and capsular attachments are detached from the metacarpal and retained. The metacarpal head along with the attached synovial tissue is removed. The synovectomy is then completed as far as possible.

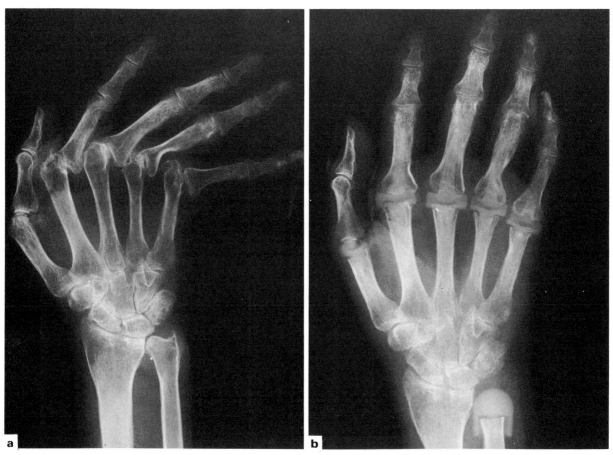

Fig. 25.32. (a) Preoperative radiograph showing a typical finding of rheumatoid arthritis in the hand and wrist, particularly the ulnar deviation of the fingers and subluxation of the metacarpophalangeal joints.

(b) Four-year postoperative radiograph showing reconstructive surgery with implants at the metacarpophalangeal joints and the distal ulna.

Complete and symmetrical soft tissue release, which may include the palmar plate, must be done in order to obtain an appropriate width of the joint space. The ulnar intrinsic tendon is pulled up into the wound with a blunt hook and if found tight, sectioned at the myotendinous junction. The abductor digiti minimi is cut on the ulnar aspect of the fifth metacarpophalangeal joint, taking care to avoid the digital nerve. The flexor digiti minimi is preserved.

Bone resection may include also the base of the proximal phalanx in presence of marginal osteophytes or severe deformity which could interfere with the implant. The medullary canals are carefully prepared by a drill with a smooth leader tip to avoid cortical perforation. The stem of the implant should fit well down both canals so that its transverse part abuts against the bone. The wound is thoroughly irrigated with saline to remove all debris and all implants are inserted with *blunt* instruments and *a no-touch technique*. When the joint is put in extension, the bones should not impinge on the transverse part of the implant, if the soft tissue release and bone resection have been adequate. The extensor hood is reefed in order to bring the extensor tendon to the midline. Reconstruction of the radial collateral ligament is carried out in the index and long fingers by suturing it to a new position on the dorsoradial aspect of the neck through small drill holes.

The capsule is also sutured to the dorsal aspect of the bone (Fig. 25.33). The sutures are placed before the implant is inserted, and tied as the finger is held in supination and radially deviated. The first dorsal interosseous fibres are relocated dorsally by this. Flexion may be limited but this is outweighed by increased stability and a better correction of the pronation deformity. The skin incision is closed and a bulky conforming dressing, including a palmar plaster splint, applied. Postoperative elevation of the limb is essential. The change of the dressing and institution of the dynamic brace and the postoperative programme takes place usually between the third and fifth postoperative days.

Proximal interphalangeal joint arthroplasty

Successful treatment of deformities of this joint is difficult.

Indications. The specific indications for arthroplasty are: (1) destroyed or subluxated joint (Fig. 25.34a, b), and (2) stiffened joint in which a soft tissue release alone would be inadequate.

In a severe disability of this joint in the index alone, implant arthroplasty is indicated. The patient would use the long finger for strong pinch and would appreciate the additional range of movement of the index. In a working

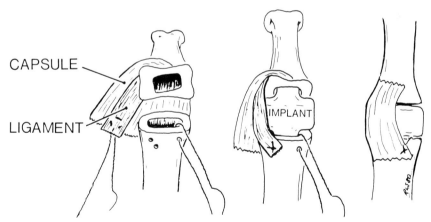

FIG. 25.33. Measures to correct pronation deformity of index finger. Proper rectangular and axial reaming of intramedullary canal is necessary to stabilize implant stems and maintain slight supination. Axis of rectangle is placed high on dorsal ulnar side of base of proximal phalanx and low on its radial palmar side.

A distally based flap made of collateral ligament and related structures is released from neck of metacarpal and sutured with 3–0 Dacron to its dorso-radial aspect through small drill holes.

Preserved radial capsule can be included in this repair.

man with disability of the proximal interphalangeal joints of both the index and long fingers, arthrodesis of the index joint in a position of 20–30° of flexion and implant arthroplasty of the long finger joint, reconstructing the radial collateral ligament are preferred. The more stable index can be used for pinch while the flexion obtained from the arthroplasty in the other finger should assist in grasp. Active flexion of the proximal interphalangeal joints of the ring and little fingers is very important for grasping and should be restored if possible.

Technique of arthroplasty. A dorsal approach with splitting of the central tendon is preferred (Fig. 25.34c, d, e). Each half of the tendon is displaced palmarward to expose the joint. If this is not possible, the head of the proximal phalanx is resected first. If the insertion of the central tendon needs to be detached to expose a severely deformed or contracted joint, this is later re-attached through drill holes in the bone. The collateral ligaments are preserved whenever possible; if released or their tension readjusted to correct lateral deviation, they must also be reattached to bone. The bone ends are prepared for the implant with small burrs and the air drill. The joint is reduced in position over the implant and the capsule and ligaments are reconstructed to allow good lateral alignment and stability. Full extension and flexion to 90° must be obtained.

In severe swan neck and boutonnière deformities (pp. 364, 371) the longitudinal digital arch must be reestablished and the distal joint should also be placed in posi-

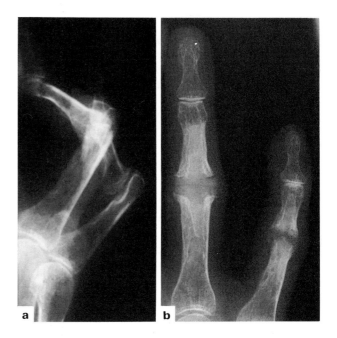

FIG. 25.34. Implant arthroplasty for proximal interphalangeal joint.

(a) Preoperative radiograph showing boutonnière deformity with severe joint destruction and dislocation in a rheumatoid patient.

(b) Radiograph 7 years after implant reconstruction.

(c) The central tendon is incised longitudinally from the base of the middle phalanx through the distal two-thirds of the proximal phalanx.

(d) and (e) Following adequate bone preparation, a 1 mm drill hole is made in the base of the middle phalanx to receive a 3–0 Dacron suture for reinsertion of the halves of the central tendon. This is especially necessary after the central tendon has been released to remove exostoses as seen in osteoarthritis, or if the central tendon has been ruptured. Wherever possible, tendons or ligaments must be sutured to bone in order to obtain a firm fixation.

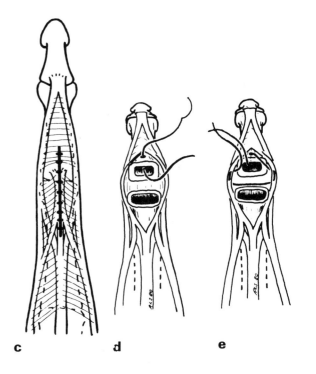

tion for the best function. Adjustment of the tension of the central and lateral tendons is essential. Simply stated, in swan-neck deformity the central tendon is relatively tight and must be released while in the boutonnière deformity the central tendon is relatively loose and must be tightened.

A small padded aluminium splint is applied with the finger straight after 2 or 3 days. The active postoperative exercises are started after 7–10 days. Splinting in extension at night is required for up to 6 weeks but passive exercises can be started at 3 weeks. In swan-neck deformity, the postoperative splint is applied with 20° flexion for 10 days and full extension is avoided for 3 to 6 weeks to obtain a slight flexion contracture of the PIP joint. In boutonnière deformity, splinting in extension is maintained throughout but the distal joint is allowed to flex freely.

The distal interphalangeal joint

Fusion procedures are the treatment of choice (p. 494) and arthroplasty of this joint is not indicated in rheumatoid arthritis.

The thumb ray

All three joints of the thumb are important in functional adaptations and each one may be primarily or secondarily affected by imbalance of the remainder. A sound understanding of the mechanism of deformities (p. 362) is important in selection of the correct treatment.

The interphalangeal joint

Instability of this joint requires arthrodesis. Occasionally a mobile hyperextension deformity of this joint occurs: the patient may be able to flex the joint actively but during strong pinch severe hyperextension is manifested. A flexor hemitenodesis prevents hyperextension and still allows flexion; in a number of patients with pain and disability and who have an adequate bony and ligamentous stability, resection arthroplasty has been performed, inserting a single- or double-stemmed silicone implant. The use of this articular spacer preserves some flexion which can be important when the other joints are disabled, but is seldom indicated.

The metacarpophalangeal joint

Fusion is indicated when there is severe joint destruction (p. 495); it may be also important in balancing a severe collapse deformity when the distal and basal joints are adequate. If possible, fusion should be limited to only one joint of the articular chain if a reasonable function is to be achieved.

Implant resection arthroplasty, using the flexible finger joint implant, is indicated for a severely destroyed joint in the presence of associated stiffness of the distal or basal joint and for boutonnière deformity in which the metacarpophalangeal joint is destroyed and the distal joint requires fusion. For good results it is essential to follow the technical considerations as for finger joint arthroplasty and to reconstruct the extensor mechanism. If the distal joint is to be fused, the extensor pollicis brevis and longus is sutured to the base of the proximal phalanx and the intrinsic muscles are reefed over the joint. A padded aluminium splint is taped on the thumb to hold the joint straight for 3–4 weeks. No special exercises are prescribed after the splint removal; normal function and avoidance of forceful activities for six to eight weeks is advised.

The carpometacarpal joint

Severe absorptive changes of the trapezium and base of the metacarpal produce a result not unlike resection arthroplasty. If the joint is reasonably stable, mobile and pain-free, *no surgery* is indicated. Some patients, however, have a dislocation of the metacarpal off the trapezium in addition to severe erosive and absorptive bony changes and ligamentous loosening at the base of the thumb: the destructive changes may be too great to allow implant or other stabilizing procedures and *a simple resection arthroplasty* is indicated.

Implant arthroplasty of this joint has a definite place in the reconstruction of the rheumatoid hand. Two different procedures have been designed: (1) trapezium implant replacement, and (2) trapeziometacarpal arthroplasty. Meticulous and firm reconstruction of the capsule and ligaments around these implants and correction of the associated thumb deformities are essential.

Trapezium implant arthroplasty

This implant is a space filler preserving the anatomical relationships after resection of the trapezium. It aids stability, prevents the tendency to subluxation which may follow simple resection and obviates the disadvantages of rigidity or poor positioning which may follow fusion. Preservation of motion at the basal joint allows stabilization or fusion of the distal joints in position of function. Satisfactory relief of pain and a good strength of grip and pinch is obtained.

Indications. In rheumatoid arthritis the implant replacement is indicated when the destruction is limited to the joints around the trapezium (p. 16), singly or in combination and when there is a sufficient bone to support the implant.

Surgical technique (Fig. 25.35). A longitudinal dorsal incision centred over the trapezium is made on the ulnar side and parallel to the extensor pollicis brevis tendon; its proximal end is continued transversely across the front of the wrist and then prolonged longitudinally and proximally in line with the flexor carpi radialis tendon. The branches of the superficial radial nerve are protected. The retinacular roof of the first dorsal compartment is incised and the dissection is carried down between the tendons of the abductor pollicis longus and extensor pollicis brevis. The radial artery is carefully mobilized and retracted (Fig. 25.35a). The capsule over the scaphoid, trapezium and the base of the first meta-

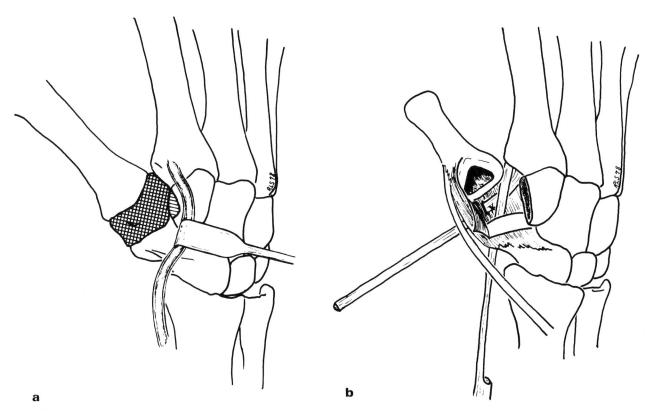

a   **b**

FIG. 25.35. Technique for trapezium implant arthroplasty.

(a) Retraction of radial artery over scaphoid bone is essential for proper exposure. Adequate excision of the trapezium including projection between the first and second metacarpals and, when necessary, trimming of the radial aspect of the trapezoid bone, are most important to obtain perfect fit of implant over the scaphoid facet. A 6–8 cm distally based slip of flexor carpi radialis tendon is used for capsular reinforcement.

(b) Excision of bone completed. Flexor carpi radialis tendon slip is dissected to its insertion on second metacarpal, passed deep to and sutured to flexor carpi radialis tendon and palmar capsule. Slip exits radially through abductor pollicis brevis muscle.

carpal is incised longitudinally and dissected carefully off the underlying bones and joints. The trapezium is removed piecemeal including the most medial portion, taking care to avoid injury to the underlying capsule and the tendon of the flexor carpi radialis. Small specks of bone with the underlying capsule may be left in order to maintain a good palmar capsular and ligamentous support. Any osteophytes or irregularities of the distal end of scaphoid or trapezoid can be trimmed. Occasionally a portion of the trapezoid should be removed to allow the implant to fit better over the scaphoid. The base of the metacarpal is squared off leaving most of the cortical and subchondral bone. The

medullary canal of the metacarpal is then carefully prepared in a triangular fashion on cross-section to receive the stem of the implant. The implant of the correct size, selected from the five available sizes, should fit the space left by the resection of the trapezium and should allow full circumduction of the thumb while remaining stable over the scaphoid. The base of the implant should fit well over the distal scaphoid facet. The collar of the implant should be seated snugly on the base of the metacarpal. It is most important to obtain a secure capsular and ligamentous support around the implant. Before its insertion the palmar capsule should be inspected for any inadvertent tears or 'holes' and if

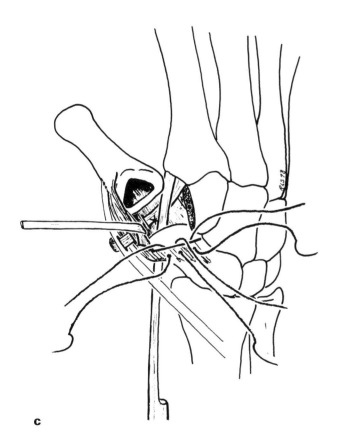

c

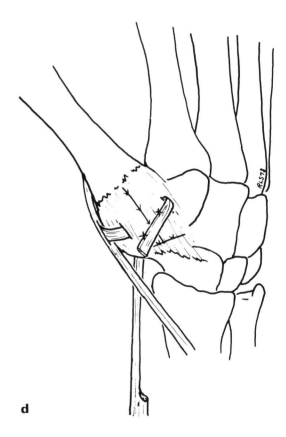

d

FIG. 25.35 *Continued*

(c) Flexor carpi radialis slip passed through abductor pollicis longus tendon and lateral capsule. Sutures passed through capsular reflections off scaphoid bone or through 1 mm drill holes made in edge of bone to secure capsular closure.

(d) After implant is inserted and the dorsal capsule sutured, the flexor carpi radialis slip is brought over and through radial capsule to exit through ulnar capsule. Slip is then pulled, folded over and across the dorsal capsule and sutured in position.   *[Continued overleaf]*

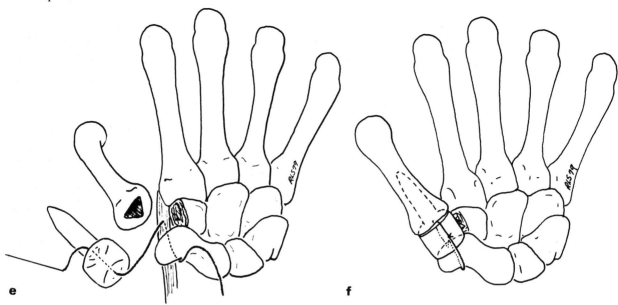

e   f

FIG. 25.35 *Continued*

(e) Temporary fixation of trapezium implant with 0 synthetic absorbable suture on TR-5 needle. As radial artery is retracted, the curved needle is passed under and around waist of scaphoid and picked up distally. Suture is passed through insertion of flexor carpi radialis tendon. Curved needle is then straightened and passed through implant from middle of concave facet to exit distally adjacent to the stem.

(f) Implant inserted, and temporary fixation suture tied securely with multiple surgical knots.

(g) Alternate method of temporary fixation with 0.045″ Kirschner wire passed through body of implant into trapezoid bone.

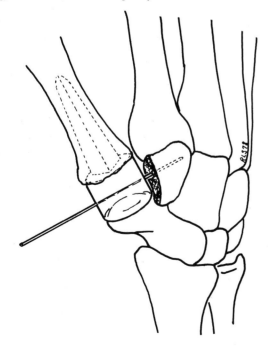

g

present, they should be repaired. The dorsal and radial capsule is sutured tightly over the implant with non-absorbable sutures, using an inverted knot technique. It is most important to secure radial capsular repair by suturing the proximal part of the capsule to the scaphoid; the sutures may be placed through 1 mm drill holes in the scaphoid. If the capsular sutures are inadequate or subluxation of the trapeziometacarpal joint was present, further reinforcement using tendon strips from the abductor pollicis longus, extensor carpi radialis longus or, preferably, from the flexor carpi radialis is provided (Fig. 25.35b, c, d). With the modern implant, its temporary fixation with either a small Kirschner wire into the trapezoid or an absorbable suture passed through the centre of the implant into the scaphoid, is permissible (Fig. 25.35e, f, g). The skin is closed and a small drain is inserted subcutaneously. A conforming dressing is applied, including an anterior plaster splint. The limb is kept elevated and below elbow plaster is applied after 4 or 5 days. If a Kirschner wire was used a small window

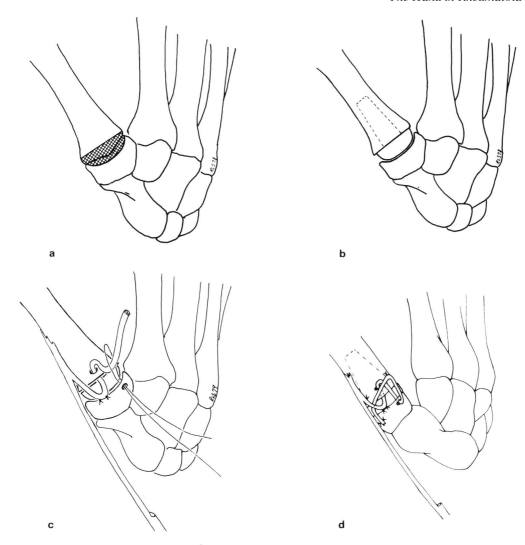

FIG. 25.36. Arthroplasty of the trapeziometacarpal joint with a convex condylar, single stem silicone implant.

(a) The resection should include the distal surface of the trapezium and its articulating projection to the second metacarpal base. A sufficient resection of the base of the metacarpal is carried out to provide an adequate joint space.

(b) The stem of the convex condylar implant is introduced into the prepared intramedullary canal of the first metacarpal. The thin implant head seats on the prepared trapezium.

(c) An 8 cm distally based slip of the abductor pollicis longus tendon is prepared and its insertion to the radial aspect of the metacarpal is preserved. The slip is then looped into the intramedullary canal and the end of the slip is extracted through a 2–3 mm hole in the radiodorsal aspect of the metacarpal. A similar hole is made in the trapezium. The end of the slip is then drawn from the inside of the bone to the outside. It can be noted that when this slip is pulled up tight, this arrangement forces the metacarpal slightly ulnarward, providing an excellent check-rein to radial subluxation of the base of the metacarpal. (Slip should be inside-out–inside-out.) The previously sized implant is inserted and the tendon slip is pulled tight.

(d) The remaining tendon slip is securely interwoven and secured to reinforce the capsular closure as noted in this illustration. The distal end of the slip is passed through or under the insertion of the abductor pollicis longus and sutured to the radial capsular structures of the trapezium.   *[Continued overleaf]*

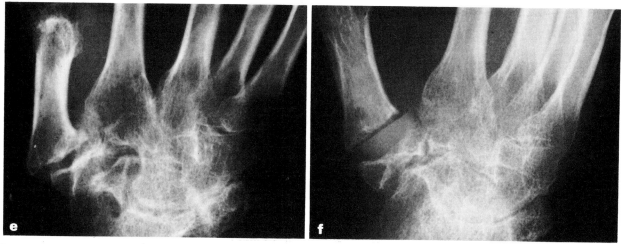

FIG. 25.36 *Continued*

   (e) Radiograph showing severe destruction of the trapeziometacarpal joint in a rheumatoid patient. Note the severity of involvement of the carpal bones in this patient.

   (f) Radiograph 1 year following trapeziometacarpal joint arthroplasty using a convex condylar implant and the abductor pollicis longus ligamentous reconstruction.

is made over its exit site; it is removed after 2 weeks and the cast after 6 weeks. The patient is instructed to start a guarded range of motion, pinch and grasp activities.

Trapeziometacarpal implant arthroplasty

Many patients with disabilities of the basal joint of the thumb show destruction of the carpal bones which makes trapezium implant replacement difficult; frequently the trapezium is fused to the scaphoid or the latter is absorbed or shifted ulnarly. Instead of excising the trapezium, *a limited resection of the base of the metacarpal and of the distal surface of the trapezium* is performed (Fig. 25.36a). Enough bone should be removed to allow the metacarpal to be abducted radially to 45°. The stem of the specially designed convex *condylar implant* (Fig. 25.36b) is inserted into the medullary canal of the first metacarpal. There is usually a tendency to subluxation which can be corrected by a firm capsular and ligamentous repair, using a slip from the tendon of the abductor pollicis longus (Fig. 25.36c). The distally based slip is interwoven through the metacarpal, trapezium and the capsule to provide an excellent stabilizing effect (Fig. 25.36d). Because of the narrow joint space in this

procedure, the usual range of motion achieved by the standard trapezium implant arthroplasty cannot be expected. However, a stable, pain-free and functioning joint can result if the recommended technique is followed (Fig. 25.36e, f).

Other deformities affecting the outcome of arthroplasties of the thumb are:

Adduction of the first metacarpal, if severe and untreated, will unbalance the thumb and affect seriously the result of the resection arthroplasties of the trapezium. If the angle between the first and second metacarpals does not reach 45° or more, the origin of the adductor pollicis muscle should be released from the third metacarpal through a separate palmar incision.

Hyperextension of the metacarpophalangeal joint contributes to the adduction tendency of the metacarpal and prevents its proper abduction and seating of the implant. If it is less than 10°, no treatment is necessary except application of the postoperative cast in such a way that it is not the proximal phalanx but the metacarpal which is abducted. With hyperextension between 10° and 20° temporary fixation with a Kirschner wire is indicated and if greater than 20°, stabilization by palmar capsulodesis or fusion is an absolute necessity; when there is 30–40° of metacarpophalangeal flexion present,

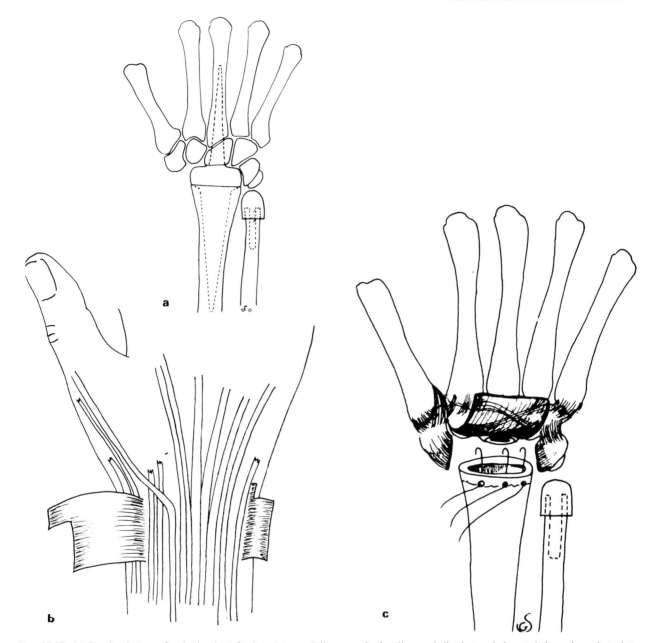

FIG. 25.37. (a) Proximal stem of wrist implant fits into intramedullary canal of radius, and distal stem is inserted through capitate into intramedullary canal of third metacarpal. Silicone ulnar head implant is also shown in place.

(b) Preparation of extensor retinaculum flap based between first and second dorsal compartments. Ulnar flap is based on ulnar aspect of the sixth dorsal compartment. Small additional flap is prepared distally to be used as pulley for relocation of extensor carpi ulnaris tendon in simultaneous implant arthroplasty of the distal radioulnar joint.

(c) Preparation of distally based radiocarpal flap made by elevating the dorsal **capsuloligamentous** structures from the underlying radius and carpal bones.   [*Continued overleaf*]

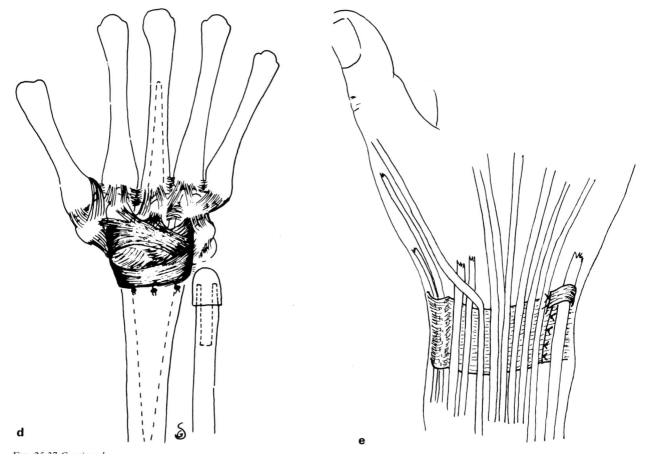

d

e

FIG. 25.37 *Continued*

(d) Radiocarpal capsuloligamentous flap is firmly sutured over the wrist implant. Sutures (3–0 Dacron) are passed through small drill holes in the dorsal cortex of radius and the knots inverted.

(e) Extensor retinacular flap is placed over wrist joint under extensor tendons. Small distal retinacular flap is used to relocate extensor carpi ulnaris tendon over distal ulna.

the joint being otherwise stable and showing good articular surfaces, capsulodesis is the operation of choice. If the swan-neck deformity is severe with no metacarpophalangeal flexion available, fusion of this joint and temporary fixation of the distal joint in extension is advised.

Radiocarpal flexible implant arthroplasty

It has been used as an adjunct to simple resection in order to maintain an adequate joint space and alignment, while at the same time supporting the reconstructed capsule and ligament. The implant is made of modern material and is available in five sizes. The degree of mobility, stability, durability and biological tolerance obtained with this technique to date has been encouraging (Fig. 25.37a).

Indications

(1) Instability of the wrist due to sublūxation or dislocation,

(2) Wrist deviation causing digital imbalance.

(3) Stiffness when movement is required for hand function,

(4) Stiffness or fusion in non-functioning position.

A fusion of the wrist could always be done if the

implant arthroplasty did not meet the functional requirements; however, it has not yet been found necessary.

Surgical technique. A longitudinal dorsal incision is made taking care to protect the superficial sensory nerves. The extensor retinaculum is incised to prepare a radially based flap over the second dorsal compartment (Fig. 25.37b). Another retinacular flap can be prepared at the same time to relocate the tendon of the extensor carpi ulnaris in associated implant reconstruction of the ulnar head. Synovectomy of the extensor compartment is performed after the remainder of the capsule and ligaments are reflected from the radius as a distally based flap. A part of the proximal carpal row is found usually destroyed; the remnants of the lunate and scaphoid are resected along with the portion of the base of the capitate. The underlying palmar tendons and neurovascular structures are protected. The end of the radius is squared off to fit against the distal carpal row; the radiocarpal subluxation should be completely reduced. The medullary canal of the radius is prepared for the proximal stem of the implant, while that of third metacarpal is identified by passing carefully a wire or a very thin broach through the capitate, the base of the third metacarpal and into its shaft, which is prepared to receive the distal stem of the implant. Reconstruction of the distal ulna is carried out if required, and the hand centralized over the radius. After inserting the radiocarpal implant the capsule and ligaments are firmly sutured over the implant through small drill holes in the dorsal cortex of the radius (Fig. 25.37c, d). The repair should be tested to ensure that approximately 45° of extension and flexion range and 10° each of ulnar and radial deviation are possible on passive manipulation. The retinaculum is then carefully repaired deep to the extensor tendons and sutured in place to provide further support (Fig. 25.37e); the wrist extensors are shortened or transferred as required in order to obtain extension without lateral deviation; the digital tendons are repaired if necessary. The wound is closed and a drain inserted subcutaneously. A bulky, conforming dressing is applied including a plaster splint with the wrist in straight position. The limb is elevated for 3–5 days when a below elbow cast with the wrist in the above position is applied and fitted with outriggers to hold the rubber-band slings in order to support the fingers in extension if the tendons have been repaired. This is worn for 2–4 weeks followed by a flexion–extension exercise programme with 50–60° of normal range as an ideal goal.

Implant arthroplasty of the distal radioulnar joint

Intramedullary cuffed implant to cap the end of the resected ulna was designed to help in preserving the anatomical relationships and function of the distal radioulnar joint following ulnar head resection.

Indications. Specific indications include pain and weakness of the wrist not improved by conservative treatment and also instability of the ulnar head with radiographic evidence of erosion and subluxation. The procedure can be also used to correct sequelae of a failed simple ulnar head resection.

Surgical technique. A longitudinal incision is centred over the ulnar head preserving the dorsal cutaneous branches of the ulnar nerve. The extensor retinaculum over the sixth dorsal compartment is incised in such a way as to preserve a narrow, radially based distal and a broad, ulnarly based proximal flap. Synovectomy of the dorsal compartment may also be carried out. The tendon of the flexor carpi ulnaris is retracted and the distal ulna sectioned at the neck; the periosteum is not stripped off the distal ulna, but muscle attachments on its anterior surface are released over the distal 2 cm. The ulnar head and attached synovial sac are removed and synovectomy of the joint completed. The bone end is smoothed so that it presents a cylindrical shape to fit the contour of the implant. The medullary canal of the ulna is prepared to receive the appropriate size implant stem which must fit snugly into the canal and the cuff should seat loosely over the end of the bone. The retinaculum of the sixth dorsal compartment is used as a check ligament to hold dorsally subluxated ulna in a reduced position: the broad, ulnarly based proximal flap is placed under the extensor carpi ulnaris tendon and sutured with non-absorbable material over the ulna to the remaining ligaments of the distal radioulnar joint, to the soft tissues around the radius and to the retinacular fibres of the fifth dorsal compartment; sutures may be placed through drill holes in the radius if necessary. The extensor carpi ulnaris tendon is mobilized proximally and distally; the narrow, radially based distal retinacular flap is looped under and around the tendon and sutured to itself to act as a pulley maintaining this tendon over the ulnar head implant. The digital extensors are repaired if they are ruptured. The incision is closed and the wound drained. A bulky, conforming dressing, including a palmar plaster splint, is applied with the hand in slight dorsiflexion. The drain is removed on the third postoperative day and, if there is no swelling, a below elbow cast or splint is applied in the same position for three to four weeks.

REFERENCES

[1] ANSELL, B. AND HARRISON, S. A five year follow-up of synovectomy of the proximal interphalangeal joint in rheumatoid arthritis. *The Hand*, 1975, **7**, 34.

[2] ARTHRITIS AND RHEUMATISM COUNCIL AND BRITISH ORTHOPAEDIC ASSOCIATION. Controlled trial of synovectomy of knee and metacarpophalangeal joints in rheumatoid arthritis. *Annals of Rheumatic Diseases*, 1976, **35**, 437.

[3] ELLISON, M. R., KELLY, K. J. AND FLATT, A. E. The results of surgical synovectomy of the digital joints in rheumatoid disease. *Journal of Bone and Joint Surgery*, 1971, **53A**, 1041.

[4] SOUTER, W. A. Planning treatment of the rheumatoid hand. *The Hand*, 1979, **11**, 3.

[5] FLATT, A. E. *The Care of the Rheumatoid Hand*, 3rd ed., St. Louis, Mosby, 1974.

[6] BACKDAHL, M. The caput ulnae syndrome in rheumatoid arthritis. *Acta rheumatologica Scandinavica*, 1963, Supplement, **5**, 1.

[7] KELLGREN, J. H. AND BALL, J. Tendon lesions in rheumatoid arthritis. *Annals of Rheumatic Diseases*, 1950, **9**, 48.

[8] BACKHOUSE, K. M., KAY, A. G. L., COOMES, E. N. AND KATES, A. Tendon involvement in the rheumatoid hand. *Annals of Rheumatic Diseases*, 1971, **30**, 236.

[9] STRAUB, L. R. AND RANAWAT, C. S. The wrist in rheumatoid arthritis. Surgical treatment and results. *Journal of Bone and Joint Surgery*, 1969, **51A**, 1.

[10] SAVILL, D. L. Combined management of rheumatoid arthritis. *Manitoba Medical Review*, 1966, **46**, 527.

[11] VAUGHAN-JACKSON, O. J. Rupture of extensor tendons by attrition at the inferior radio-ulnar joint. *Journal of Bone and Joint Surgery*, 1948, **30B**, 528.

[12] VAUGHAN-JACKSON, O. J. Attrition ruptures of tendons as a factor in the production of deformities in the rheumatoid hand. *Proceedings of the Royal Society of Medicine*, 1959, **52**, 132.

[13] VAUGHAN-JACKSON, O. J. Rheumatoid hand deformities considered in the light of tendon imbalance. *Journal of Bone and Joint Surgery*, 1962, **44B**, 764.

[14] ABERNETHY, P. J. AND DENNYSON, W. G. Decompression of extensor tendons in rheumatoid arthritis. *Journal of Bone and Joint Surgery*, 1979, **61B**, 64.

[15] CLAYTON, M. L. Surgical treatment at the wrist in rheumatoid arthritis. A review of thirty-seven patients. *Journal of Bone and Joint Surgery*, 1965, **47A**, 741.

[16] SAVILL, D. L. The use of splints in management of the rheumatoid hand. In *La Main Rheumatoide*, p. 219, Groupe D'Etude de la Main Monograph No. 3, ed. R. Tubiana. Paris, L'Espansion, 1969.

[17] LAINE, V. A. I. AND VAINIO, K. J. Spontaneous rupture of tendons in rheumatoid arthritis. *Acta orthopaedica Scandinavica*, 1955, **24**, 250.

[18] SAVILL, D. L. Surgery of the rheumatoid hand. *Journal of Bone and Joint Surgery*, 1972, **54B**, 559.

[19] VAUGHAN-JACKSON, O. J. Egg-cup erosion. *The Hand*, 1969, **1**, 9.

[20] RANAWAT, C. S., FREIBERGER, R. H., JORDON, L. R. AND STRAUB, L. R. Arthrography in the rheumatoid wrist joint. A preliminary report. *Journal of Bone and Joint Surgery*, 1969, **51A**, 1269.

[21] SHAPIRO, J. S. The etiology of ulnar drift: a new factor. *Journal of Bone and Joint Surgery*, 1968, **50A**, 634.

[22] STACK, H. G. AND VAUGHAN-JACKSON, O. J. The zig-zag deformity in the rheumatoid hand. *The Hand*, 1971, **3**, 62.

[23] PAHLE, J. A. AND RAUNIO, P. The influence of wrist position on finger deviation in the rheumatoid hand. *Journal of Bone and Joint Surgery*, 1969, **51B**, 664.

[24] LANDSMEER, J. M. F. Studies in the anatomy of articulation: the equilibrium of the intercalated bone. *Acta morphologica neerlando-Scandinavica*, 1960, **3**, 287.

[25] LINSCHEID, R. L. AND DOBYNS, J. H. Rheumatoid arthritis of the wrist. *Orthopaedic Clinics of North America*, 1971, **2**, 649.

[26] MANNERFELT, L. AND MALMSTEN, M. Arthrodesis of the wrist in rheumatoid arthritis. A technique without external fixation. *Scandinavian Journal of Plastic and Reconstructive Surgery*, 1971, **5**, 124.

[27] RANA, N. A. AND TAYLOR, A. R. Excision of the distal end of the ulna in rheumatoid arthritis. *Journal of Bone and Joint Surgery*, 1973, **55B**, 96.

[28] SAVILL, D. L. Personal communication, 1966.

[29] NICKEL, V., PERRY, J. AND SNELSSON, R. *Hand Book of Hand Splints*. Rancho Los Amigos Hospital, Downey, California.

[30] KESSLER, I. AND VAINIO, K. Posterior (dorsal) synovectomy for rheumatoid involvement of the hand and wrist. A follow-up study of sixty-six procedures. *Journal of Bone and Joint Surgery*, 1966, **48A**, 1085.

[31] CRACCHIOLO, A. AND MARMOR, L. Resection of the distal ulna in rheumatoid arthritis. *Arthritis and Rheumatism*, 1969, **12**, 415.

[32] JACKSON, I. T., MILWARD, T. M., LEE, P. AND WEBB, J. Ulnar head resection in rheumatoid arthritis. *The Hand*, 1974, **6**, 172.

[33] LAUENSTEIN, C. Zur Frage der Derangement Interne des Kniegelenks. *Deutsche Medizinische Wochenschrift*, 1890, **16**, 169.

[33a] GONÇALVES, D. Correction of disorders of the distal radioulnar joint by artificial pseudoarthrosis of the ulna. *Journal of Bone and Joint Surgery*, **56B**, 462.

[34] SWANSON, A. B. Implant arthroplasty for disabilities of the distal radio-ulnar joint. Use of a silicone rubber capping implant following resection of the ulnar head. *Orthopaedic Clinics of North America*, 1973, **4**, 373.

[35] BUNNELL, S. *Surgery of the Hand*, 2nd ed., Philadelphia, Lippincott, 1948.

[36] FERNANDEZ-PALAZZI, F. AND VAINIO, K. Sinovectomia das articulaçoes carpais na artrite reumatoide. Observaçao de 47 casos. *Archives interamericanos de reumatologia*, 1965, **8**, 238.

[37] LIPSCOMB, P. R. Synovectomy of the wrist for rheumatoid arthritis. *Journal of the American Medical Association*, 1965, **194**, 655.

[38] VAINIO, K. Synovectomies of the hand and wrist in rheumatoid arthritis. In *La Main Rheumatismale*, p. 22, Groupe D'Etude de la Main Monograph, No. 1, ed. R. Tubiana. Paris, L'Expansion, 1966.

[39] SAVILL, D. L. Synovectomy of the wrist joint. In *Early Synovectomy in Rheumatoid Arthritis*, p. 100, ed. W. Hijmans, W. D. Paul and H. Herschel. Proceedings of the Symposium on Early Synovectomy in Rheumatoid Arthritis, Amsterdam, Excerpta Medica, 1969.

[40] SOUTER, W. A. Splintage in the rheumatoid hand. *The Hand*, 1971, **3**, 144.

[41] ALBRIGHT, J. A. AND CHASE, R. A. Palmar shelf arthroplasty of the wrist in rheumatoid arthritis. A report of nine cases. *Journal of Bone and Joint Surgery*, 1970, **52A**, 896.

[42] CARROLL, R. E. AND DICK, H. M. Arthrodesis of the wrist for rheumatoid arthritis. *Journal of Bone and Joint Surgery*, 1971, **53A**, 1365.

[43] MILLENDER, L. H. AND NALEBUFF, E. A. Arthrodesis of the rheumatoid wrist. An evaluation of sixty patients and a description of a different surgical technique. *Journal of Bone and Joint Surgery*, 1973, **55A**, 1026.

[44] SWANSON, A. B. Flexible implant arthroplasty for arthritic disabilities of the radiocarpal joint. A silicone rubber intramedullary stemmed flexible hinge implant for the wrist joint. *Orthopaedic Clinics of North America*, 1973, **4**, 383.

[45] MEULI, H. C. Total wrist joint replacement. In *Joint Replacement in the Upper Limb*. Institute of Mechanical Engineers Conference Publications, 1977, **5**, 117.

[46] GSCHWEND, N., SCHEIER, H. AND BAHLER, A. (1977) GSB elbow, wrist and PIP joints. *Institute of Mechanical Engineers Conference Publications*, 1977, **5**, 107.

[47] JACKSON, I. T. Interpositional arthroplasty of the wrist. Paper presented to combined meeting of American and British Hand Societies in Edinburgh, May 1977.

[48] NALEBUFF, E. A. Surgical treatment of tendon rupture in the rheumatoid hand. *Surgical Clinics of North America*, 1969, **49**, 811.

[49] SHANNON, F. T. AND BARTON, N. J. Surgery for rupture of extensor tendons in rheumatoid arthritis. *The Hand*, 1976, **8**, 279.

[49a] HARRISON, S. H., SWANNELL, A. G. AND ANSELL, B. M. Repair of extensor pollicis longus using extensor pollicis brevis in rheumatoid arthritis. *Annals of the Rheumatic Diseases*, 1972, **31**, 490.

[50] RIDDELL, D. M. Spontaneous rupture of the extensor pollicis longus. *Journal of Bone and Joint Surgery*, 1963, **45B**, 506.

[51] BOYES, J. H. *Bunnell's Surgery of the Hand*, p. 448. Philadelphia, Lippincott, 1964.

[52] SAVILL, D. L. Some aspects of rheumatoid hand surgery. In *La Main Rheumatismale*, p. 27, Groupe D'Etude de la Main Monograph No. 1, ed. R. Tubiana, Paris, L'Expansion, 1966.

[53] BREWERTON, D. A. Hand deformities in rheumatoid disease. *Annals of Rheumatic Diseases*, 1957, **16**, 183.

[54] VAINIO, K. Carpal canal syndrome caused by tenosynovitis. *Acta rheumatologica Scandinavica*, 1957, **4**, 22.

[55] BARNES, C. G. AND CURREY, H. L. F. Carpal tunnel syndrome in rheumatoid arthritis. A clinical and electrodiagnostic survey. *Annals of Rheumatic Diseases*, 1970, **26**, 226.

[56] SOUTER, W. A. Synovectomy of flexor tendons in rheumatoid arthritis. A review of 80 cases. Paper presented to combined meeting of American and British Hand Societies in Edinburgh, May 1977.

[57] WISSINGER, H. A. Digital flexor lag in rheumatoid arthritis. *Plastic and Reconstructive Surgery*, 1971, **47**, 465.

[58] SAIRANEN, E. The trigger finger as a rheumatic manifestation. *Acta rheumatologica Scandinavica*, 1957, **3**, 266.

[59] NALEBUFF, E. A. Nature and management of flexor tendon nodules in the rheumatoid hand. In *La Main Rheumatoide*, p. 123, Groupe D'Etude de la Main Monograph No. 3, ed. R. Tubiana. Paris, L'Expansion, 1969.

[60] HELAL, B. Distal profundus entrapment in rheumatoid disease. *The Hand*, 1970, **2**, 48.

[61] MANNERFELT, L. AND NORMAN, O. Attrition ruptures of flexor tendons in rheumatoid arthritis caused by bony spurs in the carpal tunnel. *Journal of Bone and Joint Surgery*, 1969, **51B**, 270.

[62] HARRISON, S. H., ANSELL, B. AND HALL, M. A. Flexor synovectomy in the rheumatoid hand. *The Hand*, 1976, **8**, 13.

[63] CLAYTON, M. L. AND FERLIC, D. C. Flexor tenosynovectomy in rheumatoid arthritis. Paper presented to combined meeting of American and British Hand Societies in Edinburgh, May, 1977.

[64] SWANSON, A. B. Silicone rubber implants for replacement of arthritic or destroyed joints in the hand. *Surgical Clinics of North America*, 1968, **48**, 1113.

[65] HUESTON, J. T. AND STRANG, R. F. A. Flexor tendon synovectomy. *Medical Journal of Australia*, 1973, **2**, 371.

[66] JACKSON, I. T. AND PATON, K. C. The extended approach to flexor tendon synovitis in rheumatoid arthritis. *British Journal of Plastic Surgery*, 1973, **26**, 122.

[67] DAHL, E., MIKKELSEN, O. A. AND SORENSEN, J. U. Flexor tendon synovectomy of the hand in rheumatoid arthritis. A follow-up study of 201 operated hands. *Scandinavian Journal of Rheumatology*, 1976, **5,** 103.

[68] BUNNELL, S. *Surgery of the Hand*, 5th ed., p. 247. Philadelphia, Lippincott, 1970.

[69] FINOCHIOTTO, R. Retracion Isquemica de les intersers de la mano per traumetismo, Buenos Aires, Bilitines y Trabajos de la Societat de Ciringia, 1920.

[70] PARKES, A. R. Traumatic ischaemia of peripheral nerves with some observations on Volkmann's ischaemic contracture. *British Journal of Surgery*, 1945, **32,** 403.

[71] HARRIS, C. AND RIORDAN, D. Intrinsic contracture in the hand and its surgical treatment. *Journal of Bone and Joint Surgery*, 1959, **36A,** 10.

[72] LITTLER, J. W. Restoration of the oblique retinacular ligament. G.E.M. No. 1. Paris, 1966.

[73] NALEBUFF, E. A. Surgical treatment of finger deformation in rheumatoid arthritis. *Surgical Clinics of North America*, 1969, **49,** 833.

[74] BACKHOUSE, K. M. The mechanics of normal digital control in the hand and an analysis of the ulnar drift of rheumatoid arthritis. *Annals of the Royal College of Surgeons of England*, 1968, **43,** 154.

[75] BREWERTON, D. A. Hand deformities in rheumatoid disease. *Annals of Rheumatic Diseases*, 1957, **16,** 183.

[76] FLATT, A. E. Some pathomechanics of ulnar drift. *Plastic and Reconstructive Surgery*, 1966, **37,** 295.

[77] HAKSTIAN, R. W. AND TUBIANA, R. Ulnar deviation of the fingers. *Journal of Bone and Joint Surgery*, 1967, **49A,** 299.

[78] SMITH, R. J. AND KAPLAN, E. B. Rheumatoid deformities at the metacarpophalangeal joints of the fingers. *Journal of Bone and Joint Surgery*, 1967, **49A,** 31.

[79] KUCZYNSKI, K. The synovial structures of the normal and rheumatoid digital joints. *The Hand*, 1971, **3,** 41.

[80] KUCZYNSKI, K. The variations in the insertion of the first dorsal interosseous muscle and their significance in rheumatoid arthritis. *The Hand*, 1972, **4,** 37.

[81] SHAPIRO, J. S. The etiology of ulnar drift. A new factor. *Journal of Bone and Joint Surgery*, 1968, **50A,** 634.

[82] STACK, H. G. AND VAUGHAN-JACKSON, O. J. The zig-zag deformity in the rheumatoid hand. *The Hand*, 1971, **3,** 62.

[83] NICOLLE, F. Personal communication, 1976.

[84] KEMBALL, H. Paper presented Meeting British Society for Surgery of the Hand, London, 1976.

[85] HARRISON, S. H. Reconstructive arthroplasty of the metacarpophalangeal joints using the extensor loop operation. *British Journal of Plastic Surgery*, 1971, **24,** 307.

[86] HARRISON, S. H. The importance of middle (long) finger realignment in ulnar drift. *Journal of Hand Surgery*, 1976, **1,** 87.

[87] RATLIFF, A. H. C. Deformities of the thumb in rheumatoid arthritis. *The Hand*, 1971, **3,** 138.

[88] NALEBUFF, E. A. Restoration of balance in the rheumatoid thumb. Meeting of British Society of Surgery of the Hand, Lausanne, 1967.

[89] KESSLER, I. Contracture of the thumb in rheumatoid arthritis. *The Hand*, 1973, **5,** 170.

[90] CLAYTON, M. L. Surgery of the thumb in rheumatoid arthritis. *Journal of Bone and Joint Surgery*, 1962, **44A,** 1376.

[91] SWANSON, A. B. *Flexible Implant Resection Arthroplasty in the Hand and Extremities*. St. Louis, Mosby, 1973.

[92] LEACH, R. E. AND BAUMGARD, S. H. Correction of swan neck deformity in rheumatoid arthritis. *Surgical Clinics of North America*, 1968, **48,** 661.

[93] NALEBUFF, E. A., POTTER, T. A. AND TOMASELLI, R. Surgery of swan neck deformity of the rheumatoid hand: a new approach. *Arthritis and Rheumatism*, 1963, **6,** 289.

[94] NALEBUFF, E. A. Surgical treatment of finger deformities in the rheumatoid hand. *Surgical Clinics of North America*, 1969, **49,** 833.

[95] NALEBUFF, E. A. AND MILLENDER, L. H. Surgical treatment of the swan neck deformity in rheumatoid arthritis. *Orthopedic Clinics of North America*, 1975, **6,** 653.

[96] SWANSON, A. B. Surgery of the hand in cerebral palsy and the swan neck deformity. *Journal of Bone and Joint Surgery*, 1960, **42A,** 951.

[97] LITTLER, J. W. Restoration of the oblique retinacular ligament for correction of hand. G.E.M. No. 1. Paris, L'Expansion, 1966.

[98] LITTLER, J. W. Intrinsic contracture in the hand and its surgical treatment. *Journal of Bone and Joint Surgery*, 1954, **36A,** 10.

[99] SWANSON, A. B. Silicone rubber implants for replacement of arthritic or destroyed joints in the hand. *Surgical Clinics of North America*, 1968, **48,** 1113.

[100] SWANSON, A. B. Flexible implant arthroplasty for arthritic finger joint. *Journal of Bone and Joint Surgery*, 1972, **54A,** 435.

[101] SWANSON, A. B. *Flexible Implant Resection Arthroplasty in the Hand and Extremities*. St. Louis, Mosby, 1973.

[102] FOWLER, S. B. In *The Care of the Rheumatoid Hand*, ed. A. E. Flett. St. Louis, Mosby, 1963.

[103] HEYWOOD, A. W. B. Correction of the rheumatoid boutonnière deformity. *Journal of Bone and Joint Surgery*, 1969, **51A,** 1309.

[104] LITTLER, J. W. AND EATON, R. G. Redistribution of forces in the correction of the boutonnière deformity. *Journal of Bone and Joint Surgery*, 1967, **49A,** 1267.

[105] MATEV, I. The boutonnière deformity. *The Hand*, 1969, **1,** 90.

[106] NALEBUFF, E. A. Surgical treatment of finger deformities in the rheumatoid hand. *Surgical Clinics of North America*, 1969, **49,** 833.

[107] DOLPHIN, J. A. Extensor tenotomy for chronic boutonnière deformity of the finger. Report of two cases. *Journal of Bone and Joint Surgery*, 1965, **17A,** 161.

[108] SWANSON, A. B. Flexible implant arthroplasty for arthritic finger joints. *Journal of Bone and Joint Surgery*, 1972, **54A,** 435.

[109] NALEBUFF, E. A. AND MILLENDER, L. H. Surgical treatment of the boutonnière deformity. *Orthopedic Clinics of North America*, 1975, **6,** 753.

[110] SWANSON, A. B. Finger joint replacement by silicone rubber implants and the concept of implant fixation on encapsulation. *Annals of Rheumatic Disease*, 1969, **28,** 47.

[111] SWANSON, A. B. Silicone rubber implants for replacement of arthritic or destroyed joints of the hand. *The Hand*, 1969, **1,** 38.

[112] SWANSON, A. B. Disabling arthritis at the base of the thumb: treatment by resection of the trapezium and flexible (silicone) implant arthroplasty. *Journal of Bone and Joint Surgery*, 1972, **54A,** 456.

[113] SWANSON, A. B. Flexible implant arthroplasty for arthritic finger joints: rationale, technique and results of treatment. *Journal of Bone and Joint Surgery*, 1972, **54A,** 435.

[114] SWANSON, A. B. *Flexible Implant Resection Arthroplasty in the Hand and Extremities*. St. Louis, Mosby, 1973.

[115] SWANSON, A. B. Flexible implant arthroplasty in the hand. *Clinics in Plastic Surgery*, 1976, **3,** 141.

[116] SWANSON, A. B. Reconstructive surgery in the arthritic hand and foot. Clinical Symposia, Vol. 31, No. 6. New Jersey, CIBA Pharmaceutical Co., 1979.

[117] SWANSON, A. B., DE GROOT SWANSON, G. AND LEONARD, J. Postoperative rehabilitation program in flexible implant arthroplasty of the digits. In *Rehabilitation of the Hand*, pp. 477–495, ed. J. M. Hunter, L. H. Schneider, E. J. Mackin and J. A. Bell. St. Louis, Mosby, 1978.

CHAPTER 26

Nerve Compression Syndromes

J. CHALMERS

Impaired dysfunction of peripheral nerves due to mechanical causes has been recognized for at least a century [1]. These lesions usually arise where nerves pass through narrow anatomical tunnels, which have become further constricted by some space-occupying lesion or by distortion resulting from trauma or arthritis. Such compression lesions or 'entrapment neuropathies' have been described involving all the main nerves supplying the forearm and hand.

Pathomechanism

As the title indicates the main cause is mechanical compression. Traction and friction are less important although these factors may operate in cervical rib syndrome and a subluxating ulnar nerve. Pressure may affect the nerve fibres directly but inevitably also interferes with the local blood supply. The relative importance of each varies but Gilliatt and Sunderland make it clear that both play a part [2, 3]. Transient mild compression causes venous stasis leading to anoxia, with rapid recovery when the compression is relieved and the circulation restored. Sustained and increased pressure leads to a local dispersal of myelin and conduction delay or block [4]. Motor fibres appear more susceptible than sensory fibres although there is much variability depending on the intraneural arrangement of nerve bundles and their size [3].

If the pressure is not relieved Wallerian degeneration may result producing a second degree nerve injury with slow recovery after release of pressure. More prolonged compression may result in marked narrowing of the nerve with extensive intraneural fibrosis, leading to obliteration of the endoneural tubes and irreversable loss of function. The pathological changes associated with nerve compression have been well reviewed by Spinner and Spencer [5]. The vulnerability of peripheral nerves to compression appears to be increased in some individuals who may develop lesions in several nerves. Patients with diabetes are particularly susceptible [6, 7], and a familial liability to pressure palsies has also been reported [8, 9].

Investigations

Most common compression lesions can be diagnosed from the patient's history coupled with meticulous clinical examination which will reveal motor and sensory changes which point to a specific nerve and frequently indicate the level of involvement. Careful palpation along the course of the nerve for abnormal swellings, pulsations or a point of tenderness on percussion can help to localize the lesion. If the findings are confined to the territory of a specific nerve the probability of a local mechanical cause of dysfunction is high. If the neurological deficit extends beyond the territory of a peripheral nerve then the lesion is likely to be more proximal although the possibility of anomalous distribution must be borne in mind. A radiograph may be of value in identifying cervical spondylosis, cervical rib, arthritis or previous fracture at elbow or wrist. Delay of nerve conduction of both sensory and motor fibres (p.

TABLE 26.1 Sites of involvement of peripheral nerves supplying forearm and hand

Nerve	Anatomical tunnel
Median Proximal	Beneath ligament of Struthers Between two heads of pronator teres Deep to the fibrous arch of origin of flexor digitorium sublimis
Distal	Carpal tunnel Thenar tunnel (motor branch only)
Anterior interosseous	Anomalous bands or muscles in proximal forearm
Ulnar	
At elbow	cubital tunnel
At wrist	Guyon's tunnel
Motor branch	Deep palmar tunnel
Radial	Deep to lateral head of triceps
Posterior interosseous	Arcade of Frohse Supinator muscle
Musculocutaneous	Coracobrachialis

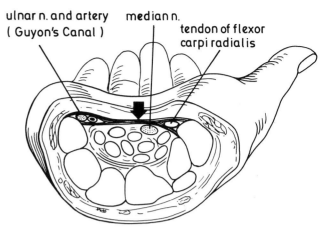

FIG. 26.1. Relationships within the carpal tunnel. Site for division of the transverse carpal ligament is arrowed.

181) may also help to localize the site of compression and has been widely used for this purpose [10, 11, 12]. It has an accuracy of about 90 per cent but such tests are not necessary in the majority of cases. Surgical decompression is followed by recovery if done before degeneration of the nerve endings has taken place. Failure to recover would suggest incorrect diagnosis or incomplete decompression. The sites of involvement of the peripheral nerves supplying the forearm and hand are listed in Table 26.1.

Carpal tunnel syndrome

By far the most common and familiar compression syndrome involves the median nerve within the carpal tunnel. Decompression of the carpal tunnel is the fourth most common operation done in one orthopaedic hospital (following hip arthroplasty, meniscectomy and Keller's arthroplasty). The condition was described by Paget [13], and surgical decompression first performed by Learmonth [14], but credit for the definitive description which brought general recognition must go to Brain, Wright and Wilkinson, and Cannon and Love [15, 16].

Anatomical consideration (Fig. 26.1) (pp. 9, 25)

The anatomy of the carpal tunnel and its contents has been well described by Robbins [17]. The transverse carpal ligament is a dense structure varying in thickness from 2–4 mm [9]. Its fibres are transversely orientated. Proximally it blends with the deep fascia of the forearm. At its radial attachment there is a separate tunnel which contains the tendon of flexor carpi radialis and at its ulnar attachment another tunnel, Guyons canal, allows the passage of the ulnar nerve and vessels. The capacity of the carpal tunnel is narrowest at its mid-point and is further reduced by extreme positions of flexion and extension of the wrist [9].

Clinical features

The age distribution of the author's cases is shown in Fig. 26.2. Occurrence during childhood is rare [18]. The peak incidence in this and all other series is among women in their forties and fifties, the mean age being 54. Women outnumber men in all series, by a ratio of four to one [7, 19, 20, 21]. Both hands are affected in the majority of cases but usually the dominant hand suffers more [22].

The typical history of nocturnal pain in one or both hands occurring at about the same time each night, is so characteristic as to be diagnostic. The pain is variously described as a burning or bursting sensation and the

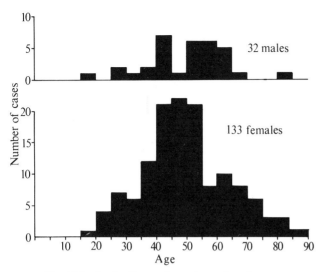

FIG. 26.2. Age incidence of carpal tunnel syndrome.

symptoms linked with physical activity may be the only complaint. Occasionally progressive sensory loss may occur without the development of pain and rarely thenar paralysis may develop without sensory loss [23], and with minimal disability.

Clinical signs

Sensory or motor impairment may be found on detailed testing but it is important to remember that about one quarter have no demonstrable loss of function [7], but the history should enable the diagnosis to be made. Percussion over the median nerve at the wrist (Tinel's sign) is positive in 60 per cent of cases and swelling of the nerve or synovium proximal to the carpal tunnel may be felt in 20 per cent.

TABLE 26.2 Systemic conditions contributing to carpal tunnel syndrome

Conditions	Local effect	References
ENDOCRINE RELATED		
Menopause	? Fluid retention	
Pregnancy	,,	35, 38, 100, 101
Contraceptive pill	,,	33, 41
Diabetes	Increased vulnerability of nerve	6, 7, 22, 33
Acromegaly	Narrowed tunnel	16, 35, 102, 103
Myxoedema	Fluid retention	19, 33
Hyperthyroidism	?	7, 22, 27
Hyperparathyroidism	Calcium deposits	104
METABOLIC		
Obesity	Fat deposition	7
Gout	Uric acid deposit	7, 27, 46, 105
INFECTIVE		
Leprosy	Enlarged nerve	106
COLLAGEN DISEASE		
Rheumatoid arthritis	Narrowed tunnel synovitis	7, 19, 22, 32, 33
Lupus erythematosis	? Vascular	27
STORAGE DISORDERS		
Amyloid disease	Amyloid accumulation	107
BLOOD DISORDERS		
Myeloma	Amyloid accumulation	7, 19
Leukaemia	Haematoma	108
Haemophilia	Haematoma	109
MISCELLANEOUS		
Rubella immunization	Fluid retention	110

hand feels numb, stiff and swollen. The symptoms may be restricted to one or more digits within the median territory but frequently the whole hand appears involved and the discomfort may extend proximally to the elbow. The apparent involvement of all the digits may be due to simultaneous compression of the ulnar nerve within Guyon's tunnel [7] but is more usually due to inaccurate observation by the patient. The nocturnal pain may be explained by venous congestion and oedema due to the vasodilitation associated with carbon dioxide retention during sleep and delayed venous return due to diminished muscle activity. Lying on the arm or holding the wrist in flexion may also contribute. The patient learns to perform some activity such as elevating or shaking the hand, holding it under a cold tap or making a cup of tea which brings relief within a few minutes, the activity restoring the venous circulation.

In the morning the affected hand frequently feels clumsy or swollen due to residual numbness and thenar weakness so that the patient may have difficulty in doing up buttons or in holding a cup. But these symptoms soon recover and may not return during the day unless the patient engages in heavy or repetitive manual activity particularly with the wrist flexed [9].

Only when the condition has persisted for long periods does subjective sensory loss or motor weakness persist throughout the day. Variations from the typical pattern are not uncommon. Among men in particular diurnal

Associated conditions (Tables 26.2 and 26.3)

Association with other disorders involving the connective tissues suggests a systemic connective tissue disorder

TABLE 26.3 Local conditions contributing to carpal tunnel syndrome

Conditions	Local effect	References
SYNOVITIS		
Acute pyogenic	Inflammatory products	111
Tuberculous	,,	27, 112
Rheumatoid	,,	7, 19, 22, 27, 32, 33
Traumatic and non specific	,,	7, 27, 33
CHRONIC ARTHRITIS		
Rheumatoid	Narrowed tunnel	7, 19, 22, 27, 33
Osteoarthritis and post traumatic arthritis	,,	7, 16, 19, 33, 113
Leri's pleonosteosis	Thickened carpal ligament	114, 115
TRAUMA		
Colles fracture	Narrowed tunnel	27, 33, 116
Carpal fractures and dislocation	,,	27, 33, 113
Soft tissue trauma	Oedema and haematoma	33
Use of cane or crutches	External pressure	27
Insect sting	Oedema	117
Surgical	Tendon graft prosthesis	118
VASCULAR CAUSE		
Arteriovenous shunt		
Traumatic	Venous stasis	109
Surgical (for renal dialysis)	? Vascular steal	119, 120, 121
Raynaud's disease	Probably association rather than cause	7, 19, 22, 26
Anomalous median artery	Local pressure	
Patent		7, 122
Thrombosed		123
Spontaneous intraneural haemorrhage		124
ANOMALOUS MUSCLE	Space encroachment	9, 27, 33, 125
LOCAL TUMOURS		
Ganglion	Space encroachment	3, 7, 126
Osteoid osteoma	,,	127
Lipoma	,,	27, 33, 91
Synovial chrondromatosis	,,	27
Haemangioma of median nerve	,,	128
Calcific deposit	,,	7, 20
Neuroma	,,	7, 16
Lipofibroma of median nerve	,,	129, 130
Benign mesodermal	,,	131

in some cases. Murray and Wright found tennis elbow present in 33 per cent of carpal tunnel patients compared with 7 per cent of controls [24]. Lishman and Russell suggested an association between cervical spondylosis and peripheral neuritis postulating that pathological changes at one level may influence vulnerability at others [25].

Raynaud's phenomenon and acrocyanosis co-existing with carpal tunnel syndrome were reported in 28 patients many of whom had systemic collagen disease [26]. Surgical decompression had a beneficial effect on both the vascular and neurological symptoms although vascular improvement was sometimes incomplete. Other disorders frequently associated are de Quervain's disease, trigger finger and thumb and perarthritis of the shoulder [7, 22, 27].

Diagnostic tests and investigations

A number of diagnostic tests have been described which may help to confirm the diagnosis. None of these tests is absolutely diagnostic and in the typical case none is needed, nevertheless these tests are of interest in that they shed light on the pathomechanics of the disorder.

Wrist flexion test

Unforced complete flexion of the wrist for 30–60 seconds reproduces or aggravates the symptoms of carpal tunnel syndrome in 80 per cent of cases [7, 28].

Tourniquet tests

(1) Gilliatt and Wilson inflate the cuff around the upper arm to above the systolic pressure [29]. The painful symptoms are reproduced with 60 seconds and sensory impairment can be detected within 10 minutes, whereas the normal nerve takes longer to show such changes. The basis of this test lies in the increased susceptibility of the median nerve in carpal tunnel syndrome to ischaemia [30]. Heathfield found this test to be of limited value [31].

(2) Vainio, inflating the cuff to occlude the venous circulation only, reproduced the symptoms in a high proportion of cases [32, 33].

The splint test

Splinting the wrist in a neutral position [34] brings temporary relief in about 75 per cent of patients [31, 35, 36], and may be used at night as a method of treatment in mild or transient cases. It succeeds because it holds the wrist in a position in which the capacity of the tunnel is at its greatest.

Hydrocortisone injection test

The injection of 50 mg of hydrocortisone with local anaesthetic into the carpal tunnel brings temporary relief in more than two-thirds of cases [35], but only a few gain lasting benefit. The test must be carefully performed to avoid damage to the median nerve. The

injection is made just medial to the palmaris longus tendon at the level of the distal wrist crease and the needle aimed distally to enter the carpal tunnel (Fig. 26.3).

Electrodiagnostic tests (see also p. 181)

Diminished nerve conduction velocity is a characteristic of all nerve compression syndromes and has been widely used for identifying and localizing the lesion. Simpson first described delay in motor nerve conduction across the wrist in carpal tunnel syndrome [10]. The usual normal terminal latency is 3m/sec with a maximum of 5m/sec. Increase in latency is found in about 90 per cent of patients with carpal tunnel syndrome [11], although a higher proportion of negative results has been reported [7].

Delay in conduction and reduced amplitude of sensory nerve action potentials also occurs [37], and is a more sensitive indicator than motor fibre delay [36].

Natural history of carpal tunnel syndrome

Experience suggests that the prognosis is infinitely variable ranging from cases which recover almost immediately the causal factor is relieved, for example by the completion of pregnancy or by discontinuance of an aggravating physical activity, to patients with lasting severe discomfort. One patient in the author's experience had been awakened nightly for twenty years with relentless pain. Many of the menopausal patients and those associated with Colles fracture have relatively mild symptoms which regress spontaneously within a few months, and surgical treatment should be delayed in these cases until time and conservative measures have been given a chance.

Treatment

Conservative measures include diuretic drugs, oestrogens, systemic or local corticosteroids and splintage. Diuretics are appropriate where fluid retention is likely to be of limited duration, as in cases during pregnancy [38]. Success has been claimed for oestrogens in post menopausal patients [39], but has not been confirmed by others [40], and indeed the contraceptive pill with

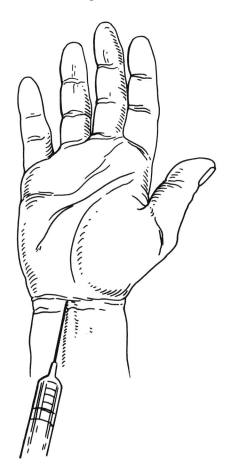

FIG. 26.3. Site for injection of carpal tunnel.

high oestrogen content has been implicated as a cause of carpal tunnel syndrome [41].

Local injection of hydrocortisone into the carpal tunnel as previously described may occasionally have lasting benefit and is always worth a trial. A night splint which holds the wrist in a neutral position may be sufficient treatment for mild cases [31]. Patients who do not have lasting benefit from these simple measures and those with objective neurological deficit should be treated by surgical decompression.

Surgical decompression

A tourniquet is necessary if damage to the median nerve and its occasional anomalous branches is to be avoided. Bier's regional anaesthesia is ideal but axillary block is also satisfactory. The incision should be planned to preserve the palmar cutaneous branch of the median nerve, injury to which can be a source of troublesome post-operative symptoms [19, 27, 42]. The anatomy of this branch (see Fig. 1.51) has been described by Carroll & Green, and Taleisnik [42, 43]. It arises usually from the radial aspect of the median nerve as it emerges from the radial margin of flexor digitorum superficialis. It separates from the main nerve but runs parallel to it along its radial border to a point about 1 cm proximal to the volar carpal ligament where it diverges to pass through its own tunnel within the ligament just medial to the flexor carpi radialis. There it divides into its terminal branches which pass through the palmar fascia to supply a variable area of skin overlying the thenar eminence and base of the palm. Das & Brown describe a number of variations from this pattern [19], but only rarely does this branch arise from the ulnar side of the median nerve. These authors also draw attention to the variations in distribution of the thenar (motor) branch of the median nerve which may occasionally arise above the wrist and pass in front or through the transverse carpal ligament. Rarely it may arise from its ulnar side. The incision should therefore allow open division of the volar carpal ligament so that damage to these branches whether of normal or anomalous distribution may be avoided.

The incision curves gently from the ulnar border of the tendon of palmaris longus where it crosses the distal wrist crease to the mid palm, running parallel on the ulnar side of the thenar crease finishing in mid palm (Fig.

26.4). This incision lies to the ulnar side of the median nerve and will avoid all but a few terminal branches of the palmar cutaneous nerve. For most cases this incision is adequate. If a proximal extension is required, for example to permit synovectomy, it should cross the wrist crease in a sinuous manner, as indicated by the dotted line of Fig. 26.4, to avoid scar contraction.

The palmar fascia which at wrist level forms the fan-shaped insertion of palmaris longus is then divided longitudinally. The inexperienced may mistake this layer for the transverse carpal ligament itself but the irregular oblique arrangement of its fibres will differentiate it from the transversely orientated carpal ligament beneath. This ligament is then divided at its mid point comfortably to the ulnar side of the median nerve (Fig. 26.1). Once

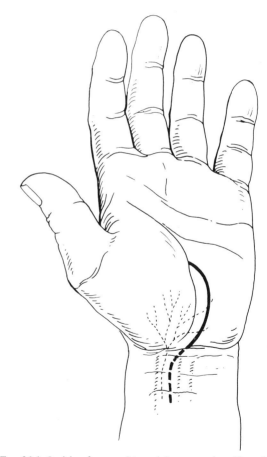

FIG. 26.4. Incision for carpal tunnel decompression. Note site of superficial palmar branch of median nerve.

an opening is made into the carpal tunnel a dissector should be passed to protect its contents during completion of the division. Incomplete division is the commonest cause of failure of the operation [45]. It is not necessary to cut out a segment of the transverse carpal ligament. Neurolysis of the median nerve should be performed if it is densely adherent to the deep surface of the flexor retinaculum or the adjacent tendons and a synovectomy may occasionally be indicated, if it is grossly hypertrophied. The flexor tendons should be retracted to allow inspection of the floor of the carpal tunnel to see if a space occupying lesion such as a ganglion is present. A median artery if present need not be removed unless it is thrombosed.

Internal neurolysis has been advocated by Curtis & Eversman who claim improved results by such a procedure [46]. They argue that intraneural fibrosis may maintain compression of the axons after the carpal tunnel is divided. This procedure, demands considerable skill and if widely practised more harm than good could result. Evidence does not yet justify the widespread use of this procedure [33]. Inspection and mobilization of the motor (recurrent) branch of the median nerve is not a necessary routine unless the motor function of the nerve is selectively impaired to a greater degree than the sensory functions, in which case the nerve should be carefully traced to its terminal branches in the thenar muscle. Isolated involvement of this branch may occur as it angles over the distal margin of the transverse carpal ligament or when it has an anomalous course through the ligament [23, 47]. Following decompression the tourniquet should be released and haemostasis secured. Only the skin is closed. It is curious that no disability appears to result from the division of such a well-defined structure as the transverse carpal ligament. A light compression bandage is applied, the arm elevated for a few hours but, thereafter, the patient may use the hand freely and can be discharged from hospital the same day.

Results of Surgery

Virtually all patients have immediate relief of pain if the operation is done within 6 months of the onset of symptoms [48]. Motor and sensory signs may recover more slowly and recovery may be incomplete [22, 33], but rarely to an extent that constitutes a handicap to the patient. Delay in nerve conductivity also improves following decompression [49], although it may take 1–2 years to do so [36, 50]. Delay in decompression beyond 6 months is associated with a lower incidence of recovery [48]. Curtis and Eversman claim that intraneural neurolysis will minimize these poor results [46].

However, the general experience is that simple decompression brings lasting relief to almost all patients in whom the diagnosis has been correctly made.

Complications

Incomplete recovery, recurrence of symptoms following surgical decompression or complications of this operation are described by Hybinette & Mannerfelt, Langloh and Linscheid and Semple and Cargill [33, 45, 48]. The commonest causes of failure are excessive delay in treatment, inadequate surgical decompression, fibrous proliferation or incorrect diagnosis. Re-operation may be successful where the original operation was inadequate. A painful scar may be a minor complaint in a third of patients [22], but significant pain due to involvement of the palmar cutaneous branch was present in four of 170 operations reported by Das and Brown [19]. Symptoms from this source diminish with time and are helped by local injection of triamcinolone. Very occasionally proximal section of the palmar cutaneous branch is required if troublesome pain persists. Hypertrophied scars and accidental division of motor or sensory branches have also been described but such complications should be avoided by careful technique.

Proximal causes of median nerve compression

Two proximal sites of compression of the median nerve have been described; one supracondylar deep to the ligament of Struthers [51] and the other in the forearm as it passes between the two heads of pronator teres or deep to the fibrous arch of origin of flexor digitorum sublimis. Both are extremely rare in contrast to the frequency of carpal tunnel syndrome.

Supracondylar compression

Supracondylar compression is caused by an anomalous ligament of Struthers which extends from a supracondylar spur arising from the antero medial aspect of the distal humerus to the medial epicondyle (Fig. 26.5). The spur and its ligament when present give origin to pronator teres. In man the incidence of the spur is about 1 per cent and is often bilateral [52].

The brachial or ulnar artery and median nerve pass under the ligament and may be hooked round the spur. Tension on these structures is increased when the elbow is extended. The clinical syndrome associated with this anomaly may have vascular or neurological features separately or together [53]. Pain, paraesthesia and weakness within the median distribution may be present and the hand may be pale and colder than the opposite side. The symptoms may be increased by extension of the elbow and hand and full extension and supination

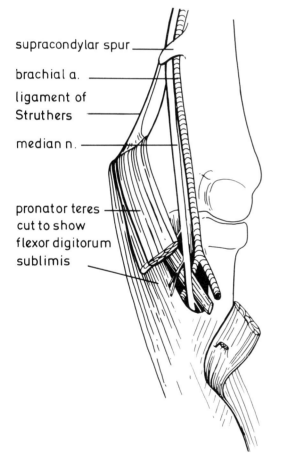

supracondylar spur

brachial a.

ligament of Struthers

median n.

pronator teres cut to show flexor digitorum sublimis

FIG. 26.5. Possible sites of proximal involvement of the median nerve.

may obliterate the radial pulse. Forearm claudication may develop with repetitive activity. Motor weakness if present may involve any or all of the muscles supplied by the nerve. Ulnar nerve involvement may occasionally occur as it is also closely related to the spur although it does not pass under the ligament [54, 55]. The spur is readily palpable and is clearly seen on radiographs. It should be looked for in all cases of median neuritis. Treatment consists of surgical excision of the spur and its ligament.

Pronator syndrome [56]

Anatomy (Fig. 26.5) (pp. 21, 33)

Variations in the relationship of the median nerve to pronator teres have been described [57], and as is frequently the case with peripheral nerve compression lesions, minor variations in anatomy may be the critical factor.

Clinical features

The pronator syndrome affects men more than women and usually occurs in the dominant arm in patients whose occupation demands strong pronation movement. Pain is not a prominent symptom and nocturnal awakening is unusual. Sensory loss and paraesthesiae may develop within the median distribution and motor weakness involves the forearm muscles supplied by the median nerve distal to pronator teres, as well as the thenar muscles. Weakness of flexor pollicis longus, flexor digitorum sublimis and flexor digitorum profundus to the radial fingers is the most valuable indication of a median nerve lesion at this level. Local tenderness at the side of compression and delayed nerve conduction in the forearm with normal terminal latency across the wrist will also help to differentiate this condition from carpal tunnel syndrome.

Treatment consists of exploration of the median nerve in the proximal forearm with division of the deep head of pronator teres and the fibrous arch of origin of flexor digitorum sublimis and any other anomalous bands or muscles which appear to be compressing the nerve. Spinner and Spencer recommend anterior transposition of the nerve in front of pronator teres [5].

Anterior interosseous nerve syndrome

This branch of the median nerve supplies flexor pollicis longus, the lateral half of profundus and pronator quadratus. The condition is recognized by weakness of one or more of these muscles. The 'square pinch' sign (Fig. 26.6) is produced by weakness of these muscles in the presence of normal flexor digitorum sublimis and flexor pollicis brevis [58]. The condition may develop spontaneously but usually arises after single or repeated powerful gripping actions.

The anterior interosseous nerve usually arises from the posterior aspect of the median just after it has passed between the heads of pronator teres and runs distally along the interosseous membrane between the deep flexors of thumb and fingers. It does not normally pass through any confined tunnels but if it has a high origin it is subject to the same hazards as the median nerve at the level of pronator teres and the origin of flexor digitorum sublimis. Vearn and Goodfellow describe a case due to an anomalous fibrous band in this region and found considerable variation in the anatomy of the muscles and fascia at this level during the course of several dissections [59]. Many of the reported cases of anterior interosseous nerve syndrome have undergone spontaneous recovery and treatment should therefore be delayed for two or three months.

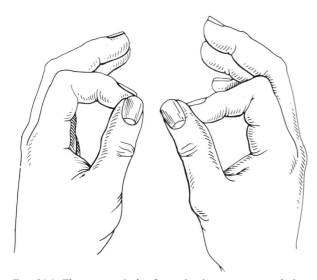

FIG. 26.6. The square pinch of anterior interosseous paralysis right.

Surgical exploration should be carried out if there is no progress at the end of that period.

Ulnar nerve compression syndromes

The incidence is one quarter that of the median. It does, however, pass through confined anatomical tunnels at elbow and wrist and is vulnerable at both sites. Ulnar nerve lesions are usually unilateral being more common in the dominant arm and in men. They may occur at any age.

Anatomy (p. 33)

At the elbow, the aponeurotic band which extends from the medial epicondyle to the medial border of the olecranon is the principle constricting agent.

These points become separated during flexion by 5 mm for every 45 degrees flexion [60, 61], so that the band which is relaxed when the elbow is extended becomes taut when it is flexed (Fig. 26.7). Proximally the band is continuous with a looser and thinner layer of fascia which extends from the medial intermuscular septum to the tendon of triceps. This fascia is not a source of compression but has the important function of restraining the ulnar nerve from subluxating forward over the medial epicondyle. About 8 cm proximal to the medial epicondyle there is a condensation of this fascia present in 70 per cent of individuals [5], first described by Struthers as an arcade [62] (not to be confused with Struthers ligament, p. 400). This arcade gives origin to some of the fibres of the medial head of triceps which may cross the nerve and could theoretically cause its compression following anterior transposition. However, compression at this level is extremely rare and the great majority of cases are involved within the cubital tunnel.

At the level of the elbow the intraneural arrangement of nerve bundles may influence their vulnerability to pressure. For example, the sensory bundles and those supplying the intrinsic muscles are the most medially placed and hence more liable to pressure from the overlying aponeurotic band [60].

Involvement or otherwise of the dorsal cutaneous branch is often the critical sign which distinguishes between proximal and distal lesions of the ulnar nerve.

At the wrist, the ulnar nerve is confined and

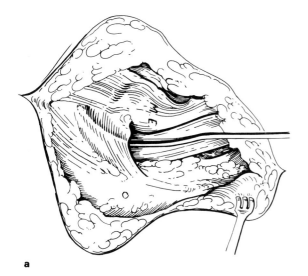

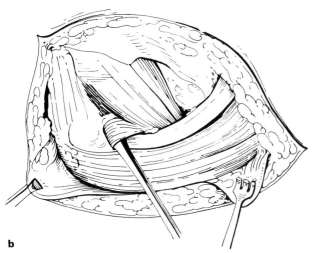

FIG. 26.7. (a) Aponeurotic band relaxed in extension, and (b) Taut when the elbow is flexed.

TABLE 26.4 Causes of ulnar nerve compression at elbow

Cause	References
Aponeurotic band of flexor carpi ulnaris (Osborne lesion)	60, 68, 69
Tardy palsy after old fracture	1, 64, 66, 67, 79, 132
Osteoarthritis	1, 65, 79, 132
Rheumatoid arthritis	133
Ganglion	60, 91, 126
Subluxating nerve	66, 67, 79
Anomalous muscle	
Anconeus epitrochlearis	60
Enlarged medial head of triceps	109
Lipoma	91
Epidermoid cyst	91
Supracondylar spur	55

vulnerable at two levels – Guyon's tunnel and the deep palmar branch tunnel – each being associated with a characteristic clinical syndrome [63].

Clinical features of lesions occurring at the elbow

The causes are listed in Table 26.4. The symptoms include paraesthesiae and numbness, which is accurately located by the patient to the medial two fingers and medial border of the hand, weakness of fine finger movements and, to a lesser extent, of grip. Rarely is pain a major complaint in contrast to carpal tunnel syndrome and sleep disturbance is uncommon. The symptoms may be increased by elbow flexion, which tightens the aponeurosis of flexor carpi ulnaris. The insidious onset and lack of acutely distressing symptoms in most patients with ulnar neuritis have the unfortunate result that many present late with extensive neurological deficits which, if present for more than 6 months, may not recover completely following decompression.

Clinical signs

These are motor and sensory deficits within the nerve territory and local signs at the elbow which may indicate the cause of the compression. The sensory impairment will include the area supplied by the dorsal cutaneous branch as well as the palmar digital branches. Ulnar sensory loss is less important than that of the median and consequently a lesser handicap to the patient. Motor involvement may include any or all of the ulnar innervated muscles but usually flexor carpi ulnaris is spared in part because some of its branches arise proximal to the compression. Involvement of other muscles depends on the relationship of the compressing agent and the intraneural disposition of nerve bundles. Occasionally, for example, a pure intrinsic paralysis may occur without involvement of the long flexors in compression lesions at the elbow which can give rise to diagnostic difficulty. Difficulty also arises due to the frequent anomalies of distribution, the commonest of which (15 per cent) is the communication between the median and ulnar nerves. Local signs may include sensitivity of the nerve to percussion at the site of compression, proximal thickening of the nerve may be palpable and the wide range of conditions listed in Table 26.4 may produce their characteristic features and help in localizing the lesion.

Tardy ulnar palsy following injury

Slowly developing ulnar neuritis many years after a fracture involving the elbow joint was first described by Panas [1]. Ununited fractures of the lateral humeral condyle occurring during childhood and leading to cubitus valgus is the most characteristic injury [64] (Fig. 26.8), but fracture of the medial epicondyle [65, 66], or any injury leading to osteoarthritic change may be the cause [60]. The common factor is narrowing of the cubital tunnel by distortion or osteophyte formation in its floor. Traction suggested by Mouchet [64], and friction postulated by Sheldon [65], are probably less important factors. The interval between injury and onset of neuritis averages 6–14 years but it may be as long as 51 years [67].

Cubital tunnel syndrome

Nerve compression by the natural boundaries of the tunnel has been recognized [68, 69], and accounts for about half of the lesions at the elbow [60]. The syndrome

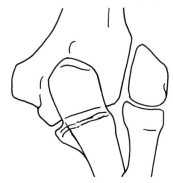

FIG. 26.8. Ununited lateral epicondyle is a cause of tardy ulnar paralysis.

occurs more commonly in men and usually affects the dominant hand and the symptoms are increased by occupational activity or elbow flexion, which may be used as a clinical test. The tunnel may become further constricted by any lesion in its vicinity so that it is somewhat artificial to separate this syndrome sharply from other causes of compression at this level. In practice excising the aponeurosis may be sufficient treatment not only for the pure cubital tunnel syndrome but also for some of the other disorders contributing to the compression. The pathological changes occurring within the ulnar nerve in cubital tunnel syndrome have been described in detail by Neary and Eames [70].

External compression lesions of the ulnar nerve at the elbow

The unconscious patient on the operating table or in a hospital bed after operation may sustain such a lesion from the weight of the arm resting on a firm surface. Individuals whose ulnar nerves tend to subluxate over the medial epicondyle (about 16 per cent of the normal population [71]) are particularly susceptible.

The nerve is particularly at risk when the forearm is pronated [72]. Conscious patients may also develop such lesions by shifting their position in bed or in an armchair by leaning on their elbows [73]. Such complications are preventable and staff should be aware of the risk and position the patient and his limbs carefully to avoid this hazard. Once the cause has been relieved recovery usually ensues although the process may take many months. In some cases, however, recovery is incomplete until the nerve has been surgically decompressed. Presumably in such cases the reaction to external pressure produces oedema and fibrosis of the tissues at this site leading to an internal compression lesion.

Treatment of compression at the elbow

Where an obvious source of compression can be relieved such as external pressure or pressure from maintenance of acute elbow flexion, treatment should be withheld for three months to allow spontaneous recovery. In all other circumstances surgical exploration should be undertaken without delay, for, sustained compression for more than 6 months may cause irreversible changes.

The surgical procedures available include simple excision of the aponeurotic band, excision of the medial epicondyle and anterior transposition of the ulnar nerve. The choice is best deferred until the cause has been exposed at operation. Excision of the aponeurotic band is sufficient treatment for the cubital tunnel syndrome, while transposition of the nerve is recommended for compression due to arthritis or deformity of the elbow joint or in cases in which no cubital tunnel lesion is found, and more extensive exploration is necessary. Excision of the medial epicondyle probably succeeds by releasing one of the attachments of the aponeurotic band [74]. It is not a procedure that has been widely adopted although favourable results are reported by Green [75].

Operation is done under tourniquet using a regional block or general anaesthesia. Bier's block is unsuitable as it is wise to release the tourniquet before wound closure to secure haemostasis. The initial incision extends from a point midway between the tip of the olecranon and the medial epicondyle and passes distally along the line of the nerve for 5 cm. The aponeurosis of flexor carpi ulnaris is defined as it overlies the nerve. Its proximal edge merges with the more tenuous fascia which invests the nerve proximally, from which it is easily distinguished. This proximal fascia is carefully preserved at this stage for if it is opened the ulnar nerve will readily subluxate forward and anterior transposition is then required. The triangular aponeurosis is then resected and the nerve carefully examined. If there is a distinct groove and proximal and distal swelling of the nerve and no other local changes, no further treatment is required. Suture of the aponeurosis deep to the nerve, a refinement suggested by Osborne has not been found necessary by others [76].

If no lesion is found a wider exposure to seek other sources of compression and anterior transposition becomes necessary. The incision is extended proximally and distally along the course of the nerve. The nerve is exposed proximally as far as its passage through the medial intermuscular septum by dividing the overlying fascia and distally by splitting the two heads of flexor carpi ulnaris (Fig. 26.9a). Anterior transposition is carried out by placing the nerve deep to the flexor muscles [77]. Subcutaneous or intramuscular beds are unsatisfactory and expose the nerve to further trauma

and scar contracture [78]. Mobilization of the nerve is restricted by its sensory branches to the elbow joint which may be sacrificed and by one of its branches to flexor carpi ulnaris, which may be freed by intraneural

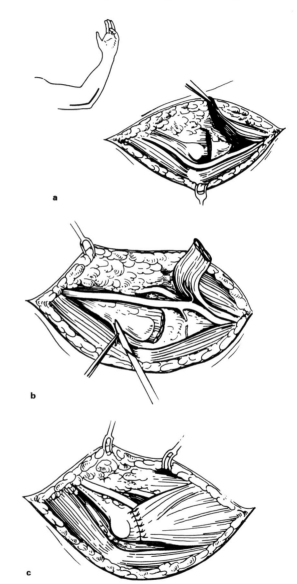

FIG. 26.9. Technique of anterior transposition.

(a) Division of the flexor origin.

(b) Excision of the intermuscular septum. The transposed nerve lies in the same plane as the median.

(c) The flexor origin repaired superficial to the nerve.

dissection, or may sometimes have to be divided. The medial intermuscular septum is then resected above the medial epicondyle so that the nerve will not be kinked over it. The flexor origin is then divided 1 cm below the epicondyle and reflected distally until a smooth soft muscle bed is reached consisting of brachialis proximally and the deep flexors distally. The ulnar nerve is then brought forward to lie in this plane alongside the median nerve (Fig. 26.9b) and the flexor muscles are re-attached superficial to the nerve (Fig. 26.9c). The elbow is a very vascular region and it is wise to release the tourniquet before wound closure. A plaster back slab is applied for 3 weeks to allow healing of the flexor muscles.

Sensory recovery is usually more rapid and complete than motor recovery [79, 80]. Full recovery may be anticipated in lesions of less than six months duration and in incomplete lesions of longer duration. Complete lesions of longer than 6 months may not recover entirely and operation is probably not worthwhile in complete lesions present for more than a year unless there are continuing sensory symptoms. Because most ulnar lesions are painless the symptomatic response to surgery is less dramatic than is usually the case with median nerve lesions and it may be several weeks or months before evidence of recovery is apparent. Patients with irrecoverable lesions seldom require reconstructive surgery. The fact that they have presented late with their condition is an indication that they have adapted well to the slowly progressive disability.

Ulnar nerve compression at the wrist

Compression in Guyon's tunnel occurs much less frequently than at the elbow. The causes of nerve compression at this level are listed in Table 26.5. Ganglia are the most common cause and tend to arise either from the inferior radioulnar joint or from carpus especially the pisotriquetral joint. The clinical presentation varies according to the exact relationship of the ganglion to the nerve. Thus there may be motor or sensory deficits alone or in combination [81]. Sparing of the dorsal cutaneous branch is a most important sign, and the long flexors are also spared but this can be so with lesions at the elbow so it is of less diagnostic help. The ganglion is usually palpable at this level and local tenderness may be elicited. Treatment consists of surgical

TABLE 26.5 Causes of ulnar nerve compression in relation to Guyon's canal

Cause	References
Ganglion	60, 85, 126, 134
Lipoma	135
Desmoid tumour	136
Thrombosed ulnar artery	137, 138, 139, 140
Osteoarthritis of radioulnar joint or piso-triquetral joint	60, 141
Rheumatoid arthritis	142
Post-traumatic fibrosis	137, 143–145
Anomaly of hamate	103
Anomalous muscles	146
Accessory ossicle	60
Haemophilic pseudocyst	147

removal of the compressing agent. The incision commences 3 cm proximal to the pisiform and passes distally along the lateral border of the tendon of flexor carpi ulnaris to curve laterally at wrist level and then distally along the lateral border of the hypothenar eminence. The nerve is identified proximally at the radial border of flexor carpi ulnaris and traced distally dividing the thin fascia covering Guyon's canal (see Fig. 1.19) until the compressing lesion is identified and removed. Complete recovery is the rule.

Deep palmar branch compression

This uncommon lesion presents a characteristic clinical syndrome which enables a precise and confident diagnosis to be made. The branch is purely motor and there are therefore no sensory symptoms or signs. All the ulnar innervated intrinsics may be involved but usually the nerve to abductor digiti minimi which arises before the nerve enters the deep tunnel is spared, producing an abducted attitude of the little finger (Fig. 26.10) [63, 82]. The patient's complaint is of difficulty with fine movements and of clumsiness of the hand. Table 26.6 lists the causes of deep palmar branch compression. By far the most common agent is a ganglion arising deeply in the carpus and emerging through the deep tunnel alongside the nerve. The ganglion is rarely palpable. Occupational trauma has long been regarded as a causal factor [83, 84], but trauma may simply be an additional insult to a nerve already threatened by a

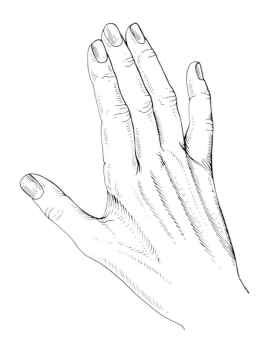

FIG. 26.10. Abducted attitude of the fifth finger in deep palmar branch paralysis.

ganglion [60, 85]. If the paralysis does not rapidly recover following cessation of the occupation, surgical exploration should not be delayed. The nerve is explored through a palmar extension of the incision described for wrist lesions. The ulnar nerve is identified in Guyon's canal and traced to its terminal branches.

The deep palmar branch is identified and followed deeply by dividing the fibrous arch which gives origin to the hypothenar muscles. The ganglion is then apparent and is removed. Sometimes the fibrous arch by itself appears to be the constricting agent. Rapid recovery follows decompression.

TABLE 26.6 Causes of deep palmar branch compression

Cause	Reference
Ganglion	60, 63, 82, 85, 126, 148
Anomalous muscles	149–152
Occupational trauma	83, 84, 153–155
Synovioma	88

Differential diagnosis of ulnar neuropathies

Many neurological disorders enter into the differential diagnosis. Intrinsic weakness of the hand is found in syringomyelia, motor neurone disease, Charcot–Marie–Tooth disease and leprosy. In each of these *all* the intrinsics, including those supplied by the median, are involved and usually bilaterally. Brachial plexus lesions such as those produced by a fibrous band extending from an elongated transverse process of C7 to the first rib may compress the lowest roots or trunk of the brachial plexus leading to intrinsic weakness of the hand. Usually all the intrinsics are involved to some extent although selective wasting of the lateral thenar pad may be prominent and some weakness of the long flexor muscles may be present. The sensory loss in this syndrome includes the inner aspect of the forearm, as well as the medial fingers, whereas the ulnar sensory supply is confined to the hand [86, 87]. Accurate localization of the lesion depends on meticulous clinical examination. Nerve conduction studies are of value in difficult cases but are unnecessary as a routine [88, 89].

Compression lesions of the radial nerve

Entrapment lesions of the radial nerve are excessively rare, although compression lesions of the nerve from external causes such as the use of crutches, a tourniquet or lying on the arm ('Saturday night palsy') are common and familiar, as is involvement of the radial nerve in acute injury such as humeral fracture. Lotem *et al.* describes three cases of radial palsy arising after vigorous muscular activity. All recovered spontaneously after a few days [90]. They postulate compression of the nerve within the spiral groove as it passes deep to the lateral head of triceps where they describe a fibrous arch which gives part origin to the lateral head.

Pressure by benign tumours, chiefly lipomas, at various points along the course of the nerve has been reported by Barber [91].

Isolated neuropathy of the cutaneous branch has been described [92, 93], but most of these lesions result from trauma and recover spontaneously; no internal entrapment lesion has been described. A tender thickening of the nerve may be felt at watch strap level. Local injections of hydrocortisone may hasten recovery.

Occasionally resection of the thickened nerve is indicated. It has been suggested that entrapment of the radial nerve in front of the elbow can be a cause of tennis elbow, and Roles and Maudsley describe an operation to release the nerve, but this has not gained wide acceptance [94].

Posterior interosseous nerve compression

The posterior interosseous nerve is narrowly confined as it enters and passes through the supinator muscle and there have been a number of reports of nerve entrapment at this level.

Anatomy (p. 34)

The nerve passes distally deep to the brachioradialis and extensor carpi radialis longus and brevis which may compress the nerve during pronation [95]. At the level of the head of the radius the nerve enters the supinator muscle by passing under the arcade of Frohse which is regarded by Spinner [95] as the main compressing agent. This arcade is formed by the most proximal tendinous

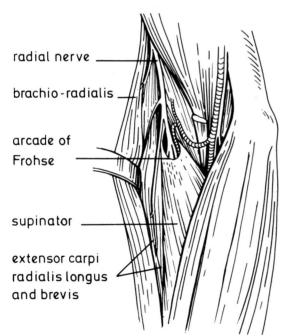

radial nerve

brachio-radialis

arcade of
Frohse

supinator

extensor carpi
radialis longus
and brevis

Fig. 26.11. The posterior interosseous nerve may be involved beneath the arcade of Frohse or within supinator.

part of the superficial head of supinator. It arises from the tip of the lateral epicondyle and arches downwards and laterally to be attached to the medial aspect of the lateral epicondyle. In 30 per cent of limbs it is a distinct fibrotendinous structure close to the capitulum (Fig. 26.11).

Clinical presentation

There is weakness or paralysis of the extensors of finger and thumb and abductor pollicis longus. There is no wrist drop and no sensory symptoms. The various conditions which have been described as contributing to the nerve compression are listed in Table 26.7. Local signs of these disorders or the low radiographic density of lipomas may help to confirm the diagnosis [96]. Cases of posterior interosseous nerve palsy due to compression by rheumatoid synovitis may easily be confused with spontaneous rupture of the tendons of extensor digitorum which is also a feature of rheumatoid arthritis (p. 346). The important diagnostic points are the gradual onset of the paralysis and the fact that it is usually incomplete and may also involve extensor carpi ulnaris, whereas the tendon rupture is usually abrupt, complete and does not involve extensor carpi ulnaris [97].

Treatment

Cases which appear to have been precipitated by acute or repetitive muscular activity should be observed for

TABLE 26.7 Causes of compression lesions of the posterior interosseous nerve

Cause	Reference
Arcade of Frohse and supinator muscle	56, 95
Lipoma	91, 96, 156–158
Ganglion	159
Post traumatic adhesions and fibrosis	99, 160
Rheumatoid arthritis	97, 161
Tardy palsy following Monteggia fracture	162
Fibroma	160
Neuroma	163
Traumatic aneurysm	164
Anomalous course	165

6 weeks to allow spontaneous recovery to take place. Cases which do not recover within this period or cases which develop insidiously or have evidence of a local pathology should be surgically explored and the nerve decompressed. If the lesion is thought to be near the arcade of Frohse an anterior incision is made extending from the elbow in front of the radius and passing distally for 6 cm. The fibres of brachioradialis are separated exposing the cutaneous branch of the radial nerve. The posterior interosseous is found by retracting extensor carpi radialis longus and brevis radially and it is followed to its disappearance behind the arcade of Frohse (Fig. 26.11). Any constricting bands, adhesions and the arcade of Frohse are divided. If the compressing agent lies more distally within supinator the posterior approach of Henry gives better access. The incision extends distally along the posterior aspect of the radius from the posterior aspect of the lateral epicondyle. The extensor carpi radialis brevis and extensor digitorum muscles are separated to expose supinator. The nerve is looked for about 3 cm below the neck of the radius by making a careful separation of the fibres of the superficial layer of supinator. Having identified the nerve it is exposed proximally and distally by extending the muscle incision along the course of the nerve. As with other entrapments the success of surgery depends on duration of paralysis. Delayed operation may not achieve recovery [98, 99].

Musculocutaneous nerve compression

This is the rarest of all the compression lesions in the upper limb. The author has personal experience of one case in which the nerve was compressed as it passed through coracobrachialis producing paralysis of biceps, weakness of brachialis and numbness over the radial border of the forearm in the distribution of the lateral cutaneous nerve. The nerve recovered following division of the superficial part of coracobrachialis.

REFERENCES

[1] PANAS, J. Sur une cause peu connue de paralysis du nerf cubital. *Archives Générales de Médecine*, 1878, **2** (VII serie).

[2] GILLIATT, R.W. Peripheral nerve compression and entrapment. In: *11th Symposium on Advanced Medicine*, Lane, A. F., ed. London, Pitman Medical, 1975.

[3] SUNDERLAND, S. The nerve lesion in the carpal tunnel syndrome. *Journal of Neurology, Neurosurgery and Psychiatry*, 1976, **39**, 615.

[4] NEARY, D., OCHOA, J. AND GILLIATT, R. W. Subclinical entrapment neuropathy in man. *Journal of the Neurological Sciences*, 1975, **24**, 283.

[5] SPINNER, M. AND SPENCER, P. S. Nerve compression lesions of the upper limb—a clinical and experimental review. *Clinical Orthopaedics*, 1974, **104**, 46.

[6] GILLIATT, R. W. AND WILLISON, R. G. Peripheral nerve conduction in diabetic neuropathy. *Journal of Neurology, Neurosurgery and Psychiatry*, 1962, **25**, 11.

[7] PHALEN, G. S. The carpal tunnel syndrome. Clinical evaluation of 598 hands. *Clinical Orthopaedics*, 1972, **83**, 29.

[8] EARL, C. J., GULLERTON, P. M., WAKEFIELD, G. S. AND SCHUTTA, H. S. Hereditary neuropathy with liability to pressure palsies. *Quarterly Journal of Medicine*, 1964, **33**, 481.

[9] TANZER, R. C. The carpal tunnel syndrome, a clinical and anatomical study. *Journal of Bone and Joint Surgery*, 1959, **41A**, 626.

[10] SIMPSON, J. A. Electrical signs in the diagnosis of carpal tunnel and related syndromes. *Journal of Neurology, Neurosurgery and Psychiatry*, 1956, **19**, 275.

[11] CAMPBELL, E. D. R. The carpal tunnel syndrome: Investigation and assessment of treatment. *Proceeding of the Royal Society of Medicine*, 1962, **55**, 401.

[12] PAYAN, J. Electrophysiological localisation of ulnar nerve lesions. *Journal of Neurology, Neurosurgery and Psychiatry*, 1969, **32**, 208.

[13] PAGET, J. *Lectures on Surgical Pathology*, p. 43. London, Longman, Brown, Green & Longman, 1853.

[14] LEARMONTH, J. R. The principle of decompression in the treatment of certain diseases of peripheral nerves. *Surgical Clinics of North America*, 1933, **13**, 905.

[15] BRAIN, W. R., WRIGHT, A. D. AND WILKINSON, M. Spontaneous compression of both median nerves in the carpal tunnel. *Lancet*, 1947, **i**, 277.

[16] CANNON, B. W. AND LOVE, J. C. Tardy median palsy, median neuritis, median thenar neuritis amenable to surgery. *Surgery*, 1946, **20**, 210.

[17] ROBBINS, H. Anatomical study of the median nerve in the carpal tunnel and etiologies of the carpal tunnel syndrome. *Journal of Bone and Joint Surgery*, 1963, **45A**, 953.

[18] LETTIN, A. W. F. Carpal tunnel syndrome in childhood. *Journal of Bone and Joint Surgery*, 1965, **47B**, 556.

[19] DAS, S. K. AND BROWN, H. G. In search of complications in carpal tunnel decompression. *The Hand*, 1976, **8**, 243.

[20] MANGINI, U. Some remarks on the etiology of the carpal tunnel compression of the median nerve. *Bulletin of the Hospital for Joint Surgery*, 1961, **22**, 56.

[21] YAMAGUCHI, D. M., LIPSCOMB, P. R. AND SOULE, E. H. Carpal tunnel syndrome. Minnesota Medicine, 1965, **48**, 22.

[22] CSEUZ, K. A., THOMAS, J. E., LAMBERT, E. H., LOVE, J. G. AND LIPSCOMB, P. R. Long term results of operation for carpal tunnel syndrome. *Mayo Clinical Proceedings*, 1966, **41**, 232.

[23] WARTENBERG, R. Partial thenar atrophy. A clinical entity. *Archives of Neurology and Psychiatry*, 1939, **42**, 373.

[24] MURRAY, L. C. T. AND WRIGHT, V. Carpal tunnel syndrome, humeral epicondylitis and the cervical spine: a study of clinical and dimensional relationship. *British Medical Journal*, 1976, **1**, 1439.

[25] LISHMAN, W. A. AND RUSSELL, W. R. The brachial neuropathies. *Lancet*, 1961, **ii**, 941.

[26] LINSCHEID, R. L., PETERSON, L. F. A. AND JUERGENS, J. L. Carpal tunnel syndrome associated with vasospasm. *Journal of Bone and Joint Surgery*, 1967, **49A**, 1141.

[27] INGLIS, A. E., STRAUB, L. R. AND WILLIAMS, C. S. Median nerve neuropathy at the wrist. *Clinical Orthopaedics*, 1972, **83**, 48.

[28] PHALEN, G. S. Spontaneous compression of the median nerve at the wrist. *Journal of the American Medical Association*, 1951, **145**, 1128.

[29] GILLIATT, R. W. AND WILSON, T. G. A pneumatic tourniquet test in the carpal tunnel syndrome. *Lancet*, 1953, **ii**, 595.

[30] FULLERTON, P. M. The effect of ischaemia on nerve conduction in the carpal tunnel syndrome. *Journal of Neurology, Neurosurgery and Psychiatry*, 1963, **26**, 385.

[31] HEATHFIELD, K. W. G. Acroparaesthesiae and the carpal tunnel syndrome. *Lancet*, 1957, **ii**, 663.

[32] VANIO, K. Carpal canal syndrome caused by tenosynovitis. *Acta Rheumatologica Scandinavica*, 1958, **4**, 22.

[33] HYBBINETTE, C. H. AND MANNERFELT, L. The carpal tunnel syndrome—a retrospective study of 400 operated patients. *Acta Orthopaedica Scandinavica*, 1975, **46**, 610.

[34] ROAF, R. Compression of the median nerve in carpal tunnel. *Lancet*, 1947, **i**, 387.

[35] CROW, R. S. The treatment of the carpal tunnel syndrome. *British Medical Journal*, 1960, **1**, 1611.

[36] GOODWILL, C. J. The carpal tunnel syndrome. Long term follow up showing of latency measurement to response to treatment. *Annals of Physical Medicine*, 1965, **8**, 12.

[37] GILLIATT, R. W. AND SEARS, T. A. Sensory nerve action potentials in patients with peripheral nerve lesions. *Journal of Neurology, Neurosurgery and Psychiatry*, 1958, **21**, 109.

[38] WOOD, C. Paraesthesia of the hand in pregnancy. *British Medical Journal*, 1961, **2**, 681.

[39] REID, S. F. Tenovaginitis stenosans at the carpal tunnel. *Australia and New Zealand Journal of Surgery*, 1956, **25**, 204.

[40] KREMER, M., GILLIATT, R. W., GOLDING, J. S. R. AND WILSON, T. G. Acroparaesthesiae in the carpal tunnel syndrome. *Lancet*, 1953, **ii**, 590.

[41] SABOUR, M. S. AND FADEL, H. E. The carpal tunnel syndrome—a new complication ascribed to the "pill". *American Journal of Obstetrics and Gynecology*, 1970, **107**, 1265.

[42] CARROLL, R. E. AND GREEN, D. P. The significance of the palmar cutaneous nerve at the wrist. *Clinical Orthopaedics*, 1972, **83**, 24.

[43] TALEISNIK, J. The palmar cutaneous branch of the median nerve and the approach to the carpal tunne. *Journal of Bone and Joint Surgery*, 1973. **55A,** 1212.

[44] ENTIN, M. A. Carpal tunnel syndrome and its variations. *Surgical Clinics of North America*, 1968, **48**, 1097.

[45] LANGLOH, N. D. AND LINSCHEID, P. L. Recurrent and unrelieved carpal tunnel syndrome. *Clinical Orthopaedics*, 1972, **83**, 41.

[46] CURTIS, R. C. AND EVERSMAN, W. W. Internal neurolysis as an adjunct to the treatment of the carpal tunnel syndrome. *Journal of Bone and Joint Surgery*, 1973, **55A**, 737.

[47] HUNT, J. R. The thenar and hypothenar types of neural atrophy of the hand. *American Journal of the Medical Sciences*, 1911, **141**, 224.

[48] SEMPLE, J. C. AND CARGILL, A. O. Carpal tunnel syndrome. Results of surgical decompression. *Lancet*, 1969, **i**, 918.

[49] HONGELL, A. AND MATTSON, H. S. Neurographic studies before, after and during operation for median nerve compression in the carpal tunnel syndrome. *Scandinavian Journal of Plastic and Reconstructive Surgery*, 1971, **5**, 103.

[50] GOODMAN, H. V. AND GILLIATT, R. W. The effect of treatment on median nerve conduction in patients with the carpal tunnel syndrome. *Annals of Physical Medicine*, 1961, **6**, 137.

[51] STRUTHERS, J. On a peculiarity of the humerus and humeral artery. *Monthly Journal of Medical Science*, 1849, **9**, 264.

[52] BARNARD, L. B. AND MCCOY, S. M. The supracondyloid process of the humerus. *Journal of Bone and Joint Surgery*, 1946, **28**, 845.

[53] KESSEL, L. AND RANG, M. Supracondylar spur of the humerus. *Journal of Bone and Joint Surgery*, 1966, **48B**, 765.

[54] GOULON, M., LORD, G. AND BEDOISEAN, M. L'atteinte du médian et du cubital par apophyse susepitrochléene. *Presse Medicale*, 1963, **71**, 2355.

[55] FRAGIADAKIS, E. G. AND LAMB, D. W. An unusual case of ulnar nerve compression. *The Hand*, 1970, **2**, 14.

[56] KOPELL, H. P. AND THOMPSON, W. A. L. Pronator syndrome. *New England Journal of Medicine*, 1958, **259**, 713.

[57] BEATON, L. E. AND ANSON, B. J. The relationship of the median nerve to the pronator teres muscle. *Anatomical Record*, 1939, **75**, 23.

[58] SPINNER, M. The anterior interosseous nerve syndrome. *Journal of Bone and Joint Surgery*, 1970, **52A**, 84.

[59] FEARN, C. B. d'A AND GOODFELLOW, J. W. Anterior interosseous nerve palsy. *Journal of Bone and Joint Surgery*, 1965, **47B**, 91.

[60] VANDERPOOL, D. W., CHALMERS, J., LAMB, D. W. AND WHISTON, T. B. Peripheral compression lesions of the ulnar nerve. *Journal of Bone and Joint Surgery*, 1968, **50B**, 792.

[61] APFELBERG, D. B. AND LARSON, S. J. Dynamic anatomy of the ulnar nerve at the elbow. *Plastic and Reconstructive Surgery*, 1973, **51,** 76.

[62] STRUTHERS, J. On some points in the abnormal anatomy of the arm. *British and Foreign Medico-chirurgical review*, 1854, **14,** 224.

[63] HAYES, J. R., MULHOLLAND, R. C. AND O'CONNER, B. T. Compression of the deep palmar branch of the ulnar nerve. *Journal of Bone and Joint Surgery*, 1969, **51B,** 469.

[64] MOUCHET, A. Paralysies tardives du nerf cubital à la suite des fractures du condyle externe de l'humérus. *Journale de Chirurgie*, 1914, **12,** 437.

[65] SHELDON, W. D. Tardy paralysis of the ulnar nerve. *Medical Clinics of North America*, 1921, **5,** 499.

[66] PLATT, H. The pathogenesis and treatment of traumatic neuritis of the ulnar nerve in the post-condylar groove. *British Journal of Surgery*, 1926, **13,** 409.

[67] RICHARDS, R. L. Traumatic ulnar neuritis. The results of anterior transposition of the ulnar nerve. *Edinburgh Medical Journal*, 1945, **52,** 14.

[68] OSBORNE, G. V. The surgical treatment of tardy ulnar neuritis. *Journal of Bone and Joint Surgery*, 1957, **39B,** 782.

[69] FEINDEL, W. AND STRATFORD, J. The role of the cubital tunnel in tardy ulnar paralysis. *Canadian Journal of Surgery*, 1958, **1,** 287.

[70] NEARY, D. AND EAMES, R. A. The pathology of ulnar nerve compression in man. *Neuropathology and Applied Neurobiology*, 1975, **1,** 69.

[71] CHILDRESS, H. M. Recurrent ulnar nerve dislocation at the elbow. *Journal of Bone and Joint Surgery*, 1956, **38A,** 978.

[72] WADSWORTH, T. G. AND WILLIAMS, J. R. Cubital tunnel external compression syndrome. *British Medical Journal*, 1973, **1,** 627.

[73] WOLTMAN, H. W. Pressure as a factor in the development of neuritis of the ulnar and common peroneal nerves in bedridden patients. *American Journal of Medical Science*, 1930, **179,** 528.

[74] KING, T. AND MORGAN, F. P. Late results of removing the medial humeral epicondyle for traumatic ulnar neuritis. *Journal of Bone and Joint Surgery*, 1959. **41B,** 51.

[75] GREEN, D. P. Paper read at the Combined Meeting of the American and British Societies for Surgery of the Hand (Edinburgh), 1977.

[76] OSBORNE, G. Compression neuritis of the ulnar nerve at the elbow. *The Hand*, 1970, **2,** 10.

[77] LEARMONTH, J. R. A technique for transplanting the ulnar nerve. *Surgery of Gynecology and Obstetrics*, 1942, **75,** 792.

[78] SEDDON, H. J. *Surgical Disorders of the Peripheral Nerves*, 2nd ed. Edinburgh, Churchill Livingstone, 1975.

[79] MCGOWAN, A. J. The results of transposition of the ulnar nerve for traumatic ulnar neuritis. *Journal of Bone and Joint Surgery*, 1950, **32B,** 293.

[80] LEVY, D. M. AND APFELBERG, D. B. Results of anterior transposition for ulnar neuopathy. *American Journal of Surgery*, 1972, **123,** 304.

[81] SHEA, D. AND MCLAIN, E. J. Ulnar nerve compression syndromes at and below the wrist. *Journal of Bone and Joint Surgery*, 1969, **51A,** 1095.

[82] URIBURU, I. J. F., MORCHIO, F. J. AND MARIN, J. C. Compression syndrome of the deep motor branch of the ulnar nerve. Piso-hamate hiatus syndrome. *Journal of Bone and Joint Surgery*, 1976, **58A,** 145.

[83] HUNT, J. R. Occupation neuritis of the deep palmar branch of the ulnar nerve: a well defined clinical type of professional palsy of the hand. *Journal of Nervous and Mental Disease*, 1908, **35,** 673.

[84] HARRIS, W. Occupational pressure neuritis of the deep palmar branch of the ulnar nerve. *British Medical Journal*, 1929. **1,** 98.

[85] SEDDON, H. J. Carpal ganglion as a cause of paralysis of the deep branch of the ulnar nerve. *Journal of Bone and Joint Surgery*, 1952, **34B,** 386.

[86] BONNEY, G. The scalenus medius band. *Journal of Bone and Joint Surgery*, 1965, **47B,** 268.

[87] GILLIATT, R. W., LE QUESNE, P. M., LOGUE, V. AND SUMNER, A. J. Wasting of the hand associated with a cervical rib or band. *Journal of Neurology, Neurosurgery and Psychiatry*, 1970, **33,** 615.

[88] EBELING, P., GILLIATT, R. W. AND THOMAS, P. K. A clinical and electrical study of ulnar nerve lesions in the hand. *Journal of Neurology, Neurosurgery and Psychiatry*, 1960, **23,** 1.

[89] GILLIATT, R. W. AND THOMAS, P. K Changes in nerve conduction with ulnar lesions at the elbow. *Journal of Neurology, Neurosurgery and Psychiatry*, 1960, **23,** 312.

[90] LOTEM, M., FRIED, A., LEVY, M., SOLZI, P., NAJENSON, T. AND NATHAN, H. Radial palsy following muscular effort. *Journal of Bone and Joint Surgery*, 1971. **53B,** 500.

[91] BARBER, K. W. Jun., BIANCO, A. J., SOULE, E. H. AND MACCARTY, C. S. Benign extraneural soft tissue tumours of the extremities causing compression of nerves. *Journal of Bone and Joint Surgery*, 1962, **44A,** 98.

[92] SPROFKIN, B. E. Cheiralgia paraesthetica—Wartenberg's disease. *Neurology*, 1954, **4,** 857.

[93] BRAIDWOOD, A. C. Superficial radial neuropathy. *Journal of Bone and Joint Surgery*, 1975, **57B,** 380.

[94] ROLES, N. C. AND MAUDSLEY, R. H. Radial tunnel syndrome. *Journal of Bone and Joint Surgery*, 1972, **54B,** 499.

[95] SPINNER, M. The arcade of Frohse and its relationship to posterior interosseous nerve paralysis. *Journal of Bone and Joint Surgery*, 1968, **50B,** 809.

[96] RICHMOND, D. A. Lipoma causing a posterior interosseous nerve lesion. *Journal of Bone and Joint Surgery*, 1953, **35B,** 351.

[97] MILLENDER, L. H., NALEBUFF, E. A. AND HOLDSWORTH, D. E. Posterior interosseous nerve syndrome secondary to rheumatoid synovitis. *Journal of Bone and Joint Surgery*, 1973, **55A,** 753.

[98] WOLTMAN, H. W. AND LEARMONTH, J. R. Progressive paralysis of the nervus interosseous dorsalis. *Brain*, 1934, **57,** 25.

[99] MULHOLLAND, R. C. Non-traumatic progressive paralysis of

the posterior interosseous nerve. *Journal of Bone and Joint Surgery*, 1966, **48B**, 781.

[100] NICHOLAS, G. G., NOONE, B. AND GRAHAM, W. P. Carpal tunnel syndrome in pregnancy. *The Hand*, 1971, **3**, 80.

[101] WILKINSON, M. The carpal tunnel syndrome in pregnancy, *Lancet*, 1960, **i**, 453.

[102] SCHILLER, F. AND KOLB, F. O. Carpal tunnel syndromes in acromegaly. *Neurology*, 1954, **4**, 271.

[103] WOLTMAN, H. W. Neuritis associated with acromegaly. *Archives of Neurology and Psychiatry*, 1941, **45**, 680.

[104] WEINSTEIN, J. D., DICK, H. M. AND GRANTHAM, S. A. Pseudogout, hyperparathyroidism and carpal tunnel syndrome. *Journal of Bone and Joint Surgery*, 1968, **50A**, 1669.

[105] WARD, L. E., BICKEL, W. H. AND CORBIN, K. B. Median neuritis (carpal tunnel syndrome) caused by gouty tophi. *Journal of the American Medical Association*, 1958, **167**, 844.

[106] MURLEY, A. H. G. Orthopaedic surgery in the treatment of leprosy. *Journal of Bone and Joint Surgery*, 1964, **463**, 503.

[107] LAMBIRD, P. A. AND HARTMANN, W. H. Hereditary amyloidosis, the flexor retinaculum and the carpal tunnel syndrome. *American Journal of Clinical Pathology*, 1969, **52**, 714.

[108] McLAIN, E. J. AND WISSINGER, H. A. The acute carpal tunnel syndrome: nine case reports. *Journal of Trauma*, 1976, **16**, 75.

[109] CHALMERS, J. 1977. Unreported observation.

[110] HALE, M. S. AND RUDERMAN, J. E. Carpal tunnel syndrome associated with rubella immunisation. *American Journal of Physical Medicine*, 1973, **52**, 189.

[111] LANZ, V. AND VOLTER, J. Das Akute carpal tunnel syndrome. *Chirurgie*, 1975, **46**, 32.

[112] KLOFKORN, R. W. AND STEIGERWALD, J. C. Carpal tunnel syndrome as the initial manifestation of tuberculosis. *American Journal of Medicine*, 1976, **60**, 4.

[113] NEWMAN, P. H. Median nerve compression in carpal tunnel. *Postgraduate Medical Journal*, 1948, **24**, 264.

[114] WATSON-JONES, R. Leri's pleonosteosis, carpal tunnel compression of the median nerve and Morton's metatarsalgia. *Journal of Bone and Joint Surgery*, 1949, **31B**, 560.

[115] YEOMAN, P. M. Leri's pleonosteosis. *Proceedings of the Royal Society of Medicine*, 1961, **54**, 275.

[116] ABBOTT, L. C. AND SAUNDERS, J. B. DE C. M. Injuries of the median nerve in fracture of the lower end of the radius. *Surgery, Gynecology and Obstetrics*, 1933, **57**, 507.

[117] LAZARO, L. Carpal tunnel syndrome from an insect sting. *Journal of Bone and Joint Surgery*, 1972, **54A**, 1095.

[118] DELUCA, F. N. AND COWEN, N. J. Median nerve compression complicating a tendon graft prosthesis. *Journal of Bone and Joint Surgery*, 1975, **57A**, 1975.

[119] HARDING, A. E. AND FANU, J. LE. Carpal tunnel syndrome related to antebrachial cimino-brescia fistula. *Journal of Neurology, Neurosurgery and Psychiatry*, 1977, **40**, 511.

[120] UNGARRO, M. A., CORRES, J. J. AND DISPALTRO, F. Median carpal tunnel syndrome following a vascular shunt procedure in the forearm. *Plastic and Reconstructive Surgery*, 1976, **51**, 96.

[121] WARREN, D. J. AND OTIENO, L. S. Carpal tunnel syndrome in patients on intermittent haemodialysis. *Postgraduate Medical Journal*, 1975, **51**, 450.

[122] BUNNELL, S. Discussion. *Journal of the American Medical Association*, 1951, **145**, 1128.

[123] JACKSON, I. T. AND CAMPBELL, J. C. An unusual cause of carpal tunnel syndrome. *Journal of Bone and Joint Surgery*, 1970, **52B**, 330.

[124] HAYDEN, J. W. Median neuropathy in the carpal tunnel caused by spontaneous intraneural haemorrhage. *Journal of Bone and Joint Surgery*, 1964, **46A**, 1242.

[125] BACKHOUSE, K. M. AND DAVIDSON, D. C. Anomalous palmaris longus muscle producing carpal tunnel like compression. *The Hand*, 1975, **7**, 22.

[126] BROOKS, D. M. Nerve compression by simple ganglia. *Journal of Bone and Joint Surgery*, 1952, **34B**, 391.

[127] HERNDON, J. H., EATON, R. G. AND LITTER, J. W. Carpal tunnel syndrome. An unusual presentation of osteoid osteoma. *Journal of Bone and Joint Surgery*, 1974, **56A**, 1715.

[128] KOJIMIA, T., IDE, Y., MARUMO, E., ISHIKAWA, E. AND YAMASHITA, H. Haemangioma of the median nerve causing carpal tunnel syndrome. *The Hand*, 1976, **8**, 62.

[129] JOHNSON, R. J. AND BONFIGLIO, M. Lipofibromatous hamartoma of the median nerve. *Journal of Bone and Joint Surgery*, 1969, **51A**, 984.

[130] YEOMAN, P. M. Fatty infiltration of the median nerve. *Journal of Bone and Joint Surgery*, 1964, **46B**, 737.

[131] TOMKINS, D. G. Median neuropathy in the carpal tunnel caused by tumour like conditions. *Journal of Bone and Joint Surgery*, 1967, **49A**, 737.

[132] GAY, J. R. AND LOVE, J. G. Diagnosis and treatment of tardy paralysis of the ulnar nerve. Based on a study of 100 cases. *Journal of Bone and Joint Surgery*, 1947, **29**, 1087.

[133] PULKKI, T. AND VAINIO, K. Compression of the ulnar nerve due to rheumatoid arthritis of the elbow. *Annales Chirurgiae et Gynaecologiae Fenniae*, 1962, **51**, 327.

[134] JENKINS, S. A. Solitary tumours of peripheral nerve trunks. *Journal of Bone and Joint Surgery*, 1952, **34B**, 401.

[135] McFARLAND, G. B. AND HOFFER, M. M. Paralysis of the intrinsic muscles of the hand secondary to lipoma in Guyon's tunnel. *Journal of Bone and Joint Surgery*, 1971, **53A**, 375.

[136] RITTER, M. A., MARSHALL, J. L. AND STRAUB, L. R. Extra abdominal desmoid of the hand. *Journal of Bone and Joint Surgery*, 1969, **51A**, 1641.

[137] DUPONT, C., CLOUTIER, G. E., PREVOST, Y. AND DION, M. A. Ulnar tunnel syndrome at the wrist. *Journal of Bone and Joint Surgery*, 1965, **47A**, 757.

[138] JACKSON, J. P. Traumatic thrombosis of the ulnar artery in the palm. *Journal of Bone and Joint Surgery*, 1954, **36B**, 438.

[139] TEECE, L. C. Thrombosis of the ulnar artery. *Australian and New Zealand Journal of Surgery*, 1949, **19**, 156.

[140] ZWEIG, J., LIE, K. K., POSCH, J. L. AND LARSEN, R. D. Thrombosis of the ulnar artery following blunt trauma to the hand. *Journal of Bone and Joint Surgery*, 1969, **51A**, 1191.

[141] JENKINS, S. A. Osteoarthritis of the pisiform-triquetral joint. *Journal of Bone and Joint Surgery*, 1951, **33B**, 532.

[142] TAYLOR, A. R. Ulnar nerve compression at the wrist in rheumatoid arthritis. *Journal of Bone and Joint Surgery*, 1974, **56B**, 142.

[143] CAMERON, B. M. Occlusion of the ulnar artery with impending gangrene of the fingers relieved by section of the volar carpal ligament. *Journal of Bone and Joint Surgery*, 1954, **36A**, 406.

[144] HOWARD, F. M. Ulnar nerve palsy in wrist fractures. *Journal of Bone and Joint Surgery*, 1961, **43A**, 1197.

[145] STEIN, A. H. Jun. AND MORGAN, H. C. Compression of the ulnar nerve at the level of the wrist. *American Practitioner*, 1962, **13**, 195.

[146] SWANSON, A. B., BIDDULPH, S. L., BAUGHMAN, F. A. AND GROOT, G. DE. Ulnar nerve compression due to an anomalous muscle in the canal of Guyon. *Clinical Orthopaedics*, 1972, **83**, 64.

[147] BAYER, W. L., SHEA, J. D., CURIEL, D. C., SZETO, I. L. F. AND LEWIS, J. H. Excision of a pseudocyst of the hand in a haemophiliac. *Journal of Bone and Joint Surgery*, 1969, **51A**, 1423.

[148] TOSHIMA, Y. AND KIMATA, Y. A case of ganglion causing paralysis of the intrinsic muscles innervated by the ulnar nerve. *Journal of Bone and Joint Surgery*, 1961, **43A**, 153.

[149] JEFFERY, A. K. Compression of the deep palmar branch of the ulnar nerve by anomalous muscle. *Journal of Bone and Joint Surgery*, 1971, **53B**, 719.

[150] MULLER, L. H. Anatomical abnormalities at the wrist causing neurological symptoms in the hand. *Journal of Bone and Joint Surgery*, 1963, **45B**, 431.

[151] SCHJELDERUP, H. Aberrant muscle in the hand causing ulnar nerve compression. *Journal of Bone and Joint Surgery*, 1964, **46B**, 361.

[152] MAGEE, K. R. Neuritis of deep palmar branch of the ulnar nerve. *Archives of Neurology and Psychiatry*, 1955, **73**, 200.

[153] BAKKE, J. L. AND WOLFF, H. G. Occupational pressure neuritis of the deep palmar branch of the ulnar nerve. *Archives of Neurology and Psychiatry*, 1948, **60**, 549.

[154] RUSSELL, W. R. AND WHITTY, C. W. M. Traumatic neuritis of the deep palmar branch of the ulnar nerve. *Lancet*, 1947, **i**, 828.

[155] WORSTER-DROUGHT, C. Pressure neuritis of the deep palmar branch of the ulnar nerve. *British Medical Journal*, 1929, **1**, 247.

[156] CAMPBELL, C. S. AND WULF, R. F. Lipoma producing a lesion of the deep branch of the radial nerve. *Journal of Neurosurgery*, 1954, **11**, 310.

[157] CAPENER, N. The vulnerability of the posterior interosseous nerve of the forearm. *Journal of Bone and Joint Surgery*, 1966, **48B**, 770.

[158] MOON, N. AND MARMOR, L. Parosteal lipoma of the proximal part of the radius. *Journal of Bone and Joint Surgery*, 1964, **46A**, 608.

[159] BOWEN, T. L. AND STONE, K. H. Posterior interosseous nerve paralysis caused by a ganglion at the elbow. *Journal of Bone and Joint Surgery*, 1966, **48B**, 774.

[160] SHARRARD, W. J. W. Posterior interosseous neuritis. *Journal of Bone and Joint Surgery*, 1966, **48B**, 777.

[161] MARMOR, L., LAWRENCE, J. F. AND DUBOIS, E. L. Posterior interosseous nerve palsy due to rheumatoid arthritis. *Journal of Bone and Joint Surgery*, 1967, **49A**, 381.

[162] LICHTER, R. L. AND JACOBSEN, T. Tardy palsy of the posterior interosseous nerve with Monteggia fracture. *Journal of Bone and Joint Surgery*, 1975, **57A**, 124.

[163] WHITELEY, W. H. AND ALPERS, B. J. Posterior interosseous palsy with spontaneous neuroma formation. *Archives of Neurology*, 1959, **1**, 226.

[164] DHARAPAK, C. AND NIMBERG, G. A. Posterior interosseous nerve compression. Report of a case caused by traumatic aneurysm. *Clinical Orthopaedics*, 1974, **101**, 225.

[165] HUSTEAD, A. P., MULDER, D. W. AND MACCARTY, C. S. Non-traumatic progressive paralysis of the deep radial (posterior interosseous) nerve. *Archives of Neurology and Psychiatry*, 1958, **79**, 269.

[166] FENNING, J. B. Deep ulnar nerve paralysis resulting from an anatomical abnormality. *Journal of Bone and Joint Surgery*, 1965, **47A**, 1381.

[167] HENRY, A. K. *Extensile Exposure*, 2nd ed. Edinburgh, E. & S. Livingstone, 1957.

[168] KOPELL, H. P. AND THOMPSON, W. A. L. *Peripheral Entrapment Neuropathies*, 2nd ed. Baltimore, Williams & Wilkins, 1976.

[169] THOMAS, C. G. Clinical manifestation of an accessory palmaris muscle. *Journal of Bone and Joint Surgery*, 1958, **40A**, 929.

CHAPTER 27

The Hand in Quadriplegia

D. W. LAMB

This chapter refers to the management of the hand following injury to the cervical spinal cord, but the principles described are applicable to severe bilateral upper limb paralysis from other causes.

Complete cervical cord damage is frequently sustained in a vehicle accident or at some sporting activity. The victims tend to be young and previously active in every way, and this catastrophe of the greatest magnitude alters completely and permanently their whole mode of living. Because of the astonishing developments in the management of such patients over the past few years, it is now commonplace for them to survive this serious injury and to have a life expectancy of 20 or 30 years.

Approximately 500 spinal cord injuries occur in Britain every year—an incidence of 1/100 000 population. The incidence of patients with cervical injury is at least equal to that of dorsolumbar injuries and thus the numbers of cervical injuries is considerable. A significant group of young people are left with impaired ability to look after their own needs. The quality of their lives can be improved immensely by provision of some upper limb function and grasp of the hand [1–13]. In a recent survey by Moberg [14], a group of young quadriplegics were asked to put in order of preference their wish for the following:

(1) normal use of legs,
(2) normal bladder and bowel function,
(3) normal use and feeling of sexual organs, and
(4) normal use of arms and hands.

Seventy-five per cent rated (4) as their top requirement. The possible benefits of reconstructive procedures should be known to those responsible for the care of these unfortunate individuals in order to obtain where possible, optimal functional efficiency in a home environment.

Any injury of the cervical spinal cord may result in some degree of impairment of function in the upper limbs. The higher the level of the cord injury the more extensive is the paralysis.

Injuries of the cervical spine are due mainly to forced flexion, in which the cord injury tends to be complete, or to hyperextension with a greater incidence of the partial cord damage.

In the immediate care of the patient, considerations other than the management of the upper limb necessarily take precedence, but it is important that those responsible for primary care should prevent joint contractures. Even if the paralysis appears complete, there may have been root escape with a possibility of some recovery of muscle power. If the joints have been allowed to stiffen, this power will be of course much less effective.

Initial management of the upper limbs

There is no necessity for splintage but all joints should be put gently through a passive range several times daily to *prevent contractures*: patients are not infrequently seen with adducted shoulder, elbow flexed, metacarpophalangeal joints stiff in extension and the thumb web contracted. If this is allowed to occur, no spontaneous recovery nor any surgery is going to be of practical use in restoration of function.

An early accurate *assessment of the motor and sensory impairment* is necessary.

All upper limb *muscles must be tested* in orderly sequence; this requires knowledge of the usual spinal segmental level of supply (Fig. 27.1). Complete cord injuries above the fourth segment are rare and seldom compatible with survival while injuries below the first thoracic segment do not involve the upper limb. Injuries between these levels result in some degree of upper limb impairment, but three-quarters of these will show survival of the sixth cervical segment in part or whole with good shoulder control and normal elbow flexion but no extension. Active pronation and supination are usually present although their power varies with the level of the lesion. The only other motor function is found in the radial carpal extensors and the brachioradialis, although the flexor carpi radialis is occasionally active [9].

There is usually satisfactory *sensation* along the lateral aspect of the limb.

Functional deficiencies are:

(1) lack of grasp and release in the hand due to paralysis of the digital flexors, extensors and the intrinsic muscles, and

(2) lack of lateral pinch (key grip).

These deficiencies are bilateral, the pattern being similar on both sides, although this is not invariable.

Methods of improving upper limb function and self-care activities

The life style of a quadriplegic depends predominantly on a wheelchair, thus anything which can help to control the movements of the wheelchair is most valuable. Moberg has shown how elbow extension can be restored very effectively by transfer of the posterior third of the deltoid and elongating this into the lower triceps [10]. The bilateral loss of active elbow extension is very serious and its effects have been underestimated as it prevents the use of the arms for balance and support while sitting. The restoration of elbow extension is very much appreciated and allows the ability to stretch out the arm against gravity and increases the functional range available to the hand.

Any measures undertaken to improve the hand function can be divided into conservative and surgical.

Conservative measures

Simple but valuable measures can be devised by the *occupational therapist* to permit holding pens and pencils, knives and forks and other necessary implements. Many patients become adept at holding objects in a bimanual fashion, between the bases of the thumbs and palms, giving a limited degree of self-care, e.g. washing the face, shaving with an electric razor, dressing and undressing.

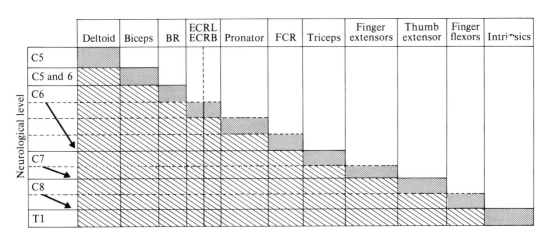

FIG. 27.1. The normal spinal segmental level of innervation to the muscles of the upper limb. The dotted areas show the main segmental muscle supply. Note the large number of muscles supplied from the sixth segment and its typical descending arrangement despite the very small total area of the segment.

Splintage, such as the wrist-operated flexor hinge splint [15, 16] may provide functional improvement [17]. With this splint, as the wrist is dorsiflexed, the digits flex, meet and can grip and hold objects which in turn are released by palmar flexion of the wrist. Splints powered by external means, (e.g. CO_2, electric) can provide a considerable degree of independence [15, 18] but are so sophisticated that, while used successfully in a hospital environment, are usually discarded on returning home.

Surgical measures

The possibility of improving upper limb function by surgery should always be considered. Knowledge of the available procedures is vital but of equal importance is the care with which surgical treatment is carried out. A selection of patients with poor motivation, or surgery which has been badly performed will produce poor results and lead to apathy and opposition to surgical treatment in this condition.

Tendon transfers to restore grasp or release in the hand have been used for a wide variety of conditions but the first report of significance for quadriplegics was published in 1957 [9] describing a two-stage operation in which an attempt was made to provide extension and flexion of the digits.

Zancolli reported his experience over 25 years of tendon transfers for restoration of grasp in quadriplegics at the C_6 survival level [13]. He also tried to provide both active digital extension and flexion but in some of his patients clawing of the fingers resulted from overaction of the transfer into the digital extensors.

This chapter is based on experience in the past 20 years in assessment and management of over 200 quadriplegic patients. Just under three-quarters have come into the group with survival of the sixth cervical segment. Great care is made in the selection of patients likely to benefit by operation [6, 7, 8]. No surgery is recommended in a complete lesion until at least 6 months after injury. If there is any recovery in a muscle previously completely paralyzed, operation is not contemplated until further improvement has stopped. Presence of considerable spasm, particularly if variable, is an absolute contra-indication to tendon transfer in this group as it may lead to fixed flexion contractures. In the older age groups and particularly with anterior spinal damage from extension injuries, there is a tendency to spasticity, but in the young person with complete cord damage from a flexion injury spasm is seldom a problem, unless there is a complication from urinary infection or pressure sores. The presence of sufficient sensation in the hand is necessary to make the surgery worthwhile. It is essential to retain mobility of the wrist; arthrodesis of the wrist is absolutely contraindicated.

Preoperative assessment should be done with the patient in the wheel chair, not while lying in bed. It must be made clear that operation cannot restore hand function approaching normality, but that it should improve the ability to grip. To the patient who has nothing, even a little is a lot; more than eight out of every ten on whom operation has been performed request operation on the other hand.

Operative procedure

The initial procedure used was that of Lipscomb [9], but it soon became apparent that an attempt to restore both extension and flexion of the digits was too ambitious. Grasp is provided by the transfer of the extensor carpi radialis longus into the tendons of the flexor digitorum profundus and of the brachioradialis tendon into the

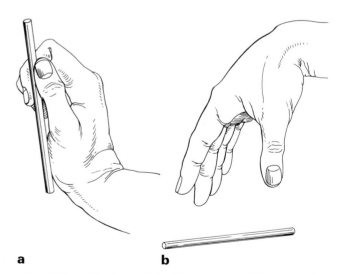

a　　　　　　　　**b**

FIG. 27.2. (a) The type of lateral key-pinch for picking up and holding an object after tendon transfers. (b) Release of object by dropping wrist. Full extension of digits is possible by the tenodesis effect of the extensors.

flexor pollicis longus. Following the principle of the wrist-operated flexor hinge splint where dorsiflexion of the wrist is used for grasp which in turn is released by palmar flexion of the wrist, no attempt is made to provide active extension of the digits, a natural extensor tenodesis effect being considered sufficient for the purpose (Fig. 27.2).

The second aim is to provide *a lateral key pinch of the thumb* against the radial aspect of the middle phalanx of the index finger (Fig. 27.2).

Operation [7, 8]

General anaesthesia is not advised as the operation can be done adequately under a Biers intravenous regional technique (see Chapter 7). A curved incision convex distally and centred on the radial styloid is used (Fig. 27.3). The insertions of the extensor carpi radialis longus and brachioradialis are identified, freed and dissected proximally to the musculotendinous junction. Care should be taken of the lateral cutaneous nerve of the forearm which lies closely along the anterior border of the brachioradialis tendon which is particularly well invested with fascia. At least one other transverse incision is required on the radial side of the forearm (Fig. 27.3); the tendons are transferred round the radial side of the forearm to the front where the brachioradialis is interwoven through the tendon of the flexor pollicis longus and the extensor carpi radialis longus through each separate slip of the flexor digitorum profundus from radial to ulnar side (Fig. 27.3).

When suturing the transferred tendon it is of prime importance to adjust its tension so that, with the wrist fully dorsiflexed the fingers are semiflexed and the thumb rests against the radial side of the middle phalanx of the index and on palmar flexion of the wrist the digits are capable of full passive extension (Fig. 27.2). It has not been found necessary to immobilize the wrist postoperatively. The extensor carpi radialis brevis, which is left intact, serves to dorsiflex the wrist and in only two patients has there been any weakening of dorsiflexion of the wrist postoperatively. It is difficult to isolate individual function of both radial carpal extensors but if there is any doubt about the power of the short extensor, operation should be avoided.

Usually within a month of operation, the transfers can be felt working and steady recovery and improve-ment of function will continue for about 6 months. Transfer of the long carpal extensor of the wrist to the flexor digitorum profundus is a procedure using

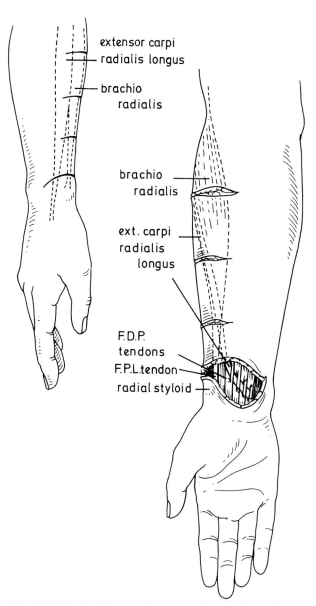

FIG. 27.3. The incisions used to expose the musculotendinous units of extensor carpi radialis longus and brachioradialis for transfer to the front of the wrist into the tendons of flexor digitorium profundus and flexor pollicis longus.

synergistic muscles and thus dorsiflexion of the wrist potentiates its effect. The amplitude of excursion provides very strong movement with the fingers flexing fully into the palm and is an entirely different and more effective procedure than elective tenodesis of the flexor tendons [11, 12].

In some patients premature flexion of the thumb into the palm obstructs finger flexion but this can be overcome by the patient learning to stretch the thumb against the side of the chair or table before flexing the fingers. Moberg meets this problem by stabilizing the interphalangeal joint of the thumb with a Kirschner wire [10], while Zancolli carries out arthrodesis of the basal joint of the thumb [13]. A recent report attempts to stabilize the thumb for 'Key' pinch by transfer of the brachioradialis as motor into the transposed tendon of the ring finger superficialis to provide an adduction-opponens plasty [5].

In summary, the transfers provide: (1) mass finger flexion for grasp, and (2) independent thumb flexion against the middle phalanx of the index. Consistently satisfactory results have been obtained by these simple procedures [6, 7] and it is a mistake to attempt to restore too many sophisticated functions at the same time.

The management of the young patient with traumatic quadriplegia is interesting and rewarding work. The general care of the patient is paramount but the possibilities of improving upper limb function, and therefore the ability for self-care, must not be neglected.

With careful selection of patients the results of tendon transfers can be a great help.

REFERENCES

[1] CURTIS, R. M. Tendon transfers in the patient with spinal cord injury. *Orthopedic Clinics of North America*, 1974, **5**, 415.

[2] FREEHAFER, A. A. Care of hands in cervical spinal cord injuries. *Paraplegia*, 1969, **7**, 118.

[3] FREEHAFER, A. A. AND MAST, W. A. Transfer of the brachioradialis to improve wrist extension in high spinal cord injury. *Journal of Bone and Joint Surgery*, 1967, **49A**, 648.

[4] FREEHAFER, A. A., VON HAAM, E. AND ALLEN, V. Tendon transfers to improve grasp after injuries to the cervical spinal cord. *Journal of Bone and Joint Surgery*, 1974, **56A**, 951.

[5] HOUSE, J. H., GWATHMEY, F. W. AND LUNDSGAARD, D. K. Restoration of strong grasp and lateral pinch in tetraplegia due to cervical spinal injury. *The Journal of Hand Surgery*, 1976, **1**, 152.

[6] LAMB, D. W. The management of the upper limb in cervical cord injuries. Proceedings of a Symposium held in the Royal College of Surgeons, Edinburgh, Morrison and Gibb, 1963.

[7] LAMB, D. W. AND LANDRY, R. The hand in quadriplegia. *The Hand*, 1971, **3**, 31.

[8] LAMB, D. W. AND LANDRY, R. The hand in quadriplegia. *Paraplegia*, 1972, **9**, 204.

[9] LIPSCOMB, P. R., ELKINS, D. C. AND HENDERSON, E. D. Tendon transfer to restore function of the hands in tetraplegia, especially after fracture dislocation of the sixth cervical vertebra on the seventh. *Journal of Bone and Joint Surgery*, 1958, **40A**, 1071.

[10] MOBERG, E. Surgical treatment for absent single hand grip and elbow extension in quadriplegia, principles and preliminary experience. *Journal of Bone and Joint Surgery*, 1975, **57A**, 196.

[11] STREET, D. M. AND STANBAUGH, H. T. Finger flexor tenodesis. *Clinical Orthopaedics*, 1959, **13**, 155.

[12] WILSON, J. N. Providing automatic grasp by flexor tenodesis. *Journal of Bone and Joint Surgery*, 1956, **38A**, 10.

[13] ZANCOLLI, E. Surgery for the quadriplegic hand with active strong wrist extension preserved—a study of 97 cases. *Clinical Orthopedics*, 1975, **112**, 101.

[14] MOBERG, E. (1977) Personal communication.

[15] NICKEL, V. L., PERRY, J. AND GARRETT, A. L. Development of useful function in the severely paralyzed hand. *Journal of Bone and Joint Surgery*, 1963, **45A**, 933.

[16] ENGEL, W. II., KINIOTEK, M. A. AND HOOF, J. P. A functional splint for grasp driven by wrist extension. *Archives of Physical Medicine*, 1967, **48**, 43.

[17] KAY, H. W. Clinical evaluation of the Engen plastic hand orthosis. *Artificial Limbs*, 1969, **13**, 13.

[18] STAUFFER, E. S. Orthotics for spinal cord injuries. *Paraplegia*, 1969, **7**, 118.

CHAPTER 28

The Upper Limb in Cerebral Palsy

G. E. FULFORD

Cerebral palsy is not a disease entity but is the name given to a number of chronic, non-progressive disorders of the brain in children which impair motor function. The causes are very varied: developmental malformations, encephalopathies in early childhood, brain damage from vascular disease and trauma. The impairment of motor function can affect power, tone and co-ordination. Often there are associated disabilities such as epilepsy, mental retardation and, probably most important when considering function in the upper limb, disturbances of sensibility.

Classification by neurological presentation

An understanding of the causes of cerebral palsy is important for prevention but, because in any particular patient the cause may be ill-understood or multiple, an aetiological classification has not proved useful in treatment. Neurologists prefer to classify cerebral palsy, primarily by distribution of the motor deficit (hemiplegia, bilateral hemiplegia, diplegia, ataxic diplegia, ataxia and dyskinesia) with subdivisions by nature (hypotonic, dystonic, rigid or spastic) and extent (right, left, hemi, mono, di, tri, tetra and paraplegic) [1]. This classification allows discussion with colleagues, helps understanding of associated problems and, in general terms, divides patients into groups related to the benefit obtained from orthopaedic surgery. However, it is not helpful in selecting surgical procedures for any particular patient.

Neurological classification and associated upper limb function

Hemiplegia

Hemiplegia involves the upper and lower limbs on the same side, with the upper limbs apparently more severely involved, and is usually associated with spasticity. The apparent greater involvement of the upper limb is because it performs finer functions than the lower limb, and these are the first to be lost.

The characteristic posture is: shoulder adduction with internal rotation, elbow flexion and forearm pronation with the wrist palmar-flexed and the fingers flexed over the adducted thumb (Fig. 28.1).

In mild involvement this posture may not be apparent at rest but appears on strenuous activities.

The degree of involvement can be:

(1) *Mild*, when the hand is used spontaneously, but lacks full voluntary supination and thumb abduction.

(2) *Moderate*, when the affected hand is only used to assist the normal upper limb because of further loss of voluntary control, including full extension of the fingers.

(3) *Severe*, where there is no useful hand function and the upper limb is only used to hold objects against the trunk. The tone is increased (spasticity) as are the tendon reflexes. There is commonly an associated athetosis, a slow writhing movement in the fingers, best seen when the hand is being used.

The most important loss associated with these motor alterations is a sensory loss of 'cortical type' which is present in about half the patients. Whilst light touch and temperature appreciation are commonly preserved there

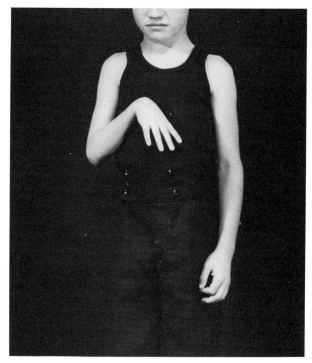

FIG. 28.1. The characteristic position of an upper limb affected by a spastic hemiplegia: shoulder adduction with internal rotation, elbow flexion and forearm pronation with the wrist palmar flexed and the thumb in the palm of the hand.

is impairment of kinaesthetic and two point discrimination and often loss of positional sense. Neglect of the affected limb and dyspraxia occurs more frequently in acquired than in congenital hemiplegia [2].

A hemiplegic at worst has one normal and one ugly and functionless upper limb. These patients have little functional disability so that any surgery to the affected limb must produce considerable improvement in function to be useful. In contrast, the appearance of the limb is often a considerable embarrassment and surgery which improves this may be greatly appreciated and, therefore, well worthwhile.

Bilateral hemiplegia

This is a tetraparesis with more severe involvement of the upper than the lower limbs. The handicap is greater than one would expect from two hemiplegias, for there is involvement of the bulbar muscles.

The patient presents with loss of voluntary control as in the hemiplegic, but affecting both sides and commonly asymmetrical. The limbs usually show greatly increased stretch reflexes (spasticity). Associated problems are difficulties with feeding and dysarthria due to the involvement of the bulbar muscles, and often epilepsy and severe mental retardation.

These patients have poor function in both upper limbs and may be totally dependent. Anything that can be done surgically to improve function will be a help, but often the physical and mental involvement is so severe that it precludes this.

Diplegia

Diplegia describes a more or less symmetrical paresis in the limbs, more severe in the lower than the upper limbs and commonly associated with spasticity or rigidity. There may also be involvement of bulbar muscles, but less severe than in bilateral hemiplegia. Both upper limbs show the same pattern of loss of voluntary control as in a hemiplegic upper limb, but generally less severe. The commonest problem is the flexed adducted thumb often with loss of finger extension so that the fingers remain flexed over the thumb. There is loss of voluntary supination, elbow extension and shoulder abduction/external rotation in the more severely involved patients. Abnormalities of sensation are less common than in the hemiplegics.

Ataxia

Ataxia is associated with generalized weakness, hypotonia and incoordination of movement, causing an intention tremor and unsteadiness. The tendon reflexes are diminished. By the time the child can sit with support a coarse intention tremor is obvious on reaching for an object. These patients cannot be helped by surgery to their upper limbs but luckily they steadily improve so that whilst their motor milestones are delayed the majority of these patients become independent. They often appear to deteriorate during the adolescent growth spurt but they improve again once they have stopped growing.

Ataxic diplegia

Such patients show ataxia with superimposed signs of diplegia; spasticity and exaggerated tendon reflexes in the lower limbs whilst the upper limbs tend to be hypotonic with sluggish reflexes. Surgery to the upper limbs is not indicated if they are mainly affected by the ataxic element but may be indicated for the diplegic element if this is predominent.

Dyskinesia

Dyskinesia is the impairment of voluntary movement by involuntary movement. These involuntary movements have been subdivided by their distribution and pattern. Athetosis is a slow writhing movement of the distal part of the limb, most obvious when a voluntary movement is attempted. Choreoid movements are relatively rapid movements predominantly in the proximal segments of the limb whilst dystonic movements are slow involuntary movements of the proximal parts of the limbs usually involving the trunk. Tremor is a regular alternating involuntary movement.

The more precise the voluntary movement the more likely it is to be disturbed by involuntary movements. Dyskinesia is, therefore, more likely in the upper limb and can particularly interfere with hand function. Peripheral surgery cannot help although the presence of dyskinetic movements is not a contra indication to surgery when there are other indications such as hemiplegia with associated athetosis.

Mixed cerebral palsy

This group includes patients with a diplegia or ataxic diplegia with a superimposed hemiplegia or diplegia with dyskinesia.

Associated sensory impairment

Touch, pain and temperature are usually not affected but the synthesis of these modalities by the parietal cortex into perception giving, for example, stereognosis, is commonly impaired. Amongst hemiplegics one-half show impaired stereognosis, one-third impaired two-point discrimination and one-sixth impaired position sense [3]. Lesny showed similar impairment of two-point discrimination which was more severe distally and also significantly impaired in the apparently normal limb [4].

As a general rule an upper limb with a motor deficit is more likely to lead to poor hand function if there is also poor sensation, but this is not inevitable. Similarly improvement in function following surgery to alter the motor control is less likely to be successful if there is poor sensibility but this by itself does not contraindicate surgery.

Orthopaedic classification

Although cerebral palsy includes many different disorders of the central nervous system the peripheral effects have a number of common features. The orthopaedic surgeon can only alter the motor aspect of these peripheral effects which are:
(1) muscle weakness,
(2) altered muscle tone,
(3) muscle incoordination, and
(4) involuntary movements.
Surgery on the upper limb is only helpful in the first two groups although it is possible that problems caused by muscle incoordination and involuntary movements may be helped by neurosurgery.

It is when muscle weakness results in an imbalance between agonists and antagonists that deformity occurs, with shortening of the stronger muscles, giving rise to a fixed deformity.

Muscle tone can either be decreased (hypotonia) or increased (hypertonia). Hypotonia is associated with joint laxity but this rarely causes problems in the upper limb except when it allows 'locking' of the proximal interphalangeal joints associated with the 'swan-neck' deformity. Hypertonia, or the 'spastic' element causes dynamic deformities. These deformities, unlike fixed deformities, are not permanent and can be temporarily eliminated by passive stretching sufficient to overcome the stretch reflex. The differentiation between a dynamic and a fixed deformity can be difficult, particularly when the reflex resistance to stretch is painful, so that the absolute test is carried out with the muscles relaxed by anaesthesia when only the fixed deformity will persist. Although fixed and dynamic deformities have been described as separate entities, it will be found that they commonly co-exist and any particular deformity will contain an element of both. They should be considered as the extremes of a spectrum with a mixture in the middle and an increasing element of one or other types as one moves towards the extremes.

Gravity affects the position of the limb and if it results in one position being held for a long period then muscles will adjust their length to this position; a positional deformity. This is more commonly seen in the lower limb but does occur in the upper limb when the muscle weakness is so severe that the limb cannot be moved against gravity.

Assessment

The particular problems limiting function must be established so that appropriate procedures can be chosen. Accurate assessment of function is necessary before operation, and repeated after surgery to determine whether the aims have been achieved. The upper limb is assessed under the following headings:

Appearance

The appearance is particularly important to the adolescent girl but can cause problems at any age. The adolescent is usually sufficiently mature to express feelings about appearance, but the younger child, suffering from taunting at school, is not able to ask for something to be done. The appearance can vary with the patient's emotional state so that a limb in a relaxed patient can rest in an entirely normal position yet when the same patient is under stress the limb can appear grossly abnormal being held in the characteristic deformed position (Fig. 28.1). This change is due to reflex activity and is a dynamic deformity.

Range of passive movements

The passive movements at all joints are recorded to determine fixed deformities and thereby decide how much of any abnormal appearance is fixed and how much dynamic deformity. The amount of fixed deformity is an indication of the extent of the muscle imbalance.

Muscle power

This is assessed and recorded using the Medical Research Council grading of muscle power [5]. Because of the associated increase in tone accurate assessment can be difficult requiring both experience and perseverance. The power of a muscle may appear stronger when part of a mass action, but functionally the strength during isolated action is what matters.

Tone

This is the resistance to a passive movement as a result of the stretch reflex. It varies with the mental stress upon the patient as well as the speed and force with which the local stretch is applied to the muscle. It is, therefore, very variable but usually it is possible to grade the tone as normal, increased or greatly increased.

Range of voluntary movements

These are recorded for the same movements as passive movements, but generally the range is less. Comparison of the range of active movements before and after surgery is a useful assessment of the surgical procedure.

Sensory function

The method developed by Baker is used [6]. This consists of six different shapes and six different surfaces, each in duplicate. The patient sees and feels these and then, out of vision, a test shape or texture is put into the hand. If the patient is unable to manipulate the object it is moved across the hand by the examiner. The patient points to the piece that he thinks is the same in the duplicate set of pieces.

Two-point discrimination is also recorded for the fingers and has been found to be useful as a quick method of assessment.

Tests of function and speed

Functional assessment charts developed by occupational therapists are based on the activities required for independence. This is most important when considering the patient as a whole but these charts tend to become lengthy and yet do not give the detailed information that is required to plan any particular surgical procedure.

A limited number of tests each selected to show a particular aspect of hand function are used. The appropriate test can be timed.

Writing. This shows the type of grip and the position of the fingers.

The writing movement is noted, whether it is a gross movement of the whole upper limb or a fine movement from the fingers.

Picking up a ball. This shows the ability to open the hand and in particular the thumb position. The ability can vary with different sized balls.

Using a hammer. This is another test of grip particularly of the ulnar side of the hand, as well as a test of wrist and forearm movement.

Picking up pegs from a peg-board. This test, with two sizes of pegs, allows an assessment of pinch grip. The patient is asked to try and store the pegs in the palm of the hand whilst picking up another peg. This requires independent function of the ulnar fingers as well as supination.

Screwing and unscrewing nuts and bolts. This requires the use of both hands, one to hold the bolt while the other screws on the nut, either by using a fine finger movement or pronation–supination.

Diagnostic splints

Temporary splints, either plaster of Paris or thermoplastic, are made to hold the position to be obtained by surgery and then an assessment is made whether function is improved. Splints are used to control palmar flexion of the wrist, adduction and flexion of the thumb and swan-neck deformity of the fingers. Splinting the wrist is particularly useful as it shows whether finger movement is related to wrist movement by a tenodesis effect.

Photography

Photographs are taken from the dorsal aspect to show the alignment of the hand to the forearm and from the radial side with the hand closed and open (Fig. 28.2a). Cine-photography provides the permanent record of function and speed and is used to record the above tests of function.

Intelligence and 'drive'

'Drive' or determination is independent of intelligence and when present can be a considerable factor influencing the success of a surgical procedure.

Age

Surgery is rarely indicated before seven years as before this the normal neurological maturation can produce changes in both function and deformity. If surgery is performed to improve function it is best done before 10 years, before the patterns of use become too well established.

Electromyography

Electromyography shows whether a muscle is active, and to some extent the degree of activity, but it cannot decide whether this is voluntary or part of a mass action reflex. Electromyography determines the phasic activity of a muscle and, therefore, it's likely action if it is transferred, for the phase of action does not change.

Nerve blocks

Selective nerve blocks with a local anaesthetic can be helpful in assessing which muscles are causing a deformity and may also reveal improved activity in the antagonists.

Principles of correction of deformity

Before deciding how to correct a deformity the cause must be understood. As already described two main types of deformity occur in cerebral palsy.

Fixed deformity results from imbalance of power produced by voluntary activity and is treated by release of the shortened muscle, commonly by tendon lengthening. To prevent recurrence of deformity muscle balance must be restored, either by weakening the strong muscles, or

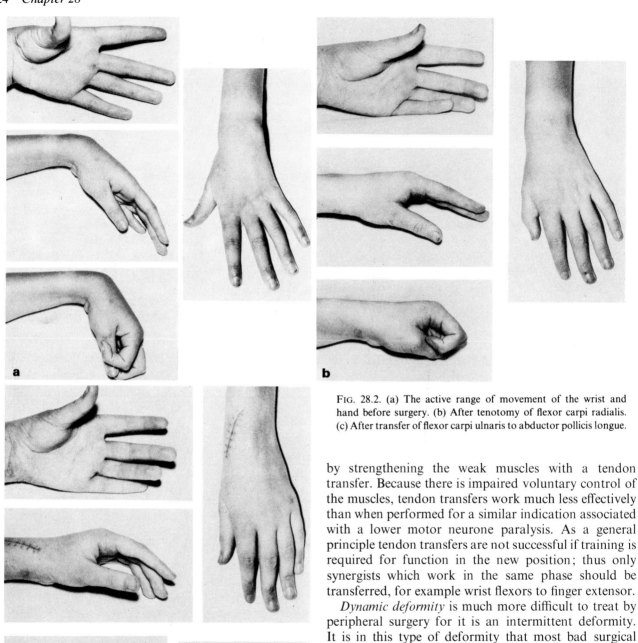

Fig. 28.2. (a) The active range of movement of the wrist and hand before surgery. (b) After tenotomy of flexor carpi radialis. (c) After transfer of flexor carpi ulnaris to abductor pollicis longue.

by strengthening the weak muscles with a tendon transfer. Because there is impaired voluntary control of the muscles, tendon transfers work much less effectively than when performed for a similar indication associated with a lower motor neurone paralysis. As a general principle tendon transfers are not successful if training is required for function in the new position; thus only synergists which work in the same phase should be transferred, for example wrist flexors to finger extensor.

Dynamic deformity is much more difficult to treat by peripheral surgery for it is an intermittent deformity. It is in this type of deformity that most bad surgical results occur. Attempts have been made to reduce this reflex activity by tendon lengthening, tenotomy and denervation. These procedures all weaken the muscle which may lead to the development of a fixed deformity in the reverse direction. An alternative approach is to transfer one of the muscles with increased reflex activity into its antagonists where, because these muscles do not change their phasic activity, the transfer continues to act in the same phase and it becomes a reflex antagonist to the muscle group from which it has been taken.

Based on an understanding of the causes of deformity the general principles of surgery of the upper limb in cerebral palsy are:

(1) Existing movements may appear to improve as a result of removing fixed deformity or over-riding dynamic activity.

(2) Function may be improved by altering the arc of movement without altering the range.

(3) New movements and improved range can only be obtained by tendon transfer.

(4) Only muscles under good voluntary control should be transferred to restore voluntary activity.

(5) The phasic activity of a transfer for voluntary control should be the same as the movement it is reinforcing.

(6) Dynamic deformity can be corrected by transferring a muscle with reflex activity in the same phase as an antagonist to the deformity because the transfer continues to act reflexly in the same phase.

Surgical procedures

The affected upper limb is held in the position previously described (Fig. 28.1). Taking into account the cause of the deformity and whether the proposed surgery is to improve function or appearance the following procedures are amongst the more useful.

Shoulder

If the shoulder deformity is so severe that surgical correction is required then it is likely that the control at the periphery of the limb is so impaired that there is no useful function and there is, therefore, no indication for surgery at the shoulder.

Elbow

Fixed flexion deformity at the elbow is common but rarely is of such a degree that it interferes with function. Lengthening of biceps and brachialis has been described but are seldom indicated [7].

Dynamic flexion deformity of the elbow can be troublesome, particularly in the very severely involved child, where it makes nursing and feeding difficult. Tenotomy of biceps brachii may be sufficient but where there is marked reflex activity transfer of biceps to triceps is indicated.

Forearm

Active pronation and supination are necessary for good hand function. In cerebral palsy the forearm is held in pronation and lacks active supination. Release of pronator teres from it's insertion corrects much of the fixed deformity that may be present, and can increase the range of voluntary supination. Once the fixed pronation deformity has been released transfer of flexor carpi ulnaris around the ulnar aspect of the forearm into a radial wrist extensor will also assist active supination [8]. For dynamic deformity crushing of the motor nerve to pronator teres has produced dramatic, but temporary improvement of voluntary supination.

Wrists

The wrist held in flexion–ulnar deviation is most worrying to the patient, both functionally and cosmetically. Function with the wrist splinted in the neutral position should be assessed before surgical correction. This will show any tightness in the finger flexors and also how much finger movement is due to a tenodesis effect of wrist movement. Usually immobilizing the wrist causes loss of both active and passive finger extension with loss of function.

Tenotomy or tendon lengthening of wrist flexors

This is indicated where there is good hand function but the wrist is held in some flexion. If passive correction of the wrist deformity does not interfere with the finger function then tenotomy which, providing the tendon sheath is left intact, allows the tendon to heal with a lengthened state will often be sufficient to restore the normal position and balance at the wrist (Fig. 28.2b).

Pronator teres to extensor carpi radialis brevis [9]

The indications for this transfer are similar to those of tenotomy of the wrist flexors but this procedure also reinforces wrist extension. Volitional grasp and release must be associated with and impeded by wrist drop, so that when the wrist is held in a neutral position the grasp is improved and the capacity to release unimpaired.

Flexor carpi ulnaris transfer to wrist extensors [8]

Flexor carpi ulnaris is carried around the ulnar aspect of the forearm to extensor carpi radialis longus so that it reinforces supination as well as wrist extension. There must be a full range of passive supination and wrist dorsiflexion before using the transfer. This transfer is not within the same phase and is successful because of its reflex activity which opposes that in the remaining wrist flexors.

Brachioradialis to extensor carpi radialis longus and brevis [10]

Brachioradialis appears usually to be under relatively good voluntary control. It is, therefore, a useful muscle to transfer in order to gain an increase in voluntary motor power and can be used to strengthen wrist dorsiflexion by transfer into the radial wrist extensors.

Flexor muscle slide [11]

This will transfer the arc of movement of muscles that are under good voluntary control into a more normal range without loss of power or range (Fig. 28.3a & b). For success the common flexor origin must be released from the medial epicondyle and the rest of the muscular origins from the radius, ulna and interosseus membrane by dissection carried down into the lower third of the forearm. The wrist is held in 30° of dorsiflexion and the fingers in full extension for 3 weeks and a night splint worn for 4 months after this. If the cause of the deformity was muscle imbalance at the wrist the extensors may have to be reinforced by a tendon transfer to prevent a recurrence of deformity. This slide is also useful to release a wrist flexion contracture often present in an otherwise functionless hand before undertaking arthrodesis of the wrist to improve the appearance. It is not infrequently found that the improved position after the slide is maintained without need for arthrodesis [12].

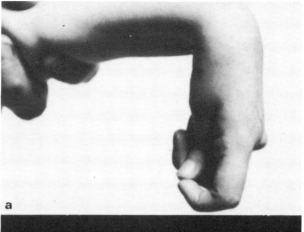
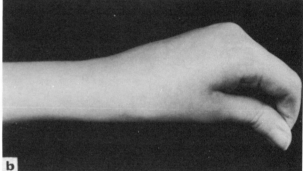

FIG. 28.3. (a) Wrist and finger movement before surgery. (b) After flexor muscle slide.

Wrist arthrodesis

Wrist movement is often important in producing finger movements by a tenodesis effect on the long finger muscles and arthrodesis of the wrist should be undertaken with caution. Finger function should be assessed with the wrist held in a corrected position by a splint when tightness of the finger flexors may become apparent. This shortening is best treated by a flexor muscle slide after which arthrodesis may be unnecessary or if still required it can be performed without shortening the forearm. If wrist arthrodesis is undertaken when there is only slight shortening of the finger flexors this can be allowed for by shortening of the forearm by spiking the distal radius into the carpus [13] or by removing the proximal row of carpal bones.

When a spike arthrodesis is performed the dorsal cortex on the distal radius should be retained and made into the shape of a gouge [14] as it makes the spike stronger and puts the wrist in slight dorsiflexion in the same way as does the Seddon modification of the Smith Peterson technique [15]. Setting the hand in ulnar deviation helps to pull the thumb out of the palm [16].

Fingers

Flexor muscle slide [11]

Often there is good voluntary control of the fingers, but the range of movement is only satisfactory with the wrist in flexion. The wrist position can be improved without losing any finger movement by a flexor origin slide (see wrist) (Fig. 28.3).

Tenodesis of flexor digitorum sublimis [17]

Swan-neck deformity can cause considerable disability as well as being unsightly. The finger 'locks' in hyperextension at the proximal interphalangeal joint, so that the finger flexors cannot flex the joint (Fig. 28.4a).

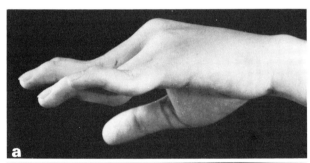
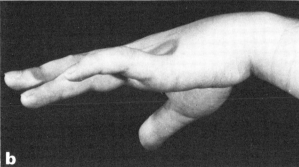

FIG. 28.4. (a) Extension of the fingers showing the swan-neck deformity. (b) After a Swanson tenodesis of flexor digitorum sublimis.

The joint has to be unlocked by an external force, often the other hand, or pushing the back of the fingers against a firm surface. The cause of the deformity is still debated, but it is possibly due to an imbalance of the long finger muscles rather than intrinsics. It is successfully treated by tenodesis of flexor digitorum sublimis to the proximal phalanx (Fig. 28.4b). The tenodesis should be made tighter than eventually required as it always stretches particularly in people who have a tendency towards joint laxity. Immobilization in flexion must be maintained by using a 'boxing glove' dressing and a plaster of Paris back slab for 3 weeks followed by a below elbow plaster cast with a hood over the flexed fingers to prevent extension at the metacarpophalangeal and interphalangeal joints for 5 weeks.

Thumb

Typically the thumb lies adducted across the palm of the hand so that, as well as being incapable of abduction and opposition, it gets in the way of the fingers when they are used for gripping. The first aim of surgery is to allow free use of the fingers by removing the thumb from the palm. The second aim is to gain useful function from the thumb. Passive correction of the thumb can be obtained by intrinsic release, but a tendon transfer is usually required to augment voluntary abduction and extension. In practice true opposition is rarely obtained and at best a lateral pinch against the index finger is the best that can be hoped for. Van Rensburgh describes five different types of thumb deformities, the straight adducted thumb, the flexed adducted thumb, the opposed straight thumb, the opposed flexed thumb and the 'W' thumb [18]. The best results of intrinsic release are obtained in the first two types. The 'W' thumb may also occur after any corrective surgery on the thumb and is treated by metacarpophalangeal fusion.

Intrinsic release [19]

Many methods of releasing the short muscles have been described but release of the origins of adductor pollicis from the shaft of the third and the base of the second metacarpal, release of the origins of flexor pollicis brevis and the distal two-thirds of abductor pollicis brevis allows the thumb to be passively abducted and extended without usually encouraging hyper-extension at the metacarpophalangeal joint. Active extension usually has to be re-inforced by a tendon transfer.

Brachioradialis to extensor pollicis longus [10]

Many transfers have been used to reinforce extension and abduction of the thumb after the intrinsic muscles have been released. Flexor carpi ulnaris can be used if it is not required for correction of the wrist deformity (Fig. 28.2c).

Brachioradialis is a suitable muscle for transfer because it is usually under good voluntary control, and providing its tendon is adequately released proximally has a good excursion. It is inserted into the tendon of extensor pollicis longus which has been rerouted by release from under the extensor retinaculum so that the transfer has a direct line of action on the thumb.

Intermetacarpal bone graft

Maintaining the thumb in full abduction and opposition by this method is successful when there is paralysis of abductor brevis and opponens pollicis [20]. The same procedure can be used with the spastic thumb, but the results are much less satisfactory. Because of the sensory impairment, particularly in the hemiplegic, the affected hand is mainly used for coarse grasp with the fingers and is seldom used for accurate manipulation associated with a pinch grip.

The thumb-in-palm deformity prevents the fingers being used for grasp, but the thumb fixed in abduction and opposition by an intermetacarpal bone graft is just as much an obstruction. If the graft has to be used then the thumb should be positioned in extension with the first metacarpal in the plane of the other metacarpals. Frequently the first metacarpophalangeal joint must be stabilized at the same time.

REFERENCES

[1] INGRAM, T. T. S. *Paediatric Aspects of Cerebral Palsy.* Edinburgh, Livingstone, 1964.

[2] INGRAM, T. T. S. (1973). Disorders of the central nervous system. In *Textbook of Paediatrics,* ed. Forfar, J. O. and Arneil, G. C. Edinburgh, Churchill Livingstone.

[3] TACHDJIAN, M. O. AND MINEAR, W. L. Sensory disturbances in the hands of children with cerebral palsy. *Journal of Bone and Joint Surgery,* 1958, **40A,** 85.

[4] LESNY, I. Disturbance of two-point discrimination sensitivity in different forms of cerebral palsy. *Developmental Medicine and Child Neurology,* 1971, **13,** 330.

[5] MEDICAL RESEARCH COUNCIL. *Aids to the Investigation of Peripheral Nerve Injuries,* 1942. Medical Research Council War Memorandum, No. 7, London, HMSO.

[6] BAKER, R. H. Personal communication, 1971.

[7] MCKISSOCK, W. AND NISSEN, K. I. The orthopaedic rehabilitation of a patient after excision of a cerebral tumour. *Postgraduate Medical Journal,* 1950, **26,** 166.

[8] GREEN, W. T. Tendon transplantation of the flexor carpi ulnaris for pronation-flexion deformity of the wrist. *Surgery, Gynecology and Obstetrics,* 1942, **75,** 337.

[9] COLTON, C. L., RANSFORD, A. D. AND LLOYD-ROBERTS, G. C. Transplantation of the tendon of pronator teres in cerebral palsy. *Journal of Bone and Joint Surgery,* 1976, **58B,** 220.

[10] MCCUE, F. R., HONNER, R. AND CHAPMAN, W. C. Transfer of the brachio-radialis for hands deformed by cerebral palsy. *Journal of Bone and Joint Surgery,* 1970, **52A,** 1171.

[11] PAGE, C. M. An operation for the relief of flexion contractures in the forearm. *Journal of Bone and Joint Surgery,* 1923, **5,** 233.

[12] WHITE, W. F. Flexor muscle slide in the spastic hand. *Journal of Bone and Joint Surgery,* 1972, **54B,** 453.

[13] EVANS, D. L. Wedge arthrodesis of the wrist. *Journal of Bone and Joint Surgery,* 1955, **37B,** 126.

[14] NISSEN, K. I. Personal communication, 1978.

[15] BROOKS, D. M. Tendon transplantation in the forearm and arthrodesis of the wrist. *Proceedings of the Royal Society of Medicine,* 1949, **42,** 838.

[16] COOPER, W. Surgery of the upper extremity in spastic paralysis. *Quarterly Review of Paediatrics,* 1952, **7,** 139.

[17] SWANSON, A. B. Treatment of the swan-neck deformity in the cerebral palsied hand. *Clinical Orthopaedics and Related Research,* 1966, **48,** 167.

[18] VAN RENSBURGH, W. Thumb-in-palm in cerebral palsy. *South African Medical Journal,* 1972, **46,** 373.

[19] MATEV, I. Surgical management of spastic 'thumb-in-palm' deformity. *Journal of Bone and Joint Surgery,* 1963, **45B,** 703.

[20] BROOKS, D. M. Inter-metacarpal bone graft for thenar paralysis. *Journal of Bone and Joint Surgery,* 1949, **31B,** 511.

CHAPTER 29

Upper Extremity Surgery Following Stroke

R. L. WATERS, V. L. NICKEL and D. GARLAND

Upper extremity surgery in the stroke patient is most commonly performed to relieve pain or correct deformity caused by spasticity. Surgery to improve hand function is performed on the patient who has relatively intact motor control and sensation, and in whom extension at the wrist, fingers, or thumb is restricted by mild flexor spasticity. Patients with bilateral hemiplegia due to multiple strokes are usually not considered for surgery in order to improve function because they have a poor rehabilitation prognosis.

In the stroke patient, hemiplegic dysfunction is usually the result of an infarction in the region of the cerebral cortex which is supplied by the middle cerebral artery or one of its branches. An ascending frontal branch supplies the anterior central gyrus (motor cortex) and an ascending parietal branch is distributed to the posterior central gyrus (sensory cortex). Most hemiplegics have motor and sensory involvement.

Motor recovery

Motor recovery in the paralyzed upper extremity follows a consistent recovery pattern with most of the recovery occurring during the first six weeks [1]. Recovery depends upon the extent of the lesion and the amount of collateral circulation. An extremity that is flaccid for more than four weeks signifies a poor prognosis.

In the flaccid extremity shoulder flexion appears as a first voluntary movement. With further recovery, flexion occurs at the more distal joints of the limb. Willed movement at this time results in flexion of all joints accompanied by forearm supination. Flexor spasticity is greatest at this time, and if no further recovery occurs, contractures are common unless the joints are passively extended during a daily exercise programme.

Extension movement at the shoulder and elbow generally occurs by the time the flexor synergy includes the wrist and fingers. The ability to extend the fingers selectively without evoking a mass extensor response in the proximal joints gradually develops with marked improvement in motor control and a reduction in flexor spasticity.

Mass flexion or extension of all fingers occurs simultaneously before the ability to flex and extend one finger independently is regained. Thumb opposition is at first to the side of the index finger (key pinch) with opposition to the finger tips returning later.

The hemiplegic patient will not use the hand in routine activities unless he can open selectively the fingers or thumb without eliciting a mass extensor response at the shoulder and elbow.

Sensory impairment

Functional use of the hand is as dependent on sensation as on motor function [2]. If the cerebral infarct involves the entire sensory cortex, the patient will respond to the basic modalities (touch, temperature, pain), but will be unable to appreciate the more discriminative aspects of sensation (shape, size, texture, proprioception). The patient may use his affected hand on request, relying on visual feedback, but will not routinely use that hand to assist the other. If the infarct extends posteriorly to the parietal lobe, the patient has additional perceptual problems involving space, motion of the limb in space, and awareness of the limb itself (body image).

Spontaneous use of the affected hand is not observed in hemiplegic patients when proprioception is absent and two point discrimination distance is greater than one centimetre at the fingertip or palm. Patients prefer to perform activities one-handed rather than grope with a hand that lacks sensation. Most patients will use the hand for assistance if motor function is intact and two point discrimination distance is less than 5 mm.

Procedures to improve hand function

The following rules will aid in selecting hemiplegics who will benefit reliably from surgery:

(1) nine months should have elapsed since the CVA and good cognition and motivation should be present,

(2) selective extension of finger or thumb has been regained,

(3) spontaneous use of hand for some functional activity is present,

(4) proprioception is intact and two point discrimination distance is less than 10 mm and preferably is 5 mm in the palm or fingers, and

(5) fixed joint contractures are absent.

These rules can be disregarded if surgery is intended for pain relief or correction of contractures.

The thumb

Some patients with voluntary key pinch between the thumb and side of the index finger may have restricted abduction and extension due to adductor pollicis or flexor pollicis longus spasticity. Unless the deformity is long standing, contracture of the first web space is uncommon. If movement is significantly improved following an ulnar nerve block, release of the adductor is indicated. The release is performed distally at the metacarpophalangeal joint; the thumb is splinted in abduction and extension for three weeks. A significant loss of key pinch strength or late metacarpophalangeal instability is not a problem after this procedure.

If the interphalangeal joint of the thumb is flexed during attempted extension, the flexor pollicis longus is restricting terminal extension and should be lengthened in the forearm by Z-plasty and the interphalangeal joint fused at neutral position to ensure stability.

Fusion of the interphalangeal joint of the thumb is also helpful in patients with paresis of the flexor pollicis longus and with hyperextension and instability of the joint hindering pinch.

The fingers

Active finger extension is often restricted by spasticity. This can be determined by anaesthetic block of the median and ulnar nerves. If the block improves extension the patient will benefit from surgery. Common flexor origin release has been advocated as a method for treatment of spastic wrist and finger flexors in the past [3]. This procedure requires extensive dissection and, in our experience, supination deformity often occurs as its complication. Individual tendon lengthening in the forearm is a more reliable procedure.

Lengthening of spastic flexor tendons results in some loss of voluntary flexor strength. Therefore, at surgery, the amount of tendon lengthening is one-half of the amount necessary to extend the finger from the point of voluntary restriction to full extension [4]. Frequently passive extension of the fingers reveals spasticity only in the superficialis muscle; however, lengthening of the superficialis tendons alone often unmasks restrictive spasticity in the profundus. Consequently, both tendons are lengthened an equal amount.

Tendon lengthening is performed either by multiple Z-plasty of the individual tendons or fractional lengthening [5]. The hand is splinted for three weeks prior to active movements.

The wrist

Inadequate wrist extension may be present despite satisfactory finger extension. If the finger flexors are spastic, or contracted, finger extension range may be lost after the wrist flexion deformity is corrected. Therefore, a pre-operative check of finger extension is performed with the wrist in corrected position. If the fingers extend, wrist flexor tendon lengthening may be safely performed. Manual palpation usually reveals a tight flexor carpi ulnaris; by performing ulnar nerve block, the contribution of this muscle can be judged. If satisfactory extension occurs after the block, the flexor carpi ulnaris only is lengthened; if the wrist remains flexed, the flexor carpi radialis is also lengthened and the palmaris longus is divided.

Transfer of the wrist flexors to the wrist extensors in hemiplegics is not necessary. The degree of spasticity, active range of excursion, and pattern of activity of the individual tendons varies in each patient. There are no accurate guidelines to determine the proper tension of the transferred tendon; if it is too tight, a wrist hyperextension deformity will ensue. Most patients with intact finger extension, who will benefit from surgery, have sufficient wrist extensor strength providing the wrist flexors are lengthened.

Surgery in the non-functional upper extremity

Surgery is indicated in the non-functional extremity to correct spastic deformities which cause pain or prevent adequate hygiene.

The hand

The surgeon should resist the temptation to release all finger and wrist flexors in the severely flexed hand and wrist. If any extensor tone is present, the wrist will be hyperextended post-operatively and may even dislocate dorsally on the radius. When excessive finger flexion is present without wrist flexion, sufficient tendon lengthening can be obtained by multiple Z-plasties or fractional tendon lengthening.

The superficialis to profundus (STP) transfer is a reliable method of achieving the necessary amount of tendon lengthening when severe wrist and finger flexion deformities are present [6]. Through a volar approach in the distal forearm all superficialis tendons are divided distally and all profundus tendons proximally. The proximal ends of the superficialis tendons are then sutured en masse to the distal ends of the profundus tendons. Sufficient lengthening is performed in order that the fingers and wrist can be extended to neutral. The wrist flexor tendons and the flexor pollicis longus may be lengthened through the same incision provided the wrist and interphalangeal joint of the thumb were flexed prior to surgery. Unless the finger flexion

deformities are long standing, and the skin contracted, fixed contractures of the finger joints are corrected by passive manipulation. The wrist and fingers are splinted in extension for 3 weeks.

Spasticity of the intrinsic muscles of the fingers and thumb is commonly associated with spastic extrinsic flexors. If only the flexor tendons are lengthened or superficialis to profundus transfer performed, the fingers will assume the intrinsic plus posture. Evidence of spasticity in the intrinsic muscles should be sought pre-operatively. If the intrinsic muscles of the thumb are spastic, the intrinsic muscles of the fingers are also presumed to be spastic. The cosmetic appearance of the fingers will be improved if neurectomy of the motor branch of the ulnar nerve is performed at the time of surgery. This will also relieve adductor spasticity of the thumb.

Because some patients lack extensor tone the wrist may remain in a flexed position postoperatively. A wrist splint may be applied or tenodesis of the wrist extensors may be performed at a second operation. The wrist extensors are divided longitudinally and half of each tendon is inserted through drill holes on the dorsum of the radius and sutured to themselves providing an extensor tenodesis. The wrist is protected in $20°$ of dorsiflexion by a splint for 8 weeks.

The elbow

Now that most stroke patients are placed on a preventive exercise programme elbow flexion contractures are rare and often signify a neglected patient. Fixed myostatic contracture is differentiated from spasticity by a musculocutaneous nerve block and when significant improvement is obtained, musculocutaneous neurectomy is performed. The loss of elbow flexion strength is of little consequence in stroke patients with elbow flexor spasticity because they have nonfunctional hands. The brachioradialis will allow some elbow flexion postoperatively.

Surgery is performed through a longitudinal incision made in the interval between the short head of the biceps and the coracobrachialis muscle. Most commonly the nerve is found in this interval. The incision may be extended proximally or distally if further dissection is necessary to locate the nerve. If the fixed elbow flexion deformity is greater than 75°, release of the elbow flexor muscles is also performed. A lateral longitudinal incision is placed over the origin of the brachioradialis and following release of this muscle the biceps muscle is divided. Only 30–40° of correction is generally obtainable at surgery due to associated contracture of the neurovascular bundle. Further correction of any residual deformity can be obtained postoperatively by serial casts.

The shoulder

Shoulder contractures are as rare as those at the elbow provided patients receive early passive movement.

Surgery is indicated when a severe contracture is present and is causing pain or preventing axillary hygiene.

Four muscles are responsible for adduction and internal rotation of the shoulder and kinesiologic electromyography may demonstrate all these muscles to be spastic and contributing to the deformity [7]. These are the pectoralis major, subscapularis, latissimus dorsi, and teres major and all but the subscapularis are palpable when the shoulder is abducted. Resistance to external rotation, with the arm at the side, is presumed secondary to shortening of the subscapularis.

Surgery is performed through a short incision in the deltopectoral groove and the tendons of pectoralis major, subscapularis, teres major and latissimus dorsi are released. A postoperative physiotherapy programme is essential for success.

REFERENCES

[1] TWITCHELL, T. E. The restoration of motor function following hemiplegia in man. *Brain*, 1951, **74,** 443.

[2] TWITCHELL, T. E. Sensory factors in purposive movement *Journal of Neurophysiology*, 1954, **17,** 239.

[3] CALDWELL, C. B., WILSON, D. J. AND BRAUN, R. M. Evaluation and treatment of the upper extremity in the hemiplegic stroke patient. *Clinical Orthopaedics*, 1969, **63, 69**.

[4] PERRY, J. AND WATERS, R. L. Orthopedic evaluation and treatment of the stroke patient. In: *Instruction Course Lectures— The American Academy of Orthopedic Surgeons*, pp. 51–55,

XXIV, St. Louis, Mosby, 1975.

[5] TACHDJIAN, M. O. *Pediatric Orthopedics*, pp. 842–845. Philadelphia: Saunders, 1972.

[6] BRAUN, R. M., VISE, G. T. AND ROPER, B. Preliminary experience with superficialis-to-profundus tendon transfer in the hemiplegic upper extremity. *Journal of Bone and Joint Surgery*, 1974, **56A,** 466.

[7] ZARINS, B. Evaluation of the painful shoulder in hemiplegia using EMG. In: *Orthopedic Seminars*, Vol. V, 1972, pp. 459–462. Downey, California, Rancho Los Amigos Hospital.

CHAPTER 30

Infections of the Hand

GENERAL INFECTIONS
M. ELIZABETH SHELSWELL

Hand infections still cause the loss of many working days each year even with modern antibiotic treatment. Some patients have permanent disability as a result of severe infections in which treatment has been delayed or is inadequate.

Many cases respond to conservative treatment and are successfully managed by the general practitioner, whereas in others who present for treatment too late or, when the infecting organism is not sensitive to the antibiotic given, surgery is required. The vast majority of these patients are treated as out-patients. Because of its seriousness a separate section is devoted to infection of tendon sheaths (p. 440).

Cause

Most hand infections occur after trivial injury which may seem unimportant at the time. Minor scratches, small penetrating wounds and even blisters can provide a portal of entry for infection. Surprisingly, severe injuries of the hand do not often become infected provided careful surgical toilet is carried out with excision of all devitalized tissue. Bites, both by animals and humans, frequently go septic. Foreign bodies can be a source of infection and small or even large foreign bodies may be missed if they are not radio-opaque.

The staphylococcus is the most common infecting organism [1]. Streptococcal infections, although less often seen, cause a more serious spreading infection with severe general symptoms. *E. coli* and other bacteria are found in a small proportion of cases. Mixed infection occurs in about a quarter of all cases of hand infection [2].

Conditions which predispose to or may be associated with hand infections

Diabetes

Occasionally an undiagnosed diabetic presents with a septic lesion. A routine test for glycosuria in all cases of hand sepsis is desirable and should certainly be carried out when the infection is slow to respond to treatment (Fig. 30.1).

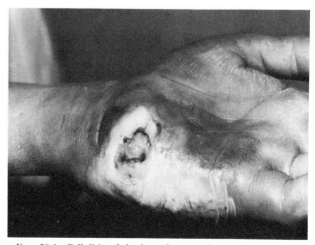

Fig. 30.1. Cellulitis of the hypothenar eminence in a diabetic.

Ischaemic conditions

Conditions such as Reynauds disease, arteriosclerosis and scleroderma may be associated with hand infections especially around the finger tips.

Neurological disorders

Those which cause impaired sensibility in the fingers predispose to infection. Minor trauma which is unnoticed causes breaches in the skin through which organisms can enter and the early warning sign of pain is absent.

Leprosy can be included in this group. Brand has pointed out that infections occurring in the insensitive hands of leprosy patients contribute to the absorption of digits [3].

Steroid therapy

This is well known to predispose to infection.

Drug addiction

Intravenous injection of drugs by addicts quite frequently produces severe infections [4]. When the arm veins are used up, injections are made into the veins of the fingers. It should be remembered that a number of these patients are carriers of infective hepatitis.

Anatomy and spread of infection

Kanavel made a detailed study of the anatomy of the hand with special reference to the way infection can spread [5]. Although this is less important than it was forty years ago it is still a useful classification. The following description is based partly on it.

There are three main pathways by which infection can spread but they may overlap:
  (1) tendon sheaths,
  (2) fascial spaces, and
  (3) lymphatics.

Tendon sheath infections (See also later section)

The anatomy of the synovial flexor sheaths is well known (pp. 10, 25, 41). Infection within a sheath spreads rapidly.

From the tendon sheath of the index finger pus can spread to the thenar space, while pus in the sheaths of the middle and ring fingers may spread to the mid-palmar space (see Fig. 32.2). If the little finger is involved pus can spread into the common flexor sheath (ulnar bursa), and if the sheath of flexor pollicis longus is infected pus extends proximally under the transverse carpal ligament (radial bursa).

Nail and fascial space infections

Paronychia. The infection begins in the nail fold and spreads round the side and deep to the nail. Sometimes the whole nail is lifted from its bed. In advanced cases it may extend to the terminal pulp space.

Subungual abscess (apical pulp space infections). Pus forms at the tip of the finger and spreads beneath the distal part of the nail.

Pulp space. On the flexor surface of each finger there are three pulp spaces separated by the flexor creases, at which point the skin is attached to the underlying fibrous flexor sheath (see Fig. 1.13).

Owing to the arrangement of the fibro-fatty tissue in the terminal pulp space pressure can build up rapidly leading to necrosis of the soft tissue (Fig. 30.2), and sloughing of the overlying skin. If left unrelieved osteitis of the terminal phalanx may occur (Fig. 30.3).

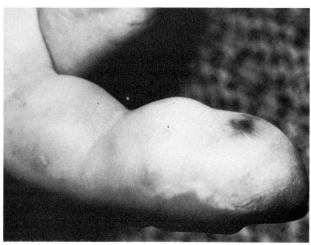

Fig. 30.2. Terminal pulp space infection.

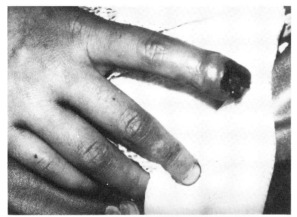

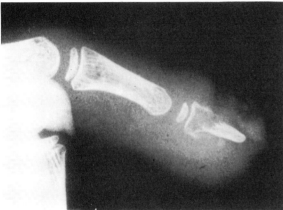

FIG. 30.3. Osteomyelitis of the terminal phalanx.

In severe cases the distal two-thirds of the phalanx can sequestrate. Kanavel thought this was due to thrombosis of the vessels from pressure [5], the proximal third being spared because its blood supply is from a branch of the digital artery arising more proximally. However, Pilcher and his colleagues thought that the staphylococcal exotoxin was responsible for the vascular thrombosis [6]. Possibly both factors are involved.

Pus in the middle and proximal pulp spaces can spread round the sides of the finger and from the proximal space it may extend into the web space.

Web space. This area of loose connective tissue between the bases of the fingers communicates with the subcutaneous tissue at the sides of the fingers, the dorsum of the hand and fingers and the spaces around the lumbrical muscles. Infections may spread into it from

these areas or come from cracks in the overlying skin. Swelling separates adjacent digits (Fig. 30.4) and oedema of the dorsum is pronounced.

The mid-palmar space (Fig. 30.5). This lies deep in the palm between the interossei and the flexor tendons and extends from the third to the fifth metacarpal bone. Infection may spread into it along the tendon sheaths of the middle and ring fingers or from the lumbrical canals. Oedema of the dorsum of the hand is severe.

The thenar space (see Fig. 30.5). This is anterior to the adductor pollicis and extends from the third metacarpal to the thenar eminence. Infection reaches it from the tendon sheath of the index finger or the lumbrical canal. Marked swelling is seen on the dorsum. (Infection of the mid-palmar and thenar spaces is now very rare.)

The palmar subaponeurotic space (see Fig. 30.5). This space is most often infected following penetrating wounds. Pus lies deep to the palmar aponeurosis usually without involvement of the flexor tendon sheath. There is deep swelling of the palm and oedema of the dorsum. The fingers can be partially extended although with considerable pain.

Thenar and hypothenar compartments. Infection in these spaces remains localized and points superficially.

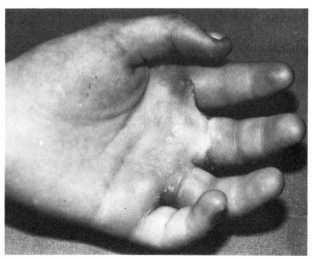

FIG. 30.4. Web space infection.

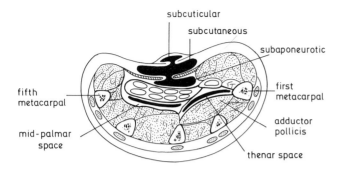

subcuticular

subcutaneous

subaponeurotic

fifth metacarpal

first metacarpal

adductor pollicis

mid-palmar space

thenar space

FIG. 30.5. Section through the middle of the hand to show the position of palmar abscesses.

Dorsal Infections. Hair follicle infection occurs on the dorsum of the hand and fingers. Pus in the subcutaneous space can spread easily and swelling is obvious. The dorsal subaponeurotic space deep to the extensor tendons is infrequently involved.

Lymphatic

Lymphatic spread may accompany a relatively trivial inflammation. Lymphangitis is seen as red lines which run up the flexor aspect of the forearm and there may be adenitis of the epitrochlear or axillary glands. It is associated with pyrexia and general malaise. It is usually due to Streptococcal infection.

Prevention

A recent wound should be thoroughly cleaned and ingrained dirt carefully removed. Many minor wounds on the hand and fingers do not require formal excision as long as the tissues can be cleaned carefully and are viable. More extensive wounds should be explored under general anaesthesia with a tourniquet so that all foreign matter can be removed and all dead and badly crushed tissues excised. Great care should be taken not to damage viable important structures such as tendons or nerves.

Tetanus toxoid should be given. This does not give immediate protection in those who have not been immunized before therefore antibiotics must also be administered. For those already actively immunized a booster dose of tetanus toxoid is required and it is wise to give antibiotics as well.

Treatment

Conservative treatment

Rest, if necessary by splintage in the safe position (see p. 2), elevation and antibiotics often cure early infections if treatment is started before tissue necrosis has occurred. At this stage the choice of antibiotic is empirical because the sensitivity of the infecting organism is not known. The causal organism is usually a staphylococcus or streptococcus. Penicillin is satisfactory in the majority of streptococcal infections, whereas staphylococcal infections are more effectively treated with ampicillin, flucloxacillin or tetracycline. Sensitivities, however, vary enormously with time and place. Once the infecting organism has been cultured and sensitivities tested the correct antibiotic should be given.

If definite signs of clinical improvement are not seen within 24–48 hours and if it is thought that pus has not yet formed, a change of antibiotic may still be successful, but if the symptoms persist pus is usually present. The length of antibiotic treatment will vary but must be continued until all signs of inflammation have subsided.

Operative treatment

When pus has formed drainage is required. Antibiotics circulating in the blood stream do not enter a walled off abscess cavity, but after incision and removal of the pus, blood containing antibiotic will spread into the cavity and eliminate residual infection. It has been suggested that recovery is more rapid if the skin is sutured but it is wiser to leave the wound open.

If the infection is in the distal part of the digit, surgery is possible under digital nerve block but where possible general anaesthesia and the benefit of a tourniquet is advisable. The limb should be exsanguinated by elevation for a few minutes before a pneumatic tourniquet is placed around the upper arm. It is better not to use an Esmarch's bandage in the presence of infection. A bloodless field facilitates exploration and efficient drainage of the whole abscess. Fine instruments should be used and great care taken not to damage important structures. With antibiotic cover, extensive incisions with through drains are not necessary. In most cases an incision can be made in or close to a skin crease where an abscess is pointing or over the area of maximum tenderness. If all pus is removed and if the abscess cavity collapses, drainage is not necessary but in larger thicker walled cavities a gauze or rubber drain may be used.

Collar stud abscesses are sometimes overlooked and not completely drained. In these pus in the subcutaneous tissues bursts through the deeper layers of the epithelium and produces a septic blister. When the blister is cut away a hole in the dermis is revealed through which pus can be squeezed. For good drainage this should be enlarged and the whole cavity explored and cleaned out.

It is wise to remove the tourniquet before applying the dressings and to wait for a few minutes while gentle pressure over the wound controls the initial bleeding. The dressings are then less likely to become stuck. If the abscess is small and there is not much oozing from the wound after incision, the dressing may be left for two to three days but where there is much bleeding or continued purulent discharge the dressing should be changed daily.

If a recent wound in the hand becomes infected removal of the sutures will frequently provide sufficient drainage.

Where an infection is due to a retained foreign body, this must be removed. In the case of wooden splinters care should be taken to extract all the pieces for which a tourniquet is essential.

Common types and sites of staphylococcol infection

Acute paronychia

An incision is made where the abscess points and, if there is subungual pus, part or whole of the nail should be removed. Sometimes it is necessary to take the nail fold back as a flap to facilitate excision of the proximal part of the nail.

Subungual abscess
(Apical pulp space infection)

Enough nail should be removed to allow good drainage.

Terminal pulp space infection

The pulp of the finger becomes tense, swollen, red and painful (Fig. 30.2).

Antibiotics are effective only if given within 48 hours of the onset of infection. Drainage should be instituted before tissue destruction or skin necrosis occurs and certainly before the blood supply to the terminal phalanx is affected. The classical signs of abscess formation are not seen in the early stages and the diagnosis rests on a tense swelling of the pulp and a history of a sleepless night due to pain. The incision is made over the point of maximum tenderness and with efficient drainage pain is relieved at once. Healing occurs rapidly but pockets of undrained pus will delay recovery.

In later cases, where sloughing of tissues has occurred, all dead tissue must be removed otherwise it will keep infection going. Collar stud abscesses may occur and it is essential to eliminate deep cavities.

Middle and proximal pulp space infections

These are less common than terminal pulp space infection. Pus formation is easier to diagnose than in the terminal space because there are no fibrous septa within the space to contain it.

A longitudinal incision is made over the point of maximum tenderness or where an abscess is pointing. Healing is usually rapid.

Web space infection (Fig. 30.4)

Incision is made where the abscess is pointing, preferably in a skin crease and the depth of the space is explored.

Infections in the palm (Fig. 30.5)

These are now uncommon. The patient usually presents early and antibiotics control the infection in a large number of cases. Sneddon found that only 52 per cent of palmar and web space infections required incision [7]. This is a much lower percentage than for pulp infections and paronychia.

Subcuticular pus is drained by cutting away the blister. This will reveal any subcutaneous abscess which should be cleaned out by enlarging the existing aperture in the dermis or incising in a skin crease.

Blunt probing will indicate any extension to the subaponeurotic space and if this exists the aponeurosis must be incised in the line of a skin crease and the depth of the cavity explored.

A mid-palmar space abscess is approached through an incision in the web and follows the line of the lumbrical canal.

The thenar space is drained through a dorsal incision along the radial border of the first dorsal interosseous muscle.

Boils and carbuncles

These occur in the hair bearing parts of the hand and fingers. Once the slough has separated, healing occurs. Incision is not often necessary unless a subcutaneous abscess develops.

Osteomyelitis (Fig. 30.3)

This is most common in the terminal phalanx following a neglected pulp space infection or a severe paronychia. It should be suspected if a pulp infection fails to resolve. The earliest radiographic sign is rarefaction and, later, sequestration of the distal two thirds of the terminal phalanx.

In the early stages, gentle curettage of the terminal phalanx with removal of all dead tissue from the pulp space combined with a course of several weeks or months of antibiotics should control the infection. In the later stages, part of the terminal phalanx may have to be removed which leads to deformity and shortening of the finger tip.

Suppurative arthritis

Acute arthritis may follow a penetrating wound of a joint. It sometimes occurs after injudicious attempts to prick a ganglion which is associated with degenerative arthrosis of the joint. The joint becomes swollen, hot and painful.

Treatment in the early stages is conservative. Splintage in the safe position (p. 2), elevation of the limb (p. 120) and antibiotics, especially lincocin may be successful [8]. If pus has formed the joint should be drained and necrosed bone and cartilage removed. With severe infection a fibrous ankylosis or bony fusion will occur. At the terminal interphalangeal joint this is not a great disability, but a fixed metacarpophalangeal or proximal interphalangeal joint leads to an awkward stiff finger which may justify amputation.

Streptococcal infections

These are poorly localized in the early stages. An area of redness and induration forms on the hand or fingers or there may be multiple septic blisters. Lymphangitis and adenitis are common. The patient feels ill with fever and toxaemia.

These infections should not be incised unless there is a definite abscess because early incision may spread the infection. The limb should be rested and elevated and the patient confined to bed if the toxaemia is severe. Penicillin is usually very effective.

Chronic infections

Chronic paronychia

This is often due to a fungal infection of the nail fold. It occurs in bakers and others who handle yeast or it may be associated with infections elsewhere in the body such as monilial vaginitis. Removal of the nail or base of the nail should not be done. Careful attention to hygiene, protective gloves to keep the hands dry and regular painting of the nail fold with an antiseptic solution such as tincture of penotrane or nystatin cream usually clears the infection. However, recurrence is common and any other source of infection such as vaginitis must also be treated. An anti-fungal drug such as Griseofulvin may also be used.

Chronic pyogenic arthritis

This can arise from acute arthritis which fails to resolve completely or may follow a chronic course from the start.

Like acute arthritis it is more liable to occur in joints which are the seat of degenerative change. The joint remains slightly swollen, warm and tender. Movement is painful and limited and there may be instability.

Continued splintage and a prolonged course of lincocin may eradicate the infection but, in some cases, arthrodesis of the joint gives a better result. Amputation may also have to be considered.

Pyogenic granuloma (Fig. 30.6)

This is a chronic staphylococcal infection which follows a trivial penetrating injury. Chronically inflamed granula-

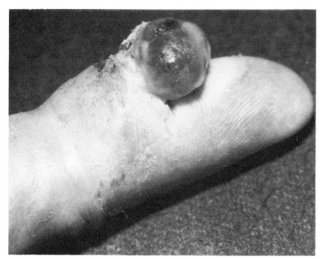

Fig. 30.6. Pyogenic granuloma.

tion tissue forms as a small tumour which bleeds easily. This is deceptive as much of the granulation tissue lies below the skin. If the protruding part only is removed it will recur. Careful dissection and removal of all the infected tissue will cure the condition.

Differential diagnosis

This should be made from:

(1) Other infections

Tuberculosis. Dactylitis, tenosynovitis and infection in abrasions of the fingers occur rarely in this country. Occasionally a rapid onset of tuberculous dactylitis may look like a pyogenic infection. Axillary adenitis is frequently associated with tuberculous disease.

Erysipeloid. This is a self limiting specific infection which may be mistaken for cellulitis. It is due to the organism which causes swine fever (Erysipelothrix rhusiopathiae), and occurs in people who handle meat or fish. It appears as a dusky red irritable swelling in the skin with a well marked edge. Its course can be shortened by the administration of Penicillin.

Orf. This is a virus infection which appears as a pink circumscribed swelling in the skin. Later an ulcer forms which may become secondarily infected. It is self limiting and lasts from 6 to 8 weeks. It occurs in people who handle sheep.

Herpes simplex. This starts like a pulp infection but later vesicles form which become purulent. It is contracted usually by dentists and nurses from patients with oral herpes. Like oral herpes it subsides in 7 to 10 days, but recurrent infection may occur which is difficult to eradicate.

Accidental vaccinia. Following a primary vaccination the virus may infect the finger gaining entry through cracks in the skin or invading a chronic paronychia; vaccinia may be grown from the lesions.

(2) Other local conditions

Inclusion dermoids. These are common on the fingers. They can become infected and unless a careful history is taken the diagnosis may not be made. Complete excision is necessary to cure the condition.

Subungual malignant melanoma. This can be mistaken for a chronic infection. The tumour starts as a painless pigmented lesion under the nail. As it grows it may become secondarily infected. Pigmentation is not always obvious but careful examination shows some pigmentation at the edges. The diagnosis is of the utmost importance so that the correct treament can be given straight away (see Chap. 31).

Conditions associated with generalized disease

Rheumatoid arthritis (see Chap. 25). This is only likely to confuse the diagnosis in the early proliferative stage.

Gout (see p. 484). Gout may present with a hot, swollen, inflamed finger, similar to a septic arthritis. Later other joints are affected. The serum uric acid is raised.

Psoriatic arthropathy. This usually affects the terminal digital joints. The condition often occurs in the absence of the typical skin lesions.

Sarcoid. This can produce a red, swollen finger suggestive of subacute infection. A radiographic examination aids diagnosis by showing the typical mosaic pattern.

Metastasis (see Chap. 31). A secondary deposit in a phalanx or metacarpal causes swelling which may be severe. Pain may be absent but a radiograph suggests the diagnosis.

Conclusion

The discovery of antibiotics has revolutionized hand infections. Whereas in the past extensive incisions were required and severe septicaemia sometimes resulted in the loss of limb or life, now hand infections rarely require admission to hospital and most make a complete recovery. However, there is still room for improvement. Prevention of accidents and careful attention to the initial treatment of wounds to avoid infection is most important. The recognition and efficient treatment of those conditions which lead to the more severe complications of osteomyelitis and septic arthritis will reduce still further the number of patients left with permanent disability.

ACUTE TENDON SHEATH INFECTION
A. G. POLLEN

Acute infection of the flexor synovial sheaths of the hand in this country now is a relatively uncommon condition. It accounts for 1–2 per cent of all hand infections so that even in a busy hand clinic only a few cases will be treated annually. Although uncommon it is important because function is likely to be gravely impaired if treatment is inadequate or delayed, whereas prompt treatment should lead to a good recovery.

Before antibiotics this condition had a high morbidity. The usual outcome was a stiff useless digit and subsequent amputation was not uncommon. Occasionally a patient died from an overwhelming streptococcal infection.

Spread of infection

Although the sheath for the little finger is continuous with the ulnar bursa (pp. 10, 25, 41, and Figs. 1.41–43), in practice infection of the bursa by this route is rare, probably because the little finger is least commonly involved. Conversely, infection of the thumb sheath spreads proximally to the radial bursa frequently. Despite the anatomical communication between the two bursae, spread of infection from one to the other must be exceedingly unusual. Spread from primary infection of the ulnar bursa to the digits is equally uncommon. Spread to the deep compartments of the hand and to the space of Parona in the forearm are not now reported as in the era before antibiotics [9].

Surgical pathology

The digital synovial sheath forms a closed, relatively indistensible cavity and thus its response to infection is rapid. Hyperaemia of the synovium is followed by an effusion at the site of the injury within a few hours, and this may extend the length of the sheath within 24 hours. The increased tension within the sheath impedes the blood supply to the tendon and particularly its venous drainage. The oxygen requirement of tendon is low so that it is able to withstand the effects of hypoxaemia for a long period without undergoing necrosis. The subsequent progress of infection depends upon the nature of the bacteria as well as the speed with which adequate treatment is instituted. Staphylococcal infections produce a fibrinous exudate which may delay the extension of infection along the tendon sheath. Streptococci produce fibrinolysins and hyaluronidases which may have a profound effect on the progress of the infection: the former dissolves fibrin so preventing localization of the infection, the latter break down the mucopolysaccharides of the ground substance and so damage the structure of the tendon. Necrosis of the tendon occurs late and only in the untreated or neglected case, by which time virtually all the soft tissues will have been destroyed. The chief problem in the treated case is stiffness from intrathecal adhesions which form as part of the repair process and are more likely to occur after a staphylococcal infection.

Bacteriology

The principal organisms are the staphyloccus aureus and streptococcus pyogenes but mixed infections are not uncommon. In the early part of the century streptococcal infections were commoner than staphylococcal (Table 30.1). A very severe infection occurred associated with lymphangitis, endangering limb and life. Butler recorded the deaths of two patients with streptococcal tendon sheath infection, out of a total of eight cases [10]. In recent decades staphylococcal infection has predominated, reflecting the general fall in incidence of all kinds of streptococcal infections.

TABLE 30.1. Bacteriology of 125 patients [12].

Organisms	Numbers
Streptococcus	45
Staphylococcus	39
Streptococcus + Staphylococcus	13
No culture	28

Sensitivity to antibiotics

For two decades benzyl penicillin was the antibiotic of choice in hand infections because streptococcus pyogenes and the non-hospital staphylococci remained sensitive to it. Unfortunately in recent years an increasing number of 'domestic' staphylococci produce penicillinase (Table 30.2), and it has become necessary to use other antibiotics, particularly the newer antibiotics (Table 30.2). In a recent series cultures were sterile in nearly half of the cases (13 out of 29) [11]. Twelve patients were given antibiotics before attending the hand clinic which suggests that the concentration of antibiotic within the synovial sheath was sufficient to exert a bacteriostatic effect *in vitro*, though inadequate *in vivo*.

TABLE 30.2. Bacteriology of 29 patients 1964–74 (author's series).

Organisms	Numbers	Penicillin resistant
Streptococcus	5	0
Staphylococcus	9	3
Streptococcus + Staphylococcus	2	0 / 2
Sterile culture	13	—

Classification

There are two groups depending on the route of infection.

(1) *Primary* when the organisms are implanted directly into the sheath, and

(2) *Secondary* when the sheath is involved as a result of the spread of infection from an adjacent lesion.

Primary infections arise commonly from a penetrating wound, the majority being near a flexion crease (Fig. 30.7) because the sheath is particularly vulnerable where the skin of the crease is bound down to the fibrous sheath which is thin in this area. A variety of agents are responsible for the initial injury: in industry wooden splinters and metal turnings, at home needles, splinters and garden thorns. Lacerations are less common as a source of tendon sheath infection. This is so because these wounds are usually treated surgically at an early stage whereas a patient with a needle prick will not seek treatment unless infection supervenes. In a minority of patients no history of injury is obtained nor is there evidence of a wound on examination, so that the route of infection is uncertain. It is possible that organisms reach the synovial sheath through a minute breach in the skin; alternatively one may postulate that the infection is blood borne in a manner comparable to that of acute osteomyelitis.

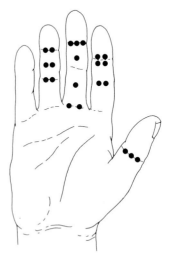

FIG. 30.7. Diagram to show the position of 22 wounds of the digits in 29 patients. Only 4 were remote from the flexion creases. In 7 patients no wounds were present.

Secondary infection is rare today but in the first half of the century accounted for nearly half of all cases. Grinnell reported 46 per cent of secondarily infected cases [12] and Flynn [13] 41 per cent.

Secondary infections arise in two ways: (1) by direct spread from an adjacent lesion, or (2) by accidental puncture of the synovial sheath during the surgical drainage of an adjacent abscess. The fibrous sheath acts as an effective barrier to the spread of infection. An extensive proximal pulp infection may surround the tendon sheath by pus and yet the sheath and tendons remain intact. It requires a long period of sepsis with complete destruction of the pulp tissue before necrosis of the sheath will occur.

In the preantibiotic era the control of virulent hand infections was difficult, pulp space infections were drained by the traditional lateral 'through and through' incisions which could endanger the sheath; anaesthesia was often primitive so that operations were performed hurriedly, without a bloodless field, and often by inexperienced surgeons. Small wonder that under such conditions secondary tendon sheath infection was common.

Cases of secondary infections are now rare and usually occur in pulp infections treated for long periods with oral antibiotics. In these cases the *pain* subsides though the swelling persists, the lack of acute symptoms and signs deceiving the doctor into thinking that the infection has subsided. Only when it is apparent that no active flexion of the digit is possible is the patient referred to hospital.

The rarity of secondary infection today is due to the improved standards of surgery of the infected hand, the correct use of antibiotics and the establishment of hand clinics in many hospitals.

Clinical presentation

The classical picture of acute tendon sheath infection is well known. Pain, throbbing and unrelenting in character, makes sleep impossible. The digit is diffusely swollen, held in a position of slight flexion (Fig. 30.8). All movements cause pain, but passive extension at the proximal interphalangeal joint is intensely painful. Extreme local tenderness along the course of the sheath may be elicited by blunt pressure.

This presentation, however, is seldom seen today

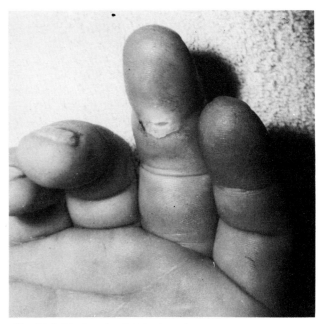

Fig. 30.8. Tendon sheath infection of left ring finger caused by a needle prick at the distal flexion crease 5 days earlier.

because treatment with oral antibiotics has usually been commenced before attending hospital, which modifies the clinical picture considerarly. In particular, the digit may be moved appreciably without severe discomfort. However, two reliable signs are present:

(1) *localized tenderness* along the length of the sheath; this must be sought with great care and gentleness using a blunt ended probe, and

(2) *passive extension* of the proximal interphalangeal joint will produce pain even though flexion of the digit, active or passive may be performed without undue discomfort.

Involvement of the synovial bursae

Infection of the *ulnar bursa* causes intense pain in the hand and digits, often in the thumb, index and middle fingers due to compression of the median nerve within the carpal tunnel. The fingers and hand show a considerable swelling extending as a fullness above the wrist for several centimetres. The fingers are held immobile in semiflexion (Fig. 30.9), and any attempt to move them is accompanied by severe pain and resisted.

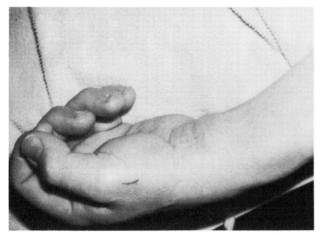

Fig. 30.9. Infection of the ulnar bursa showing the characteristic position of the fingers. Note the swelling extending above the wrist.

Involvement of the *radial bursa* is associated with proximal extension of infection within the sheath of flexor pollicis longus tendon. The thumb, thenar eminence and first web space are swollen, the thumb being held in flexion (Fig. 30.10).

Differential diagnosis

Only a few conditions may cause difficulty:

Acute infective arthritis of an interphalangeal joint. Although there is restriction of movements, the pain and swelling are localized around the joint and the maximal tenderness is found on the dorsal aspect of the joint.

'Collar stud' abscess of the web space. Although digital movements are inhibited by pain, maximal tenderness lies between the fingers not along the tendon sheath, the swelling is around the base of the fingers and extends onto the dorsum of the hand.

Acute calcareous deposits in the digits. These occur around joints or within the distal portion of the flexor tendons and may mimic a tendon sheath infection. However, the tenderness is very sharply localized to the site of the lesion; radiography will reveal a discrete radio-opaque deposit in a typical position.

Acute cellulitis. Although the digit may be diffusely swollen, movements are not so restricted as in the tendon sheath infection, there is usually an associated lymphangitis and lymphadenopathy characteristic of streptococcal infections of the hand.

Treatment

This has changed radically since the advent of antibiotics. Previously treatment was largely by long lateral incisions into the digital sheaths. The wounds were packed or 'through and through' drains inserted. In many patients a stiff finger was the inevitable sequel, in others the digit was amputated as an emergency procedure or removed subsequently because it was painful as well as useless. A few patients died from overwhelming infection [10]. Grinnell reviewed 125 patients treated during a 17-year period: in only 21 (17 per cent) was good recovery achieved [12]. Yet less than one decade later there came a dramatic improvement in the results. Curr reported good results in 19 out of 25 patients [14], and Gordon obtained good function in over 80 per cent of his patients [15].

This rapid improvement of prognosis resulted from
(1) the use of penicillin, and
(2) the advance in surgical technique.

The beneficial effect of antibiotics has led to a change of emphasis in the treatment of this condition. Controversy still exists as to the role of surgery in its management and even more so with regard to its timing.

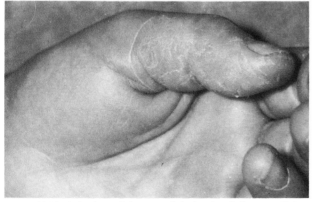

Fig. 30.10. Infection of the synovial sheath of flexor pollicis longus. Note that the swelling extends into the thenar eminence.

Some surgeons advocate a conservative approach [7], the patient being admitted for observation, the hand splinted, and antibiotics administered systemically. In early cases the infection may subside but should the symptoms and signs increase surgical drainage must then be undertaken. The difficulty of this method is to decide *when* it is necessary to operate. Antibiotics may modify and mask the progress of infection until so much necrosis has occurred that surgical intervention cannot restore good function.

Thus the treatment by the author is:

(1) operation as soon as possible after the diagnosis has been made,

(2) synovial sheath is exposed through small proximal and distal volar incisions,

(3) a fine catheter is inserted into the proximal end of the sheath which is thoroughly washed out with saline, and

(4) the sheath is irrigated with an antibiotic solution of 1 per cent cloxacillin which is continued during the post-operative stage; systemic antibiotics are administered concurrently.

Operative technique

Haemostasis is obtained by a pneumatic cuff around the arm. An Esmarch bandage is not used, instead the limb is elevated for several minutes before the cuff is inflated.

Infection confined to the digital sheath. Its proximal end is exposed through a short transverse palmar incision; in the little, ring and middle fingers it is made at the distal palmar flexion crease (Fig. 30.11), but for the index finger the radial end of the proximal palmar crease is used. After locating and retracting the digital nerves, the fibrous sheath is incised transversely 1 cm from its end; the synovium, often thickened, bulges through the incision, is picked up with fine-toothed forceps and opened with fine-pointed scissors. Fluid emerges, usually not under pressure, and it can be squeezed into the wound by gentle pressure over the digit. A sample should be collected for bacteriological study. The character of the fluid may give an indication of the nature of the infection: if it is cloudy but without fibrinous deposits, the infection may be streptococcal; more commonly it is slightly turbid with small flakes of fibrin present, which suggests a staphylococcal infection.

A fine nylon catheter 1 mm in external diameter is introduced into the synovial sheath distally for a distance of about 2 cm (Fig. 30.11). It will be used for washing out the synovial sheath and for postoperative irrigation. The sheath is then explored distally at the site of the wound: the skin around the wound is excised in a circular fashion about 1 cm in diameter so that the fibrous sheath is displayed. A small 'window' is cut in the fibrous layer of the sheath and the synovium is picked up and cautiously opened with fine scissors. A small quantity of fluid may emerge at this point and should be collected for culture. The tendons should be inspected for damage by the original injury. The synovial cavity is now washed with isotonic solution of saline until clear fluid emerges. A small amount of a 1 per cent solution of cloxacillin in saline is then introduced into the synovial sheath through the catheter, which is secured in position by a stitch through the skin of the

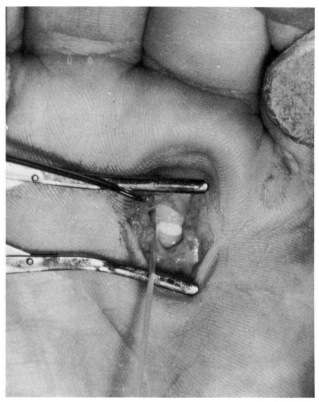

FIG. 30.11. The proximal end of the digital sheath has been opened and a catheter placed within the synovial sheath.

palm at some distance from the palmar wound (Fig. 30.12). This wound is sutured loosely around the catheter which emerges from the dressing and is secured to the forearm with adhesive dressing. No attempt is made to close the wound in the distal part of the finger; it is dressed with several layers of gauze to allow the excess fluid from the irrigation to soak into this dressing.

Postoperative management. The hand should be elevated in a roller towel and active finger movement encouraged to avoid formation of inflammatory adhesions. Cloxacillin 250–500 mg 6 hourly is given by intramuscular injection for 3 days, followed by oral flucloxacillin for 7 days. The synovial sheath is irrigated

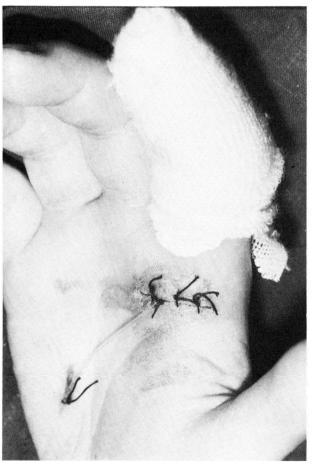

Fig. 30.12. At the conclusion of the irrigation the catheter is secured in position by a stitch through the skin of the palm.

with a 1 per cent solution of cloxacillin in isotonic saline 6 hourly, using 0.5–1.0 ml of the solution, which should be freshly prepared on each occasion. As this is painful, a preliminary instillation of 0.25 ml of 1 per cent lignocaine is made into the sheath. A few minutes later the cloxacillin can be run into the sheath slowly without causing pain. This intermittent irrigation destroys remaining bacteria within the synovial sheath and washes away fibrin deposits. It should be continued for 48 hours by which time the results of the bacteriological studies should be available. If the organism is proved to be sensitive to cloxacillin, the irrigation can be discontinued and the catheter removed. The day following removal of the catheter the patient is allowed home with strict instructions to move fingers actively.

Infection of the ulnar bursa. A volar longitudinal incision over the swelling is used extending distally 5 cm into the palm and proximally above the wrist for about 8 cm, care being taken when the deep fascia is incised because the median nerve is compressed tightly underneath. The flexor retinaculum is divided under direct vision so that the ulnar bursa is displayed completely and opened along its entire length with scissors. A sample of fluid within is sent for bacteriological investigation. The flexor tendons are lifted gently and the cavity and its contents washed out thoroughly with isotonic saline solution, removing the fluid by suction. The sheath of flexor pollicis longus must be inspected to ensure that it is not involved in the infection. Should any finger sheath be infected, it must be irrigated in the same manner. Closing the wound may be difficult because of the swelling present and it is much safer to approximate the skin edges loosely rather than attempt a formal closure.

Infection of the radial bursa. The proximal end of the synovial sheath of flexor pollicis longus tendon is exposed by a vertical incision ulnar to flexor carpi radialis tendon and continued distally into the hand for 3–4 cm. The median nerve and flexor digitorum superficialis tendons are retracted medially so that the flexor pollicis longus tendon can be exposed. Its synovial sheath will be distended making it visualized with ease. The flexor retinaculum should be divided to afford adequate decompression of the carpal tunnel contents. A small hole is cut in the synovial sheath and any fluid emerging is sent for culture. A fine catheter is then inserted into the sheath for several centimetres. The distal part of the sheath is exposed by excising the puncture wound of the thumb, a window is cut into the fibrous sheath and the tendon inspected. Irrigation of the sheath with saline injected through the catheter is carried out, but sometimes it is difficult to establish a free flow. It may be necessary to pass a second catheter in a retrograde fashion from the distal end and flush out the sheath from both ends until a satisfactory flow is achieved. A final irrigation with 1 per cent cloxacillin solution is made and the distal catheter is removed, leaving the proximal one in situ. It can be secured in position and the wrist incision closed around the catheter. The thumb wound is not sutured but allowed to heal by secondary intention.

Postoperative management. The two most important aspects are:

(1) reduction of oedema of the hand by elevation, and

(2) re-establishment of active movements of the digits. Fortunately the relief from pain is so dramatic after operation that patients are able to move their digits with surprising ease. For the first few days there is often a considerable amount of exudate from the wound which requires absorptive dressings. Once the exudate has ceased only a light dressing is needed. Wound healing may take several weeks but secondary suture should not be necessary.

Antibiotic therapy. Staphylococcal infections are treated by cloxacillin 250–500 mg, given intramuscularly 6-hourly for 7–10 days, while in streptococcal infection benzyl penicillin 0.5 mega-unit is administered 6-hourly for 7 days, followed by a suitable long-acting penicillin preparation for a further 7 days.

Treatment of the late or neglected cases. Severe tendon sheath infection with gross necrosis is fortunately rare in Britain today. When present, however, the surgeon may be confronted with a digit distended with pus, very little left intact apart from the phalanges and the neuro-vascular bundles. The volar skin must be incised the length of the digit in order to remove completely the remnants of tendons and the sheath. Usually all pulp tissue has been destroyed. Provided that the skin has retained a blood supply the digit may heal but it will be stiff and useless and the patient will be better off without it. If the digit retained good passive movement it may be possible to restore active flexion at a later date by a two-stage procedure using the silastic rod technique and subsequently a free tendon graft.

Summary

The results of treatment by the method described have been gratifying provided operation is undertaken as soon as the diagnosis is made [11]. The majority regain full movements of the affected digit. A few may have a slight restriction of extension of the proximal interphalangeal joint and others may lose the last few degrees of flexion of the distal joint. Even those with bursal infection regain good function although the healing time may be appreciably longer than when infection is confined to one digit.

This method of treatment has three distinct advantages:

(1) the diagnosis is confirmed at operation,

(2) the infecting organism can be identified and its sensitivity to antibiotics can be tested in the laboratory, and

(3) a high concentration of antibiotic is delivered to the site of infection.

REFERENCES

[1] BELL, M. S. The changing pattern of pyogenic infections of the hand. *The Hand*, 1976, **8**, 298.

[2] EATON, R. C. Antibiotic guidelines for hand infections. *Surgery, Gynaecology and Obstetrics*, 1970, **130**, 119.

[3] BRAND, P. W. *The Hand in Leprosy*. Clinical Surgery. The Hand. London, Butterworths, 1966.

[4] PETRIE, P. W. R. AND LAMB, D. W. Severe hand problems in drug addicts following self administration of injections. *The Hand*, 1973, **5**, 130.

[5] KANAVEL, A. B. *Infections of the Hand*. Philadelphia, Lea and Febiger, 1933.

[6] PILCHER, R. S., DAWSON, R. L. G., MILSTEIN, B. B. AND

RIDDELL, A. G. Infections of the fingers and hand. *Lancet*, 1948, **1,** 777.

[7] SNEDDON, J. *The Care of Hand Infections*. London, Edward Arnold, 1970.

[8] SNEDDON, J. Sepsis in hand injuries. *The Hand*, 1970, **2,** 58.

[9] BAILEY, H. *Emergency Surgery*, 5th Edition, pp. 757–759. Bristol, Wright, 1945.

[10] BUTLER, E. C. G. AND BARCLAY, G. A. *Penicillin*, ed. Sir A. Fleming, pp. 225–229. London, Butterworth, 1950.

[11] POLLEN, A. G. Acute infections of the tendon sheaths. *The Hand*, 1974, **6,** 21.

[12] GRINNELL, R. S. Acute suppurative tenosynovitis of the flexor tendon sheaths of the hand. A review of 125 cases. *Annals of Surgery*, 1937, **105,** 97.

[13] FLYNN, J. E. Acute suppurative tenosynovitis of the hand. *New England Journal of Medicine*, 1950, **242,** 241.

[14] CURR, J. F. The use of penicillin in acute infections of the hand. *Edinburgh Medical Journal*, 1945, **52,** 469.

[15] GORDON, I. Expectant treatment of pyogenic infections of the hand with special reference to infection of the flexor aspect of the fingers. *British Journal of Surgery*, 1950, **38,** 331.

CHAPTER 31

Tumours

J. CHALMERS

Included here are not only true neoplasms but also a wide range of similarly presenting non-neoplastic lumps. Interpreted in this way the tumours of the hand are very common, accounting for 30 per cent of orthopaedic referrals [1] and varied in their pathological features, but *the great majority are benign*. The rare malignant tumours tend to have a favourable prognosis as they come to notice early. There have been many series published on hand tumours [1–13]. The incidence in the above series varies according to the particular interest of the authors and also to the geographical location. Table 31.1 lists some of the more important tumours and indicates their relative frequency

Warts

Warts are very common, can affect any part of the body, but occur most frequently in the hands, feet and genitalia. Warts of the hands are commonest in childhood. They are contagious and the infectious agent has been identified recently as a papova virus. Occupational transmission is recorded. They consist of localized benign papillomatous hyperplasia with hyperkeratosis which gives them a horny character. They have been well reviewed by Bunney [13]. Although unsightly, they are usually painless unless traumatized. They tend to undergo spontaneous resolution, 25 per cent within 6 months of appearance and almost all within 5 years. Natural cure is due to the development of a cell-mediated immune response; patients on immuno-suppressive drugs tend to get resistant widespread warts. Malignant change does not arise in warts of the hands

and feet. The natural tendency towards recovery makes it difficult to evaluate the benefits of therapy. Cryotherapy with carefully applied liquid nitrogen or carbon dioxide snow, repeated if necessary at intervals of 3 weeks, is effective in two-thirds of patients. Collodion paint containing 15 per cent salicylic acid (a keratolytic agent) is as successful as cryotherapy, causes less discomfort, but may take longer. Surgical curettage and cauterization of the residual cavity under local or general anaesthesia is the most effective treatment when conservative measures fail.

Epidermoid inclusion cysts (inclusion dermoid)

These are due to the traumatic subcutaneous implantation of a fragment of skin, resulting in a cystic swelling lined with squamous epithelium and occupied by a creamy fluid containing cholesterol crystals and keratin flakes. The vulnerability of the hand to minor injury renders it a common site, particularly on the palmar aspect. Like ganglia they are firm, round and if large, fluctuant, but they differ from ganglia in their more superficial subcutaneous position where their yellow content may show through the skin. Rarely they are more deeply placed and occasionally may occupy and expand the terminal phalanx [14] (Fig. 31.1). Epidermoid cysts are painless but may cause discomfort because they get in the way or are unsightly and in that event should be excised. They have no firm attachment and are very simply enucleated through a small incision. They do not recur.

TABLE 31.1. Tumours and tumour-like conditions of the hand. XXXX, Very Common; XXX, Common; XX, Uncommon; X, Rare.

Tissue	Benign	Frequency	Malignant	Frequency
Skin	Wart	XXXX	Squamous carcinoma	XXX
	Epidermoid cyst	XXX	Basal cell carcinoma	X
	Pyogenic granuloma	XXX	Malignant melanoma	XX
Vascular tissues	Glomus	XX	Angiosarcoma	X
	Angioma	XX	Lymphosarcoma	X
	Aneurysmal bone cyst	X		
Fat	Lipoma	XX	Liposarcoma	X
Fibrous tissue	Fibroma	XX	Fibrosarcoma	X
	Juvenile aponeurotic fibroma	X		
	Digital fibrous tumour	X		
Nerves	Neurilemmoma	X		
	Neurofibroma	X		
	Neurofibromatosis	XX		
	Traumatic neuroma	XXX		
Muscle	Leiomyoma	X	Rhabdomyosarcoma	X
Tendon	Xanthomas	X		
Joint capsule and tendon sheath	Ganglion	XXXX	Synovial sarcoma	X
	Mucous cyst	XXX		
	Pigmented nodular synovitis	XXXX		
Cartilage	Chondroma	XXX	Chondrosarcoma	X
	Osteochondroma	XX		
Bone	Osteoid osteoma	XX	Osteosarcoma	X
	Subungual exostosis	X		
Unknown			Epithelioid sarcoma	X
Miscellaneous	Hamartoma	XX	Metastases	X

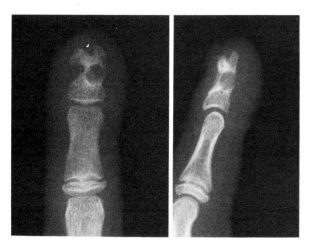

FIG. 31.1. Inclusion dermoid arising within the terminal phalanx following a compound fracture.

Pyogenic granuloma

As its name implies, this is not a true tumour but an inflammatory reaction commonly found in the hand following a minor wound. Healing is delayed because of continued use of the hand and exposure to trauma and contamination. Infection produces a highly vascular granulomatous lesion which grows from the site of injury like a mushroom (Fig. 31.2). It occurs most commonly on the volar aspect of the finger or palm and is acutely painful. It responds readily to surgical excision or application of silver nitrate.

Glomus tumour

This is a small benign lesion thought to derive from the glomus body which is widely distributed in the stratum reticulum of the skin particularly of the digital tips.

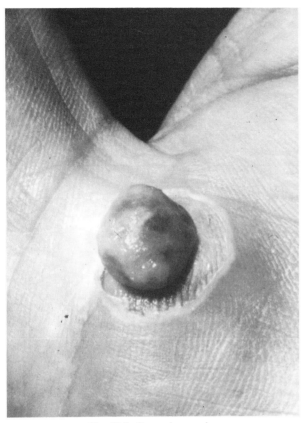

FIG. 31.2. Pyogenic granuloma.

Fifty per cent occur in the hand and of these half are subungual and most of the rest are within the terminal segments of the digits. Collectively they are uncommon accounting for only 1.6 per cent of 500 soft tissue tumours of the extremity reported from the Mayo Clinic.

Glomus tumours are always less than 1 cm in diameter and are well-defined, encapsulated, purple lesions. They consist of hypertrophied and disorganized elements normally found in the glomus body. Enlarged and tortuous arteries are surrounded by the characteristic rounded uniform (epithelioid) glomus cells; myelinated and non-myelinated nerve endings are present and may account for the pain. Acute tenderness, pain and cold sensitivity are the classic symptoms. The pain may be so severe that the patient becomes reluctant to use the finger and may wear a protective glove or finger stall. Despite the compelling character of the symptoms delayed diagnosis is common, sometimes for many years [15]. In the common subungual situation the purple colour of the tumour may be seen through the nail (Fig. 31.3), and ridging of the nail may occur. Otherwise the small tender lump may be palpable in the pulp or in the subcutaneous tissue elsewhere, but even if no lump is detected the characteristic symptoms and localized acute tenderness justify surgical exploration. Glomus tumours may occur at any age but are uncommon in childhood. Radiographs may show scalloping of the terminal

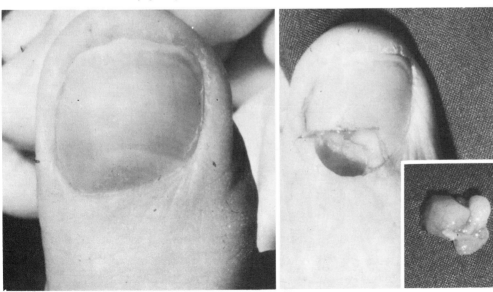

FIG. 31.3.
Subungual glomus tumour.

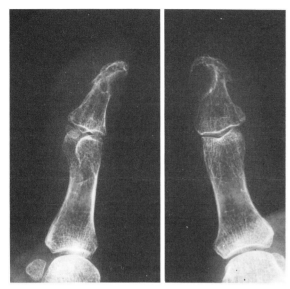

FIG. 31.4. Scalloping of the terminal phalanx by glomus tumour.

rare [20], but show the usual appearance of coarsened trabeculae arranged in a honeycomb manner on radiographs. Within a soft tissue mass radiography may show round calcified phleboliths. Many of the soft tissue lesions appearing in infancy regress spontaneously, thus treatment should not be contemplated until at least the age of six years. Thereafter, cosmetic reasons or troublesome swelling may indicate surgical treatment. Complete excision is rarely possible because of the diffuse complexity of the malformation, but occasionally local enlargement, painful because of thrombosis, justifies local removal. These malformations do not become malignant in spite of an aggressive histological appearance. Haemangiosarcoma which is rare in the hand, arises *de novo*. Maffucci's syndrome is a rare disorder in which a diffuse haemangioma is associated with multiple enchondromatosis (Fig. 31.5).

phalanx from pressure by the tumour [16] (Fig. 31.4), and wholly intraosseous glomus tumours within the terminal phalanx have been described [17]. Angiography which reveals a highly vascular lesion with rapid venous return may occasionally be of diagnostic value. The only treatment is excision which may require preliminary avulsion of the nail. The lesion usually can be shelled out easily from its false capsule. Recurrence is rare and indicates incomplete removal. Excision brings immediate relief from pain.

Haemangioma

This may affect the hand as it may any part of the body. The lesion may be discrete and localized but more often is associated with widespread haemangiomatous change affecting the arm or trunk [18]. Haemangiomata range from the capillary telangiectasis of the skin to extensive and more deeply sited cavernous lesions which may involve any or all tissues of the hand. The deeper lesions can be diagnosed by their soft compressibility. Gigantism of the limb, hand or one or two digits may occur if there is significant arteriovenous fistula and is known as Klippel-Trenaunay-Weber syndrome [19]. Haemangiomas arising in the bones of the hand are very

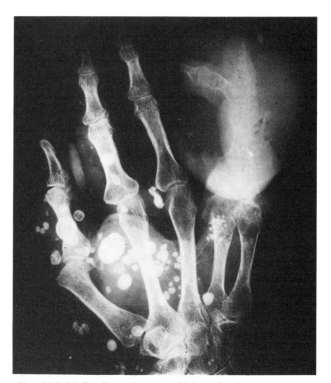

FIG. 31.5. Maffucci's syndrome: multiple enchondromata associated with diffuse haemangioma indicated by the calcified phleboliths.

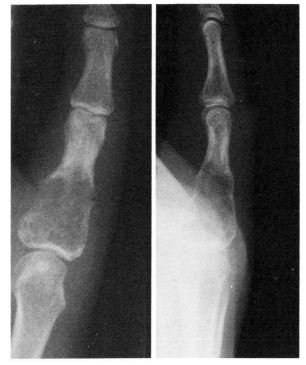

FIG. 31.6. Aneurysmal bone cyst. This lesion would be hard to distinguish from the more common enchondroma on its radiographic appearance alone. Courtesy of Mr W. J. Gillespie.

Aneurysmal bone cyst

This is rare in the hand [21]. The diagnosis is suggested by the thinned and expanded cortex (Fig. 31.6), which unless it is markedly eccentric would be hard to distinguish radiographically from a chondroma. Involvement of the terminal phalanx has been reported [22]. Local swelling or pathological fracture is the usual presentation. Treatment consists of curettage and if large, replacement by bone graft.

Lipoma

This is comparatively rare among the benign tumours of the hand—less than 5 per cent in most series and yet there have been several reports of large numbers [23, 24]. They are more common after middle age and are most frequent in the palm where there may be subcutaneous or subfascial. Most present as painless

swellings (Fig. 31.7); occasionally they may cause peripheral nerve compression [25]. If superficial, their smooth, soft, fluctuant character indicates their nature. Subfascial lesions may be hard to diagnose before operation although radiographically they may be suspected from the relative radiolucency of fat. If they give rise to symptoms or cosmetic concern they may be simply shelled out by blunt dissection. Recurrence is rare.

Intraneural lipoma (lipofibroma of the median nerve)

Intraneural lipoma and fatty infiltration producing massive enlargement of the median nerve within the hand has been described [26, 27]. These lesions can seldom be excised without damaging the nerve and once their nature is recognized they are best left alone, simple decompression being adequate treatment [28]. An ossifying lipofibroma of the median nerve has been described [29].

Fibroma

Fibroma is rare in the hand and is most commonly found in the skin as a small firm nodular swelling. Elsewhere it presents as nonspecific swelling easily mistaken for a ganglion. If it causes symptoms it may be simply excised. Non-ossifying fibroma of bone did not occur in the hand in the large series recorded by Dahlin [30].

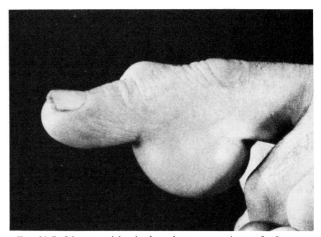

FIG. 31.7. Lipoma arising in the subcutaneous tissue of a finger.

Recurring digital fibrous tumour of childhood

This is a rare and curious benign tumour which develops in the fingers, and toes, in early childhood. It consists of a proliferation of fibroblasts within the dermis and may involve several digits producing diffuse cutaneous swellings. Intracytoplasmic inclusion bodies have been described and a viral origin is postulated but unproved. Reported cases indicate a variable natural history ranging from spontaneous regression to local progression necessitating amputation. Initial treatment should be conservative consisting of local excision and skin grafting. Complete surgical excision is difficult and may have to be repeated because of local recurrence. Malignant transformation has not been reported [31, 32].

Juvenile aponeurotic fibroma [33]

This is another fibrous tumour largely confined to children and occurring most commonly in the palms and soles. It consists of an ill-defined highly cellular fibrous proliferation involving the subcutaneous tissue, deep fascia and sometimes muscle. Foci of bone and cartilage may occur. It may suggest a sarcoma histologically because of its invasive tendency, but although it may recur locally it never becomes malignant and treatment should be conservative, consisting of local excision with preservation of important structures [34].

Nerve tumours

Benign nerve tumours such as neurilemmoma, neurofibroma and intraneural lipofibroma may occur in the hand as elsewhere. They present as slowly growing tumours and may be associated with symptoms or loss of function within the distribution of the affected nerve. It is of utmost importance to remember that although not common they do occur and may be misdiagnosed prior to surgery as a ganglion or similar lesion. If their true nature is unrecognized at operation because of the inexperience of the surgeon or of inadequate surgical exposure irreparable harm may be done to the nerve.

Neurilemmoma (Schwannoma)

White [35] reported ten of these tumours occurring in the nerves of the hand. They arise in the nerve sheath and are usually solitary, round, white lesions. They may occur on the surface of the nerve or be contained within the sheath with compression of the nerve fibres. Larger tumours may develop cystic change. Characteristic histological feature consists of bundles of spindleshaped Schwann cells often orientated with their nuclei in parallel rows. Neurilemmomas are said to remain discrete from the nerve fibres and may be shelled out without damage to the nerve if great care is exercised in separating overlying nerve fibres under magnification. Neurilemmomas may occasionally involve the bones of the hand [36].

Neurofibromas

These are rarely solitary and more commonly present as multiple lesions in neurofibromatosis (Von Recklinghausen's disease). The lesions consist of a diffuse proliferation of Schwann cells and other neural elements. They are not encapsulated and are so intimately involved with the conductive elements that surgical removal without damage to the nerve is rarely possible. The solitary lesions cannot be distinguished from neurilemmomas except at surgery when the lack of encapsulation becomes apparent. Excision is best abandoned at this stage unless the nerve is expendable. Plexiform neurofibroma is a variant in which a length of nerve and its branches are occupied by multiple nodular and fusiform swellings; it has been described in the median nerve [4]. It cannot be treated without sacrifice of the nerve.

Multiple neuromas (neurofibromatosis)

These are inherited as an autosomal dominant disease in which multiple neuromas are associated with widespread disorders affecting many tissues of the body. It has been well reviewed by McCarroll [37] and Hunt and Pugh [38]. In the hand the chief manifestation is megalodactyly which may involve one or several digits (Fig. 31.8). It is due to hamartomatous overgrowth of all digital tissues including the phalanges which are increased in length and thickness often with osteophytic outgrowth which may limit joint movement (Fig. 31.8). The enlarged digital nerves, vessels and fat hypertrophy contribute to the gigantism which may be gross and unsightly. Treatment of megalodactyly is extremely difficult. Epiphysiodesis to arrest growth has been described

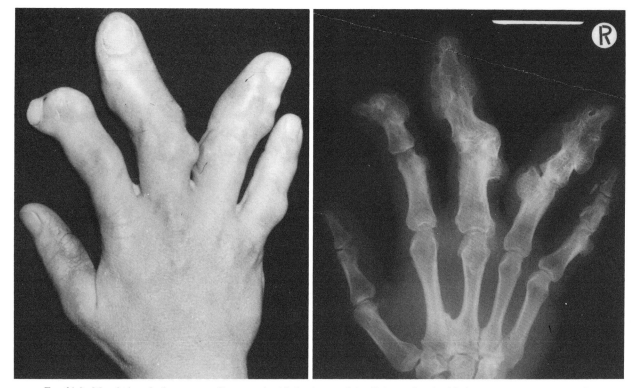

Fig. 31.8. Megalodactyly due to neurofibromatosis. All the tissues of the digits are involved in hamartomatous overgrowth.

[39], and some improvement may be effected by the surgical reduction of the hypertrophied soft tissues but the results of these procedures are rarely very satisfactory and amputation of a severely deformed digit may be preferred by the patient.

Traumatic neuromas

These are considered on p. 429.

Xanthomas

As the name implies, these are yellow frequently multiple tumours found within tendons and other tissues, including the skin, but rarely bone [40], in patients some of whom are affected by familial hypercholesterolaemia [41]. The tendo Achilles is the usual site where the tumor may be very large, but multiple smaller lesions in the extensor tendons and the skin of the hand may also occur. Their yellow colour is usually apparent through the skin. They are important only in that they draw attention to

the raised cholesterol level and the consequent susceptibility to ischaemic heart disease. If the level is corrected the xanthomas tend to disappear, for they are not true neoplasms but cholesterol accumulations. Multiple xanthomas of disordered lipid metabolism must be distinguished from pigmented nodular synovitis (p. 456). The two conditions are entirely distinct in their aetiology, clinical presentation and histology.

Ganglion

This, the most common hand 'tumour', presents as a cystic swelling consisting of a fibrous capsule with a content of clear viscous material similar to synovial fluid. Their common close relationship to joints or synovial tendon sheaths indicates a possible origin from herniation of synovial tissue, which has been strongly supported by arthrography showing a tortuous narrow duct linking the wrist joint and the ganglion in two-thirds of the cases [42]. Attempts to demonstrate such a communication in the reverse direction by injecting the ganglion invariably failed [43], suggesting a one-way valvular mechanism. Other theories, which include mucoid degeneration of fibrous tissue, benign neoplasm akin to myxomas or metaplastic transformation, could explain the occasional cystic lesions of similar character developing remotely from joints.

Clinical presentation

Seventy-five per cent occur in the hand and most of these about the wrist especially on the dorsoradial aspect. Their peak incidence is in the young adult. Trauma or occupational activity does not seem to have any part in their development. In older patients they may be associated with degenerative arthritis. They present as round or occasionally lobular swellings varying in consistency from soft fluctuant to tense and firm. Large ganglia may reach up to 4 cm or more in diameter but most are 1 cm or less. They tend to be fixed to deeper structures. Most are symptomless; occasionally they become painful particularly after hard manual activity. Nerve compression due to ganglia is described on p. 406. Spontaneous disappearance or fluctuation in size is not uncommon.

Ganglia of fibrous flexor sheaths

About 10 per cent of ganglia in the hand arise from the digital flexor tendon sheaths, either opposite the middle of the proximal phalanx or opposite the metacarpophalangeal joint [44]. They are small and hard like a dried pea, are fixed to the tendon sheath and do not move with the underlying tendon. They are exposed to pressure whenever the patient grips a hard object and hence they tend to be painful unlike most larger ganglia elsewhere which come to notice for aesthetic reasons.

Intraosseous ganglia

Subchondral bone cysts similar in nature to ganglia have been reported increasingly in recent years [45–48] and may involve the carpal bones or distal radius and ulna. They are commonly seen radiographically as incidental findings, but sometimes present with pain following a minor injury. Pathological fractures may occur (Fig. 31.9). These cysts are rounded and unilocular with

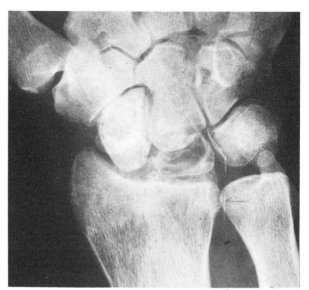

FIG. 31.9. Interosseous ganglion of lunate presenting with spontaneous fracture.

a clearly defined border, which at some point is in close contact with the articular surface. They are distinguished from osteoarthritic cysts or the rheumatoid geodes in that they arise in otherwise normal joints. Although their nature is uncertain, histological resemblance to ganglia suggests a similar origin [48].

Treatment

As more than 50 per cent of ganglia disappear spontaneously, treatment is not indicated unless there is some clear indication such as persistent discomfort or justifiable cosmetic concern or because of evidence of peripheral nerve compression. Rupture by firm pressure or aspiration with or without injections of cortisone, hyaluronidase and a variety of sclerosing agents, are attended by a high recurrence rate, although a cure of two-thirds of treated ganglia by pressure rupture alone has been reported [49] and certainly this simple measure is always worth a try. Ganglia of the fibrous flexor sheath respond particularly well to closed rupture by needling under local anaesthesia. Injections of cortisone or hyaluronidase do not improve the success rate, and sclerosing agents are potentially dangerous and should not be used. Excision is the most widely adopted treatment and its success depends on the care exercised. The operation is often more extensive than anticipated. Tourniquet is essential and regional local anaesthesia such as Bier's block (p. 113) is ideal. Incisions should allow extension if required and cutaneous nerves, e.g. terminal branches of the radial nerve, should be preserved to avoid discomfort worse than the ganglion itself. The ganglion is mobilized by sharp dissection, care being taken to identify any communications with a joint or synovial sheath as failure to remove them will be followed by rapid recurrence. The communication may be directly under the ganglion, attached to the joint capsule part of which should be removed with the lesion, or it may present as a long pedicle which has to be traced to its origin; the latter can make the operation difficult and accounts for most recurrences. Lesions occupying the carpal bones or ends of radius and ulna may be curetted if they cause pain or fracture; if the resulting cavity is large it should be packed with cancellous chips.

Differential diagnosis of ganglia

A common misdiagnosis is the *carpal boss* (p. 483), a bony swelling at the second and third carpometacarpal joints on the dorsal aspect. This minor developmental anomaly may cause cosmetic concern in girls and occasionally may be large enough to justify removal. Anomalous muscles such as extensor digitorum manus brevis can be mistaken for a ganglion [50].

Mucous cysts arise from the osteoarthritic terminal interphalangeal joints commonly in older women. They present on the dorsal aspect on either side of the extensor tendon. Histologically they resemble ganglia [51], but they deserve to be differentiated because of their specific clinical presentation with respect both to site and age. They may discharge intermittently through the skin and secondary infection can occur. They are best left alone unless symptomatic, large and unsightly. Excision involves careful search for the communication with the joint if recurrence is to be avoided. Adherence to the overlying skin may require a skin graft.

Pigmented nodular synovitis (pigmented nodular tenosynovitis, giant cell tumour of tendon sheath, fibrous xanthoma of synovium, benign synovioma)

These are just a few of the many names given to this, the second most common tumour in the hand in many series. The variety of names reveals the uncertain origin of the lesion and its variable presentation which ranges from a small nodular lesion arising from a synovial lining of tendon or joint to a widespread villonodular involvement of these structures sometimes associated with erosion of the bone ends. Aetiological theories include reaction to trauma, infection or true neoplasm. Some support for the latter is given by the rare occurrence of malignant behaviour with metastases [52] although Enzinger suggests that this case may have been an epithelioid sarcoma [53]. Tendon sheath lesions appear as firm, lobular, rarely villous, tumours of any size from 5 mm upwards. They are usually grey, with yellow or brown areas due to lipid or haemosiderin present in the histiocytes which are probably the basic cells. Multinuclear giant cells are also common, hence the name giant cell tumour of tendon sheath; a name best abandoned as the giant cells are not a constant or essential feature of the lesion and the name suggests analogy with giant cell tumours of bone which is misleading. Areas of fibrosis may also occur. Pigmented nodular synovitis of the hand is of the same nature as the less common pigmented villonodular synovitis of major joints.

Clinical features

It occurs at any age but is most common after middle age and uncommon in childhood. Women are affected twice as often as men. It presents as a painless lobular swelling usually on the flexor aspect of the fingers which are all equally susceptible; the lesion may occupy any part of the flexor sheath or it may involve any of the digital joints but most commonly the distal interphalangeal joint (Fig. 31.10) and in these cases the swelling may present dorsally. Affected joints show frequently evidence of pre-existing degenerative arthritis. Occasionally two or more fingers may be involved (Fig. 31.11). Bone erosion of adjacent phalanges may give a false impression of malignancy.

Treatment

If there is discomfort or concern the tumour may be removed. The lesions of the flexor sheath lie deep to the fibrous flexor sheath which is thinned and stretched over them and may have to be excised in part to allow access to the tumour. It is important to ensure that sufficient pulleys for the flexor tendons are left. If removal of the lesion is incomplete it may recur.

Leiomyoma (dermal angiomyoma)

These benign tumours arising in the subcutaneous tissues occur with comparative frequency in the hand.

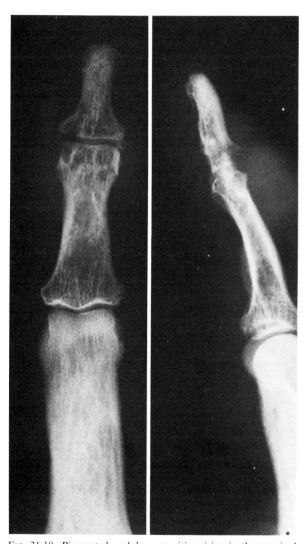

Fig. 31.10. Pigmented nodular synovitis arising in the terminal interphalangeal joint. Note the cystic erosion of the bone ends and the soft tissue tumour on the extensor aspect. Note also the coincidental involvement of the proximal phalanx with Paget's disease.

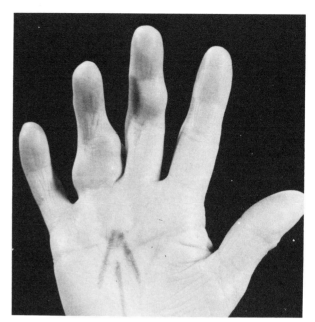

Fig. 31.11. Pigmented nodular synovitis involving the flexor sheaths of two digits. Such multiple lesions are uncommon.

Neviaser and Newman report twelve cases [54]. The lesion presents in adult life as a slowly growing and usually painless swelling of non-specific appearance [55]. At operation they are encapsulated white tumours consisting of smooth muscle fibres surrounding numerous blood vessels, and it is probable that they have a vascular origin. Recurrence following excision is rare.

Benign tumours of bone and cartilage

Chondroma

Chondroma is the most common tumour involving bone in the hand. About 50 per cent of all chondromas occur there. Most are solitary lesions but multiple chondromas are found in Ollier's disease (dyschondroplasia) (p. 338) and Maffucci's syndrome (pp. 339, 451). The proximal phalanges and the metacarpals are the usual sites, but they may occur in any bone although rarely in the carpus [56]. There have been several reports of large series [56, 57]. Chondromas of the bones of the hand are usually centrally placed and contained within the bone which may be locally expanded. Less commonly they are eccentrically placed and sometimes they break through the cortex to produce a mass in the adjacent soft tissues (ecchondroma) which accounted for 12 per cent of the forty cases reported by Noble and Lamb [58]. Periosteal chondromas which arise beneath the periosteum and erode bone from without have been reported in the phalanges [59]. Chondromas occurring in the soft tissues of the hand apparently without bony origin have also been described [60, 61]. Chondromas are lobular bluish white cartilage masses well demarcated from the surrounding tissues. Microscopy shows a moderately cellular cartilage matrix. The degree of cellularity together with the occurrence of occasional binucleate forms might in other situations such as the proximal limb bones, suggest the probability of sarcomatous change, but in the hand malignant change in a benign cartilage tumour is so rare that these appearances may be discounted unless there is clinical evidence of malignant behaviour. Chondromas are presumed to arise from rests of cartilage left behind during the growing period. The soft tissue lesions may arise from metaplasia within synovium [61]. Many chondromas are symptomless and come to light as incidental findings in the course of radiographic examination for other purposes. Some present as smooth, hard painless swellings, usually expanding or arising from a bone, while others may give rise to pathological fracture as did two-thirds of the series of Noble and Lamb [58]. They usually show little evidence of growth once skeletal maturity is reached, but during the growing period the multiple lesions of dyschondroplasia may reach enormous size producing a grotesque appearance and interfering greatly with hand function (Fig. 31.12).

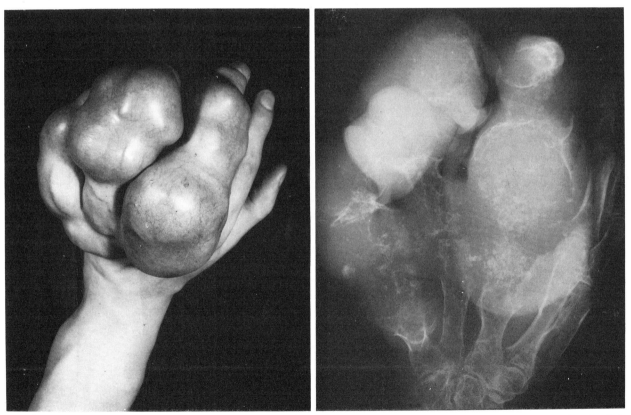

Fig. 31.12. Multiple enchondromatosis producing severe disfigurement and impairment of function in a boy with dyschondroplasia (Ollier's disease). Amputation of the medial three fingers was necessary. Fortunately the thumb and index were relatively uninvolved.

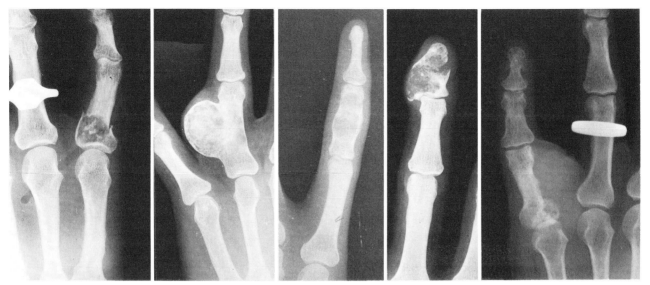

Fig. 31.13. Representative examples of chondromas.

Radiographic features (Fig. 31.13)

Circumscribed lytic areas within the long bones with the overlying cortex thinned, expanded or perforated by the tumour producing a soft tissue extension may all be seen. Irregular calcification suggests the diagnosis with reasonable certainty. Otherwise the radiographic appearances are not specific as a number of less common lesions such as inclusion dermoid and aneurysmal bone cyst enter the differential diagnosis.

Treatment

None is required for symptomless chondromas. Obviously if no biopsy is taken there may be some doubt about the diagnosis, and it is prudent therefore to repeat the radiographic examination after an interval of a few months to make sure that the lesion is not growing. Chondromas which are unsightly or a source of discomfort may be excised or curetted out of bone. Large cavities heal more rapidly if grafted. If a fracture has occurred it is easier to deal surgically with the tumour after the fracture is allowed to heal. Noble and Lamb found that if no operative treatment was given the clinical result was marginally better than that obtained either by currettage alone or with bone grafting [58]. Diaphysectomy is rarely indicated but excellent results

are reported from bone grafting of the resulting defect [62]. Occasionally amputation of the affected digits may be required in cases of multiple enchodromata (Fig. 31.12). Recurrence following curettage is rare and should arouse suspicion of malignant transformation.

Osteochondroma

This is relatively uncommon in the hand, where they rarely attain large size. Only seven of the 414 osteo-chondromas reported by Dahlin occurred there [31]. Malignant transformation of these lesions to chondro-sarcoma has not been described in the hand. When the size becomes a nuisance, as in Fig. 31.14, they should be removed.

Osteoid osteoma

The hand appears to be a relatively common site for this uncommon tumour. Carroll reported six cases and reviewed twenty-two others [63]. Any of the bones of the hand may be involved but the terminal phalanx appears to be a favoured location often associated with irregular growth of the nail and a bulbous tip to the finger [23]. The lesions in the hand do not differ from those occurring elsewhere in their clinical presentation. Both sexes are equally affected mostly in childhood or young adult life.

Well localized relentless pain often relieved by aspirin is the main symptom and localized tenderness, swelling and increased sweating may be present. Radiographs may appear normal as the lesion can be very small and is easily overlooked [64]. For this reason delay in diagnosis, often for many months, is not unusual; however, most cases eventually become visible radiographically. Edeiken describes three radiological types, one in which the nidus lies within the medulla and has minimal sclerosis, a cortical lesion with marked surrounding sclerosis which may obscure the nidus and a periosteal lesion producing a periosteal reaction [65]. Sometimes the nidus itself is radio-opaque and is sur-

rounded by a narrow lucent border. The affected bone may be thickened uniformly or only one cortex is affected depending on the location of the lesion. In cases in which diagnosis is suspected on clinical grounds and yet the radiographs are negative, a bone scan is invaluable for osteoid osteomas usually show up as intense 'hot spots' (Fig. 31.15). The nidus is a round bony pea-like structure 2–5 mm in diameter usually lying loosely within its sclerotic capsule. It may be so small that it is hard to find. It consists of irregular immature trabeculae of densely packed bone and osteoid tissue with numerous active osteoblasts in a highly vascular supporting stroma.

Treatment

Moberg reported spontaneous resolution of symptoms in an osteoid osteoma of the hand after 18 months [66], but in other cases symptoms have persisted for many years. There is no point, therefore, in delaying removal of the nidus. Relief of pain is immediate and permanent. Recurrence is rare and implies incomplete removal [67].

Subungual exostoses

These bony outgrowths from the terminal phalanx are less common in the hand than in the foot. They cause deformity of the nail and for this reason may require removal. They are probably not true tumours but reactions to trauma.

Other benign bone tumours rarely reported in the hand include benign chondroblastoma [68], and giant cell tumour [69]. The hand is a common site for the 'brown tumour' of hyperparathyroidism which histologically resembles the giant cell tumour. General clinical and radiological features of this disease and estimation of the serum calcium confirm the diagnosis.

Malignant tumours

Squamous carcinoma

Carcinoma arising from the squamous epithelium is the most common malignant tumour of the hand. Twenty per cent of all squamous carcinomas occur in the hand,

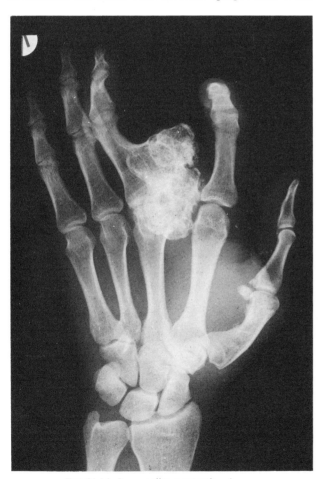
FIG. 31.14. Large solitary osteochondroma.

and men are affected three times as often as women. They tend to occur on skin surfaces exposed to sunshine particularly in the elderly and in white-skinned people living in the tropics exposed to ultraviolet radiation. X-irradiation has a similar effect, and many dentists developed squamous carcinoma of their hands as a result of holding radiographic films before this danger was recognized. Chemicals which may induce malignant change in skin include systemic arsenicals and local exposure to coal tars, shale oil, paints or indeed any chronic irritant; burn scars are also prone to malignancy [70]. Tumours arising from these causes are usually preceded for months or years by hyperkeratosis

of the skin. Others may arise spontaneously without any obvious cause or preceding lesion. The tumours occur most commonly on the back of the hand. At first they may present as an apparent hyperkeratotic nodule or a small ulcer or fissure within an area of hyperkeratosis. They enlarge slowly and ulcerate with undermining of the margin (Fig. 31.16). At other times they may present as small cauliflower-like growths. Spread to regional lymph nodes occurs in about 15 per cent of cases [71]. Biopsy shows invasion of the deeper layers of the skin by processes of squamous epithelium containing cores of keratin. More malignant tumours may be less differentiated.

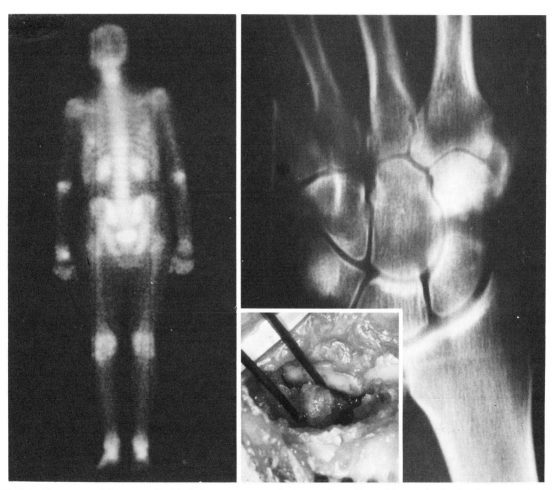

FIG. 31.15. Osteoid osteoma of the trapezoid. The lesion was not seen during routine radiographic examination but is apparent in this tomograph and is confirmed by a bone scan which shows an intense hot spot in the carpus. Inset shows the pea-sized lesion found at operation.

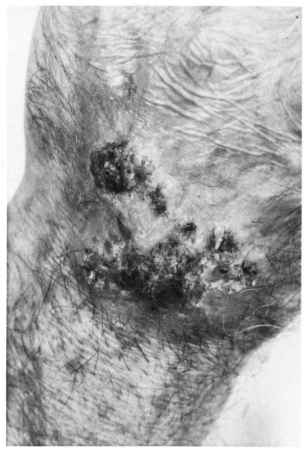

FIG. 31.16. Squamous carcinoma arising in an area of hyperkeratosis. Courtesy of Professor P. J. Hare.

Treatment

This consists of wide excision and skin grafting in most instances; the excision should include areas of skin showing premalignant hyperkeratosis. Radiotherapy is also effective but is usually reserved for cases which present difficulties in surgical excision. Removal of clinically involved regional lymph nodes coupled with radiotherapy to the drainage area should also be undertaken.

Prevention

Prevention is possible in this tumour in which the aetiological agent is so frequently known: any source of

chronic physical or chemical irritation to the skin should be avoided by wearing protective gloves.

Squamous carcinoma of the nail bed

This rare variant occurs in nail bed or fold usually following repeated trauma, chronic paronychia or epidermal dysplasia [72]. Any apparently inflammatory or traumatic ulcer in this situation which does not respond to treatment requires a biopsy to exclude or establish the presence of a squamous carcinoma or a melanotic whitlow (below). Delay in diagnosis is not uncommon owing largely to lack of awareness of their existence. Treatment consists of amputation of the terminal segment.

Basal cell carcinoma (rodent ulcer)

The great majority involve the skin of the face and neck and only rarely of the hands. Kendall reported eight basal cell carcinomas in a series of 78 malignant tumours of the hand [6]. They arise from the basal cell layer of the skin and adnexae, the tumour cells occurring in sheets and strands and rarely maturing to squamous cell formation. They are locally destructive but rarely metastasize. They present as a pale round nodule in the skin which enlarges to develop a central depression leading to ulceration with a raised smooth firm margin—the rodent ulcer. Excision or radiotherapy are both effective treatments. Excision need be less radical than for squamous carcinoma.

Malignant melanoma

This is a rare tumour which occurs most frequently in the skin of the extremities, including the hands, where the most common location is subungual or in the nail fold (Fig. 31.17). About 65 per cent of malignant melanomas arise from pre-existing benign junctional naevi, the rest appear to arise *de novo*. They are rapidly growing pigmented skin tumours which soon ulcerate and tend to form satellite lesions in the adjacent skin. In the nail fold they present as chronic paronychia resistant to treatment: the melanotic whitlow of Hutchison [73]. A border of dark pigmentation indicates its sinister nature. Amelanotic lesions can occur which contributes to the difficulty in diagnosis which is characteristic of this tumour, less than 50 per cent being correctly diagnosed [74, 75]. WHO has published a useful pamphlet on the *Clinical Diagnosis of Malignant Melanoma* [76]. Excision biopsy resolves all doubt and should be undertaken whenever the diagnosis is suspected.

The peak of incidence is in middle age; they tend to affect white races more commonly than negroes except for the subungual lesions. The maximum incidence is seen in North European stock who live in sunny areas such as Australia and South Africa. Trauma to a pre-existing benign junctional naevus appears to be an important aetiological factor and for this reason malignant melanomas tend to be more common in males. Early spread occurs to regional lymph nodes and more widely via the blood stream. Two cells are characteristic of this tumour: a large polyhedral call resembling the melanocyte, and a spindle cell with sarcomatous appearance. Both show an invasive tendency.

Treatment

Amputation of an affected digit or wide and deep surgical excision of cutaneous lesions elsewhere achieves

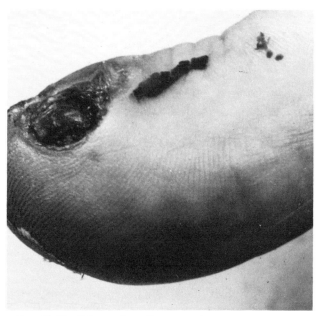

FIG. 31.17. Subungual malignant melanoma. Courtesy of Professor P. J. Hare.

5-year survival rates of 80 or 90 per cent in early and superficial tumours. Regional lymph nodes are excised if there is clinical evidence of involvement. In widespread disease chemotherapy has so far proved ineffective, and while radiotherapy may give worthwhile palliation the effects are unpredictable. Both active and passive immunotherapy are being evaluated. Promising results have been obtained in the control of disseminated disease by intralesional injection of BCG vaccine [77]. Allen and Spitz, from their very wide experience of malignant melanoma, advise a prophylactic excision of benign junctional or compound pigmented naevi from the palms or soles because of their vulnerability to malignant change [78].

Sarcoma of the hand

This is extremely rare. Marcove and Charosky draw attention to the difficulty in differentiating sarcoma from bone infection in the hand [79]. The only sarcomas which occur here with any frequency are chondrosarcoma, fibrosarcoma, osteosarcoma, rhabdomyosarcoma and epithelioid sarcoma and these alone will be described here. Other tumours more rarely reported include synovial sarcoma, liposarcoma [82], malignant schwannoma [82], lymphangiosarcoma occurring in post-mastectomy lymphoedema [83], Ewing's tumour [84], haemangiopericytoma [80], haemangioendothelioma [85], Kaposi's sarcoma [18, 86] and myeloma [87].

Epithelioid sarcoma of the hand [53]

This tumour is unique among sarcomas in showing preference for the forearm and hand and was the most common tumour in a series of 85 malignant soft tissue sarcomas of the hand collected by Bryan *et al.* [80]. They reported 10 epithelioid sarcomas in the hand and three in the forearm. They are tumours of childhood or young adult life. They grow along fascia or tendons producing multiple nodules which may ulcerate through the overlying skin or erode the underlying bones. They tend to spread in the subdermal lymphatics and may produce satellite lesions in the skin more proximally. Lymph node and lung metastases also occur. It is characteristic of this tumour that growth is slow and metastases develop late so that its malignant character may not be suspected initially.

Histological diagnosis is also difficult. The principal cells, which resemble epithelioid cells, are arranged in nodules which may show areas of necrosis. Sarcomatous spindle cells occur around the nodule and may suggest fibrosarcoma. The range of histological appearances suggested by different areas of this bizarre tumour include inflammatory granuloma, squamous cell carcinoma and even synovial sarcoma.

Treatment

This consists of wide local excision. Local recurrence should be treated by forearm amputation. Despite such treatment and despite the slow growth of the tumour, death from metastases occurred in three of the cases reported by Bryan *et al.* [80]. Two others had metastases, one 12 and the other 19 years after their initial presentation. Awareness of this rare tumour and of its inexorable course is important otherwise its undramatic presentation may lull the surgeon into inadequate surgery.

Fibrosarcoma

This was one of the most common of soft tissue sarcomas of the forearm and hand reported by Bryan [80], although, of these, only five occurred in the hand itself. Other series report few cases. The clinical presentation is non-specific. The diagnosis depends on biopsy which reveals large fibroblast-like spindle cells among which are varying amounts of collagen fibres. Highly malignant lesions may show much pleomorphism and so little collagen formation that the fibroblastic origin may be difficult to establish. Excision may involve complete or partial amputation of the hand. Butler *et al.* report prolonged survival in their three cases [4].

Rhabdomyosarcoma

Twelve cases of this tumour of the hand have been collected by Potenza and Winslow [88], including all the cases that had been reported to that date. Bryan added six more [80]. They tend to occur in childhood or young adult life. The tumours presented as painless or painful swellings involving any of the muscles of the hand. Erosion of adjacent metacarpals was noted in two cases. Diagnosis was suggested by multinucleated muscle giant cells and striations in the primitive muscle fibres. The prognosis is uniformly bad. In the cases of Potenza and Winslow death occurred within 2 or 3 years of diagnosis despite amputation or radiotherapy [88].

Chondrosarcoma

Although the most common of the malignant tumours of bone in the hand, this is still extremely rare, which contrasts with the relative frequency of benign cartilaginous tumours. Dahlin and Salvador and Roberts and Price have reported the largest series [61, 89]. They tend to occur in the older age group and involve the proximal phalanges most commonly. The clinical behaviour of the tumours may give better indication of malignancy than the histological findings. Increase in size and destruction of the cortex suggest malignant change. Few chondrosarcomas show irregular calcification on radiographic examination so commonly found in benign cartilaginous tumours. About half the chondrosarcomas arising in the hand have evidence of a preceding benign cartilaginous lesion. Treatment consists of excision which may require removal of a ray or partial hand amputation. These tumours metastasize late and the cure rate is high.

Osteosarcoma

Osteosarcoma of the hand is exceedingly rare. Carroll reported 10 cases collected from the literature and his own experience [90]. Dromp reported a unique case of bilateral osteosarcoma of the phalanges arising in bones affected by Paget's disease [91]. The radiographic features show bone destruction with extension of tumour bone into the surrounding soft tissue (Fig. 31.18). Diagnosis depends on biopsy before radical treatment is contemplated, for in the hand as elsewhere osteosarcoma may mimic other disorders such as myositis ossificans or osteomyelitis. In Carroll's cases the prognosis was little better than for osteosarcoma in general at that time, however, one would hope that with the advent of effective chemotherapy the prognosis today would be considerably improved following radical local excision of the primary tumour. One case of parosteal osteosarcoma of the hand has been described [92]. Myositis ossificans would enter into differential diagnosis of such a lesion.

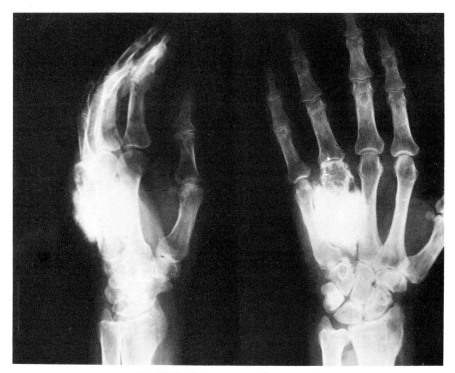

FIG. 31.18. Osteosarcoma of metacarpal.

Metastatic tumours in the hand

These are uncommon. Kerin in a review of the literature found only 23 cases and reported 7 more [93]. Uriburu's cases bring the total to 90 [94]. Table 31.2 derived from his paper lists the primary sites. Almost all metastases have arisen in bone, although a chordoma metastasis to the muscle of the thenar eminence has been reported [95] as has a chondrosarcoma metastasis to the finger pulp [96]. Metastatic tumours show a particular preference for the terminal phalanx* especially of the thumb and tend to involve the carpal bones rarely.

---

*The terminal phalanx shows a curious susceptibility to a wide range of disorders as well as to metastatic lesions. The frequency of osteoid osteomas, glomus tumours and epidermoid inclusion cysts in this site is also referred to in this chapter. Schajowicz adds aneurysmal bone cyst to this list [22]. Loss of the terminal tuft is a feature of such diverse disorders as hyperparathyroidism, pyknodysostosis, craniocleido-dysostosis, polyvinylchloride poisoning and pachydermoperiostitis.

As painful swellings they may be confused with infective lesions. Radiographs show irregular destruction of bone (Fig. 31.19), and the diagnosis is confirmed by biopsy or by identification of the primary tumour. Treatment depends on such factors as the nature of the tumour,

TABLE 31.2. Primary sites of metastatic tumours in the hand (derived from [94]).

Lung	42	Tonsil	
Breast	15	Nasopharynx	
Kidney	4	Oesophagus	
Parotid	4	Stomach	
Prostate	3	Testicle	
Colon	3	Bladder	
Rectum	3	Brain	1 each
Lymphosarcoma	2	Adrenal gland	
Oral cavity	2	Skin	
		Uterus	
		Larynx	
		Thyroid	

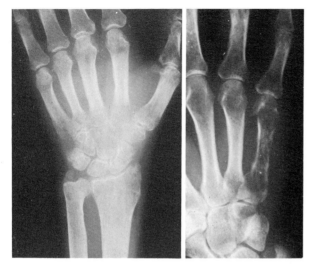

FIG. 31.19. Two examples of metastases to the hand both arising from carcinoma of the lung. Carpal lesions shown in the left radiograph are unusual.

the extent of dissemination, the radiosensitivity of the lesion and the patient's general condition. In general, surgery should be conservative although amputation of an affected digit or ray may be a useful palliative procedure.

Miscellaneous pseudo-tumours of the hand

A wide range of systemic and local diseases (Chap. 33) may be associated with tumour-like swellings of the hand. In general the systemic disease is apparent and the hand lesion is often a minor and unimportant manifestation. Occasionally it may suggest the diagnosis. Several of these conditions are illustrated in Fig. 31.20. These examples are by no means exhaustive and to them might be added thorn granuloma [97], and haemophilic pseudotumour [98]. Most readers could add to this list from their own experience.

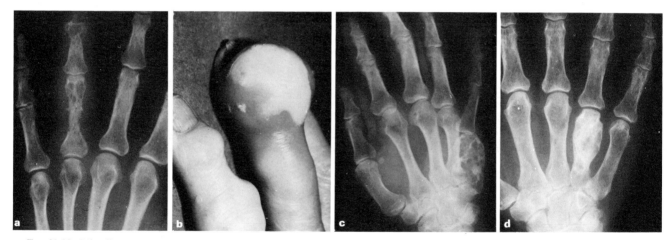

FIG. 31.20. Miscellaneous tumour-producing lesions of the hand. (a) sarcoid dactylitis, (b) gout, (c) fibrous dysplasia, (d) hyperparathyroid brown tumour.

REFERENCES

[1] STACK, H. G. Tumours of the hand. *Postgraduate Medical Journal*, 1964, **40**, 290.

[2] ALTER, A. W. AND HABER, M. H. Hand tumours—a review. *Hawaii Medical Journal*, 1967, **26**, 403.

[3] BOYES, J. H. *Bunnell's Surgery of the Hand*, 5th Edition. Philadelphia, J. B. Lippincott, 1970.

[4] BUTLER, E. D., HAMILL, J. P., SEIPEL, R. S. AND LORIMER, A. Tumours of the hand, a ten-year survey and report of 437 cases. *American Journal of Surgery*, 1960, **100**, 293.

[5] HOWARD, J. M. Tumours of the hand. *Surgical Clinics of North America*, 1951, **31**, 1307.

[6] KENDALL, T. E., ROBINSON, D. W. AND MASTERS, F. W.

Primary malignant tumours of the hand. *Plastic and Reconstructive Surgery*, 1969, **44**, 37.

[7] MANGINI, U. Tumours of the skeleton of the hand. *Bulletin of the Hospital for Joint Diseases*, 1967, **28**, 61.

[8] MASON, M. L. Tumours of the hand. *Surgery, Gynaecology and Obstetrics*, 1937, **64**, 129.

[9] PACK, G. T. *Tumours of the Hand and Feet*. Mosby, St Louis, 1939.

[10] POSCH, J. L. Tumours of the hand. *Journal of Bone and Joint Surgery*, 1956, **38A**, 517.

[11] SALIB, P. I. Tumours of the bones of the hand. *American Journal of Orthopedic Surgery*, 1966, **8**, 114.

[12] WOODS, J. E., MURRAY, J. E. AND VAWTER, G. F. Hand tumours in children. *Plastic and Reconstructive Surgery*, 1970, **46**, 130.

[13] BUNNEY, M. H. Warts. *British Journal of Hospital Medicine*, 1975, **13**, 565.

[14] BYERS, P., MANTLE, J. AND RALM, R. Epidermal cysts of phalanges. *Journal of Bone and Joint Surgery*, 1966, **48B**, 577.

[15] CARROLL, R. E. AND BERMAN, A. T. Glomus tumours of the hand. Review of the literature and report on 28 cases. *Journal of Bone and Joint Surgery*, 1972, **54A**, 691.

[16] MATHIS, W. H. AND SCHULTZ, M. D. Roentgen diagnosis of glomus tumours. *Radiology*, 1948, **51**, 71.

[17] SUGIURA, I. Intraosseous glomus tumour. *Journal of Bone and Joint Surgery*, 1976, **58B**, 245.

[18] BOOHER, R. J. Tumours arising from blood vessels in the hand and the feet. *Clinical Orthopaedics*, 1961, **19**, 71.

[19] BROOKSALER, F. The angio-osteohypertrophy syndrome. Klippel-Trenaunay-Weber syndrome. *American Journal of Diseases of Childhood*, 1966, **112**, 161.

[20] GUTIERREZ, R. M. AND SPJUT, H. J. Skeletal angiomatosis. Report of 3 cases and review of the literature. *Clinical Orthopaedics*, 1972, **85**, 82.

[21] TILLMAN, B. P., DAHLIN, D. C., LIPSCOMB, P. R. AND STEWART, J. R. Aneurysmal bone cyst: an analysis of 95 cases. *Mayo Clinical Procedures*, 1968, **43**, 478.

[22] SCHAJOWICZ, F., AIELLO, C. L. AND SLULLITEL, I. Cystic and pseudocystic lesions of the terminal phalanx. *Clinical Orthopaedics*, 1970, **68**, 84.

[23] CARROLL, R. E. AND DOYLE, J. R. Lipoma of the hand. *Journal of Bone and Joint Surgery*, 1967, **49A**, 581.

[24] PAARLBERG, D., LINSCHEID, R. L. AND SOULE, E. H. Lipomas of the hand. *Mayo Clinical Proceedings*, 1972, **47**, 121.

[25] PHALEN, G. S., KENDRICK, J. I. AND RODRIGUEZ, J. M. Lipomas of the upper extremity. A series of 15 tumours in the hand and wrist of 6 tumours causing nerve compression. *American Journal of Surgery*, 1971, **121**, 298.

[26] PULVERTAFT, R. G. Unusual tumours of the median nerve. *Journal of Bone and Joint Surgery*, 1964, **46B**, 731.

[27] YEOMAN, P. M. Fatty infiltration of the median nerve. *Journal of Bone and Joint Surgery*, 1964, **46B**, 737.

[28] JOHNSON, R. J. AND BONFIGLIO, M. Lipofibromatous harmar-
toma of the median nerve. *Journal of Bone and Joint Surgery*, 1969, **51A**, 984.

[29] LOUIS, D. S. AND DICK, H. M. Ossifying lipofibroma of the median nerve. *Journal of Bone and Joint Surgery*, 1973, **55A**, 1082.

[30] DAHLIN, D. C. *Bone Tumours, General Aspects and Data on 3987 Cases*, 2nd Edition. Springfield, Charles C. Thomas, 1969.

[31] BLOEM, J. J., VUZEVSKI, V. D. AND HUFFSTADT, A. J. C. Recurring digital fibroma of infancy. *Journal of Bone and Joint Surgery*, 1974, **56B**, 746.

[32] POPPEN, N. K. AND NIEBAUER, J. J. Recurring digital fibrous tumour of childhood. *The Journal of Hand Surgery*, 1977, **2**, 253.

[33] KEASBY, L. E. Juvenile aponeurotic fibroma (calcifying fibroma): a distinctive tumour arising in the palms and soles of young children. *Cancer*, 1953, **6**, 338.

[34] SPECHT, E. E. AND STAHELI, L. T. Juvenile aponeurotic fibroma. *The Journal of Hand Surgery*, 1977, **2**, 256.

[35] WHITE, N. B. Neurilemmomas of the extremities. *Journal of Bone and Joint Surgery*, 1967, **49A**, 1605.

[36] MORTON, K. S. AND VASSAR, P. S. Neurilemmoma in bone. *Canadian Journal of Surgery*, 1964, **7**, 187.

[37] MCCARROLL, H. R. Clinical manifestations of congenital neuro-fibromotosis. *Journal of Bone and Joint Surgery*, 1950, **32A**, 601.

[38] HUNT, J. C. AND PUGH, D. G. Skeletal lesions in neuro-fibromatosis. *Radiology*, 1961, **76**, 1.

[39] JONES, K. G. Megalodactylism. *Journal of Bone and Joint Surgery*, 1963, **45A**, 1704.

[40] HAMILTON, W. C., RAMSEY, P. L. AND HANSON, S. M. Osseous xanthoma and multiple hand tumours as a complication of hyperlipidemia. *Journal of Bone and Joint Surgery*, 1975, **57A**, 551.

[41] WESSLER, S. AND AVIOLI, L. A. Classification and management of familial hyperlipoprotinaemia. *Journal of American Medical Association*, 1969, **207**, 929.

[42] ANDREN, L. AND EIKEN, O. Arthrographic studies of wrist ganglions. *Journal of Bone and Joint Surgery*, 1971, **53A**, 299.

[43] MCEVEDY, B. V. Simple ganglia. *British Journal of Surgery*, 1962, **49**, 585.

[44] MATTHEWS, P. Ganglia of the flexor tendon sheaths in the hand. *Journal of Bone and Joint Surgery*, 1973, **55B**, 612.

[45] FELDMAN, F. AND JOHNSTON, A. Intraosseous ganglion. *American Journal of Roentgenology*, 1973, **118**, 328.

[46] KAMBOLIS, C., BULLOUGH, P. G. AND JAFFE, H. L. Ganglionic cystic defects in bone. *Journal of Bone and Joint Surgery*, 1973, **55A**, 496.

[47] NIGRISOLI, P. AND BELTRAMI, P. Subchondral cysts of bone. *Lo Scapello*, 1971, **1**, 65.

[48] SIM, F. H. AND DAHLIN, D. C. Ganglion cysts of bone. *Mayo Clinic Proceedings*, 1971, **46**, 484.

[49] NELSON, C. L., SAWMILLER, S. AND PHALEN, C. S. Ganglion of the wrist and hand. *Journal of Bone and Joint Surgery*, 1972, **54A**, 1459.

[50] ROSS, J. A. AND TROY, C. A. The clinical significance of the

extensor digitorum brevis manus. *Journal of Bone and Joint Surgery*, 1969, **51B**, 473.

[51] KLEINERT, H. E., KUTZ, J. E., FISHMAN, J. H. AND McGRAQ, L. H. Etiology and treatment of the so-called mucous cyst of the finger. *Journal of Bone and Joint Surgery*, 1972, **54A**, 1455.

[52] BLISS, B. O. AND REED, J. R. Large cell sarcoma of tendon sheath. Malignant giant cell tumours of tendon sheath. *American Journal of Clinical Pathology*, 1968, **49**, 776.

[53] ENZINGER, F. M. Epithelioid sarcoma. A sarcoma simulating a granuloma or a carcinoma. *Cancer*, 1970, **26**, 1029.

[54] NEVIASER, R. J. AND NEWMAN, W. Dermal angiomyoma of the upper extremity. *The Journal of Hand Surgery*, 1977, **2**, 271.

[55] STOUT, A. P. Solitary cutaneous and subcutaneous leiomyoma. *American Journal of Cancer*, 1937, **29**, 435.

[56] TAKIGAWA, K. Chondroma of the bones of the hand. *Journal of Bone and Joint Surgery*, 1971, **53A**, 1591.

[57] JEWUSIAK, E. M., SPENCE, K. F. AND SELL, K. W. Solitary benign enchondroma of the long bones of the hand. *Journal of Bone and Joint Surgery*, 1971, **53A**, 1587.

[58] NOBLE, J. AND LAMB, D. W. Enchondromata of bones of the hand. A review of 40 cases. *Hand*, 1974, **6**, 275.

[59] ROCKWELL, M. A., SAITER, E. T. AND ENNEKING, W. F. Periosteal chondroma. *Journal of Bone and Joint Surgery*, 1972, **54A**, 102.

[60] LICHTENSTEIN, L. AND GOLDMAN, R. L. Cartilage tumours in soft tissue particularly in the hand and foot. *Cancer*, 1964, **17**, 1203.

[61] DAHLIN, D. C. AND SALVADOR, A. H. Cartilagenous tumours of the soft tissues of the hand and feet. *Mayo Clinic Proceedings*, 1974, **49**, 721.

[62] MOSHER, J. F. Multiple enchondromotosis of the hand. *Journal of Bone and Joint Surgery*, 1976, **58A**, 717.

[63] CARROLL, R. E. Osteoid osteoma in the hand. *Journal of Bone and Joint Surgery*, 1953, **35A**, 888.

[64] SULLIVAN, M. Osteoid osteoma of the fingers. *Hand*, 1971, **3**, 175.

[65] EDEIKEN, J., DePALMA, A. F. AND HODES, P. S. Osteoid osteoma. *Clinical Orthopaedics*, 1966, **49**, 201.

[66] MOBERG, E. The natural course of osteoid osteoma. *Journal of Bone and Joint Surgery*, 1951, **33A**, 166.

[67] DUNLOP, J. A. Y., MORTON, K. S. AND ELLIOTT, G. B. Recurrent osteoid osteoma. *Journal of Bone and Joint Surgery*, 1970, **52B**, 128.

[68] NEVIASER, R. J. AND WILSON, J. N. Benign chondroblastoma in the finger. *Journal of Bone and Joint Surgery*, 1972, **54A**, 389.

[69] GOLDENBERG, R. R., CAMPBELL, C. J. AND BONFIGLIO, M. Giant cell tumour of bone. An analysis of 218 cases. *Journal of Bone and Joint Surgery*, 1970, **52A**, 619.

[70] TAYLOR, G. W., NATHANSON, J. T. AND SHAW, D. T. Epidermoid carcinoma of the extremities. *Annals of Surgery*, 1941, **113**, 268.

[71] JOHNSON, R. E. AND ACKERMAN, L. V. Epidermoid carcinoma. *Cancer*, 1950, **3**, 657.

[72] CAMPBELL, C. J. AND KEOKARN, T. Squamous cell carcinoma in the nail bed in epidermal dysplasia. *Journal of Bone and Joint Surgery*, 1966, **48A**, 92.

[73] HUTCHISON, J. Melanotic whitlow. *British Medical Journal*, 1886, **1**, 491.

[74] COCHRAN, A. J. The biology and treatment of malignant melanoma. *European Journal of Cancer*, 1976, **12**, 585.

[75] LEPPARD, B., SANDERSON, K. V. AND BEHAU, F. Subungual malignant melanoma. Difficulty in diagnosis. *British Medical Journal*, 1974, **1**, 310.

[76] WHO. *Clinical Diagnosis of Malignant Melanoma.* Milan, WHO International Reference Centre for the Evaluation of Methods of Diagnosis and Treatment of Melanoma, 1974.

[77] MORTON, D. L., EILBER, F. R., HOLMES, E. C., HUNT, J. S., KETCHAM, A. S., SILVERSTEIN, M. J. AND SPARKS, F. C. BCG immunotherapy of malignant melanomas: summary of a seven year experience. *American Surgery*, 1974, **180**, 635.

[78] ALLEN, A. C. AND SPITZ, S. Malignant melanoma. *Cancer*, 1953, **6**, 1.

[79] MARCOVE, R. C. AND CHAROSKY, C. B. Phalangeal sarcomas simulating infections of the digits. Review of the literature and report of 4 cases. *Clinical Orthopaedics*, 1972, **83**, 224.

[80] BRYAN, R. S., SOULE, E. H., DOBYNS, J. H., PRITCHARD, D. J. AND LINSCHEID, R. L. Primary epithelioid sarcoma of the hand and forearm. *Journal of Bone and Joint Surgery*, 1974, **56A**, 458.

[81] CROKER, D. W. AND STOUT, A. P. Synovial sarcoma in children. *Cancer*, 1959, **12**, 1123.

[82] POSCH, J. L. In *Hand Surgery*, Chapter 19, pp. 999–1026. Editor J. E. Flynn. Baltimore, William & Wilkins, 1966.

[83] SCOTT, R. B., UYDICK, I. AND CONWAY, H. Lymphangiosarcoma arising in lymphedema. *American Journal of Medicine*, 1960, **28**, 1008.

[84] DICK, H. M., FRANCIS, K. C. AND JOHNSTON, A. D. Ewing's sarcoma of the hand. *Journal of Bone and Joint Surgery*, 1971, **53A**, 345.

[85] McCARTHY, W. D. AND PACK, G. T. Malignant blood vessel tumour. *Surgery, Gynaecology and Obstetrics*, 1950, **91**, 465.

[86] DUTZ, W. AND STOUT, A. P. Kaposis sarcoma in infants and children. *Cancer*, 1960, **13**, 684.

[87] GRIFFITHS, D. W. Orthopaedic aspects of myelomotosis. *Journal of Bone and Joint Surgery*, 1966, **48B**, 703.

[88] POTENZA, A. AND WINSLOW, D. Rhabdomyosarcoma of the hand. *Journal of Bone and Joint Surgery*, 1961, **43A**, 700.

[89] ROBERTS, P. H. AND PRICE, C. H. G. Chondrosarcoma of the bones of the hand. *Journal of Bone and Joint Surgery*, 1977, **59B**, 213.

[90] CARROLL, R. E. Osteogenic sarcoma in the hand. *Journal of Bone and Joint Surgery*, 1957, **39A**, 325.

[91] DROMPP, B. W. Bilateral osteosarcoma of the phalanges of the hand. *Journal of Bone and Joint Surgery*, 1961, **43A**, 199.

[92] STARK, H. H., JONES, F. E. AND JERNSTROM, P. Parosteal osteogenic sarcoma of a metacarpal bone—a case report. *Journal of Bone and Joint Surgery*, 1971, **53A,** 147.

[93] KERIN, R. Metastatic tumours of the hand. *Journal of Bone and Joint Surgery*, 1958, **40A,** 263.

[94] URIBURU, I. V. F., NORCHIO, F. J. AND MARIN, J. C. Metastases of carcinoma of the larynx and thyroid gland to the phalanges of the hand. *Journal of Bone and Joint Surgery*, 1976, **58A,** 134.

[95] CHALMERS, J. AND HEARD, B. E. A metastasing chordoma.

Journal of Bone and Joint Surgery, 1972, **54B,** 526.

[96] FROIMSON, A. I. Metastatic chondrosarcoma of the hand. Report of a case. *Clinical Orthopaedics*, 1967, **53,** 155.

[97] GERLE, R. D. Thorn-induced pseudo-tumours of bone. *British Journal of Radiology*, 1971, **44,** 642.

[98] BAYER, W. L., SHEA, J. D., CURIEL, D. C., SYETO, I. L. F. AND LEWIS, J. H. Excision of a pseudocyst in the hand in a haemophiliac. *Journal of Bone and Joint Surgery*, 1969, **51A,** 1423.

CHAPTER 32

Dupuytren's Disease

D. W. LAMB

This condition produces its main effect on the hand, although it may occasionally involve the foot and owes its name to Dupuytren who described it in 1834 [1]. It had been previously recognized in an excellent description by Astley Cooper who thought it due to flexor tendon contracture [2].

It affects the palmar fascia, the anatomy of which is now described.

ANATOMY

K. KUCZYNSKI

The deep palmar fascia [3–6]

The following layers can be recognized:

Superficial anchoring fibres which run from the palmar aponeurosis to the palmar skin forming a mesh in which the subcutaneous tissue is firmly held in position for the purpose of gripping.

Superficial layer of the palmar aponeurosis continuous with the thinner parts of the deep palmar fascia covering the thenar and hypothenar muscle compartments. This layer of the palmar aponeurosis is mostly longitudinal and the mode of its termination distally will be discussed later. At its proximal end it is continued with the tendon of the palmaris longus muscle, when present (Fig. 32.1).

Deep layer of the palmar aponeurosis (Fig. 32.1) composed mostly of the transverse fibres [5] and continuous with the flexor retinaculum.

Deep anchoring fibres derived from the deep aspect of the palmar aponeurosis. These fibres at the ulnar and radial sides of the hand form marginal septa separating the hypothenar compartment from the midpalmar space and the midpalmar space from the adductor space (Fig. 32.2). In the distal palm these deep fibres form septa which lie on each side of the flexor tendons and form tunnels for the lumbricals and neurovascular bundles.

Anterior interosseous fascia which covers the palmar aspect of the interossei muscles and the metacarpal bones and is continuous distally with the palmar plates of the metacarpophalangeal joints and with the Cleland's ligaments, proximally with the floor of the carpal tunnel

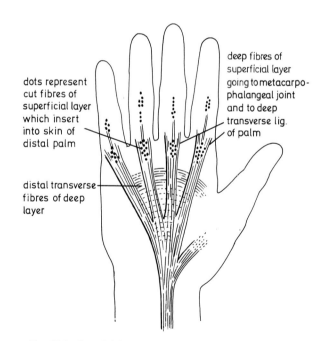

FIG. 32.1. Superficial and deep layers of palmar aponeurosis.

470

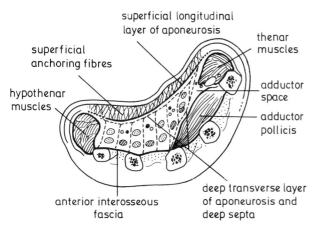

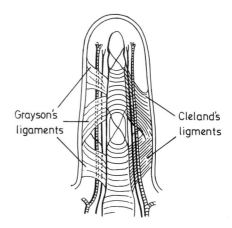

FIG. 32.2. An oblique section through the palm showing elements of the palmar aponeurosis.

Two deep septa (marginal), ulnar and radial (oblique) separate the midpalmar space from the hypothenar compartment and from the adductor space respectively. This specimen shows a split in the well developed oblique radial marginal septum.

FIG. 32.4. The digital ligaments.

and laterally with the dorsal fascia of the first dorsal interosseous muscle.

In *the fingers* the deep fascia is organized into fibrous flexor sheaths (Fig. 32.3) and digital ligaments (Fig. 32.4) (Cleland's posterior to the neurovascular bundle and Grayson's anterior to it).

The superficial layer of the palmar aponeurosis

It is triangular in shape with its apex towards the wrist (Fig. 32.1). As it approaches the distal part of the

palm it divides into four longitudinal slips overlying the line of the flexor tendons. A fifth slip is found quite often branching for a variable distance from the radial side of the proximal part of the palmar aponeurosis towards the metacarpophalangeal region of the thumb. This slip usually has no connections with the deeper structures and fades away inside the thenar fascia. The four slips of the distal part of the palmar aponeurosis terminate by sending most of the fibres into the skin of the distal palm (Fig. 32.5). Some fibres however, continue in their course towards the fingers and the mode

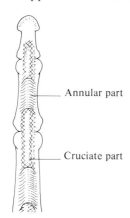

FIG. 32.3. Components of the fibrous flexor sheath.

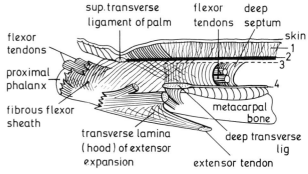

FIG. 32.5. A parasagittal section of the hand demonstrating the distal termination of the fibres of the palmar aponeurosis. Modified from Bojsen-Møller and L. Schmidt.

(1) superficial anchoring fibres.

(2) superficial longitudinal layer of palmar aponeurosis,

(3) deep transverse layer of palmar aponeuris and deep anchoring fibres, (septa) and

(4) anterior interosseous fascia.

of their termination is complex. Some of them run dorsally and distally on both sides of the metacarpophalangeal joints and reach the deep transverse ligament of the palm, the capsule of the metacarpophalangeal joint, the fibrous flexor sheath and become continuous with the Cleland's ligaments. Some fibres contribute to the deep septa in the distal palm derived from the transverse deep layer of the palmar aponeurosis, while the most distal fibres run in a superficial direction (skin fibres) and are attached to the superficial transverse ligament of the palm, the skin over the palmar aspect of the fingers and become continuous with the Grayson's digital ligaments.

The deep layer of the palmar aponeurosis (Fig. 32.1)

It is composed of predominantly transverse fibres, which during dissection of the palm become visible at the distal part of the palm in the intervals between the slips of the superficial layer. These distal transverse fibres of the deep layer of the aponeurosis quite often extend for a variable distance (sometimes as far proximally as the level of the trapezium) into the thenar fascia. Again this transverse slip to the thumb (like the superficial slip) is not attached to any deep structures but fades away gradually without leaving the layer of the thenar fascia. In many broad hands the deep aspect of

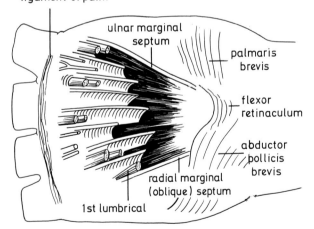

FIG. 32.6. Lateral oblique view of left hand showing shape and extent of the deep septa (deep anchoring system of the palmar aponeurosis). After Bojsen-Møller and Schmidt.

the palmar aponeurosis provides a very considerable area of attachment for the white strong fibres of the aponeurotic origin of the flexor pollicis brevis muscle just distal to the flexor retinaculum.

The deep aspect of the palmar aponeurosis also gives rise to the septa (deep anchoring fibres) which extend to the anterior interosseous fascia (Figs. 32.5 and 32.6). The two marginal septa are attached as follows: (1) the ulnar one to the shaft of the fifth metacarpal bone, and (2) the radial one to the shaft of the third metacarpal. These marginal septa are shown in an oblique section of the palm in Figure 32.2. Superficially they are attached to the ulnar and radial edges of the palmar aponeurosis. The remaining deep septa do not extend as far proximally as the marginal ones and are to be found in the distal palm only. They contribute to formation of the eight tunnels: four for the flexor tendons to the fingers and four for the lumbricals and accompanying digital nerves and vessels.

The digital ligaments

Cleland's ligament [7] lies posteriorly to the neurovascular bundle and is attached to the sides of the shafts of the phalanges and to the skin of the lateral and medial aspects of the fingers. It serves to retain the dorsal skin in position during flexion of the fingers and provides part of the support for the gripping pads of the fingers. Opposite the proximal interphalangeal joint the oblique retinacular ligament (Landsmeer) passes through the opening between the proximal and distal parts of the Cleland's ligament (Fig. 32.7). Fibres of this ligament can be traced proximally to the deep transverse ligament of the palm and to the deep anchoring fibres from the four slips of the superficial part of the palmar aponeurosis.

Grayson's ligament [8]. The fibres of this ligament are much thinner than those of the Cleland's ligament; their attachment is rather inconstant and quite often they seem to be incorporated into the fibres of the gripping pad and the 'skin fibres' of the distal attachment of the four slips of the palmar aponeurosis into the digital palmar skin. These ligaments lie anteriorly to the neurovascular bundles. The fibres of these ligaments can be traced proximally into the superficial transverse ligament of the palm.

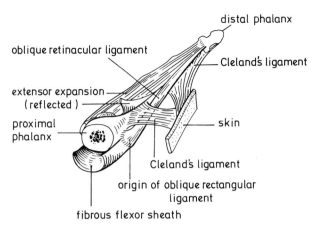

FIG. 32.7. The relationship of the oblique retinacular ligament to the proximal and distal parts of the Cleland's ligament.

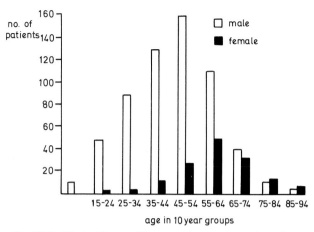

FIG. 32.8. The incidence of Dupuytren's contracture in various age groups. Note that the peak occurs in the male between 35 and 64 years of age. In the female, the relative incidence increases after middle age. Over the age of 65 the condition is as common in the female as in the male.

Aetiological and genetic factors

For many years an association with other diseases such as epilepsy, liver disease, alcoholism and tuberculosis was claimed, but it is probably just coexistence of this common condition with others equally frequent. Dupuytren's contracture and idiopathic epilepsy are both genetically determined and a linked inheritance from adjacent genes may account for the occurrence of the two conditions in the same patient. It was also suggested that its relationship with epilepsy might be due to the drugs which were given in the treatment of that condition but this is no longer felt to be valid [9].

It is only in recent years that its inheritance has been appreciated. Population studies by Early [10] and by Hueston [11] showed its frequency; and Ling [12] followed up the families of patients attending the Edinburgh clinic and found a family history in over two-thirds of those studied. This raised the possibility of some underlying chromosomal factor and preliminary studies to this end have been initiated [13]. This condition, so common in Northern Europe, is equally common in countries such as Australia where the population is predominantly of European descent. It does not appear that environmental factors, such as diet, climate, or occupation have any influence on its development.

The possible influence of injury on the development of Dupuytren's contracture may have medicolegal implications. Trauma, by itself, is not responsible for its development but injury to the hand may be followed by Dupuytren's contracture in a person genetically predisposed to this disease, and it is possible that, in some circumstances, the injury may accelerate its appearance.

Dupuytren's contracture is so common in the British Isles that it has been estimated to be manifest in 25 per cent of men over the age of 65 [9]. There may be some differences in the pattern of progress of the disease between the sexes, and, while it is less common than in the male, it is by no means rare in the female hand after the age of 40 years (Fig. 32.8).

The condition is extremely rare in the Chinese, Indian and Negro compared with populations of European descent. There is no known reason for this difference and, at the present time, the etiology of Dupuytren's disease remains obscure.

The contracture may affect any part of the fascia but usually involves only the longitudinal elements and rarely the transverse fibres [5]. The commonest early site is on the ulnar side of the distal palm and initially, tends to be nodular (Fig. 32.9). The nodules coalesce to form linear bands (Fig. 32.10) and it is the shortening of these that leads to the characteristic deformities (Figs. 32.11 and 32.12). Very careful studies of the palmar fascia and its relationship to Dupuytren's disease have been made by many authors. The monographs by Hueston [14] and Stack [6] are recommended for fuller

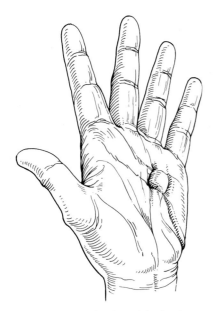

FIG. 32.9. An example of early nodular involvement in the palm. The typical site is on the ulnar side in the region of the head of the fourth metacarpal.

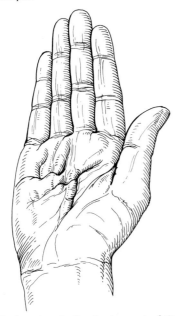

FIG. 32.10. A further stage in the development of Dupuytren's contracture in the palm. The nodules are coalescing into longitudinal linear bands, orientated towards the bases of the long, ring and little fingers. There is as yet no evidence of digital involvement, and therefore no contracture of the fingers.

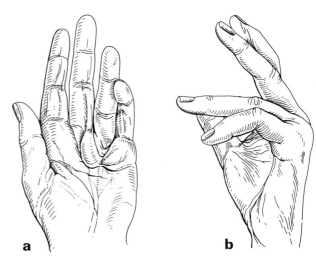

a   **b**

FIG. 32.11. A typical example of Dupuytren's contracture affecting the ulnar two digits of the left hand.

(a) Note the puckering of the skin, the contracted band of fascia extending from the base of the palm towards the ring finger and the flexion contracture affecting the ring and little fingers.

(b) The metacarpophalangeal joints are mainly affected but there is also a contracture of about 45° affecting the proximal interphalangeal joint of the little finger. The fingers are being extended as much as the contracted band will allow. Full flexion from this position is possible.

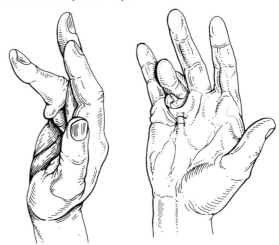

FIG. 32.12. The contracted pretendinous longitudinal band runs towards the ring finger with a flexion contracture of the metacarpophalangeal joint and commencing contracture of the proximal interphalangeal joint. There is a large nodule at the distal end of the longitudinal band overlying the proximal interphalangeal joint.

reading about the fascia and the clinical implication of its involvement.

Pathological changes

The essential early feature is the development of aggregations of fibroblasts in the palmar fascia although some authorities [15, 16, 17] believe that the condition originates superficial to the fascia in pads of fat between the fascia and skin and that the fascia is secondarily involved. Recent studies by electron microscopy [18] have suggested that the main cell in the nodular stage is the contractile fibroblast. The early nodules are rather fleshy in character and may be tender. Gradually, the cellular infiltration becomes less evident and is followed by progressive collaginization and the collagen may be of an abnormal type.

The progress of the disease is often slow and the onset of clinical manifestations rare before the fourth decade. It is for this reason presumably that the inherited nature of the condition was not appreciated for so long and why it may be difficult to trace a history of family involvement. Occasionally, the disease becomes evident at an earlier age, usually indicating a very actively progressive condition with a strong inheritance.

Clinical features

While there are certain classic features in the fully developed condition of Dupuytren's contracture (Fig. 32.12), there are numerous variants of its effects on the hand due to the extensive nature of the palmar fascia.

As Dupuytren originally described, the condition begins, proceeds and reaches its climax without any pain. There is extreme diversity in its clinical presentation and, while the palm of the hand bears the brunt of the disease and is the site of paramount clinical importance, it may also reveal itself in other sites, sometimes before there is any involvement of the palmar fascia. The most characteristic of these sites is the dorsum of the proximal interphalangeal joints where nodules develop resulting in so-called 'knuckle pads' which, in the early stages, can be quite tender. These nodules are seldom troublesome enough to require treatment but often appear as early as the late teens and twenties in those predisposed to

Dupuytren's disease. The histological features are the same as in the early palmar nodules and the pads often disappear as the palmar aspect of the disease unravels.

Another site which should always be examined is the plantar fascia. Skoog [19] estimated that 10 per cent of patients with Dupuytren's contracture had plantar involvement. The nodules may occur at an early age as a type of plantar fibromatosis and become quite large and tender. They tend to become less fleshy and troublesome and, where possible, surgical treatment should be avoided as recurrence is not uncommon. Histological examination at the early stages of nodular formation may be confused for a fibrosarcoma and cases where this mistaken diagnosis has been made are on record.

Peyronie's disease, an odd condition with nodular formation and contracture of the penis, has been described in association with Dupuytren's contracture.

Once the contracture has become apparent in the hand, the rate of progress is difficult to forecast. In some people, particularly women, the condition can remain localized to the palm for a very long period and sometimes extend no further. At other times, a contracture which has been evident for many years without progression, may suddenly deteriorate rapidly during a few months. While the ulnar side of the palmar fascia tends to bear the brunt of the disease, involvement of its radial part may not be infrequent and contractures of middle finger and the band extending onto the radial aspect of the index finger are also commonly seen. Involvement of the thumb is by no means unusual and dense bands in the fascia covering the thenar eminence can extend into the radial aspect of the thumb causing marked flexion contractures, particularly of the metacarpophalangeal joint, and also adduction contracture of the thumb web (Fig. 32.13).

As the disease progresses, there are three main areas which may contract and lead to digital flexion deformities.

(1) The central longitudinal pre-tendinous band (Fig. 32.1) may contract, leading to flexion deformity, both of the metacarpophalangeal and of the proximal interphalangeal joints (Figs. 32.11 and 32.12). This contracted band, which may affect one or more digits, may occur in isolation or be associated with contractures of deeper bands. In isolation, its removal will always allow correction of the metacarpophalangeal joint and very

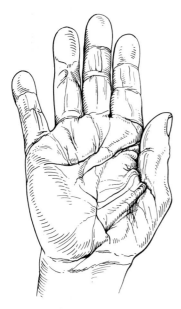

FIG. 32.13. Dupuytren's contracture affecting the palm of the right hand. The main involvement is on the radial side. Note the tight band in the thumb web which has produced an adduction contracture of the thumb; and also the tight band passing along the volar aspect of the thenar eminence and extending along the anteroradial aspect of the thumb with contracture of the metacarpophalangeal joint.

often significant improvement in the contracture of the proximal interphalangeal joint.

(2) Contractures may develop in bands blending with the deep transverse intermetacarpal ligaments (Figs. 32.1 and 32.5) or joining the digital ligaments [7, 8], (Fig. 32.4) around the neurovascular bundle and passing round this in a spiralling manner to become attached to the capsule of the proximal interphalangeal joint and to the base of the middle phalanx. Involvement of these fibres is responsible for severe flexion contractures of the proximal interphalangeal joint, the effects of which are most difficult to correct. The neurovascular bundle may be markedly displaced from its usual position.

(3) Involvement of the deep transverse intermetacarpal ligament (Fig. 32.5) may lead to severe web contractures preventing satisfactory abduction of the fingers. Rarely, the condition may involve the superficial transverse ligament (Fig. 32.5) in the webs with a similar effect.

In the little finger, there are special factors which make this the most difficult digit to correct. Very often the fibrous contracture involves the tendon of the abductor digiti minimi and this produces not only a marked flexion contracture at the metacarpophalangeal joint but also an abduction contracture. Unless this band is carefully removed, sometimes with ablation of the abductor tendon, there will be a strong tendency to recurrence. Also in the little finger, there is a peculiar linear contracture which may affect the finger without palmar involvement and, in the author's experience, has been most frequently seen in the female. It affects particularly the ulnar side of the digit, although occasionally an isolated band may be present on the radial side and may cross the distal interphalangeal joint producing its flexion deformity.

Another deformity, found most commonly in the little finger, is where, possibly due to involvement of Landsmeer's oblique retinacular ligament (Fig. 32.7) as it passes between the two portions of Cleland's ligament, in addition to flexion deformities of the metacarpophalangeal and proximal interphalangeal joints there is also hyperextension deformity of the distal joint (Fig. 32.14). This is a most difficult deformity to correct.

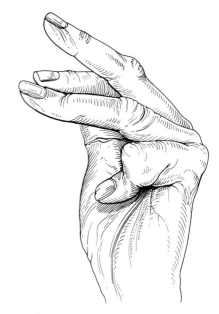

FIG. 32.14. Deformity of the little finger with hyper-extension at the terminal joint. This is not unusual in the little finger but rarely affects other digits.

It has been stated that Dupuytren's contracture does not develop in the absence of a palmaris longus but there are authenticated cases in which the tendon was absent. There may also be involvement of the palmaris brevis area of the base of the hypothenar eminence and extending above the wrist crease [20].

Prognosis and treatment

The prognosis is difficult to determine as no two patients progress in the same way. The condition is usually bilateral, although one side may become evident many months or even years before the other hand; and it is seldom that the disease is of identical or even similar pattern in both hands. There is no evidence, even in heavy workers, that the dominant hand is any more frequently involved. As a general rule, the older the patient when the disease becomes evident, the more benign its course but when the condition develops in the second or third decade with a strong family history or co-existence of epilepsy, it tends to progress more rapidly and to be predisposed to recurrence and relapses after treatment.

No treatment other than operation is known to be effective. There was a vogue for vitamin E therapy which proved ineffectual. Attempts to dissolve the contracted tissue by local injection of a mixture of trypsin, hyaluronidase and local anaesthetic [21], may give temporary improvement but is unlikely to give long-term correction. It may be indicated, however, in the very elderly patient or where operation is ill advised because of the state of the general health.

Patients are sometimes referred for treatment because they have pain in the hand. Dupuytren's contracture, by itself, does not cause pain and another cause must be sought. There may be some discomfort, particularly in the early stages, but the only impairment of function is due to the deformity induced.

The mere presence of Dupuytren's disease in the palm is not an indication by itself for surgery and it is only when the fingers are being pulled into flexion that surgery should be contemplated. This applies particularly where flexion contractures are developing at the proximal interphalangeal joint as contractures of the metacarpophalangeal joints alone need not necessarily justify surgery until there is interference with the function of the hand. The reason for this is based on anatomical grounds as flexion deformity of the metacarpophalangeal joints occurs in a safe position as far as the joint capsule and collateral ligaments are concerned and where the metacarpophalangeal joints alone are flexed operation inevitably leads to recovery of extension in the joint. On the other hand, once flexion contracture of the proximal interphalangeal joint occurs, there is a serious danger of its becoming permanent and not being relieved by removal of Dupuytren's tissue.

Surgical intervention in Dupuytren's contracture can be delayed until: (1) Proximal interphalangeal joints are being pulled into flexion, (2) Deformities interfere with function and appearance sufficiently for the patient to request treatment, and (3) Skin is becoming obviously infiltrated and involved by the Dupuytren's tissue.

In the absence of these criteria the patient should be seen at not more than six monthly intervals and told to report back if there is rapid progression of the deformity in the interval.

As a consequence of bad results which were too frequently seen following extensive radical surgery, there has been a reluctance of many doctors to refer their patients for consultation until long past the time when effective treatment can be given.

While many patients may not require surgery, doctors must be made aware of the need to refer their patients for consideration of operation before fixed flexion contractures, particularly of the proximal interphalangeal joint, have developed.

Unless surgery is carefully planned, performed with meticulous attention to surgical detail and postoperative management, a stiff and useless hand often results.

Operative treatment

In general, there are three methods of operative treatment.

Subcutaneous fasciotomy

This is very seldom required or justified and only for a longitudinal band in a very elderly patient or where general health precludes more extensive surgery. It can occasionally be used for correction of severe digital contractures which prevent proper toilet of the hand as a preliminary step to more radical surgery. The operation should be limited to the palmar portion of the fascia as the nerves are too intimately related to the digital fascial bands for this blind fasciotomy to be a safe procedure in the fingers [22].

Local fasciectomy

Local fasciectomy has gained increasing favour in recent years and means that only affected contracted fascia is excised [23 and 24]. It is usually followed by a much more rapid recovery of the hand than from a more extensive operative procedure but should be done only with the patient aware that extension of the disease may occur in other sites and may necessitate further treatment in the future.

Radical fasciectomy

Radical fasciectomy was the procedure favoured for very many years in the belief that, by removing the palmar fascia as comprehensively as possible, it would prevent recurrences and extensions. Unfortunately, this very extensive dissection often led to severe reactive swelling, followed by stiffness in the hand with disappointing functional results [25–27]. The ramifications of the palmar fascia are so wide that it is not practical to attempt removal of the whole of the fascia and current thought is in favour of localized and limited removal of the diseased tissue.

Operative technique

A wide variety of surgical approaches has been described. In the main, these can be grouped into those longitudinally orientated and transverse incisions (Fig. 32.15).

The transverse incisions have the advantage of being in the skin creases or parallel to them and were developed for this reason. The main disadvantage is an incomplete exposure of the affected fascia and, in particular, the difficulty in displaying adequately the neurovascular bundles during the dissection. Dupuytren, in the first case on which he operated in 1831, used short transverse incisions for removing the longitudinal band and various other similar techniques have been proposed. During the past thirty years the

transverse incision parallel to the distal palmar crease [28] allowing a wide exposure of the fascia in the palm and its complete removal has been used most commonly for the radical type of fasciectomy. Digital extensions of this incision were made in the mid-lateral lines, but, because the skin is often adherent to the underlying contracted fascia, McIndoe introduced his Z-plasty technique using a volar mid-line longitudinal incision over the proximal segment of the digit and converting it into a Z for closure (Fig. 32.15). While

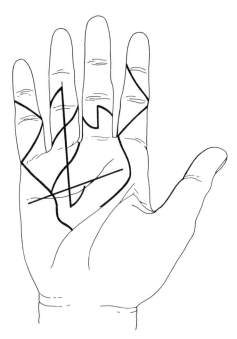

Fig. 32.15. Incisions suitable for removal of the tissue of Dupuytren's disease.

The transverse distal palmar incision described by McIndoe is shown. Digital exposure may be carried out through mid-lateral incisions (not shown in this diagram, see Fig. 7.3). The other incisions are longitudinally orientated in the index and little fingers. A volar zig-zag incision (Bruner) extending proximally in the palm in a sinuous fashion is shown.

In the long finger, the proximal segment has been opened by a Z-plasty. The triangular flaps are curved at the apex with an angle of between 45 and 60°.

In the ring finger, a straight longitudinal incision to expose a longitudinal band has been used. It is closed by converting it into multiple Z-plasty so that the transverse limbs are situated on the distal palmar crease, the crease at the base of the finger and over the proximal interphalangeal joint.

this technique and its variants can give satisfactory access, it is not easy to obtain complete exposure of the digital nerves in the difficult area where they become superficial near the web and inadvertent division was all too common.

To display the neurovascular bundle from the distal palm into the affected digits, it is natural to use a longitudinal skin incision. Straight incisions across transverse skin creases are most unsatisfactory and are frequently followed by scar contractures. However, use of the Z-plasty in order to break up the longitudinal line, results in a very effective way of dealing with the contracted fascia, particularly if there is any co-existent contracture of the skin (Fig. 32.15). Since the introduction of the volar zig-zag incision [29] (Fig. 32.15), it has been used increasingly for Dupuytren's contracture as it gives an extremely good exposure which enables the fascia to be dissected free with full visualization and protection of the neurovascular bundles. There is a strong tendency for the scar to contract unless care is taken to extend the zig-zag to the dorsal end of the transverse digital skin creases.

Whatever skin exposure is used, it is essential that it is planned for each individual problem and that a careful removal of all affected fascia is carried out.

McCash [30], noted that there was a frequent tendency to skin necrosis associated with the transverse distal palmar incision and considered this was due to three factors:

(1) the devitalization of the skin dissected off the adherent fascia,

(2) the tension on the suture line, following correction of the deformities, and

(3) the tendency to formation of haematoma.

After excision of the necrotic skin, the wound often healed extremely well and this prompted him to introduce his technique in which, following the transverse distal palmar incision and resection of the fascia, the wound is left open. This results in an oval skin defect but, as there is no skin tension and any haematoma drains freely, there is a striking absence of postoperative pain and swelling. The defect heals very satisfactorily in the course of a few weeks and eventually leaves a linear scar undetectable from one where the incison has been sutured. The McCash technique has gained increasing popularity and is now used widely by many experienced surgeons. However, no long-term follow-up of a large

series has yet been reported and the method must still remain under trial.

As Dupuytren's disease is such a diverse condition, no two cases being exactly the same, it is important that the surgeon dealing with this problem should be skilful in a variety of techniques, selecting the best available for the individual problem.

Following wide removal of fascia, most surgeons consider it advisable to release the tourniquet in order to obtain complete haemostasis.

Postoperative management

While successful removal of all affected fascia requires a delicate surgical technique and excellent knowledge of anatomy in order to prevent damage to the digital nerves and vessels, the most important part of the further management is the immobilization and postoperative care. If this is neglected, the results will inevitably be unsatisfactory. The most important complication that can develop after surgery for Dupuytren's disease is severe and uncontrolled oedema. This is most likely to develop where there has been extensive dissection and particular in those with vasomotor instability, which can often be anticipated when finding hyperreactive sweating of the hand on preoperative examination, and in those with the broad 'spade' type of hand often found in the heavy labourer. If oedema is allowed to develop, particularly if associated with palmar haematoma, stiffening of the hand and poor function will follow almost inevitably [31]. Oedema should be prevented by careful compression bandaging at the completion of operation and by elevation of the limb for 48–72 hours. A compression bandage of the boxing-glove type (Fig. 8.6) is applied with the metacarpophalangeal joints flexed and the thumb abducted. Compression is applied to the palm through fluffed gauze with orthoband wool and a crepe bandage. This must be applied firmly but not so tightly as to increase the oedema by obstructing venous return or to embarrass circulation. The arm should be elevated postoperatively in a roller towel with the elbow flexed just less than a right angle resting on a pillow and the forearm vertical (Fig. 8.5). If, 48 hours after operation, there is no evidence of swelling of the fingers and good circulation is present, the elevation in bed can be stopped and the patient allowed up but it is important that he walks about with the hand elevated. Severe pain is unusual after operation and it usually indicates either haematoma formation or that the bandage is too tight. In these circumstances, the wound must be inspected and if any haematoma is found, it must be evacuated. The patient is allowed home 48–72 hours after operation. The compression bandage is worn for two weeks following which the stitches are removed and active movements are instituted under the supervision of a physiotherapist. If there is any evidence of skin necrosis the stitches are left in for a further week but the presence of some wound break-down does not preclude active movement. Following operation, the fingers usually extend satisfactorily and the main problem facing the physiotherapist is to induce the patient to regain full active flexion as quickly as possible. This usually occurs within 2 weeks of operation, provided the patient co-operates fully during postoperative mobilization. If the hand becomes stiff and swollen, this usually indicates a lack of active use by the patient who has either been afraid to move the hand as instructed in case the wound opens or, because of pain, has stopped using the hand. It must be stressed to the patient that it is only by working hard with his hand that full active movement will be quickly regained. If it is obvious during the postoperative period that the hand is swelling and that the patient is not achieving satisfactory recovery of movement, it is wise to re-admit to hospital for a further period of elevation.

In some patients, particularly where there has been flexion contractures of the proximal interphalangeal joints for several months or years, it is often impossible to straighten the joints out at operation despite careful removal of all affected fascia [32]. Under these circumstances, capsulotomy or release of collateral ligaments is not advisable as any further gain in extension is likely to be obtained at the expense of flexion for which the patient will not be grateful. This adverse result is particularly liable to occur in a patient who develops uncontrolled oedema of the hand or who has no proper postoperative supervision and physiotherapy.

In the age group in which operation on Dupuytren's contracture is commonly performed, osteoarthritic change in the proximal interphalangeal joints is not unusual and a combination of this with oedema will lead to prolonged stiffness which may become permanent.

In some patients partial correction of contracted proximal interphalangeal joints may be obtained at operation but there is a tendency for the original contracture to recur during the postoperative phase. In these patients, it is wise to apply a splint, which should be worn particularly at night, to extend the fingers as fully as possible (Fig. 32.16).

The other main complication which may prevent a good result is accidental division of a digital nerve or nerves during the difficult dissection. This may be unavoidable in certain difficult cases, particularly in those who had previous surgery but should not be a frequent complication when due care is exercised. If this should happen, the nerve should be repaired immediately.

Where the proximal interphalangeal joint has been flexed for a prolonged period and it is impossible to improve this, the joint may either be arthrodesed after resection of a suitable amount of bone, or, particularly in the case of the little finger, amputation carried out.

To produce good results, operation must be carried out before severe fixed joint contracture develops, and operation before this stage usually preserves a supple hand with an excellent range of movement and function. Skin excision and grafting is seldom required but occasionally, where there has been recurrence and obvious extensive involvement of skin by the Dupuytren's disease, it may be necessary to resect the skin, together with the fascia and replace it by a full thickness skin graft. It is only in exceptional circumstances that a pedicle flap is required for skin replacement. Hueston [33], has stated that where there has been skin replacement, recurrence of the contracture does not occur deep to the graft.

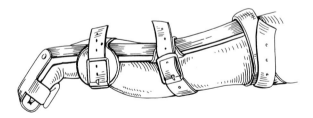

FIG. 32.16. A padded metal splint applied to the dorsum and secured by straps or velcro adjustments, is used essentially at night but can also be worn for periods during the day provided it does not interfere with active exercising. It is used postoperatively for several weeks to prevent recurrence of joint contractures.

Summary

It must be appreciated that the condition is extremely common in many countries, and there is no known treatment other than surgery. A limited fasciectomy, confined to removal of the affected fascia through whichever incision appears most appropriate for the individual patient, is recommended. It is followed by a much quicker recovery of hand function than in the more radical operations. Delicate dissection of all affected fascia with protection of the digital nerves, haemostasis and careful application of a compression bandage with elevation of the limb are essential to success. The care with which the compression bandage is applied and the patient supervised in the postoperative period are probably the two most important factors is ensuring a successful result.

REFERENCES

[1] DUPUYTREN, BARON. Permanent retraction of the fingers produced by an affection of the palmar fascia. *Lancet*, 1834, **2**, 22.

[2] COOPER, A. *A Treatise on Dislocations and Fractures of the Hand*. London, Longmans, 1822.

[3] BOJSEN-MØLLER, F. AND SCHMIDT, L. The palmar aponeurosis and the central spaces of the hand. *Journal of Anatomy*, 1974, **117**, 55.

[4] RITTER, M. A. The anatomy and function of the palmar fascia. *The Hand*, 1973, **5**, 263.

[5] SKOOG, T. The transverse element of the palmar aponeurosis in Dupuytren's contracture. *Scandinavian Journal of Plastic and Reconstructive Surgery*, 1967, **1**, 51.

[6] STACK, H. G. *The Palmar Fascia*. Edinburgh, Churchill Livingstone, 1973.

[7] CLELAND, J. On the cutaneous ligaments of the phalanges. *Journal of Anatomy and Physiology*, 1878, **12**, 526.

[8] GRAYSON, J. The cutaneous ligaments of the digits. *Journal of Anatomy*, 1941, **75**, 164.

[9] JAMES, J. I. P. The relationship of Dupuytren's contracture and epilepsy. *The Hand*, 1969, **1**, 47.

[10] EARLY, P. Population studies in Dupuytren's contracture. *Journal of Bone and Joint Surgery*, 1962, **44B**, 601.

[11] HUESTON, J. T. Incidence of Dupuytren's contracture. *Medical Journal of Australia*, 1960, **2**, 999.

[12] LING, R. S. M. The genetic factor in Dupuytren's disease. *Journal of Bone and Joint Surgery*, 1963, **45B**, 709.

[13] NOBLE, J., BOWSER-RILEY, S., BAIN, A. D. AND LAMB, D. W. Chromosome abnormalities in Dupuytren's disease. *The Lancet*, 1975, **0**, 1282.

[14] HUESTON, J. T. *Dupuytren's Contracture*, Edinburgh, Livingston, 1963.

[15] MACCALLUM, P. AND HUESTON, J. T. The pathology of Dupuytren's contracture. *Australian and New Zealand Journal of Surgery*, 1962, **31**, 241.

[16] MEYERDING, H. W., BLACK, J. R. AND BRODERS, A. C. Etiology and pathology of Dupuytren's contracture. *Surgery, Gynecology and Obstetrics*, 1941, **72**, 582.

[17] MEYERDING, H. W. Dupuytren's contracture. *Archives of Surgery*, 1936, **32**, 320.

[18] HUESTON, J. T. The contracting fibroblast as a clue to Dupuytren's contracture. *The Hand*, 1976, **8**, 10.

[19] SKOOG, T. Dupuytren's contracture: special reference to etiology and improved surgical treatment. *Acta Chirurgica Scandinavia*, 1948, **96**, Supplement, 139.

[20] BOYES, J. H. *Bunnell's Surgery of the Hand*, 5th Edition, Philadelphia, Lippincott, 1970.

[21] HUESTON, J. T. Enzymic fasciotomy. *The Hand*, 1971, **3**, 38.

[22] LUCK, J. V. Dupuytren's contracture. *Journal of Bone and Joint Surgery*, 1959, **41A**, 635.

[23] HUESTON, J. T. Dupuytren's contracture, the trend to conservatism. *Annals of Royal College of Surgeons*, 1965, **36**, 134.

[24] CARR, T. L. Local radical fasciectomy for Dupuytren's contracture. *The Hand*, 1974, **6**, 40.

[25] BRUNER, J. M. The selective treatment of Dupuytren's contracture. *Transactions of the International Society of Plastic Surgeons*, 244, Edinburgh, Livingstone, 1960.

[26] SHAW, M. H. AND BARCLAY, T. L. Dupuytren's contracture: the results of radical fasciectomy. *Transactions of International Society of Plastic Surgeons*, Baltimore, Williams & Wilkins, 1957.

[27] WAKEFIELD, A. R. Dupuytren's contracture. *Surgical Clinics of North America*, 1960, **40**, 183.

[28] MCINDOE, A. H. AND BEARE, R. L. B. The surgical management of Dupuytren's contracture. *American Journal of Surgery*, 1953, **95**, 197.

[29] BRUNER, J. M. Incisions for plastic and reconstructive surgery of the hand. *British Journal of Plastic Surgery*, 1954, **4**, 48.

[30] MCCASH, C. R. The open palm technique in Dupuytren's contracture. *British Journal of Plastic Surgery*, 1974, **27**, 211.

[31] BARCLAY, T. L. Oedema following operation for Dupuytren's contracture. *Plastic and Reconstructive Surgery*, 1959, **23**, 348.

[32] HONNER, R., LAMB, D. W. AND JAMES, J. I. P. Dupuytren's contracture—long-term effects after fasciectomy. *Journal of Bone and Joint Surgery*, 1971, **53B**, 240.

[33] HUESTON, J. T. Digital Wolfe grafts in recurrent Dupuytren's contracture. *Plastic and Reconstructive Surgery*, 1962, **29**, 342.

CHAPTER 33

Miscellaneous Conditions of the Hand

J. C. SEMPLE

A number of conditions commonly seen in the out-patient department are grouped together for convenience in this chapter. As a group they tend to produce relatively minor discomfort and disability. However, the symptoms are often persistent and resistant to or only temporarily relieved by conservative measures such as physiotherapy, splintage or hydrocortisone injections.

Triggering of fingers and thumb (tenosynovitis stenosans)

Catching of fingers or locking of joints is a common problem [1, 2], and may follow minor trauma, be associated with inflammatory synovitis, or occur quite spontaneously.

Flexion deformity of the thumb is seen in neonates and infants [3], and is due to the flexor pollicis longus tendon being swollen and stuck at the proximal opening of the fibrous sheath. It is debatable whether the tendon is swollen, or the sheath narrowed, but the treatment (surgical release of the narrowed sheath) is simple and curative.

Triggering of flexor tendons is not again common until the fourth and fifth decades when the condition occurs spontaneously, particularly in the ring and middle fingers, and in the thumb. The clinical features are quite characteristic, with the patient complaining of pain when the digit is flexed and of a painful snap or click when it is straightened (the trigger finger) which may progress to the state when the digit remains flexed and cannot be extended at all. The pathology is similar to the neonatal situation, with a swollen tendon jammed at the narrowed

mouth of the fibrous flexor sheath. Most cases appear to arise spontaneously, although repetitive work with a finger or thumb accentuates the problem, and it may also be related to the flexor tendon synovitis of rheumatoid disease (see Chapter 25).

De Quervain's tenovaginitis stenosans [4–7]

A similar condition may affect the dorsal tendons to the thumb when the patient complains of pain around the base of the thumb or radial styloid on using the thumb. There is commonly localized swelling and tenderness over the radial styloid. Forced passive flexion of the thumb across the palm reproduces pain at the radial styloid [2], and confirms narrowing of the tendon sheaths of abductor pollicis longus and extensor pollicis brevis.

This condition and triggering of the flexors may respond to simple splintage and rest or the cautious injection of local steroids around the stenosed tendon sheath. If these measures are ineffective, which is common, the affected tendon sheath should be released via a small transverse incision in the distal palm of the hand, volar aspect of base of thumb or over the radial styloid [4, 8]. Care must be taken in approaching these tendon sheaths, to preserve the digital nerves to the finger and thumb, and on the wrist, the terminal branches of the radial nerve.

Unfortunately nerve damage is by no means un-common in these operations and often leads to symptoms much more distressing than the original complaint.

In De Quervain's disease it must be appreciated that

multiple tendons may be present with several compartments which need to be released [5].

A related condition which may affect the tendon sheath of the flexor carpi radialis and cause pain on the volar radial aspect of the wrist has been described by Fitton [9].

Locking joints

The metacarpophalangeal joints, particularly of the index and long fingers, are occasionally prone to spontaneous locking. This is not at all common, but when it occurs, it is very characteristic; the patient presents with the finger held flexed at between 60° and 90° at the metacarpophalangeal joint, which cannot be extended actively or passively. This is quite different from the stuck trigger finger which is acutely flexed at the interphalangeal joints. A number of causes have been described [10–14], but the most likely is broadening of the affected metacarpal head, or an abnormally hooked volar aspect of the condyle, e.g. due to an osteophyte, allowing the volar plate and/or sesamoid bone to catch under the metacarpal head. Forcible manipulation is unlikely to be effective, may do harm, and either conservative splintage, that is resting the whole finger and hand while the joint relaxes itself, or surgical exploration from the lateral or volar aspect of the joint, will reveal the trapped volar plate and allow its release.

Carpometacarpal bossing

An exaggeration of the bony prominences on the dorsum of the base of the second or third metacarpal bones may produce unsightly and occasionally tender bumps (carpal bossing) [15–18]. These may easily be confused with ganglia which are often remarkably hard and may appear almost anywhere on the dorsum of the carpometacarpal area. True metacarpal bosses are usually evident on lateral radiographic films of the wrist but special carpal views may be required [19, 20]. They rarely justify surgical removal, although if they are large enough to be unsightly, or if there is risk of attrition of one of the extensor tendons, removal may be warranted.

In some cases an accessory ossicle (the styloid bone [19, 21]) lies at the base of the metacarpal bone, and it is

this that causes the swelling. Symptoms of aching pain and weakness in the wrist may develop from the pull of the radial carpal extensor tendons. Persistent symptoms justify excision of the ossicle.

Osteoarthritis

Degenerative osteoarthritis mainly affects large weight bearing joints, such as the knee or hip, but certain joints in the hand are also particularly prone. Any joint, of course, can be affected by osteoarthritis following trauma or infection, and in the hand this is well seen around the scaphoid with collapse of an ischaemic proximal pole leading to osteoarthritis between the scaphoid and the lower radius.

Primary osteoarthritis, however, is characteristically seen in the hand in the distal interphalangeal joints [22], and the carpometacarpal joint of the thumb (Fig. 33.1) [23–25]. Stiffness, crepitus, and osteophyte formation in these joints is seen commonly as part of the normal ageing, but these changes may occur in younger patients in the 5th and 6th decades, particularly affecting the carpometacarpal joint of the thumb in the post-

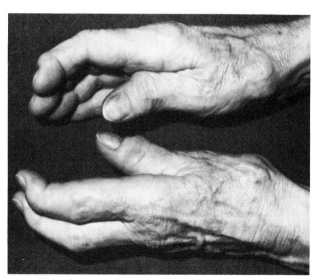

FIG. 33.1. Characteristic deformity in osteoarthritis in the hands affects the carpometacarpal joint, with adduction deformities of the first metacarpal, and narrowing of the thumb–index web space. There is also degeneration and stiffness with flexion contractures of the distal interphalangeal joints.

menopausal female [24, 25]. Osteoarthritic changes in the distal finger joints rarely cause significant symptoms, although patients are often concerned at the disfiguring effect of the osteophytes and deformity. Occasionally there is a case for fusing the joint to reduce deformity or control pain, but conservative measures, including anti-inflammatory medications, such as indomethacin or butazolidin, are generally sufficient.

Osteoarthritic changes in the basal joint of the thumb, however, can give rise to considerable problems quite apart from the pain and discomfort it produces. As degeneration continues, the carpometacarpal joint tends to sublux, with the metacarpal base moving laterally [25] and proximally and the metacarpal shaft developing an adduction contracture. This in turn may lead to a hyper-extension deformity at the metacarpophalangeal joint of the thumb, and general loss of function in the hand with a very poor thumb–index grip and loss of opposition. Correction of an adduction deformity of the first meta-carpal is difficult, and it is better to prevent this occurring by controlling the degenerative changes in the joint. In the early stages of degeneration, conservative medical treatment, and avoidance of excess strain on the joint, will suffice. When pain and weakness becomes pressing, or an adduction deformity is commencing, surgery should be considered. In some cases there may be excessive capsular laxity and a ligament–soft tissue repair is indicated [25]. When radiographs establish loss of articular cartilage, and subluxation of the joint, the choice lies between excision of the trapezium (with or without prosthetic replacement), and fusion of the carpo-metacarpal joint. Excision of the trapezium, possibly replacing its bulk with a portion of the nearby flexor carpi radialis or palmaris tendon [26], is a straight-forward operation which generally relieves the pain of osteoarthritis, but there is a definite tendency for post-operative subluxation.

Excision of the trapezium, and its replacement by a prosthesis, usually silastic [27], provides a more stable basal thumb joint and a useful degree of movement (p. 381).

In those requiring heavy work for many years, fusion of the carpometacarpal joint may be preferable. This procedure should not be carried out where there is any arthritic change in other carpal joints, especially the scaphoid/trapezium joint [27], as carpometacarpal joint fusion would simply accentuate these secondary changes.

Gout

Gout is a deposition of monosodium urate in the tissues which may affect the hand (Fig. 33.2), although more commonly the initial lesion occurs in the foot. In a sudden, acute, painful, red and swollen joint in the hand gout must, however, always be considered [28]; the diagnosis may be confirmed by a plasma uric acid concentrate of 7 mg/100 ml (6 mg/100 ml in females) and higher and by the rapid symptomatic response to colchicine or phenylbutazone. It is unusual to find radio-logical changes in the hand in early gout, although chronic cases may show erosive periarticular changes. Pseudo-gout, a less common and less acute variety of crystal deposition arthritis, in which calcium pyro-phosphate is precipitated in articular cartilage, may show radiological changes in the wrist joint, particularly in the triangular cartilage (disc) at the head of the ulna.

Acute gouty arthritis is entirely a medical problem [29], and there is no indication for surgery on the inflamed joint. Chronic gout does, however, produce urate deposits in the subcutaneous tissues, and these

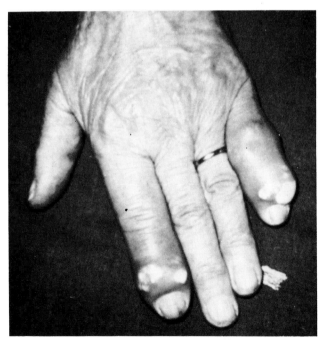

Fig. 33.2. Subcutaneous inflammation related to gouty tophi in the fingers may require a simple excision and curettage.

tophi can be large and troublesome in the digit [30]. They may require surgical removal, but are prone to recurrence, and the patient must appreciate that strict medical control by drugs is the only way to prevent further problems in the hand.

Osteochondritis in the wrist and hand

Certain bones in the hand, particularly in the carpus, are prone to ischaemic changes. These may occur following trauma as in the proximal pole of the scaphoid following fracture through the waist, or spontaneously as in Thiemann's disease (osteochondritis of the basal epiphysis of the middle phalanx of the fingers).

Kienböck's disease (avascular necrosis of the lunate bone), was described in 1910 and generally presents as a painful wrist, with no clear history of specific trauma. Rooker and Goodfellow have described its frequent occurrence in adult spastic patients who tend to hold their wrists in excessive flexion. All the carpal bones have a relatively precarious blood supply as they are largely covered by articular cartilage, and blood vessels can only penetrate through relatively small ligamentous attachments on their volar and dorsal surfaces (p. 17). The lunate appears to have a particularly fragile blood supply, and either spontaneously or following minor trauma, its vascularity is compromised and radiological changes appear. The bone becomes relatively radiodense, and collapses in a proximal–distal fashion, with eventual osteoarthritic changes occurring between the surrounding carpal bones and the radius.

A mild form of this condition may be responsible for inexplicable symptoms of pain and stiffness in the wrists of teenage girls which generally settle following a few weeks rest in a plaster.

Once the radiological changes of collapse become established (Fig. 33.3), however, a decision has to be taken regarding surgical intervention. Simple removal of the collapsed lunate bone may provide temporary improvement, but will lead to further osteoarthritic changes in the wrist. Replacement by an acrylic or silastic prosthesis is possible although care must be taken in the immediate postoperative phase to prevent dislocation, usually dorsal, of the prosthesis. In patients with heavy manual occupations, prosthetic replacement may not be strong enough for their purposes, and

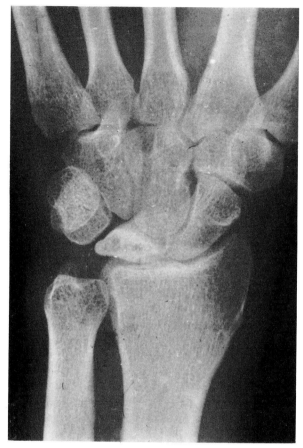

FIG. 33.3. Characteristic changes in osteochondritis of the lunate bone (Kienböck's disease) are collapse and density of the bone, with commencing osteoarthritis.

change to a lighter job or the alternative of a wrist fusion if the symptoms persist may have to be considered.

The management of foreign bodies in the hand

The introduction of foreign bodies into the hand is a common occurrence. Most of these are metallic, wooden or glass. Patients are usually, but not invariably, aware of the entry of the foreign body and a careful history will usually elicit the nature and mechanism of any wound and the likelihood of some foreign material being retained.

If there is any possibility of a retained foreign body

the care of the wound and its management are very important. If the entry wound is small then it becomes necessary to enlarge this using the type of incisions recommended in Chapter 7. It is essential that this should be done in a bloodless field using a pneumatic tourniquet and either general anaesthesia, brachial plexus block or intravenous Bier's technique.

Sometimes the entry of the foreign body is inconspicuous and the victim may initially be unaware of its presence. If the material is relatively inert the foreign body may cause no symptoms or signs and only become evident at some later date, when some low grade infection may develop, or it may track to the surface and cause local tenderness or discharge itself.

Radiography is always advisable to try and locate a suspected foreign body as many are radioopaque, particularly those of a metallic nature. Splinters of wood may occasionally show up and also pieces of glass if there is a lead element present.

The mere presence of a foreign body is no indication for its removal unless it is causing symptoms. Great care is necessary with removal as much more damage may be done by careless surgery without a tourniquet than from leaving the foreign body alone. It is important to try and localize it accurately before its removal, and if it is radioopaque this can be done by using metallic markers on the skin surface to localize it by radiography or to make use of the image intensifier.

Many metallic foreign bodies remain within the hand without any symptoms or cause for alarm. Asymptomatic foreign bodies do not require removal and this is especially the case when they are multiple as for example with lead shot.

In the case of wooden foreign bodies most are radio lucent and therefore impossible to localize by radiography. Fortunately many are relatively inert and cause little trouble but some woods have a very toxic effect on tissue, particularly if they have a high resin content or if they are covered with creosote or toxic aniline dyes. These materials may provoke quite an acute inflammatory reaction and unless the foreign material is quickly removed and the wound drained thoroughly may provoke considerable induration and fibrosis.

Sudeck's post traumatic osteodystrophy

This condition generally follows minor trauma to the upper limb or hand but may develop after medical conditions such as myocardial infarction, herpes zoster or the painful shoulder syndrome. Pain is a prominent symptom, the joints of the hand become stiff and function limited, and signs of sympathetic hyperactivity may become evident. This complication is largely preventable and in units where there is careful and early supervision of exercise and active movement of the upper limb and hand following injury and operations and where there is a good physiotherapy service, it is rare. Once the condition has developed, it is difficult to treat but minor changes respond to activity and physiotherapy. Where marked dystrophic changes have taken place and evidence of disuse osteoporosis becomes obvious, the outlook is gloomy and progress is poor. A radiograph shows the characteristic patchy rarefaction. The hand tends to remain swollen, cold to the touch and of a bluey-white colour, very sensitive to handling and without function. Many cases have thickening of the palmar fascia [31]. The cause of this condition is unknown but it appears to occur more frequently in patients who are emotionally unstable and the changes are often attributed to psychosomatic factors for this reason.

There is some evidence that, in this more advanced stage of the condition, in addition to intensive continuous physiotherapy, oral prednisolone may be helpful. Sympathetic block or sympathectomy has been recommended but is seldom fully effective. Its development handicaps any attempt at reconstructive surgery which would have to be delayed until complete recovery—often many months. Should this condition complicate reconstructive procedures the results will be very poor.

REFERENCES

[1] FAHEY, J. J. AND BOLLINGER, J. A. Trigger finger in adults and children. *Journal of Bone and Joint Surgery*, 1954, **36A,** 1200.

[2] LIPSCOMB, P. R. Tenosynovitis of the hand and wrist. In *Clinical Orthopaedics*, vol. 13, ed. A. P. De Palma. Philadelphia, Lippincott, 1959.

[3] SPREECHER, E. E. Trigger thumb in infants. *Journal of Bone and Joint Surgery*, 1949, **31A,** 672.

[4] FAITHFUL, D. K. AND LAMB, D. W. De Quervain disease. A clinical review. *The Hand*, 1971, **3,** 23.

[5] KEON-COHEN, B. De Quervain's disease. *Journal of Bone and Joint Surgery*, 1951, **33B,** 96.

[6] LAPIDUS, P. W. Stenosing tenovaginitis. *Surgical Clinics of North America*, 1953, **33,** 1317.

[7] MUCKART, R. D. De Quervain's disease. In *Clinical Orthopaedics*, vol. 33, ed. A. P. De Palma. Philadelphia, Lippincott, 1964.

[8] WOODS, T. H. E. De Quervain's disease. A plea for early operation. *British Journal of Surgery*, 1964, **51,** 358.

[9] FITTON, J. M., SHEA, F. W. AND GOLDIE, W. Lesions of the flexor carpi radialis tendon and sheath causing pain at the wrist. *Journal of Bone and Joint Surgery*, 1968, **50B,** 359.

[10] ASTON, J. N. Locked middle finger. *Journal of Bone and Joint Surgery*, 1960, **42B,** 75.

[11] BLOOM, M. H. AND BRYAN, R. S. Locked index finger caused by hyperflexion and entrapment of sesamoid bone. *Journal of Bone and Joint Surgery*, 1965, **47A,** 1383.

[12] FLATT, A. E. Recurrent locking of an index finger. *Journal of Bone and Joint Surgery*, 1958, **40A,** 1128.

[13] GOODFELLOW, J. W. AND WEAVER, J. P. A. Locking of the metacarpo-phalangeal joint. *Journal of Bone and Joint Surgery*, 1961, **43B,** 772.

[14] YANCEY, H. A., Jr. AND HOWARD, L. D., Jr. Locking of the metacarpo-phalangeal joint. *Journal of Bone and Joint Surgery*, 1963, **44A,** 380.

[15] ARTEZ, T. D. AND POSCH, J. L. The carpo-metacarpal boss. *Journal of Bone and Joint Surgery*, 1973, **55A,** 747.

[16] BOYES, J. H. *Bunnell's Surgery of the Hand*, 4th ed., pp. 292–293. Philadelphia, Lippincott, 1964.

[17] CARTER, R. M. Carpal boss: a commonly overlooked deformity of the carpus. *Journal of Bone and Joint Surgery*, 1941, **23,** 935.

[18] CURTISS, P. H. The hunchback carpal bone. *Journal of Bone and Joint Surgery*, 1961, **43A,** 392.

[19] BASSOE, E. AND BASSOE, H. H. The styloid and carpal bossing disease. *American Journal of Roentgenology*, 1955, **74,** 886.

[20] DOROSIN, N. AND DAVIS, J. G. Carpal boss. *Radiology*, 1956, **66,** 235.

[21] KOOSTRA, G., HUFFSTADT, A. C. AND KAVER, J. M. G. The styloid bone. A clinical and embryological study. *The Hand*, 1974, **6,** 185.

[22] RADEN, E. L., PARKER, H. G. AND PAUL, I. L. Pattern of degenerative arthritis, preferential involvement of distal finger joints. *Journal of Bone and Joint Surgery*, 1972, **54A,** 908.

[23] AUNE, S. Osteoarthritis of first carpo-metacarpal joint. An investigation of 22 cases. *Acta chirurgica Scandinavica*, 1955, **109,** 449.

[24] BURTON, R. I. Basal joint arthrosis of the thumb. *Orthopedic Clinics of North America*, 1973, **4,** 331.

[25] EATON, R. G. AND LITTLER, J. W. A study of the basal joints of the thumb. *Journal of Bone and Joint Surgery*, 1969, **51A,** 661.

[26] FROIMSON, A. I. Tendon arthroplasty of the trapezio-metacarpal joint. *Clinical Orthopedics*, 1970, **70,** 191.

[27] SWANSON, A. B. Disabling arthritis at the base of the thumb. *Journal of Bone and Joint Surgery*, 1972, **54A,** 456.

[28] TALBOTT, J. H. The diagnosis and treatment of gout. *Medical Clinics of North America*, 1961, **45,** 1489.

[29] WALLACE, L. The treatment of gout. *Arthritis and Rheumatism*, 1972, **15,** 317.

[30] STRAUB, L. R., SMITH, J. W., CARPENTER, G. K. AND KIETZ, G. H. The surgery of gout in the upper extremity. *Journal of Bone and Joint Surgery*, 1961, **43A,** 731.

[31] PLEWES, L. W. Sudeck's atrophy in the hand. *Journal of Bone and Joint Surgery*, 1956, **38B,** 195.

CHAPTER 34

Psychology of the Deformed Hand

R. C. B. AITKEN

The principles underlying clinical management of a patient with a deformed hand do not differ from those of one with any serious disability. Attention is required to all relevant factors, psychological and social no less than surgical. The purpose of this chapter is to encourage surgeons themselves to provide a comprehensive approach to the care of their patients.

Any disability has a psychological effect, perhaps none more than of the hands, as their deformity can have important social consequences. Functional potential of the human hand can give a full range to many activities, from the accomplishments of an artist or musician to that of an unskilled worker, from a casual greeting to signs of intimate affection, even from dependency on others for help to undertake simple everyday bodily functions right to the extremes of human endeavour.

Learning full use of the hands is an obvious feature of development and growth, the degree of attainment determining the economic and leisure activities throughout life. Capability to learn new skills influences the outcome of any disordered function; this capability is related to emotional and intellectual factors as well as to neuromuscular and orthopaedic ones. New skills to be acquired by those with cerebral degenerative disease, however mild, are so much poorer than by those with youthful brains. Novel skills can be achieved by the younger person not only in the deformed hand but in other parts of the body such as the feet and mouth.

Learning of new skills requires determination influenced by personality and motivation with success most likely in those used to face a challenge.

Hand deformity, unlike that of a lower limb, is likely to be visible unless unusually well masked. Even when using a cover, however well flesh-coloured and shaped, it is likely to be conspicuous. Distress may arise from apprehension of the responses of others to the appearance and to clumsiness of movement.

Clinical assessment of personality

It should never be said that the psychiatrist has a monopoly of skills in assessment of personality. Any doctor who knows his patient well acquires much of the necessary information, though not always appreciating its significance.

Information should always be sought systematically from more than one source. When patient and relative describe independently the same event similarly, it is likely to be true. Information should be obtained on more than one occasion; apprehension at the first interview is likely to become less, as doctor–patient confidence develops. It is chiefly for this reason that continuity of contact in clinical management is so desirable. It is best to listen to what the patient wants to say and to elicit and observe the evidence confirming the story. Patients seldom wish to deceive but some may do so unintentionally with the true significance of the information missed by the doctor.

Let us consider an example. A patient after healing of an injury experiences pain during finger movement and naturally wishes that something be done for its relief; he complains to the doctor of severe symptoms. It is not difficult to imagine that he could feel foolish if he complained of trivial pain, thinking that little might then be done for him. His wife may not confirm his story and mentions that he can still button his shirt, write his pool coupon and sleep undisturbed in front of the television. On examination he may not appear to be distressed, pain being communicated only when the hand is examined and not when making similar movements in undressing. Only in the second interview, if even then, does the patient reveal that: (1) he fears to return to work in case of further injury, (2) he is frustrated by inadequate compensation, and (3) he feels guilty for having laid aside the safety guard at the time of injury. It may well be his wife who mentions that his brother had to change from skilled to unskilled work after a road accident or that her husband has been drinking more heavily than usual and now faces financial hardship with the rent being in arrears.

In difficult cases the only way to detect relevant information is to make systematic enquiry (more detailed method can be obtained in most standard textbooks of psychiatry or in '*A Companion to Medical Studies*'). The following topics are suggested:

Personal history

The life history should be taken from birth through childhood, including early homelife. School and work record provides the facts about attainment with a comment on the financial affairs, including housing arrangements. Information on duration and harmony of the marriage and about the children can give a good indication of the quality of close personal relationships. Enquiries are made here about sexual experience and adjustment, and whether they meet the expectation of affectionate expression.

Details of the family background, particularly of contact with parents and siblings, can indicate the kind of support experienced in earlier years and what could become available now if help is needed. Medical and psychiatric history is obviously important.

Personality appreciation

Much of the information in the personal history will allow appraisal of the life-style. It will distinguish obviously an isolated vagrant from a socially successful business executive. More details however about certain aspects can be of value in order to appreciate the patient's usual way of coping with life's challenges. The keys to this lie in understanding the usual relationships the patient has with other people and the moods he experiences in various circumstances, and how he is likely to receive and use the help from medical and social services. His previous response to adversity, particularly to loss, is an important consideration. He may be prone to excessive anxiety in fearful situations or to denial of expected feelings (a not uncommon response). He may be liable to misery or apathy, or may respond to frustration with intolerance and anger. The degree to which such responses distress the patient or disturb others can be crucial in rehabilitation.

The interests a person has can indicate his social adjustment. His habits regarding sleep, food, smoking and alcohol may be very relevant to his management. While under strain, (1) hypnotics and analgesics, to which he can become addicted, can be unnecessarily prescribed, (2) overeating and underexercise can lead to troublesome obesity, and (3) increased consumption of alcohol can produce related problems, perhaps precipitated by enforced idleness.

Personality traits are little more than adjectives describing common features. For brief professional communication these may be grouped into types such as hysterical, obsessional or sociopathic but such classification renders categories that are not mutually exclusive nor an allocation known to be wholly consistent.

Expected responses to stress

Anxiety

It is normal for people to experience anxiety when faced suddenly with a catastrophic event such as a serious hand injury. Anxiety produces distractability and forgetfulness, patients often misunderstanding information conveyed while they are under strain as at the outpatient clinic or on the ward round. Sleeplessness is common.

Muscular tension and trembling, restlessness and fidgeting, incoordination and impaired performance are all relevant to hand function. Pain may be experienced at tendon insertion; indeed its threshold is influenced by the mood. Flushing, sweating (particularly of the palms and forehead) and dry mouth are common.

Palpitations, tachycardia and transient hypertension can occur. Complaints of fatigue should be no surprise. Anorexia, dyspepsia and diarrhoea are more likely to be due to mood disturbance than to organic disease. Reduced libido, impotence and mental disturbance are also to be expected in someone coping with adversity.

Depression

Apathy, self-absorption and a search for blame are common features, particularly after loss such as can occur in hand injury. The feelings are similar to bereavement, which time usually relieves. Prolonged corrective surgical programme, particularly when outcome is uncertain, will disturb even the most robust. Search for blame may go no further than the patient himself, unnecessary self-blame being a feature of depressive illness. Inner miseries may be revealed, even on specific enquiry, only to those close to the patient. Such feelings should be taken into account when planning treatment.

Hostility

In some people insecurity precipitates arrogance and aggression. The search for blame may be directed at others, not always justly. Failure to keep outpatient appointments or even just arriving perpetually late can sometimes be the way the patient expresses his annoyance. Intolerance of frustration such as in awaiting an ambulance or in undertaking a difficult task, can be conveyed more forcibly than might be expected. Criticism and complaints about the activities of others such as nurses or casualty officers, perhaps even justified, may be voiced indirectly in a way that suggests little forgiveness for the occasional imperfections of others. These hostile feelings may linger as resentment, in certain circumstances precipitating litigation. Initiation of legal proceedings may be as much in order to justify these feelings by established proof of blame as to recover compensation.

Normal defences

Everyone has some kind of defence which allows him to cope with life's unfavourable circumstances and this is likely to be required when faced with hand surgery for however trivial reasons. The importance of the use of the hand and the helplessness when its function is limited is all too apparent. Exaggeration of these defences may occur to the extent of recognizable psychiatric disorder; even at lesser degree they determine the extent and nature of the patient's distress and his progress.

Many of these defences are exaggerations of the inherent personality traits. Even should the feelings be painful, denial of the experience to the extent of stoicism is not uncommon. An *obsessional* person prone to pay excessive attention to detail, to display bigotry and litigiousness, and to be insensitive to the emotional needs of others, is likely to be even more so when coping with disability. A *hysterical* person can be somewhat uncontrollable in her/his expression of emotion, very dependent on others and yet with shallow emotional involvement and perhaps hypochondriacal. She/he is likely to behave even more so at loss of vital function, particularly one that is visible and that requires persistence to achieve recovery. Even in the most stable person, increased dependence on others for emotional support is likely.

Psychiatric disorders

Anxiety state or a depressive illness may be precipitated by injury. *Anxiety* may persist for irrational reasons and may occur in certain situations which will be avoided by the patient; he has developed a phobia. A social phobia is not uncommon, perhaps related to feelings of stigma associated with deformity or with reluctance to return to a place of injury. Intense anxiety may be associated with a mental state of depersonalization in which there are abnormal body feelings akin to psychosis.

Hysteria in pure form is rare nowadays. The relative importance of psychological versus physical factors in impairment of function and prolongation of symptoms in patients with a deformed hand is a commonly drawn distinction often questioned. For diagnostic or legal purposes this division is seldom a strict dichotomy; nor even is the distinction between hysteria and malingering. Claims for payment of compensation can be a powerful motive inhibiting improvement. Some awareness of exaggeration of functional impairment is usually present in the patient, but insight into the social circumstances and consequences is commonly deficient in one claiming compensation, such as into the true effects on himself and his family of prolonged idleness and litigious behaviour. Disturbance by social isolation or exposure to additional risk such as further surgery is rarely appreciated.

The incidence of hand injury is greater in those with psychiatric illness. *Mental deficiency* and *dementia* render the person prone to both injury and to complications resulting from neglect of its treatment. *Alcoholism* and *psychopathic states* are associated with increased rates of industrial and road traffic accidents. *Drug addiction* with intravenous agents may commonly lead to infection of the upper limb. The delusions of *schizophrenia* may lead to a patient suffering a bizarre self-injury, not uncommonly of the hand.

It should be remembered, however, that psychological factors seldom play an important part in prolonging disability in someone of undoubtedly mature and sound personality, unless psychiatric illness has intervened.

Clinical management

Motivation and morale

Many therapeutic measures require the full cooperation of the patient and his participation; when enthusiasm is lacking in either staff or patient, progress will be impaired. Apathy, perhaps due to depression or disinterest, is a sign of low motivation. Some degree of anxiety about the outcome motivates the patient's efforts, but excessive worry may restrict his activities in order to protect the hand from his imagined fears. Intolerance of frustration to the extent of perpetual annoyance with adversities will diminish the patient's attention to a set task; his thoughts can dwell so easily on irrelevancies, such as litigation or hostility directed to those trying to help. Motivation can be much enhanced when there is a positive relationship with staff who themselves radiate confidence. Feelings and behaviour which reflect apathy, excessive anxiety or anger reduce motivation; attention to these moods in clinical management should be worthwhile. Many patients are not highly motivated. Staff need to be tolerant of their foibles, not responding by chastising or rejecting those who recurrently express their annoyance, either overtly or indirectly. Staff should not allow however the patients to manipulate situations because of the disturbed feelings. Staff should be also

clear in their instructions and expectations so that patients with reduced motivation are unequivocally aware of the reasons for insufficient progress.

Learning new skills

Reduced function requires learning of new skills to compensate for the loss. While awaiting the outcome of treatment, the patient may learn better use of an existing alternative, such as of the left hand if previously right-handed; a substantial effort may be needed to write neatly with the other hand. Sometimes it is forgotten that half the population have an I.Q. less than average. Intellect influences performance of many tasks; motor ability and hand-eye coordination are impaired when intelligence is low. Brain damage suffered in adulthood affects performance, while verbal fluency and vocabulary are unaffected. Hence the effects of this damage may not be suspected on casual clinical contact as the patient speaks in the same way as before; yet the patient, particularly an elderly one, may have become slow in comprehending instructions and learning anything new. With dementia, a short-term memory disturbance prohibiting new learning and resulting in disorientation is present.

It is important to reward the desired behaviour either by appreciative smile for success or by providing something more tangible like payment in employment therapy. It should be remembered that the reward should go to the patient who is progressing rather than to the one who is less cooperative. The opposite happens often as the staff have to spend more time with more troublesome patients; they soon detect this and seek staff attention as and when they wish.

Patients can feel anxious when expected to undertake tasks which involve some risk such as when returning to the use of machinery. They should be exposed to the risk in a graded fashion so that they remain comfortable and achieve confidence sufficient to accomplish the task.

Therapeutic importance of staff–patient relationship

Any member of staff can contribute to the patient's benefit in two ways: firstly by his professional skill and secondly by his capability to relate to the patient in a way which assists his recovery. In many instances the latter may be as important as the former because the patients can become very dependent on individual members of the staff or even on the place of attendance. Some patients may make excessive demands with the result that the staff, particularly inexperienced, become overinvolved in the patient's needs, especially emotional ones.

The patient should be faced with an attitude optimal in assisting him in recovery of his independence. The skill is to help the patient help himself and not to do for the patient what he can do for himself. This may require self-discipline and almost superhuman patience and even be contrary to the caring instinct natural to the health professions.

Continuity of contact is desirable so that both patient and staff appreciate the needs of each other, certainly when the treatment programme is to be long. It is preferable that the contact should not become too intense nor on the other hand too detached. Changes of staff should not occur precipitiously otherwise patients can feel rejected.

FURTHER READING

LEVINE, S. & SCOTCH, N. *Social Stress*, Chicago, Aldine, 1970. L

MCDANIEL, J. W. *Physical Disability and Human Behaviour*, 2nd Ed. New York, Pergamon Press, 1978.

MCGRATH, J. *Social and Psychological Factors in Stress*, New York, Rinehart and Wilson, 1970.

PASSMORE, R. & ROBSON, J. S. eds. *A Companion to Medical Studies,* Vol. 3, part 2, Chap. 35. Edinburgh, Blackwell Scientific Publications, 1974.

SHORTZ, F. C. *Psychological Aspects of Physical Illness and Disability*. New York, Macmillan, 1975.

CHAPTER 35

Reconstructive Procedures in the Disabled Hand

D. W. LAMB

Planning of treatment and general principles of management [1, 2]

Planning surgical reconstruction of a disabled hand involves many factors but, in general, should concentrate first on placing the skeleton in the desired position, release of contractures and provision of good soft tissue and skin cover. Restoration of lost nerve deficit is the next priority followed where required by tendon repair, graft or transfer. Consideration of the following points is thus required.

Skeletal positioning

The joints of the wrist and hand should be positioned for optimum function and least stiffness. This position may be temporary during treatment when it is that used for early immobilization after extensive hand injuries consisting of metacarpophalangeal flexion, interphalangeal extension and abduction of the thumb (see Fig. 8.6, p. 123). If the positioning is to be permanent resulting in either ankylosis or operative fixation of the joints, then the rules governing the best position of fixation for each joint must be observed (pp. 494–496).

Skin cover

It is important that the skin cover should have good sensation in the vital tactile areas. The best skin is provided by that of the hand itself and, where possible, local flaps are used. If these are not available, con-

sideration should be given to split skin grafts except where gliding planes under skin are required for tendon function or where there is a poorly vascularized defect. Flaps from a distance would then have to be planned (see Chapter 9).

Restoration of grasp

The type of grasp which can be provided will depend on the severity of the lesion. Where possible, one tries to provide both precision and power grips. Precision handling depends for its minimal requirements on a thumb of as much length and mobility as possible and on a finger against which it can actively oppose.

In power grasping, the movement of the fingers required to wrap around the object depends on mobile interphalangeal joints. Where these objectives cannot be obtained, the more rudimentary action of pincers or of hook is all that can be provided. For a simple pincer action, two parts must be able to oppose each other, one of which must be mobile; sensation is desirable.

Sensibility

Painful or insensitive fingers are seldom used. Restoration of sensation by repair of any peripheral nerve is desirable within a year of injury. Some degree of protective sensation is obtained by late repair of nerves up to at least five years and sometimes longer with microsurgical technique and nerve grafting (pp. 192–197). When the skin of an important tactile surface has been lost, a sensitive skin flap can be transferred from less important areas, e.g. by local rotation flaps and the neurovascular island transfer (p. 503).

Physiotherapy (Chapter 36) and splintage (Chapter 37) are usually required between each stage and sufficient time must elapse to allow soft tissue induration to resolve. Following severe hand injuries, the reconstructive programme is likely to be a long and tedious one with many operations, and a change of occupation and retraining may be required. The full co-operation of the patient is necessary and a prolonged programme requires the support of many special services.

A realistic appraisal by the surgeon of the needs of the patient is essential and as Littler [3] has said: 'To commit a patient to an unreasonable series of elective surgical procedures of uncertain end is to be condemned'.

SKELETAL POSITIONING

Arthrodesis of joints of the hand [4, 5, 6]

Arthrodesis of the joints of the fingers and thumb may be required.

(1) For destruction of joints due to rheumatoid arthritis (Chapter 25), osteoarthrosis, psoriatic arthritis or in joints damaged by infection.

(2) Following severe destruction of the joint by trauma.

(3) Very occasionally for paralysis.

The choice usually lies between arthrodesis or arthroplasty (p. 496). Excellent results are obtained from arthrodesis in the distal and proximal interphalangeal joints of the fingers and the interphalangeal and metacarpophalangeal joints of the thumb and this is more suitable at the present time than arthroplasty at these sites. Arthroplasty, however, gives more satisfactory results in the metacarpophalangeal joints of the fingers and the carpometacarpal joint of the thumb.

The distal interphalangeal joint

This should be arthrodesed in a degree of flexion, increasing from radial to ulnar side from about 15–20° at the index finger to 35° at the little finger.

Technique

This should be precise and gentle. The joint is exposed by a sinuous dorsal incision with the transverse limb over the distal crease or by a T-incision (Fig. 35.1). The articular cartilage is excised to give firm bony contact between the head of the middle phalanx and the base of the distal phalanx at the required angle. It is important not to interfere with the nail bed. The position is best maintained by Kirschner wires inserted with the power drill. To ensure that the correct angle and rotation is obtained a Kirschner wire is inserted through the pulp and across the joint. Once the position has been checked, and firm contact of bony surfaces ensured, one or more oblique Kirschner wires are driven across the joint to control rotation.

If good fixation is secured by two oblique wires, the pulp pin can be removed. Kirschner wires which are to be left in should be cut off immediately deep to the skin. It is seldom that bone chips are required unless there is some bone loss.

Where bone destruction has made it difficult to get good apposition, an alternative is the use of the small

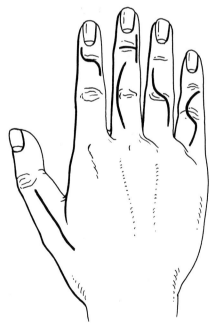

FIG. 35.1. Incisions used in arthrodesis to expose dorsum of interphalangeal joints and metacarpophalangeal joint of thumb.

polypropylene peg [7] which can be very effective and is usually followed over the course of several months by firm, bony ankylosis.

The proximal interphalangeal joint

Arthrodesis at this joint results in a very useful finger provided there is good metacarpophalangeal and terminal joint function. The index and long fingers are fused in a position to give good precision pinch to the thumb whereas the ulnar two digits require the joint slightly more flexed so as to give good power grip. The joints are therefore arthrodesed in an increasing degree of flexion from index at 30° to little finger at 45–50°.

Technique

This is similar to that for the distal joint but the straight stabilizing wire is inserted through the dorsum of the proximal or middle phalanx to cross the joint (Fig. 35.2). If the finger has been in a stiff straight position there may be difficulty with skin closure when it is brought into the flexed position and the skin incision should be planned to allow for this (Fig. 35.1).

If there is extensive bony destruction the use of the polypropylene peg of appropriate angle is very helpful [7].

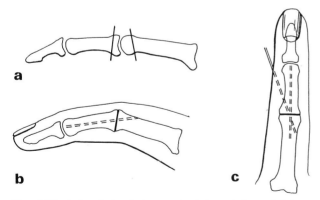

FIG. 35.2. Arthrodesis of the proximal interphalangeal joint (a) line of bone resection to get correct angle of arthrodesis. (b) Lateral view of finger showing firm co-aptation of joint surfaces with angle as for index finger and held by longitudinal Kirschner wire. (c) Dorsal view of finger showing longitudinal and oblique Kirschner wires used for fixation.

The metacarpophalangeal joints of the fingers

Arthrodesis of these joints is seldom indicated and arthroplasty gives better results (p. 377). Where necessary the joint is arthodesed about 25° flexed at index increasing to 45° at little finger.

The interphalangeal joint of the thumb

A position of 20–30° of flexion and about 10° of pronation gives a very stable thumb for pinch to the other digits and for power grasp. The technique is similar to that for the distal interphalangeal joint of the finger.

The metacarpophalangeal joint of the thumb

The normal range of flexion movement at this joint varies from 0 to nearly 90°, the average being about 20–30°. The loss of this amount of movement by arthrodesis is well compensated and the function is usually excellent. Satisfactory arthrodesis is usually easily obtained and the joint should be fixed in about 10° of flexion, 5–10° of abduction and the same degree of pronation so as to allow satisfactory pinch to the other pulps.

Technique

The joint is exposed through a dorsal straight or curved skin incision (Fig. 35.1) deepened between the short and long extensor tendons. The articular surface is removed retaining a ball and socket arrangement of the head of the metacarpal and the base of the phalanx. The use of crossed Kirschner wires gives good fixation, but if firm compression is desired the Charnley technique can be used with parallel pins through metacarpal and phalanx held in compression clamps.

Harrison has described the successful use of the straight polypropylene peg for fixation of this joint and in one hundred consecutive cases firm bony arthrodesis was obtained [8].

The carpometacarpal joint of the thumb

Arthrodesis of the trapeziometacarpal joint often relieves pain and gives stability. It will maintain strength of grip and would be indicated where heavy manual work is required [9]. However, the subsequent restriction of mobility limits overall hand function and prevents the hand being flattened in confined spaces. If other trapezial joints are affected this procedure will not be effective in relieving the pain completely. In addition sound fusion is not readily achieved. The joint is exposed by a dorsal incision, the terminal branches of the radial nerve being protected. The approach to the joint is between the extensor pollicis brevis and abductor pollicis longus tendons and the insertion of the latter is reflected. Following excision of the joint surfaces the bone ends are apposed and require some form of internal fixation to provide stability and compression. This can be achieved by cross Kirschner-wires followed by external immobilization in a plaster or by using parallel Kirschner-wires with external compression. Eaton [10] describes immobilization in the 'fist position' with the first metacarpal set at an angle of 35–40° abduction and 20° extension relative to the second metacarpal. He considers this position critical and it is maintained by cross Kirschner wires and an additional Kirschner wire between first and second metacarpals.

Postoperative routine following arthrodesis of small joints of the hand

If firm fixation by Kirschner wires is ensured external support may not be required. If there is any doubt about the care which will be exercised by the patient an additional plaster slab is advisable.

Fusion of the joint is usual within 6–8 weeks and should be checked by radiograph. The Kirschner wires are then removed under local anaesthesia.

Arthroplasty

Osteoarthrosis in the hand most frequently affects the terminal interphalangeal joints and the carpometacarpal joint of the thumb (Chapter 33).

Arthroplasty is not indicated for the terminal interphalangeal joints, arthrodesis being the procedure of choice.

Very occasionally osteoarthritic changes of sufficient severity to justify surgery occur in the metacarpophalangeal joints, particularly of the index and long fingers. This may occur spontaneously but occasionally results from injuries to the joints. If pain and disability warrant joint replacement, the operative procedure is as described in rheumatoid arthritis (Chapter 25).

The Swanson silastic prosthesis can give very satisfactory results [22]. Goldner [23] recently reported experiences with the Niebauer silicone/dacron prosthesis at the metacarpophalangeal joint. In the metacarpophalangeal joints arthroplasty is preferable to arthrodesis except where the hand is to be used for heavy manual work.

Severe derangement of the proximal interphalangeal joints may result from fractures or dislocations and lead to sufficient disability to justify arthroplasty particularly in a young person. Satisfactory results at this joint have been obtained by the use of the Niebauer prosthesis [24]. Iselin [25] has also reported good results but in most circumstances arthrodesis of the painful joint is the procedure of choice.

In the management of the painful osteoarthritic joint at the base of the thumb, however, arthroplasty is frequently required.

Osteoarthrosis at the base of the thumb

The joints of the trapezium allow the wide range of movement enjoyed by the thumb. Possibly because of this activity osteoarthrosis is very common, particularly at the carpometacarpal joint. Arthritic changes may be superimposed on previous damage from trauma but one is struck by the relative infrequency following Bennett's fracture and most cases of osteoarthrosis are of primary type and in over 90 per cent occur in the female. The reason for this is at present obscure. Eaton & Littler [10] suggested that there may be some ligamentous laxity, particularly of the volar ligament holding the base of the first metacarpal to the trapezium and second metacarpal (p. 43). This allows lateral displacement of the base of the 1st metacarpal on the trapezium and is often seen radiographically in the early stages of osteoarthrosis. Routine radiography often fails to visualize the joint surfaces accurately, but the clinical features of osteoarthrosis are characteristic and often severe prior to any marked radiological changes.

The patient complains of pain at the base of the thumb on movement, of impairment of grip and a tendency to drop objects. Swelling over the joint may be obvious and there is usually localized joint tenderness. Undue passive mobility is often evident at the joint, particularly in a dorsovolar plane, which is accompanied by a characteristic painful clicking or grating.

When the symptoms become significant and persistent surgical treatment should be considered. The choices lie between arthrodesis [9] (p. 495) and arthroplasty.

(1) *Excision arthroplasty*

Excision of the trapezium can give excellent results (Gervis) [12]. This is effective in relieving pain whether it is arising from the trapeziometacarpal or scapho-trapezial joints. There is good mobility but the thumb is shorter than normal with some loss of power of grip. For the needs of the average middle-aged woman, the results are excellent but inadequate where hard manual work is required.

Operative technique

The trapezium can be removed through the same dorsal incision used for arthrodesis or through a curved incision around the base of the thumb. The trapezium has many ligamentous attachments which have to be divided before the bone can be removed satisfactorily. The procedure may be facilitated by removal of the bone piecemeal.

It is wise to identify the radial vessels running across the floor of the anatomical snuff-box, before dividing the ligamentous attachments of the trapezium to the base of the metacarpal, trapezoid and scaphoid. As the dissection nears the volar aspect it is necessary to protect the tendon of the flexor carpi radialis in its groove.

Following removal of the bone the remaining capsule and periosteum is repaired while traction is applied to the thumb maintaining as much length as possible. The joint should be immobilized in plaster for 3–4 weeks.

It has been recommended that the space left should be filled by coiling up the palmaris longus tendon to separate the bone surfaces and maintain the length [11], but this is unnecessary.

(2) *Replacement arthroplasty*

The procedure most commonly employed is excision of the trapezium and replacement with a silastic prosthesis. Good results are reported from this procedure [13–17].

The main complication is a tendency for subluxation of the prosthesis off the scaphoid in a dorsal and radial direction. Various points in the operative technique are stressed in order to prevent this complication.

Operative technique (see also Chapter 25)

(1) The exposure and removal of the trapezium is as described for its excision, taking care to preserve the capsule.

(2) The size of cavity left is inspected and assessment made of the size of prosthesis. Five sizes are available and it is seldom that anything larger than the first three sizes is required. The metacarpal articular surface is removed by a small oscillating saw directing the cut obliquely from dorsal to volar aspect so that the angle the dorsal surface of the metacarpal makes with the cut base is just less than 90°. This reduces the tendency to subluxation subsequently [13].

The metacarpal shaft is reamed to prepare a triangular fit in the metacarpal for the stem of the prosthesis. This is made easier by using the air-powered drill. The correct size of trial prosthesis is then chosen and the permanent prosthesis inserted.

(3) An important factor in preventing subluxation is careful repair of the lateral capsule and periosteum tightly over the prosthesis. This should be reinforced by a slip of the flexor carpi radialis tendon which is split longitudinally to its insertion over a distance of 6 cm. One slip is divided proximally and passed through a drill hole in the base of the metacarpal and sutured to the insertion of the abductor pollicis longus. In this way the first intermetacarpal ligament, so important for the stability of the first metacarpal base, is re-inforced.

(4) The trapezoid may protrude and obstruct the insertion of the prosthesis, and may be trimmed to get a good fit.

The results of this operative procedure are good and the tendency to displacement of the prosthesis is much reduced by the above points in technique. Relief of pain with good mobility is usual and the normal length of thumb and power of grip should be maintained.

Results from use of the Niebauer prosthesis have also been satisfactory [18].

In an alternative procedure described by Kessler [19,

20], the base of the metacarpal is removed and one of the three sizes of prostheses inserted to replace it. The trapezium is left intact. While this procedure may be useful in the earlier stages of osteoarthrosis, in the more advanced stages, where there is instability at the carpometacarpal joint, it is less satisfactory.

Ashworth [21] has described a similar procedure using a neurosurgical burr-hole cover placed over the trapezium after limited resection of its distal joint surface and bone. Good results were claimed.

Postoperative management

The thumb is immobilized for four weeks after operation in a padded plaster of the scaphoid fracture type. Swelling is often quite marked and the hand should be elevated routinely for 48–72 hours.

Corrective osteotomy in the hand

Osteotomy may be required to correct a rotary or angulatory deformity [26] or to place a digit in a more functional position during reconstruction in a severely mutilated hand [27].

When malalignment occurs following fracture, corrective osteotomy is indicated at the site of injury.

Angulatory deformity is usually easily seen both clinically and radiologically and can be accurately assessed. Rotary malalignment, however, is much more difficult to detect, particularly when it is only a few degrees, although sufficient to cause obstruction of movement of the other digits. It is useful to remember in clinical assessment that the fingers all flex towards the scaphoid and that the fingernails lie in parallel.

Technique

Metacarpals are approached from the dorsum and phalanges either through a dorsal incision splitting the extensor tendor or from a mid-lateral incision. The bone is exposed subperiosteally and divided by the small bladed oscillating power saw.

In metacarpals the corrected position can be maintained by transverse Kirschner wire fixation to an adjacent metacarpal as for metacarpal fractures (p. 204).

For phalanges a more satisfactory method of fixation is by intraosseous wiring. Prior to division of the bone drill holes are made proximal and distal to the site of osteotomy. To correct angulatory deformity a suitable closing wedge resection is carried out at the site of osteotomy. Wire of 35 gauge is passed through the holes and tightened to maintain the corrected position. To avoid tendons fraying over the wire ends these should be buried in a drill hole in the cortex [28].

In other reconstructive procedures the position is often best maintained by Kirschner wire fixation. The ends of the wires are left protruding from the skin and rigid fixation can be obtained by bonding these in acrylic cement [29].

Bone grafting in the hand

Non-union of fractures of the hand is very rare and while bone grafting for this reason may occasionally be required, it is usually needed for reconstruction following injuries with bone loss or for bone lengthening procedures (p. 502). Unless there has been massive bone loss the hand is unlikely to be suitable for onlay or inlay bone grafts and the introduction of large amounts of cancellous chips is unlikely to be satisfactory except in destructive lesions such as enchondromata and aneurysmal bone cysts (p. 452).

In the isolated bone defect affecting a metacarpal or phalanx the most satisfactory procedure is by intramedullary fixation of the graft in the proximal and distal segments. This can best be achieved by a 'bail' type of graft cut from the iliac crest or by a small graft cut from the subcutaneous surface of the upper ulna to fit firmly into the medullary cavity.

Where cancellous chips are required these are obtained from the iliac crest [30]; a very useful source, usually sufficient to fill small cavities in the hand bones, is the lower end of the radius entered through the styloid process.

If a corticocancellous graft can be cut accurately to fit firmly into the medullary cavity no other form of internal fixation may be required. If the fixation is considered insufficient, the addition of longitudinal Kirschner wires is indicated. In the metacarpal the graft can be fixed by transverse Kirschner wires to the adjacent metacarpal.

Mobilization of stiff joints and correction of soft-tissue contractures (see Chapter 22)

SKIN COVER

The reconstructive procedures necessary to provide good skin cover are described in Chapter 9.

RESTORATION OF GRASP

Reconstruction for the partially amputated hand [31–35]

There are four basic patterns of mutilated hand resulting from partial amputation [36, 37].

Group 1. Radial hemi-amputation (i.e. absence of the thumb—partial or complete) (Fig. 35.3). (See p. 500.)

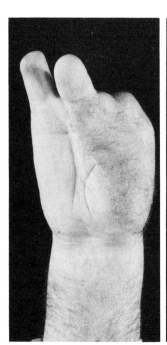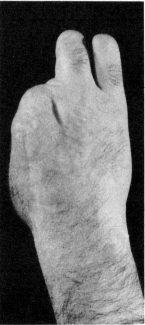

FIG. 35.3. Radial hemi-amputation.

Group 2. Ulnar hemi-amputation (i.e. absence of the ulnar side of the hand)

No treatment is required if one remaining digit or intact metacarpal remains to which the thumb can be opposed. Where amputation has been through the bases of the ulnar four metacarpals, and the thumb has no useful structure to oppose against, the management would consist of application of a prosthesis or artificial strut for the thumb to oppose. Very occasionally the reconstruction of a bone graft and flap on the ulnar side of the hand would be justified [38–40].

Group 3. Central hemi-amputation (i.e. absence of central part of the hand)

Where the radial and ulnar components of the hand are normal no treatment will be required. If these segments are so short that they cannot meet, removal of the remaining portions of the central metacarpals may be required to allow apposition of the two digits. Sometimes a rotation osteotomy through the ulnar component will bring it into better position to oppose the thumb.

Group 4. Transverse hemi-amputation (i.e. transverse loss of all digits)

Sometimes the stumps are of sufficient length to be of useful function and no treatment is required. If the thumb segment is short deepening of the thumb web may be all that is required to give the thumb a greater functional length. Proximal loss of all the digits leaves a hand of little functional use (Fig. 35.4). Provided the greater parts of the metacarpal bones remain, a useful grip can be restored by removing the central metacarpals and allowing pinch between the remnants of first and fifth metacarpals. A method of occasional application in these circumstances is to leave the third metacarpal because of its adductor attachment and to resect the second and fourth metacarpals. The third metacarpal can act as a useful prop for both the first and fifth metacarpals [41].

In those circumstances where transverse amputation is through the bases of the metacarpals considerable ingenuity is required to provide any useful function by surgical reconstruction. One such case and its successful management is shown in Figure 35.5.

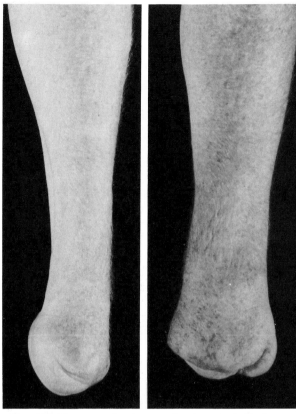

FIG. 35.4. Transverse hemi-amputation is not suitable for any useful surgical reconstruction.

In many cases of proximal transverse hemi-amputation reconstructive surgery is not possible (Fig. 35.4). In one of these a functional cosmetic wrist-operated prosthesis (Fig. 35.6) was used.

Restoration of the thumb

The importance of the thumb to the function of the hand is well recognized. Where the thumb is absent from birth, lost through injury or amputated for disease, every consideration should be given to its restoration [42–45].

Congenital absence

Where the thumb is absent or functionally useless by virtue of failure of development its replacement by reconstructive procedures should be considered. This is particularly so when the condition is bilateral but even when unilateral, there may be a place for it. As it is likely that all the structures associated with the thumb, including the muscles and tendons, are absent, a procedure designed for a total replacement of function, such as transference of one of the adjacent digits is required. The index finger is the most appropriate finger to transfer provided it shows good function with normal bone and joint structure. On occasion, it may be advisable to transpose one of the other digits.

Several methods of index finger transfer into the position of a thumb have been described [46–49], but the author has found that very satisfactory results can be obtained by a combination of the sinuous incision described by Barsky [50], with a dorsal extension along the proximal phalanx to facilitate exposure of the extensor mechanism and reattachment of the intrinsic muscles [51]. The digit is transferred on a neurovascular bundle as described by Littler [52, 54], and to prevent the tendency to hyperextension deformity at the base of the new thumb the metacarpal head is rotated as described by Buck-Gramcko [51].

Operative technique (see also p. 307)

The incision is deepened and the flap is raised until the neurovascular bundles to the index finger can be identified. In congenital cases the vessels and nerve to the radial side of the index may be absent and great care is required with the identification and preservation of the vessels to the ulnar side of the same finger. The branch of the artery to the radial side of the middle finger is ligated and divided and the common digital nerve is then separated gently into its two components using either the back of the scalpel or a fine dissector. The parts of the nerve to the index and middle fingers can be separated as far proximally as the base of the palm so that the neurovascular bundle will not be put on tension when the digit is transposed. Attention is now turned to the dorsum of the second metacarpal and the first dorsal and palmar interosseous muscles are dissected off the metacarpal. The deep transverse metacarpal ligament is divided, the metacarpal shaft is stripped of the periosteum and the proximal part of the shaft and base are removed leaving only the metacarpal head supporting the index, the finger now being ready for transfer.

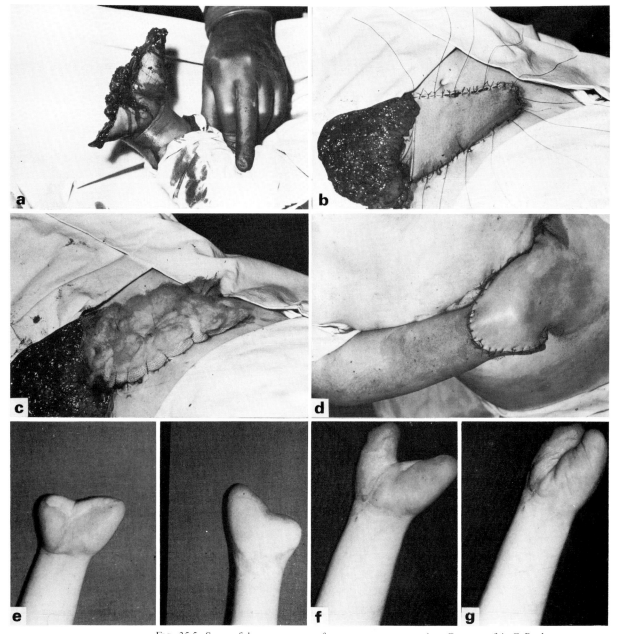

Fig. 35.5. Successful management of a transverse amputation. Courtesy of A. C. Buchan.

(a) Original injury.

(b) An abdominal flap is raised to provide skin cover. The defect is closed by free skin graft.

(c) Paraffin gauze dressing applied to skin graft with compression applied by the skin sutures tied firmly over the dressing.

(d) Abdominal flap attached over skin defect in the hand.

(e) Skin cover after separation of abdominal flap.

(f) Ulnar side of hand elongated by bone graft. Cocked-hat procedure used (Fig. 35.7) to preserve sensation over tip of ulnar components.

(g) Range of movement and apposition of radial and ulnar components.

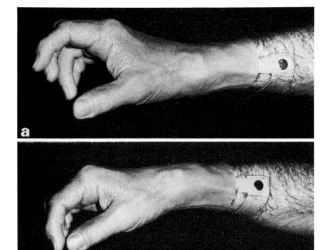

Fig. 35.6. A wrist-operated prosthesis constructed of silicone rubber. (a) The fingers and thumb are opened by dorsi-flexion of the wrist. (b) Grasp and apposition of fingers and thumb is obtained by wrist palmar flexion.

There is seldom any trapezium or scaphoid bones present and the head of the second metacarpal must now be transposed into the recess created by resection of the base of the second metacarpal. No attempt is made to get bony fixation to the third metacarpal base. The digit is rotated 150° *on its* long axis (see Fig. 1.62 in anatomy section on orientation of trapezium in relation to the plane of dorsum of the hand) and the head of the second metacarpal held in its new position by several soft tissue stitches. There is a tendency for a hyperextension deformity to develop at the base of the new thumb due to laxity of the volar capsule and this is why the head of the metacarpal should be rotated in order to tighten the volar capsule before the head is placed in position [51].

With the thumb now fixed in the desired position, the tourniquet should be released to check vascularity and haemostasis is obtained. The interosseous muscles are now reattached to the extensor tendon at the level of the proximal interphalangeal joint of the index which will now become the metacarpophalangeal joint of the new thumb. In this way the interossei boost the extensor power of the new thumb and provide some degree of its control [51, 55] similar to that of the short abductor and adductor on the dorsal expansion

of the normal thumb. The design of the original skin incision is to provide a satisfactory flap for the new thumb web. It is seldom that any additional skin is required but if the closure seems to be too tight or obstructing venous return, an appropriate split skin graft is inserted. The desired position of the thumb is usually maintained by the soft tissue sutures and the closure of skin but if there is any problem with its fixation a Kirschner wire can be inserted from the new thumb into the third metacarpal. A compression bandage and plaster slab is applied and it is advisable to continue immobilization for six weeks.

It is surprising how quickly tendon function is restored in the young particularly that of the flexor activity. Extension is often rather less efficient and if at the end of operation the extensor tendons seem unduly loose, a shortening can be carried out to tighten them up. If the structure and function of the index finger prior to operation was normal or near normal, a useful and effective thumb is usually provided in the young child (see Fig. 24.21).

Amputation following trauma or disease

The necessity to reconstruct the thumb and the method employed will depend upon the remaining length. If the portion missing is distal to the level of the middle of the proximal phalanx the remainder will provide a thumb with adequate function. Treatment should not be required provided there is good quality non-adherent skin cover with satisfactory sensation. Where the thumb is lost proximal to this point the method of management depends upon the age of the patient, whether it is the dominant hand and the remainder of the hand is normal, the work and use required from the hand and what functional disability proves to be present. A variety of surgical procedures are available:

(1) In young people lengthening of the first metacarpal has been shown by Matev [56] to be a practical proposition and an increase of length of 2–2.5 cm can be obtained.

(2) The 'cocked hat' procedure [57, 58] or the reversed 'cocked hat' procedure [59] can be used very satisfactorily to provide some length of thumb by inserting an iliac bone graft and advancing a skin flap with normal sensation over the end of the bone; the defect is closed with split skin graft (Fig. 35.7).

(3) In thumbs of shorter length, missing through the

shaft of the metacarpal, a major reconstructive procedure can be carried out involving lengthening with an iliac bone graft inserted into the stump of the metacarpal and **covering the end with a flap graft [57, 59, 60, 61]. This** procedure can provide a stump of good functional length but the results are often unsatisfactory due to lack of sensation in the flap and to poor vascularity which also may lead to bone graft resorption.

The whole situation has been revolutionized by the introduction of the neurovascular island transfer (see later). By bringing in an island flap with specialized sensation and intact blood supply, a very satisfactory state is obtained whereby there is good nourishment and sensation of the terminal part [64]. In early months after transfer, the cortical sensory appreciation will be referred into the donor finger but in time reorientation may occur although this is more likely in the younger patient.

With the introduction of free flap transfer with microsurgical anastomosis of vessels and nerve an entirely new concept of thumb reconstruction became available and the same techniques have allowed successful free trans-

fer of the great or second toe to replace the thumb [62, 63].

(4) Where the thumb is lost at the base of the metacarpal, pollicization often gives a more satisfactory result. Where there has been partial damage to other digits it is often most practical to replace the thumb by the partially damaged digit which can give very satisfactory results [60]. If there is no other digital damage, transfer of the index finger is most appropriate and the general technique is similar to that used in the congenital case [65]. Where there is sufficient stump of the first metacarpal it is preferable for the base of the second metacarpal to be fixed into the stump of the first metacarpal. On occasion transfer of a digit other than the index may be indicated [66].

Neurovascular island transfer

This procedure was introduced to transfer an area with normal skin sensibility to an important area of sensory loss in the hand [67, 68]. This applies particularly to the pulp of the thumb and the radial side of the index finger as in irrecoverable nerve damage or to improve results of reconstruction of the thumb by skin flap [64, 69]. The aim is to transpose skin together with its nerve and blood supply to the deficient area. In the case of irreparable median nerve damage this would require transfer of the ulnar side of the ring finger with its ulnar innervation to the new position in the thumb.

While the results of this procedure can be very satisfactory this is not always the case [70], the indications are few and the patients should be selected with care.

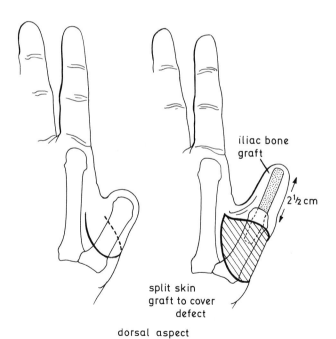

FIG. 35.7. Lengthening the thumb using the cocked-hat procedure.

Technique (Fig. 35.8)

The amount of skin tissue transferred depends upon the area of sensation required. If it is simply to restore sensation to the thumb pulp it is sufficient to remove the hemi-pulp from the ring finger but if necessary it is possible to transfer areas from the middle and proximal segments of the finger as well. The area required is outlined and then continued proximally by a midlateral digital incision and extended in a volar zig zag fashion into the palm (Fig. 35.8a). The neurovascular bundle to the fourth cleft is identified in the palm, dissected distally towards the web and the bifurcation of the artery. The branch to the radial side of the little finger is ligated and divided. The nerve to the cleft is gently separated proximally towards the base of the palm by blunt dissection so that the nerve to the ulnar side of ring finger is separated from the component to the radial side of little finger (Fig. 35.8b). The neurovascular bundle is then dissected into the digit with cauterization of any vascular side branches and followed into the segment of skin which is to be elevated. The recipient area is now exposed and in the thumb it is usual to apply the transferred skin onto the volar ulnar aspect of the pulp while in the index finger the radial aspect of the pulp is replaced. Any scarred or insensitive skin over these areas is excised to prepare a bed for the recipient skin. A subcutaneous tunnel is made to conduct the island flap to its new bed and

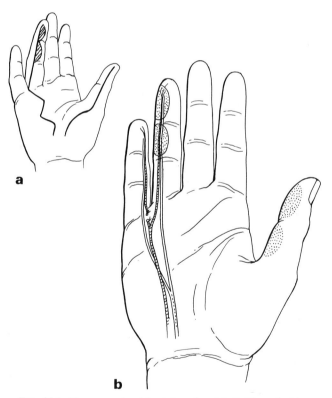

FIG. 35.8. Neurovascular island transfer. (a) Outline of skin incisions used for transfer of neurovascular island flap from ring finger to thumb. (b) Isolation of neurovascular bundle and separation of the nerve in the metacarpal space into its constituent bundles.

the transposed skin sutured in place. Split skin grafts are then applied to the donor area.

Reconstructive procedures in amputation stumps

Stump revision

Where the skin is scarred and adherent, and tender neuromata are easily palpated, resection of the neuroma, with bipolar coagulation diathermy of the nerve ends and transfer of the nerve to an environment with less scarring should be considered (see Chapter 17). If pain is of long standing, i.e. months or years, the pain pathways may be persistent and symptoms difficult to eradicate. If a careful revision of an unsatisfactory stump does not relieve symptoms amputation at a more proximal level is not advised. The use of electrical stimulation may be worthwhile.

Stump lengthening

This may be indicated in below elbow amputations where the stump is so short that it is difficult to get satisfactory prosthetic function. A skin flap is elevated as for the 'cocked hat' thumb lengthening procedure (see p. 502, Fig. 35.7) and displaced distally so as to accommodate an iliac bone graft inserted into the bone stump to provide lengthening.

The Krukenberg amputation (Fig. 35.9)

This procedure can be considered where there is a long below elbow amputation. It is seldom justified in the single amputation but where both hands have been lost, as sometimes happens in handling explosives, or where the person is blind, it is strongly indicated.

This procedure splits the forearm into its separate bony components together with those muscles arising from the radius and ulna respectively. This operation has gained little acceptance in Britain, except for the circumstances described, but has been used more frequently on the continent of Europe. It was also used with success in Vietnam [71], and it is probably indicated most frequently in those parts of the world where prosthetic replacement is difficult to provide.

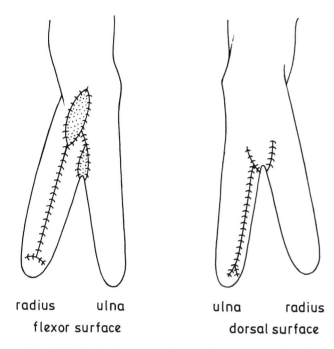

radius   ulna   ulna   radius

flexor surface   dorsal surface

FIG. 35.9. Krukenberg amputation. A forearm stump is split into the two bony components together with related muscles and covered mainly by normal skin with good sensation. The stippled areas indicate where split skin is required.

Operative technique [72]

Through radial volar and ulnar dorsal longitudinal incisions the forearm is separated into a radial component with the radius and its close muscle relations and attachments and an ulnar component with the ulna and its muscle relations and attachments. The pronator quadratus and flexor superficialis are excised. The profundus and extensor digitorum muscles are split equally between each segment. The interosseous membrane is split widely throughout the forearm. The aim is to provide two mobile segments of 10–15 cm in length, able to provide a spread of about 7.5 cm at the tips and to have sufficient strength and opposition to provide useful pincer prehension.

As the normal skin of the forearm covers the terminal parts of these segments good sensation is retained and enhances their use. There may be insufficient skin to cover the segments completely and usually split skin grafting is required to cover any de-

fects on the inner aspects. Nathan has described recently a technique to avoid the need for skin grafting [71].

The two mobile 'prongs' can be opposed to provide grip for small objects and have a spread of about 7 cms for gripping larger structures. Sensory appreciation is preserved which is of prime importance in the blind person on whom there has been bilateral amputation.

Restoration of tendon function

Tendon transfers in the upper limb and hand

Tendon transfers are indicated in the upper limb to restore some important function such as elbow flexion or extension, wrist extension or digital movement. The central nervous system is concerned not with individual muscles but with movements, in which actions of prime movers, synergists and antagonists are co-ordinated towards a common end. The emphasis should be on the restoration of specific function rather than on any individual muscle activity [73]. 'The brain knows only function—not specific muscles. It acts to provide motor function not any particular muscle action' [74]. 'Every muscle in the upper limb is synergistic with any function' and 'There is no function in the upper limb which cannot be restored by transfer of another unit even where that transfer is an antagonist' [75]. Transfers in the upper limb have a greater chance of success than in the lower limb as they do not have to contend with locomotion and weight bearing.

The transfer of healthy musculotendinous units to replace lost function may be required for a variety of conditions many of which have been described in previous chapters. The principles governing successful tendon transfer have been well described on the basis of knowledge resulting largely from experience gained in poliomyelitis [73, 75–81]. These basic principles, equally applicable to conditions such as leprosy, cord injury (Chapter 29), peripheral nerve and brachial plexus lesions (Chapter 12) and cerebral palsy (Chapter 30) require consideration of the following factors.

Power of the transposed tendons

No muscle under power of four (Table 35.1) should be considered for transfer and where possible a muscle of normal power (power five) should be used. It is

TABLE 35.1 Grading of muscle power (Medical Research Council)

Grade 0	No contraction.
Grade 1	Flicker or trace of contraction.
Grade 2	Active movement, with gravity eliminated.
Grade 3	Active movement against gravity.
Grade 4	Active movement against gravity and resistance.
Grade 5	Normal power.

Grades 4−, 4 and 4+, may be used to indicate movement against slight, moderate and strong resistance respectively.

generally considered that there may be a drop in the power of the tendon following transfer equivalent to one stage in the MRC grading.

Amplitude of transferred unit

It is important that the amplitude of excursion of the unit should be capable of the function desired. For example, a muscle of limited amplitude like the pronator teres is unlikely to be able to provide the range of movement required in a digital flexor. It should be remembered as a working rule that wrist motors have an amplitude of 3 cm, finger extensors 5 cm and finger flexors 7 cm [73]. In certain circumstances however, utilisation of a range of other movement synergistic with the function being provided will boost and enhance the range of amplitude. An example of this will be where one wrist extensor is transferred to provide flexion of the digits: the amplitude of the muscle itself would not be adequate for this task but as the other wrist extensors are left, the movement of the wrist will enhance the gliding range of the transferred tendon. By retaining wrist movement a transfer of extensor carpi radialis longus to finger flexors will double its amplitude.

Integrity of the musculotendinous unit

It is imperative that the transposed unit is not damaged during transfer and that its nerve and vascular supply should not be prejudiced. For example in the pectoralis major transfer to restore elbow flexion [82] and the transfer of the posterior third of the deltoid to provide elbow extension [83] the pectoral and circumflex nerves must be protected. Several transfers are enhanced in value by the proximal level of their neurovascular

supply, e.g. the extensor carpi radialis longus and brachioradialis which can be mobilized freely to the upper part of the muscle.

In addition no transfer should be expected to provide more than one function.

Direction of pull

The straighter the line of pull between the origin of the muscle and its new insertion, the more effective its function. The new unit should lie in a tissue plane such as between muscles or in the subcutaneous fat where it is least likely to become adherent. Occasionally it is necessary to pass tendons through tight fascial canals and these should be loosened and widened freely to allow the transferred unit to glide satisfactorily, e.g. transfer of a flexor from the forearm to the dorsum through the interosseous membrane between radius and ulna to provide a straight pull.

The best results are obtained by transfer of the tendon directly into bone but, in the upper limb, transfer of active tendon into the tendon of paralyzed muscles can prove very effective. This is best done by interweaving the donor tendon through the recipient tendon or tendons using the technique of passing a fine sharp tenotomy knife through the latter. The tip of the knife is grasped with fine crocodile forceps which is pushed through the opening in the recipient tendon to grasp the transferred tendon. An alternative method of tendon junction is that described by Brand [94] (Fig. 35.16).

Supple joints

A full range of passive movement should be ensured before any tendon transfer is performed as no muscle can move stiff contracted joints.

Expendability

It should be ascertained that the donor is expendable and its transfer leaves no significant loss of original function.

Tendons can be transferred in the upper limb to restore the following functions:
  (1) elbow flexion,
  (2) elbow extension,
  (3) extension of the wrist,
  (4) extension of the digits,

(5) flexion of the digits,

(6) abduction/opposition of the thumb,

(7) abduction of the index,

(8) adduction of the thumb, and

(9) intrinsic balance and correction of clawing of fingers.

Transfers to restore elbow flexion

The loss of elbow flexion and the ability to get the hand to the face for feeding, washing and self care activities is very serious, particularly should it be bilateral. There are various procedures to restore elbow flexion and these are described in order of preference.

Flexor origin transfer (Steindler) [75, 84, 85]

When the common flexor origin muscles are strong, its proximal transfer is a most efficient way of restoring elbow flexion.

Operative procedure

The incision is centred on the common flexor origin which is elevated from bone and transposed to the shaft of the humerus approximately at the junction of lower and middle thirds (Fig. 35.10). Attachment to the periosteum and medial intermuscular septum is often sufficient but if there is difficulty in getting satisfactory anchorage, the muscles are fixed to the bone through a drill hole.

The extensor origin, if the muscles are strong, including the brachioradialis and extensor carpi radialis longus, is elevated similarly and moved to a new position on the lateral aspect of the humeral shaft.

Pectoralis transfer [82]

The sternocostal attachment of the pectoralis major is elevated from its origin together with a strip of fascia from the anterior sheath of the rectus abdominis. The muscle is elevated proximally to the site of entry of the pectoral nerves and transferred into the upper arm to be attached to the biceps tendon where present, or if absent, as in congenital cases, the transfer has to be attached to radius direct and requires a free tendon or fascial graft to provide necessary elongation.

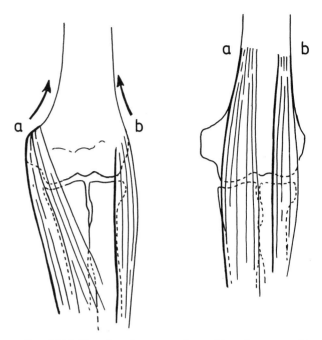

Fig. 35.10. Transfer of common flexor (a) and extensor (b) origins up the shaft of the humerus (Steindler).

Operative technique (Fig. 35.11)

Through a long, oblique incision, directed across the chest wall from the anterior fold of the axilla to the lower costal cartilages near their sternal attachment, the fascia is elevated and the muscle raised on its bed. There is considerable vascularity in this region and careful haemostasis is required. Extension onto the anterior rectus sheath may give the extra fascial length required to reach the biceps tendon or neck of radius. A tunnel sufficient to accommodate the transposed muscle and tendon is made through the anterior compartment of the upper arm. Where the biceps muscle is present but paralyzed, it is often wise to remove it to provide room. The biceps tendon should be left intact and the transposed muscle attached to it with the elbow flexed to 70°.

This transfer has produced excellent elbow flexion in lesions of the brachial plexus or musculocutaneous nerve, in poliomyelitis and in congenital absence or deficiency of the biceps. It has the disadvantage of the extensive scar on the chest wall.

A variation of this procedure [86, 87] utilises the long head of biceps, which is divided at the upper end of the

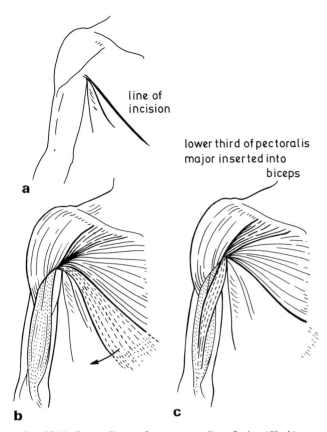

FIG. 35.11. Pectoralis transfer to restore elbow flexion (Clark).

(a) Line of incision across the chest wall from the insertion of the pectoralis to the upper part of the rectus sheath. (b) The outline of the lower third of the pectoralis major muscle is outlined ready for its transfer. (c) The pectoral is transferred into the upper arm and inserted into the biceps tendon.

bicipital groove and interwoven between the pectoral tendon and biceps insertion.

Transfer of the triceps to the biceps

This is indicated when the first two procedures are not possible [88]. In certain cases of arthrogryposis and in some cases of absence of the radius where there is deficient elbow flexion, this transfer has proved very valuable although the range of movement is usually less than that achieved by the previous two procedures. In bilateral cases of loss of elbow flexion, it would be unwise to transfer the triceps on both sides.

Operative technique

A J-shaped incision extending down the lateral aspect of the humerus to the joint line and deviating medially across the antecubital fossa is used. The triceps is isolated and freed from its insertion together with a strip of fascia on the posterior aspect of the ulna to give the extra length required to reach the neck of the radius. In elevating the muscle, the site of emergence of the radial nerve from the spiral groove must be carefully protected. Once the muscle with its tendon has been mobilized sufficiently, it is transferred round the lateral side and inserted through a drill hole in the neck of the radius, or into the tendon of biceps (Fig. 35.12b) with the elbow flexed about 70°.

An alternative which can provide excellent elbow flexion is by a complete transfer of both origin and insertion of part of the latissimus dorsi [89, 90].

Post-operative management

In all these procedures, the transfer should be attached fairly tight with the elbow flexed to 70° and this position should be maintained in a plaster for four weeks. Graduated extension is then allowed with physiotherapy

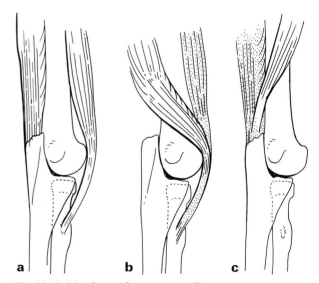

FIG. 35.12. Muscle transfers to restore elbow movement.

(a) Lateral view of the elbow region. (b) Transfer of triceps into biceps to restore flexion. (c) Transfer of biceps into triceps to restore elbow extension.

supervision, the aim being to maintain the fullest possible range of flexion. The best results are usually achieved when a flexion contracture of about 30° is established preventing full extension. It usually takes several months after operation before the final range of flexion is obtained.

Transfers to restore elbow extension

The loss of active elbow extension is usually not such a functional loss as the absence of elbow flexion, but in certain circumstances, for example in traumatic quadriplegia, the lack of elbow extension is very serious. Transfer of the posterior third of the deltoid muscle to restore elbow extension in this group [83] is successful. Through an incision along the posterior border of the deltoid (Fig. 35.13a) a strip of the muscle, about a third of its bulk, is elevated from the posterior part (Fig. 35.13b) and freed from its tendon insertion. It is elongated by strips of free tendon which are inserted into the triceps tendon (Fig. 35.13c). For good results

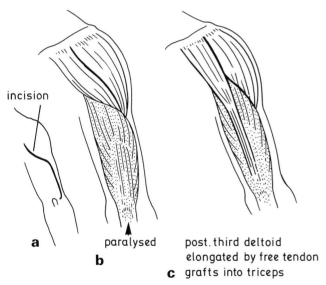

a
b paralysed
c post.third deltoid elongated by free tendon grafts into triceps

incision

FIG. 35.13. Posterior third of deltoid to triceps transfer to restore elbow extension (Moberg).

(a) Incision along the posterior border of the deltoid and down the posterolateral aspect of the upper arm. (b) Elevation of the posterior third of the deltoid muscle down to its insertion. (c) Elongation of the posterior third of deltoid by free tendon grafts into the triceps.

the postoperative regime described by Moberg must be followed strictly [83] (see also Chapter 29). It has been found that there is no impairment in the power of abduction of the shoulder as a result of this procedure and it it is one that could be used to restore elbow extension in other circumstances.

Transfer of the biceps into the triceps can also restore good extension of the elbow [89] (Fig. 35.12c).

Transfers to restore dorsiflexion of the wrist and digits

Loss of wrist extension is often associated with loss of digital extension. It is most commonly seen in irrecoverable radial nerve injuries [91] but may occur in other circumstances. In association with radial nerve lesions, the classical transfer [77] has given excellent results. The principle of this procedure is to transfer three tendons from the volar aspect to restore wrist extension, finger extension and thumb extension (Fig. 35.14). Pronator teres is transferred into the radial carpal extensors, flexor carpi ulnaris into the finger and thumb extensors and palmaris longus into long abductor of the thumb. It is always wise to leave one wrist flexor intact and the flexor carpi radialis is chosen for this purpose.

Operative procedure [92]

The following incisions are required (Fig. 35.14a).

(1) A short longitudinal incision is made over the radial aspect of the mid forearm. The superficial branch of the radial nerve lying along the anterior aspect of the mobile 'wad' [93] is protected and the radial vessels are retracted medially from the insertion of pronator teres. The muscle is disinserted and attached to the radial carpal extensors (Fig. 35.14b).

(2) A long incision on the ulnar side of the forearm exposes the flexor carpi ulnaris. It is necessary to mobilize the musculotendinous unit into the proximal forearm to free it from all fascial attachments.

(3) Through three small transverse incisions the palmaris longus is isolated and divided at its insertion.

(4) A sinuous incision on the dorsal aspect of the lower forearm and wrist is made to expose the extensors proximal to the extensor retinaculum.

The flexor carpi ulnaris is transferred round the ulnar side of the forearm and inserted into the common

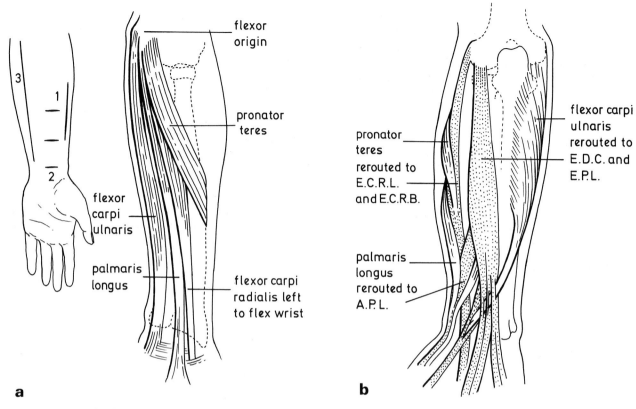

FIG. 35.14. Transfer of tendons to restore dorsiflexion of wrist and digits.
   (a) Flexor aspect of left forearm. Incisions: (1) to expose pronator teres, (2) to free palmaris longus, (3) to mobilize flexor carpi ulnaris.
   (b) Extensor aspect of left forearm following tendon transfer.

digital extensor and extensor pollicis longus proximal to the retinaculum (Fig. 35.14b). Through the lower part of the incision, the abductor pollicis longus tendon is exposed and the palmaris longus transferred into it. The interweaving technique (Fig. 35.15) is used for these transfers. An alternative method of tendon anastomosis [94] is shown in Figure 35.16.

   Boyes [73] has criticised the use of flexor carpi ulnaris which he considers to be a muscle of such importance in normal use of the wrist and hand that its integrity should not be disrupted. As an alternative, he suggests the transfer of superficial flexors to replace deficient extensor muscles. An alternative muscle which is usually available, but which requires widespread dissection to free it from all fascial attachments before it can function satisfactorily as a transfer, is the brachioradialis. It

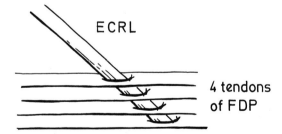

FIG. 35.15. Interweaving technique of junction of tendons. In this case the radial carpal extensor longus is woven through the flexor profundus tendons.

can be mobilized through a series of transverse incisions on the radial side of the forearm. On rare occasions mobility of the wrist may have to be sacrificed by arthrodesis to use wrist tendons to restore finger move-

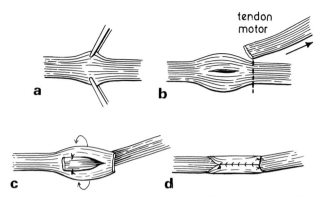

FIG. 35.16. Brand's technique of junction of tendons is especially effective when the pull of a motor unit has to be transferred through a free graft, e.g. palmaris or plantaris.

(a) The palmaris or plantaris is gripped between two forceps and spread into a sheet (b) into which a split is made through which the motor is passed. (c) The motor tendon is attached by interrupted sutures and then the expanded sheet of the free graft closed around it (d).

ment [95]. This is seldom required and priority should be given to wrist movement if possible.

Postoperative management

A plaster is applied with the wrist, fingers and thumb fully extended for a minimum of 3 weeks. Restoration of wrist and digital extension is usually excellent.

Transfer to restore extension of the thumb

Inability to extend the interphalangeal joint of the thumb may arise in combination with inability to extend the other digits as in a radial nerve palsy and the treatment of this has been described in transfers to restore extension of the digits.

Isolated loss of extension at this point is most likely to occur as a result of spontaneous rupture of the extensor pollicis longus tendon. There are two classical situations where this may occur, the first as a complication of rheumatoid disease affecting the extensor synovium and secondly as a complication of Colles fracture. In both cases the site of rupture is usually near the distal edge of the extensor retinaculum where the tendon passes round Lister's tubercle.

It is rarely possible to repair the tendon as its lesion is usually an attrition rupture, possibly associated with some ischaemia of the tendon, and as often an extensive area of the tendon is affected with the proximal end retracted. It is therefore usually advisable not to attempt repair but to transfer a healthy tendon into the distal end of the extensor pollicis longus. Various transfers have been described but one which gives consistently good results is transfer of the extensor indicis proprius tendon.

Operative procedure (Fig. 35.17)

(1) Through a short transverse incision over the distal part of the second metacarpal the indicis proprius tendon is identified lying on the ulnar side of the communis and divided transversely.

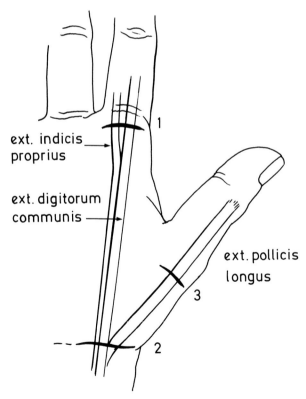

FIG. 35.17. Transfer to restore extension of the thumb. Transverse incisions (1 & 2) to expose extensor indicis proprius, (3) for tendon transfer.

(2) Through a short transverse incision just distal to the wrist the proximal part of the extensor indicis proprius is identified and the cut tendon withdrawn into this wound.

(3) Through a short transverse incision over the middle of the first metacarpal the extensor pollicis longus tendon is identified. The proximal end of the extensor indicis proprius tendon is either sutured direct to the cut distal end of the extensor pollicis longus or woven through it. The tendon junction is secured by wire sutures with the wrist in neutral position and the thumb fully extended. The wounds are closed and the wrist and thumb immobilized in the corrected position for 4 weeks.

Tendon transfers to restore digital flexion

The digital flexors have an amplitude of 7 cm and the thumb flexor of 5 cm [73]. The only tendon transfer that can restore this full range of amplitude is one of the other digital flexors.

The maintenance of active dorsi-flexion of the wrist is an essential part of successful restoration of digital flexion by tendon transfer. Attempts to provide digital movement by arthrodesing the wrist and utilizing the prime wrist movers made available in this way are generally disappointing.

If both finger and thumb flexion is required then extensor carpi radialis longus can be transferred into the long flexors [96] and brachio-radialis into the long flexor of the thumb [97].

Operative procedure (Fig. 35.18)

A curved incision convex distally and centred on the radial styloid is made on the lateral aspect of the forearm. The incision is deepened with care to preserve the distal part of the superficial radial nerve and the superficial veins.

Through the dorsal part of this incision the insertion of the radial carpal extensors is exposed and the more radial of these is identified and disinserted.

Through the central part of the incision the insertion of the brachioradialis into the lateral aspect of the radial styloid is identified and released. The tendon is very closely bound down with deep fascia and periosteum

and requires careful dissection from these attachments.

Two further transverse incisions on the radial side of the forearm, one about mid-forearm and one at the junction of the upper and middle thirds is made. Through these incisions the muscle bellies are exposed and freed by dissecting with the long-handled dissecting scissors into the upper forearm. The lateral cutaneous

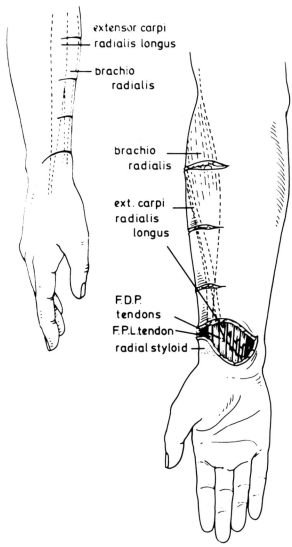

Fig. 35.18. Incisions used to expose the musculotendinous units of extensor carpi radialis longus and brachioradialis for transfer to the front of the wrist into the tendons of flexor digitorum profundus and flexor pollicis longus.

nerve of the forearm lies along the anterior border of the brachioradialis and should be protected during the dissection.

Through the volar part of the lower forearm incision the flexor pollicis longus and flexor digitorum profundus tendons are identified.

The tunneling forceps are introduced from the lower incision into the upper and a tunnel made for the passage of the tendons in the plane beneath the deep fascia. The tendon of brachioradialis is withdrawn to lie along the radial side of the flexor pollicis longus and the extensor carpi radialis longus is drawn into relationship to the profundus tendons.

The tendon of brachioradialis is interwoven through the tendon of the flexor pollicis longus at its musculotendinous junction. The tendon of extensor carpi radialis longus is interwoven through each of the profundus tendons directed from radial to ulnar side (Fig. 35.15). Individual mattress sutures of 000 nylon are used to anchor the tendons. The tension of the sutures should be such that with the wrist dorsiflexed the fingers are semi-flexed and the thumb is against the side of the middle segment of the index finger. On palmar flexion of the wrist full digital extension should be possible.

The wounds are closed, a compression bandage and a dorsal plaster slab holding the wrist in the neutral position are applied. It is not necessary to immobilize the fingers and gentle passive digital movements are carried out from the start. The plaster is removed in 3 weeks to restore wrist movement and digital flexion is encouraged under the supervision of the physiotherapist.

Transfers to restore abduction·opposition of the thumb
(Fig. 35.19)

The function of the thumb and the hand as a whole is greatly reduced by an inability to bring the thumb into pulp to pulp opposition to the other digits. This loss results from irreparable or irrecoverable median nerve lesions and is also common as a result of poliomyelitis, Charcot-Marie-Tooth muscle dystrophy, and leprosy.

Many transfers to replace this function have been described [98, 99]. Where a suitable flexor superficialis muscle is available its transfer is the procedure of choice [73] and can be relied upon to give a good result.

Bunnell procedure (Fig. 35.19)

(1) Through a transverse incision at the base of the selected finger (usually the ring) the superficialis tendon is isolated and divided.

(2) A longitudinal incision 4/5 cm in length is made along the ulnar side of the forearm to expose the

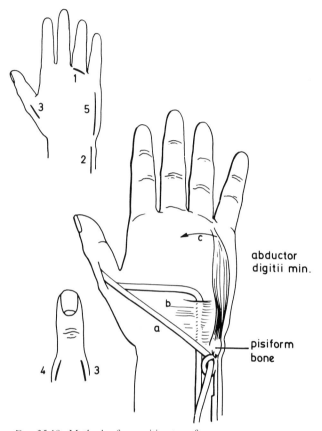

Fig. 35.19. Methods of opposition transfer.

(a) Standard opposition transfer using ring finger superficialis through pulley of FCU (Bunnell). The superficialis is inserted through the bone of the base of the proximal phalanx with fixation to the abductor pollicis brevis insertion.

(b) Transfer of ring finger superficialis left in the carpal tunnel (Thompson).

(c) Rotation transfer of abductor digiti minimi (Huber-Littler). The abductor digiti minimi is transferred into the abductor pollicis brevis insertion where this is present. If not, a new attachment to bone of base of proximal phalanx is required.

Incisions to expose (1) superficialis tendon, (2) flexor carpi ulnaris insertion (3 & 4) abductor pollicis brevis insertion and bone for fixation of transfer, (5) abductor digiti minimi.

lower part of the flexor carpi ulnaris tendon. Through the same incision the superficialis muscle is isolated and the cut tendon drawn through into the wrist. The lower 2.5 cm of the flexor carpi ulnaris tendon is then split longitudinally in two halves to its insertion and one portion separated from the main tendon proximally. This segment is utilized to provide a loop and pulley in the region of the pisiform through which the superficialis tendon can be passed (Fig. 35.19a).

(3) Two small longitudinal incisions are made on the radial and ulnar side of the metacarpophalangeal joint of the thumb, dorsal to the neurovascular bundle. The base of the proximal phalanx is exposed subperiostally and drilled transversely to accommodate the superficialis tendon.

Using the tunnelling forceps a subcutaneous passage is made from the pisiform obliquely across the base of the palm and thenar eminence to the radial thumb incision. A suitable bed and tunnel between these two sites is made and the flexor superficialis tendon having been passed through the pulley loop is drawn through this tunnel to the thumb (Fig. 35.19a). It is then passed through the drill hole in the base of the proximal phalanx from ulnar to radial side so that the tendon first crosses the dorsum of the metacarpophalangeal joint. The tendon is then tightly sutured to the tendon of the abductor pollicis brevis and then back to itself to give firm fixation, while the wrist is held in slight dorsiflexion and the thumb in full abduction.

The wounds are closed, a compression bandage and a plaster slab applied to hold the thumb in the corrected position. This is maintained for 3 weeks following which mobilization under the supervision of a physiotherapist is carried out.

A modification of this technique [100] is favoured by many. In this the superficial tendon is only withdrawn to the base of the hand but left in the carpal tunnel. It is then tunnelled across the base of the palm to its new insertion as in the Bunnell procedure (Fig. 35.19b). In this way the tendon works round the distal aspect of the flexor retinaculum for its pulley function. In the writer's experience this has given less satisfactory results than the Bunnell technique.

Where a superficial tendon is not available other alternatives must be sought but as a general rule they are less effective.

Steindler described the use of the flexor pollicis longus tendon and a modification of this method has given better results [102].

A method which has given satisfactory results is the transfer of the extensor digiti minimi tendon [103].

Operative procedure

The tendon is defined on the dorsum of the little finger and as much length as possible obtained. It is freed and withdrawn through an incision on the dorsoulnar aspect of the wrist. A tunnel is created from the ulnar side of the wrist to the insertion into the thumb. The tendon is passed through this tunnel and fixed as previously described.

Where there is an inadequate supply of tendon motors, and particularly congenital absence or hypoplasia of the thenar muscles, the hypothenar muscles can be used [104].

Procedure (Fig. 35.19).

Through an incision on the ulnar side of the hand the abductor digiti minimi is displayed from its insertion as far proximally as the carpus with care for its nerve supply.

The thumb is prepared as before and a large tunnel made across the base of the palm with tunnelling forceps. The abductor digiti minimi is led through this tunnel and is rotated like the page of a book so that its superficial surface lies deep in its new position. This prevents kinking of the neurovascular bundle and ensures a little more length. The tendon is usually not long enough to pass through a tunnel in the proximal phalanx of the thumb and has to be attached firmly to the tendon of the abductor pollicis brevis if this is present.

Transfers to restore abduction of the index, adduction of the thumb and to correct clawing of the fingers

The restoration of these functions and correction of clawing of the ulnar two digits may be required independently as an isolated feature or may be required in combination as a result of irreparable ulnar nerve lesions.

Restoration of abduction of the index [105]

Where first dorsal interosseous function is lacking due to ulnar nerve lesions or other causes the index finger cannot be stabilized in the abducted position and pinch prehension will be affected. This function may be restored by tendon transfer and depending on what motors are available the following muscles may be used:
(1) extensor indicis proprius,
(2) extensor pollicis brevis,
(3) a superficialis tendon taken round the radial side of the wrist [106].
The best results are obtained by transfer of the indicis proprius.

Operative procedure

Through a transverse dorsal incision over the head of the second metacarpal the extensor indicis proprius is identified on the ulnar side of the communis tendon and divided near its insertion. The tendon is freed proximally and then transferred in a straight line into the insertion of the first dorsal interosseous tendon. The transposed tendon is woven through the interosseous tendon and sutured as tight as possible with the finger abducted and the wrist in neutral position.

Restoration of adduction of the thumb

Loss of adduction power of the thumb is of significant effect in reducing the power of pinch grip and the absence of its function is demonstrated by Froment's sign. Replacement of its function by tendon transfer is difficult. Solonen has recommended the transfer of the extensor carpi radialis longus tendon [107]. It is elongated by a free graft taken through the second or third intermetacarpal space and along the line of the adductor and inserted into its tendon.

An alternative is to use a flexor superficialis tendon, usually to the ring finger, detached from its insertion and withdrawn through into the wrist using a longitudinal incision along the radial side of the flexor carpi ulnaris tendon. The tendon is then taken round the ulnar side of the wrist, through the second or third intermetacarpal space and inserted as with the previous tendon transfer [107]. Another method of using the superficialis tendon

[108] is to detach the insertion, leave it in the carpal tunnel and then reroute it along the adductor and into its tendon. By restoring abduction of the index and giving some adduction power to the thumb, about 50° of normal pinch grip can be obtained.

Claw hand

This may be seen in a combined median and ulnar nerve lesion when all four fingers are affected, a situation most frequently seen as a complication of leprosy. There is loss of active flexion at the metacarpophalangeal joints and active extension at the interphalangeal joints, the so-called 'intrinsic minus' hand (Fig. 35.20a). This allows the long extensors and flexors to take over control of the digits resulting in an extended position of the metacarpophalangeal joints and a tendency to a flexed position of the interphalangeal joints. Whether the metacarpophalangeal joints will adopt the position of hyperextension and therefore the true clawing of 'main en griffe' deformity will depend upon the laxity of the

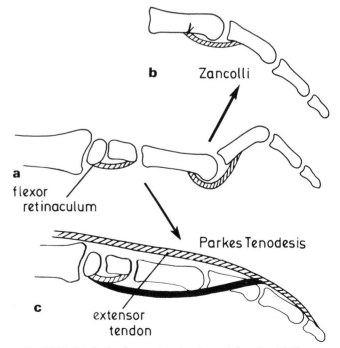

FIG. 35.20. Methods of correcting claw finger deformity. (a) The deformity, (b) Zancolli capsulodesis, (c) Parkes tenodesis.

structures on the volar aspect of the metacarpophalangeal joints. If the capsule and volar plate is tight then hyperextension and clawing will not occur. This forms the basis of Zancolli's procedure of tightening the volar plate [109] (Fig. 35.20b). This is in fact an internal 'knuckle duster' procedure analogous to the external splintage used to hold the metacarpophalangeal joints flexed to prevent their hyperextension by the long extensors and thus to bring the digits into a more balanced position.

Tendon transfers can be carried out in an attempt to replace the lost intrinsic function and to prevent or correct clawing. Transfers to replace complete abduction—adduction action of the intrinsics are not successful but, as has already been described, tendon transfer can be utilized to replace the first dorsal interosseous [105].

The history of tendon transfers to correct intrinsic weakness and clawing is long and interesting. Many transfers are more likely to work in a tenodesing manner than in true tendon gliding.

Two early attempts [73, 78] utilized the superficialis tendons to each digit divided near their insertion and transposed round the radial side of the digit along the line of the lumbrical and inserted into the extensor expansion near the proximal interphalangeal joint.

These operations were of limited success but pointed the way to other transfers passing from the volar aspect of the metacarpophalangeal joint along the lumbrical canal and inserted into the extensor.

Fowler [110] and Riordan [111] used the accessory extensors (indicis proprius and digiti minimi) which were freed as far distally as possible, each tendon split into two and taken through the intermetacarpal spaces, and along the lumbrical canal to their new attachment. The difficulty is the inadequate length and tendency of the tendons to become adherent and act more as a tenodesis.

Brand [94] introduced new techniques of tendon transfer in leprosy using as a motor either a wrist extensor or flexor, usually the extensor carpi radialis longus, or flexor carpi radialis. These motors are elongated by free tendon grafts taken through the intermetacarpal spaces and along the lumbrical canals to their new insertion. The tendons are attached with the metacarpophalangeal joints held in about 30° of flexion.

These tendon transfers have proved very effective for this purpose [112] and more normal and controlled flexion of the digits allow large objects to be held more satisfactorily.

True tendon gliding and mobility follows Brand's technique but many have felt that this is an extensive procedure and that equally good results can be obtained by a tenodesing effect as from *Parkes operation* [113] (Fig. 35.20c).

Operative procedure

Through a curved palmar incision the flexor retinaculum is displayed proximally and the lumbrical canals distally. Short longitudinal incisions are made on the dorso-radial aspect of each proximal segment of finger. Using the palmaris and plantaris or, if these are not obtainable, toe extensors, the tendons are attached firmly to the superficial surface of the flexor retinaculum. Each of four tendons is then passed through the lumbrical canal and taken through the extensor tendon to which it is firmly attached near the proximal interphalangeal joint. A pull-out wire suture is used with each tendon. The tension of the attachment is adjusted with the metacarpophalangeal joints flexed 30–40° and the proximal interphalangeal joints straight.

This tendon transfer really works as a tenodesis and is independent of any position of the wrist. When the hand is opened the long extensors straighten the metacarpophalangeal joints until the movement is checked by the tenodesis. The pull of the long extensors is then transmitted through to the interphalangeal joints.

This has proved a very effective procedure in controlling and correcting clawing of the hand, in boosting intrinsic function and allowing full activity of the long flexors and extensors in a useful range.

Tendon grafting and artificial tendons (Chapter 11)

Treatment of tendon adhesions

Conservative treatment (see also Chapters 11 & 36)

The resolution of indurated tissue following operation or injury will lead usually to a recovery of tendon gliding and movement of the tendon. Accurate measurement of the range of joint movement for which the tendon is responsible should be recorded at regular intervals and so long as this improves there would be no indication for operation.

In order to assist recovery of movement, however, a variety of conservative measures can be utilized. These include:

(1) Passive stretching and mobilizing under supervision of the physiotherapist.

(2) Serial corrective plasters or splintage and elastic traction.

(3) Gentle friction massage and the use of ultrasound.

(4) Local hydrocortisone injection.

Operative treatment (tenolysis)

Tenolysis, the freeing of an adherent tendon, may be indicated after tendon repair, tendon graft, tendon transfer or where a tendon is stuck after a fracture, joint surgery or crushing injury.

Once the range of gliding shows no further improvement a decision is made whether the functional impairment is severe enough to justify surgical release of the adhesions. If a significant increase in function can be anticipated then the timing of operation has to be carefully evaluated.

(1) *After repair*

Tenolysis should be delayed until at least six months after repair of cut tendons. Significant improvement in the range of movement may readily occur between three and six months after repair. After this period it is unlikely that there will be further improvement. Although it would be expected that adhesion would be only at the site of tendon injury it may be much more widespread, presumably due to bleeding into the tendon sheath. The development of adhesion and its extent will undoubtedly be influenced by the severity of the causal injury or by the development of any infection but also by the care and finesse of the repair procedure. With a careful technique and postoperative management (Chapter 11) tenolysis is required in about a quarter of the cases [114].

(2) *After injury*

Local tenolysis may be required where a tendon becomes adherent at the site of injury to bone or joint. A typical site for this is in fractures of the proximal phalanges where both extensor and flexor tendons are liable to get stuck. Provided joint contractures are pre-vented conservative measures should be continued while there is improvement in active range of movement. Once this has stopped improving, and where it remains significantly less than the range of passive movement, consideration should be given to tenolysis.

(3) *After transfer*

Adhesions after tendon transfers are unusual unless it has been necessary to take the transposed tendon through a scarred bed or through rigid osteofascial canals, for example, the interosseous membrane of the forearm. When the range of movement is disappointing and no progress is continuing tendon release can be considered.

(4) *After grafting*

A tendon graft is very likely to become adherent as it has to obtain an entirely new blood supply. This is largely dependent upon reaching the tendon through the adhesions along its path. The adhesions must be allowed to mature and it is the stretching of these adhesions which will eventually allow some measure of gliding of the graft. The tendency to improvement continues over a period of 6–9 months after operation. Provided the graft has been placed in a good bed and does not become adherent to unyielding structures like periosteum and joint capsule the improvement in the range of movement will often be sufficient to be functionally effective. When the graft becomes stuck and there is no useful movement tenolysis should be considered. It should not be carried out until a minimum of 9–10 months after operation. Earlier tenolysis, which inevitably will involve the whole length of the tendon, will so affect the blood supply of the tendon that rupture will be likely. It is only after a period of many months that the intratendinous vascular arrangement is such as to withstand the release of the adhesions.

It is difficult to assess how frequently tenolysis is required after tendon graft but it is probable that its judicious and selective use is responsible for a high percentage of excellent results in any large series [115]. Tenolysis is a formidable procedure which is often more difficult than the graft procedure itself and involves a very extensive release of the whole length of the tendon.

The result of tenolysis for any of the conditions

described will depend on the care with which it is carried out but also on a very careful postoperative regime of early mobilization. It is probable that the results will be improved by utilizing the technique of elastic traction [114].

Carstam [116] has shown the value of local hydrocortisone after tenolysis and James [117] uses systemic steroids for a period of three or four days to cover the operative period.

It must be appreciated that tenolysis, which requires immediate mobilization, is incompatible with other procedures at the same time that require immobilization.

The 'lumbrical plus' finger

Following amputation distal to the proximal interphalangeal joint, with resultant loss of profundus function, and after flexor tendon grafting, particularly where the graft is a little long, a most odd situation may occasionally arise. When the patient is asked to flex the finger it straightens at the proximal interphalangeal joint, a condition known as the 'lumbrical plus' finger [118]. It is considered to be due to the pull of the lumbrical muscle which, instead of working in concert with the profundus, appears as an antagonist and pulls through to its insertion into the extensor mechanism. Boyes [119] has stressed the importance of pulling the lumbrical distally on the profundus before using it to wrap round the proximal suture line of a tendon graft in order to prevent this effect. Stack [120] has described the tension in the lumbrical muscle and how this may lead to the deformity. This effect can be corrected by dividing the lumbrical tendon.

Recurrent swan neck deformity and locking of the proximal interphalangeal joint

The finger tends to adopt a swan-neck deformity on extension and easy flexion at the proximal interphalangeal joint becomes difficult. The finger may 'give' with a 'snap' as one or both lateral bands slip over the condyles of the proximal phalanx to allow flexion. The deformity may occur after injuries which have produced forced hyperextension at the proximal interphalangeal joint and torn or stretched the volar plate and capsule. This is likely to occur particularly in those that have congenital laxity of the volar structures and predisposition to hyperextension at the proximal interphalangeal joint. The disability may be slight and not require treatment but where it obstructs smooth flexion of the joint or where the snapping of the lateral bands in flexion becomes a nuisance, then the deformity should be corrected surgically. This may be achieved in various ways.

(1) A lateral band is detached proximally, dissected beyond the proximal interphalangeal joint but left attached distally. It is then brought volarwards passing across the front of the proximal interphalangeal joint and attached to the fibrous flexor sheath on the opposite side proximal to the joint which is held in about 10 degrees of flexion [121].

An alternative method described by Milford [122] is to thread the dissected lateral band through a small pulley made in the flexor tendon sheath opposite the proximal interphalangeal joint and then bring it dorsally to suture to the extensor hood under enough tension to create slight flexion contracture of the joint.

(2) If the volar plate is found to have been stretched or torn away from its bony attachment (usually to the neck of the proximal phalanx), the proximal part of the volar plate is transferred to a new attachment in the neck of the phalanx so that the joint is held rigidly in 5–10° flexion.

(3) Curtis [123] has recommended transferring half the flexor digitorum superficialis tendon which is detached proximally, threaded across the volar aspect of the proximal interphalangeal joint and attached to a drill hole in the proximal phalanx holding the joint in slight flexion.

(4) Where there is considerable joint instability, satisfactory strengthening of the volar structures can be made by a criss-cross tendon graft reconstruction fixed to bone [124].

For all these surgical procedures, access can be obtained by a mid-lateral incision centred on the proximal interphalangeal joint. It is sometimes necessary to expose the joint from each side to get satisfactory fixation. The results of these surgical procedures depend on achieving a stable repair with the joint in slight flexion. There is a tendency for the tendon reconstructions to stretch in time, and the best results are obtained where a satisfactory proximal advancement of the volar plate can be obtained.

REFERENCES

[1] MOBERG, E. The treatment of mutilating injuries of the upper limb. *Surgical Clinics of North America*, 1964, **44**, 1107.

[2] TUBIANA, R. The planning of surgical treatment. *The Hand*, 1975, **7**, 223.

[3] LITTLER, J. W. In *Reconstructive Plastic Surgery*, Ed. Converse J. M. Philadelphia, Saunders, 1964.

[4] CARROLL, R. E. AND HILL, N. A. Small joint arthrodesis in hand reconstruction. *Journal of Bone and Joint Surgery*, 1969, **51A**, 1219.

[5] MOBERG, E. Arthrodesis of finger joints. *Surgical Clinics of North America*, 1960, **40**, 465.

[6] POTENZA, A. D. A technique for arthrodesis of finger joints. *Journal of Bone and Joint Surgery*, 1973, **55A**, 1534.

[7] HARRISON, S. H. AND NICOLLE, F. F. J. A. A new intramedullary peg for arthrodesis. *British Journal of Plastic Surgery*, 1974, **27**, 240.

[8] HARRISON, S. H. The Harrison-Nicolle intra-medullary peg. Follow-up studies of 100 cases. *The Hand*, 1974, **6**, 304.

[9] EIKEN, O. AND CARSTAM, N. Functional assessment of basal joint fusion of the thumb. *Scandinavian Journal of Plastic and Reconstructive Surgery*, 1976, **4**, 122.

[10] EATON, R. G. AND LITTLER, J. W. A study of the basal joint of the thumb. *Journal of Bone and Joint Surgery*, 1969, **51A**, 661.

[11] JACKSON, I. T. AND ONGE, R. A. ST. The use of palmaris longus tendon to stabilize trapezium implants. *The Hand*, 1977, **9**, 42.

[12] GERVIS, W. H. Excision of the trapezium for osteoarthritis of the trapezio-metacarpal joint. *Journal of Bone and Joint Surgery*, 1949, **31B**, 537.

[13] HAFFAJEE, D. Endo-prosthetic replacement of the trapezium for arthrosis in the carpometocarpal joint of thumb. *Journal of Hand Surgery*, 1977, **2**, 127.

[14] LEACH, R. E. AND BOLTON, P. E. Arthritis of the carpometacarpal joint of the thumb. *Journal of Bone and Joint Surgery*, 1968, **50A**, 1171.

[15] LISTER, G. D., KLEINERT, H. E., KUTZ, J. E. AND ATESOY, E. Arthritis of the trapezial articulation treated by prosthetic replacement. *The Hand*, 1977, **9**, 117.

[16] SWANSON, A. B. Disabling arthritis at the base of the thumb. *Journal of Bone and Joint Surgery*, 1972, **51A**, 661.

[17] SWANSON, A. B. Osteoarthritis of the hand. *Journal of Bone and Joint Surgery*, 1973, **55A**, 1769.

[18] FERLIC, D. C., BUSBEE, G. A. AND CLAYTON, M. L. Degenerative arthritis of the carpometacarpal joint of the thumb. *Journal of Hand Surgery*, 1977, **2**, 212.

[19] KESSLER, I. AND AXER, A. Arthroplasty of first carpometacarpal joint with a silicone implant. *Plastic Reconstructive Surgery*, 1971, **47**, 252.

[20] KESSLER, I. Silicone arthroplasty of the trapeziometacarpal joint. *Journal of Bone and Joint Surgery*, 1973, **55B**, 285.

[21] ASHWORTH, C. R., BLATT, G., CHUINARD, R. AND STARK, H. H. Silicone rubber interposition arthroplasty of the carpometacarpal joint of the thumb. *Journal of Hand Surgery*, 1977, **2**, 395.

[22] SWANSON, A. B. Silicone rubber implants for replacement of arthritic or destroyed joints in the hand. *Surgical Clinics of North America*, 1968, **48**, 1113.

[23] GOLDNER, J. L., GOULD, J. S., URBANIAK, J. R. AND MCCALLUM, D. E. Metacarpophalangeal joint arthroplasty with silicone/dacron prosthesis (Niebauer type). Six and a half years experience. *Journal of Hand Surgery*, 1977, **2**, 200.

[24] NIEBAUER, J. J. AND LANDRY, R. M. Dacron/silicone prosthesis for the metacarpophalangeal and interphalangeal joints. *The Hand*, 1971, **3**, 55.

[25] ISELIN, F. Arthroplasty of the proximal interphalangeal joint after trauma. *The Hand*, 1975, **7**, 41.

[26] REID, D. A. C. Corrective osteotomy in the hand. *The Hand*, 1974, **6**, 50.

[27] ONNE, L. Rotary angulatory osteotomy of the metacarpal bones in mutilated hands, *Acta chirurgica Scandinavica*, 1954, **108**, 268.

[28] LISTER, G. D. Intraosseous wiring of the digital skeleton. *Journal of Hand Surgery*, 1978, **3**, 427.

[29] CROCKETT, D. J. Rigid fixation of bones of the hand using Kirschner wires bonded with acrylic resin. *The Hand*, 1974, **6**, 106.

[30] BROWN, M. Trephine techniques for small bone grafts. *The Hand*, 1974, **6**, 103.

[31] JOSHI, B. B. Sensory flaps for the degloved mutilated hand. *The Hand*, 1974, **6**, 247.

[32] KESSLER, I. Transposition lengthening of a digital ray after multiple amputations of fingers. *The Hand*, 1976, **8**, 176.

[33] MICHON, J. AND DOLICH, B. H. The metacarpal hand. *The Hand*, 1974, **6**, 288.

[34] MURAT, K. AND NAKAMURA, R. Reconstruction of the mutilated hand. *The Hand*, 1976, **8**, 78.

[35] WEKESSER, E. C. Reconstruction of a grasping mechanism following extensive loss of digits. *Clinical Orthopaedics*, 1959, **15**, 60.

[36] PULVERTAFT, R. G. Proceedings of Tenth Congress of S.I.C.O.T., 1966.

[37] PULVERTAFT, R. G. Hemi-amputation of the hand. *Journal of Royal College of Surgeons of Edinburgh*, 1969, **14**, 89.

[38] BONNEY, G. Medial component mobilisation in hemi-amputation of the hand. *Proceedings Second Hand Club*, 1975, p. 26.

[39] CLARKSON, P. Hemi-amputation of the hand. *Proceedings Second Hand Club*, 1975, p. 26.

[40] LASSAR, G. N. Reconstruction of a digit following loss of all fingers with preservation of the thumb. *Journal of Bone and Joint Surgery*, 1959, **41A**, 519.

[41] TUBIANA, R., STACK, H. G. AND HAKSTIAN, R. W. Restoration of prehension after severe mutilation of the hand. *Journal of Bone and Joint Surgery*, 1966, **48B**, 455.

[42] CLARKSON, P. W. AND CHANDLER, R. On making thumbs. *Plastic and Reconstructive Surgery*, 1962, **29**, 325.

[43] LITTLER, J. W. On making a thumb: one hundred years of surgical effort. *The Journal of Hand Surgery*, 1976, **1**, 35.

[44] TANZER, R. C. AND LITTLER, J. W. Reconstruction of the thumb. *Plastic and Reconstructive Surgery*, 1948, **43**, 533.

[45] VERDAN, C. Reconstruction of the thumb. *Surgical Clinics of North America*, 1968, **48**, 1033.

[46] BOWE, J. J. Thumb reconstruction by index transposition. *Plastic and Reconstructive Surgery*, 1963, **32**, 414.

[47] MOORE, F. T. The technique of pollicisation of the index finger. *British Journal of Plastic Surgery*, 1948, **1**, 16.

[48] ZANCOLLI, E. Transplantation of the index finger in congenital absence of the thumb. *Journal of Bone and Joint Surgery*, 1960, **42A**, 658.

[49] HARRISON, S. H. Pollicisation in children. *The Hand*, 1971, **3**, 204.

[50] BARSKY, A. J. Reconstructive surgery in congenital abnormalities. *Surgical Clinics of North America*, 1957, **39**, 449.

[51] BUCK-GRAMCKO, D. Pollicisation of the index finger—method and results in aplasia and hypoplasia of the thumb. *Journal of Bone and Joint Surgery*, 1971, **53A**, 1605.

[52] LITTLER, J. W. Neurovascular pedicle method of digital transposition for reconstruction of thumb. *Plastic and Reconstructive Surgery*, 1953, **12**, 303.

[53] LITTLER, J. W. Digital transposition. In *Current Practice in Orthopaedic Surgery, 3*, Ed. Adams, J. B. St. Louis: Mosby, 1966.

[54] LITTLER, J. W. Principles of reconstructive surgery of the hand. In *Current Practice in Orthopaedic Surgery, 3*, Ed. Adams, J. B. St. Louis: Mosby, 1966.

[55] HARRISON, S. H. Restoration of muscle balance in pollicisation. *Plastic and Reconstructive Surgery*, 1964, **34**, 236.

[56] MATEV, I. B. Thumb reconstruction after amputation at the metacarpophalangeal joint by bone lengthening. *Journal of Bone and Joint Surgery*, 1970, **52A**, 957.

[57] GILLIES, SIR HAROLD AND MILLAR, R. D. *The Principles and Art of Plastic Surgery*, Vol. 2, part 5, Chap. 23. Boston: Little, Brown, 1957.

[58] HUGHES, N. C. AND MOORE, F. T. The Gillies 'Cocked-hat' flap. *British Journal of Plastic Surgery*, 1950, **3**, 34.

[59] BARRON, J. N. Cock another hat at the thumb. *The Hand*, 1977, **9**, 39.

[60] REID, D. A. C. Reconstruction of the thumb. *Journal of Bone and Joint Surgery*, 1960, **42B**, 444.

[61] MCGREGOR, I. A. AND SIMMONETTA, C. Reconstruction of the thumb by composite bone-skin flap. *British Journal of Plastic Surgery*, 1964, **17**, 37.

[62] COBBETT, J. R. Free digital transfer. Transfer of a great toe to replace an amputated thumb. *Journal of Bone and Joint Surgery*, 1969, **51B**, 677.

[63] BURKE, H. J., MCLEAN, D. H., GEORGE, P. T. et al. Thumb replacement. Great toe transplantation by microvascular anastomosis. *British Journal of Plastic Surgery*, 1973, **26**, 194.

[64] REID, D. A. C. The neurovascular island flap in thumb reconstruction. *British Journal of Plastic Surgery*, 1966, **19**, 234.

[65] REID, D. A. C. Pollicisation—an appraisal. *The Hand*, 1969, **1**, 27.

[66] BRUCE, B. Ring finger pollicisation. *Journal of Bone and Joint Surgery*, 1964, **46A**, 1069.

[67] LITTLER, J. W. Neurovascular skin island transfer in reconstructive joint surgery. *Transactions of the International Society of Plastic Surgeons*. Edinburgh, Livingstone. 1960.

[68] TUBIANA, R. AND DUPANE, J. Restoration of sensibility in the hand by neurovascular skin island transfer. *Journal of Bone and Joint Surgery*, 1961, **43B**, 474.

[69] BUCHAN, A. C. The neurovascular island flap in reconstruction of the thumb. *The Hand*, 1969, **1**, 19.

[70] MCGREGOR, I. A. Less than satisfactory experiences with neurovascular island flaps. *The Hand*, 1969, **1**, 21.

[71] NATHAN, P. A. AND NGUYEN BUN TRUNG. The Krukenberg operation: a modified technique avoiding skin grafts. *Journal of Hand Surgery*, 1977, **2**, 127.

[72] SWANSON, A. B. The Krukenberg procedure in the juvenile amputee. *Journal of Bone and Joint Surgery*, 1964, **46A**, 1540.

[73] BOYES, J. H. *Bunnells Surgery of the Hand*, 5th Edition. Philadelphia, Lippincott. 1970.

[74] BEEVOR, A. Quoted by Boyes. *Journal of Hand Surgery*, 1976, **1**, 83.

[75] STEINDLER, A. Tendon transplantation in the upper extremity. *American Journal of Surgery*, 1939, **44**, 260.

[76] MAYER, L. The physiological method of tendon transplantation. *Surgery, Gynecology and Obstetrics*, 1916, **22**, 182.

[77] JONES, R. AND LOVETT, R. W. *Orthopedic Surgery*. New York, William Wood, 1923.

[78] STILES, H. *Treatment of Injuries of the Peripheral Nerve*. London, Hodder & Stoughton. 1922.

[79] BRAND, P. W. Biomechanics of tendon transfer. *Orthopedic Clinics of North America*, 1974, **5**, 205.

[80] CURTIS, R. M. Fundamental principles of tendon transfer. *Orthopedic Clinics of North America*, 1974, **5**, 231.

[81] OMER, G. E. The technique and timing of tendon transfers. *Orthopedic Clinics of North America*, 1974, **5**, 243.

[82] CLARK, J. M. P. Reconstruction of biceps brachii by transplantation of pectoral muscle. *British Journal of Surgery*, 1946, **34**, 180.

[83] MOBERG, E. Surgical treatment for absent single hand grip and elbow extension in quadriplegia. *Journal of Bone and Joint Surgery*, 1975, **57A**, 196.

[84] BUNNELL, S. Restoring flexion to the paralytic elbow. *Journal of Bone and Joint Surgery*, 1975, **33A**, 566.

[85] MAYER, L. AND GREEN, W. Experiences with the Steindler flexorplasty at the elbow. *Journal of Bone and Joint Surgery*, 1954, **36A**, 775.

[86] BROOKS, D. M. AND SEDDON, H. J. Pectoral transplantation for paralysis of the flexors of the elbow. *Journal of Bone and Joint Surgery*, 1959, **51B**, 37.

[87] SEDDON, H. J. Transplantation of pectoralis major for paralysis of flexion of the elbow. *Proceedings of the Royal Society of Medicine*, 1949, **42**, 837.

[88] CARROLL, R. E. Restoration of flexor power to the flail elbow by transplantation of the triceps. *Surgery, Gynecology and Obstetrics*, 1952, **95**, 685.

[89] ZANCOLLI, E. Personal communication, 1977.

[90] SCHOTTSTAEDT, E. R., LARSEN, L. J. AND BOST, F. C. Complete muscle transposition. *Journal of Bone and Joint Surgery*, 1955, **37A**, 897.

[91] BARTON, N. J. Radial nerve lesions. *The Hand*, 1973, **5**, 200.

[92] ZACHARY, R. B. Tendon transplantation for radial paralysis. *Proceedings of the Royal Society of Medicine*, 1946, **39**, 722.

[93] HENRY, A. K. *Extensile Exposure*. Edinburgh, Livingstone, 1957.

[94] BRAND, W. Tendon grafting—illustrated by a new operation for intrinsic paralysis of the fingers. *Journal of Bone and Joint Surgery*, 1961, **43B**, 444.

[95] BROOKS, D. M. Tendon transplantation in the forearm and arthrodesis of the wrist. *Proceedings of the Royal Society of Medicine*, 1949, **42**, 838.

[96] PHALEN, G. S. AND MILLER, R. C. The transfer of wrist extension muscles to restore or reinforce flexion power of the fingers and opposition of the thumb. *Journal of Bone and Joint Surgery*, 1947, **29**, 993.

[97] LAMB, D. W. AND LANDRY, R. The hand in quadriplegia. *Paraplegia*, 1972, **9**, 204.

[98] MAYER, I. Operative reconstruction of paralysed upper extremity. *Journal of Bone and Joint Surgery*, 1939, **21**, 377.

[99] GOLDNER, J. L. Tendon transfer for irreparable peripheral nerve injuries of the upper extremity. *Orthopedic Clinics of North America*, 1974, **5**, 343.

[100] THOMPSON, T. C. Modified operation for opponens paralysis. *Journal of Bone and Joint Surgery*, 1942, **24**, 623.

[101] STEINDLER, A. Flexorplasty of the thumb in thenar palsy. *Surgery, Gynecology and Obstetrics*, 1930, **50**, 1005.

[102] MAKIN, M. Translocation of the flexor pollicis longus to restore opposition. *Journal of Bone and Joint Surgery*, 1967, **49B**, 458.

[103] JOSHI, B. B. Personal communication, 1976.

[104] LITTLER, J. W. AND COOLEY, S. G. E. Opposition of the thumb and its restoration by transfer of abductor digiti quinti. *Journal of Bone and Joint Surgery*, 1963, **45A**, 1389.

[105] CLIPPINGER, F. W. AND GOLDNER, J. L. Tendon transfer as substitutes for paralysed first dorsal and ulnar interosseous muscles. *Journal of Bone and Joint Surgery*, 1965, **47A**, 633.

[106] GRAHAM, W. C. AND RIORDAN, D. Sublimis transplant to restore abduction of index finger. *Plastic and Reconstructive Surgery*, 1947, **2**, 459.

[107] SOLONEN, K. A. AND BAKALIM, G. E. Restoration of pinch grip in traumatic ulnar palsy. *The Hand*, 1976, **8**, 39.

[108] TUBIANA, R. Personal communication.

[109] ZANCOLLI, E. A. Claw hand causes by paralysis of intrinsic muscles. A simple surgical procedure for its correction. *Journal of Bone and Joint Surgery*, 1957, **39A**, 1076.

[110] FOWLER, S. B. Extensor apparatus of the digits. *Journal of Bone and Joint Surgery*, 1949, **31B**, 477.

[111] RIORDAN, D. C. Tendon transplantation in median nerve and ulnar nerve paralysis. *Journal of Bone and Joint Surgery*, 1953, **35A**, 312.

[112] WHITE, W. L. Restoration of function and balance of the wrist and hand by tendon transfers. *Surgical Clinics of North America*, 1960, **40**, 427.

[113] PARKES, A. Paralytic claw fingers—a graft tenodesis operation. *The Hand*, 1973, **5**, 192.

[114] KLEINERT, H. Personal communication.

[115] FETROW, K. O. Tenolysis in the hand and wrist. *Journal of Bone and Joint Surgery*, 1967, **49A**, 667.

[116] CARSTAM, N. Effect of cortisone on the formation of tendon adhesions and healing. *Acta chirurgica Scandinavica*, 1953 (Supp. 182).

[117] JAMES, J. I. P. The value of tenolysis. *The Hand*, 1969, **1**, 118.

[118] PARKES, A. The 'lumbrical plus' finger. *The Hand*, 1970, **1**, 164.

[119] BOYES, J. H. *Bunnell's Surgery of the Hand*, 5th Edition. Philadelphia, Lippincott, 1970.

[120] STACK, G. Tension in the lumbrical muscle. *The Hand*, 1970, **2**, 166.

[121] LITTLER, J. L. Restoration of the oblique retinacular ligament. *G.E.M.* No. 1, Paris, 1966.

[122] MILFORD, L. W. The Hand. In *Campbell's Operative Orthopaedics*, 5th Ed. Edited Krenshaw, A. H. St. Louis, Mosby, 1971.

[123] CURTIS, R. M. In *Hand Surgery*, Edited Flynn, J. F. Baltimore, Williams and Wilkins, 1966.

[124] ADAMS, J. P. Correction of chronic dorsal subluxation of the proximal interphalangeal joint by means of a criss-cross volar graft. *Journal of Bone and Joint Surgery*, 1959, **41A**, 111.

CHAPTER 36

Physiotherapy and Occupational Therapy in Rehabilitation

PATRICIA WILSON and H. MARY PEARCE

The treatment of patients with hand conditions can be most interesting and rewarding for both patient and therapist. The best results are obtained with early physiotherapy followed by combined treatment sessions later. The patient concentrates on applying the improvement gained in physiotherapy to the activities in occupational therapy [1]. We believe that attendance of the therapist at the hand clinic is most important and essential for the best results.

Department space and equipment

It is ideal for the physical and occupational therapy departments to be planned together as a comprehensive unit with an easy access to the outpatient department and ward areas.

Physiotherapy

A very large area is not required and most of the treatment can be done with several patients round a large table, working with objects such as safety pins, paper clips, dog clips, elastic bands, string, screw top bottles or jars and putty. These provide a good basis for retraining hand movements. A rollator is useful for regaining and strengthening grip, wrist movements and forearm rotation. Wax baths, ice machines and ultrasound are helpful. The expertise and facilities for provision of plaster and thermoplastic splints are essential.

Occupational therapy

Modern departments are planned with:
(1) A 'Home Unit' consisting of kitchen, bed and bath areas,
(2) A light workshop for sedentary work and
(3) A heavy workshop for carpentry, light metal work and if possible, gardening and cement work.

The emphasis on the type of activity will vary with the community in which the hospital is based.

Referral for treatment

Systems of referral will vary, but the following information is essential on the referral form:
Name, age and address of the patient.
Hospital unit number.
Name of consultant.
Diagnosis.
Full clinical details, with the dates of injury and/or operation.
Treatment requested, specifying any movement which should be restricted and whether splints may be removed during treatment.
Follow-up appointment.

Assessment

The effects of disease (e.g. rheumatoid arthritis), injury, operation and immobilization vary in degree from patient to patient, but in general may result in the following:

(1) Loss of pattern of use of the whole or part of the affected hand and of bimanual activity.

(2) Decreased range of joint movements.

(3) Decrease of power of grasp.

(4) Impaired sensation.

(5) Oedema, scarring and poor skin condition.

(6) A psychological reaction with fear and anxiety for future function and employment.

The therapist must initially assess the problem in full to form a base line for treatment. Therapists should adopt the methods of measurement used by the referring surgeon. The systems described have been used for a number of years in our combined rehabilitation clinic and have proved satisfactory.

Methods of assessment of function

Range of movement

The range of active and passive movement should be accurately recorded (see Figs. 5.5 and 5.6). Joint range should be checked at least weekly and recorded on the chart using a small goniometer so that progress can be seen readily (Fig. 5.3). To record overall flexion of a digit, the distance between the tip of the finger and the distal palmar crease is measured.

Measuring joint range using a flexible wire (The Odstock Method) is an alternative; the range is transferred to a sheet using different coloured inks for repeat measurements.

Muscle power

Accurate recordings of power grasp and pinch grip can be made using a dynamometer or sphygmomanometer (see Fig. 5.11a, b).

Sensation

Loss of sensibility to light touch, pinprick, temperature and areas of hypersensitivity or paraesthesiae should be recorded on the chart. Two point discrimination (see Fig. 5.13) is currently the best way of sensory assessment. The position of any scar should be noted on the chart of the hand. The general state of the skin and any scarring or oedema is recorded.

The occupational therapist should carry out the following more detailed assessments of sensory appreciation, the tests being carried out with the patient's eyes closed;

Shape recognition

Wooden blocks of similar size made up as a circle, square, rectangle, triangle are used.

Object recognition

A comb, spoon, pen, key, paper clip and coin are useful objects.

Texture

Cotton wool, coarse and fine sandpaper are best for this test.

Use of the hand

An objective test of grasp can be made by asking the patient to hold a hammer or brush handle and of pinch by presenting a pencil, pin and key to handle. It may be necessary to cover aspects of self-care more fully and the following list of directives will be useful to check.

Dominant hand

Eating   Pick up and grasp knife/spoon, cut food. Lift full cup.

Washing   Pick up soap/use face flannel, clean teeth, turn tap. Shave/put on make up. Brush/comb hair.

Dressing   Do up buttons/laces/zips/hooks. Pull on tights. Put on jacket/overcoat.

General   Use pencil/turn key/doorhandle.

Non-dominant hand

Eating   Pick up and grasp fork.

Washing   Squeeze tube of toothpaste, grasp soap.

Dressing   Do up buttons/laces/zips/hooks. Pull on tights. Put on jacket/overcoat.

General household. Many patients experience difficulties in performing household activities such as:

(1) Preparing food—cutting vegetables/meat.

(2) Filling and lifting kettle/saucepan. (A full 3 pint kettle weighs about 4 kg).

(3) Lifting and holding dishes, putting electric plugs into sockets.

(4) Making beds, ironing, washing.

General. Capability to use public transport and to drive a car.

Interests and hobbies. Many patients have interests or hobbies which may be used as therapeutic measures and the therapist should check that these are resumed at an appropriate stage in treatment.

Time and frequency of treatment sessions

The time may vary from minutes to an hour or more each day. Patients with serious problems should be seen every day while minor conditions may require only two or three sessions a week. A few minutes spent on instructing and checking progress may save hours of work later. The patient should be given a specific programme to carry out every hour of the day at home. Occasionally it may be necessary to give written instructions. The physiotherapist starts the initial treatment and then as progress is made, intensive occupational therapy is introduced at the appropriate stage. This should ideally be twice daily but once a day is satisfactory if the patient is prepared to carry out a programme at home.

Treatment

Physiotherapy

It is often possible to supervise several patients at the same time and group treatment can provide a useful challenge in competition between patients. However, it will be necessary to treat some patients individually, e.g. when massage is needed to loosen adherent scars or passive movements carried out to gain range before active exercises.

Skin care

As dressings can restrict movement they should be kept to a minimum and discarded as soon as possible. After operation and a period of immobilization the skin is often dry, in poor condition and its quality must be improved. If the wounds are healed sufficiently, soaks in warm water help loosen old dry skin and scabs; this is followed by local massage in the form of small circular kneadings and transverse frictions using lanoline, oil and moisturising creams. These measures may need to be repeated for the next few sessions. Any scars or indurated areas should be massaged to mobilise underlying tissues and to prevent contracture of the scars.

Oedema

When the hand is swollen, treatment is carried out with the arm in elevation; instructions should be given to continue elevation at home, if necessary sitting or lying with the hand raised above shoulder level. Slings should be avoided but the patient is taught to keep the hand elevated and the fingers moving to aid dispersal of oedema fluid.

Wax and ice

Wax and ice can both be used to stimulate the circulation prior to exercise. Wax is excellent for wrist injuries and is applied by dipping the hand and wrist in and out several times until a coat forms. The part is then wrapped in greaseproof paper or plastic bags and blankets until the heat has dispersed—about 10 to 15 minutes. The wax is then peeled off; the part feels very much freer and the range of movement can be increased with exercises. Ice is very satisfactory for finger injuries and can be given as baths or packs which help to reduce pain and spasm. When using an ice bath the hand is dipped in and out of a mixture of ice and water until the skin is flushed. This can also be used alternately with hot baths with good effect. Ice packs are very beneficial in the presence of oedema.

Ultrasonic therapy

Ultrasound is being used increasingly to help reduce oedema and to soften scars and adhesions.

Exercises

The aim of exercise is to regain a full range of movement, increase power and disperse swelling. It is important at an early stage to know if any movement should be avoided as healing tendons and nerves could be disrupted. Patients must be taught their movements and instructed to do them frequently at home, for at least five minutes every hour. Encouragement of the normal use of the hand is most important. Joints of the hand which are unaffected by operation, injury or immobilisation may easily stiffen and encouragement in their use is needed to prevent this. Care must also be taken to maintain a full range of elbow and shoulder movements. A combination of active and passive movements are usually necessary in most hand conditions. Where joints are stiff or tendon pull through is weak, concentration on mobilisation of individual interphalangeal joints is taught by holding the digit proximal to the flexor crease of the affected joint. This can become a tedious exercise but its importance must be made clear to the patient. Resisted exercises and proprioceptive neuromuscular facilitation techniques are helpful in regaining range and strength.

Contractures of the thumb web space and of the finger joints are much easier to prevent than correct. Fixed contractures of metacarpophalangeal joints are particularly difficult to improve, but contractures of the thumb web and proximal interphalangeal joints can be improved by passive movements and serial plasters [1] which are made to maintain the gain in range, and are worn between the treatments and at night. Following treatment of individual joints, other tasks are given to improve general hand function by gripping foam or putty, threading paper clips, tying knots in string, using safety pins, taking screw tops off bottles or tubes of varying diameter, picking up small pieces of paper, at first between finger and thumb and then progressing to tweezers and dog clips to add resistance. These mainly help flexion and opposition; extension can be gained by stretching elastic bands between finger and thumb and by flicking cotton wool or paper with the finger tips.

Occupational therapy

The role of the occupational therapist is to provide a planned programme of daily activities to enable recovery of potential function as quickly as possible. This implies regaining movement, power and sensation as a basis for using the hand individually and bimanually in a normal pattern. Many patients are unable to translate the improvement gained by physiotherapy to their everyday activities and occupational therapy can offer a great deal of help by the very nature of the diverse equipment in the department. Many patients avoid using the injured part through fear of experiencing further pain; lack of use of the limb over a period may result in a change in the pattern of activity, e.g. dominance may be transferred or a one handed pattern develops. Where patients are referred early, these changes can be avoided and the normal pattern reinforced.

Patients who suffer sensory loss can be trained to compensate for this by using a simple visual routine to control the use of tools and equipment.

The psychological effects of injury to the hand can be alleviated through reassurance of the patient during the treatment session and by discussing the expectation of recovery. It is surprising how many patients believe that the hand will never return to normal.

Where the injury is such that a return to previous work is impossible, an early assessment of work potential is needed for determining suitability for alternative work or retraining. A satisfactory service cannot be provided unless there is regular contact with the referring surgeon, combined attendance at follow up clinics being invaluable. The therapist learns to tailor her methods to suit the surgeon, and can give useful information on the patient's progress and identify problems which arise during treatment.

Early referral is required so that the programme has the maximum effect both physically and psychologically. The results of late referral are often unsatisfactory, and the surgeon then thinks that occupational therapy is of little value and the therapist feels that her skills are not used properly.

Many conditions present common problems and whilst the aims of treatment may be the same, programmes must be tailored to suit the patient's individual needs. These programmes are based on short periods of individual treatment, retraining pinch and gross grip, using remedial games of all kinds which are adapted to suit different conditions.

As the patient makes progress other activities are introduced; for example, daily living and household activities, light and heavy carpentry, metalwork, cord knotting, paper folding, stool seating and printing. The work is made progressively more difficult until the heaviest and most comprehensive work appropriate to the patient's job and circumstances is being used.

Common conditions of the hand requiring a combined programme of physiotherapy and occupational therapy

Crush injuries (see also Chapters 8, 9)

Crush injuries always have marked and persistent oedema and are often complicated by skin problems, fractures and tendon and nerve injuries.

Once the oedema is under control and any fractures and other injuries have had the necessary immobilisation, the physiotherapist should begin to mobilise the hand to relieve any residual swelling.

Contrast baths or ice packs in elevation followed by massage and general skin care in elevation will help to reduce swelling and mobilise scars. This is followed by active and passive exercises with stretching plasters to overcome contractures as necessary. The patient should progress to a full rehabilitation programme as soon as possible.

Fractures (see also Chapter 13)

Early attention is required by the physiotherapist to prevent stiffness of parts which do not require immobilization and then a programme of active exercises of the affected part which has been immobilized.

Lacerations

Superficial lacerations should not lead to stiff joints but if the scars become adherent, massage and skin care is given and a programme of exercises is instituted in order to mobilize the part as quickly as possible.

Tendon injuries

Following repair of flexor tendons, controlled mobilisation by the technique of Kleinert (see Chapter 11) may be practised and require the supervision of the therapist. The patient is taught to extend the finger against the traction, relaxing the elastic band if necessary by the other hand. The proximal interphalangeal joint must be fully extended to the plaster backshell, which holds the wrist and metacarpophalangeal joints each in about 40° flexion. The patient then relaxes the finger so that the elastic band returns the finger to the previous position. This is continued for 3 weeks with the patient actively moving his unaffected fingers to prevent stiffness. The plaster is then removed and active flexion of the affected digit started. The traction is retained for a further week between exercises. At this stage the traction is removed and the patient can mobilise fully.

Flexor tendon grafts (see also Chapter 11)

Prior to operation, full passive joint range must be gained and then maintained by the patient, with occasional check visits in the department.

Following operation the hand is immobilized for three weeks but full elbow and shoulder movements are maintained until the following programme of mobilization to the hand is started.

First week

(1) Passive flexion exercises of all joints of involved finger to recover passive range.

(2) Active flexion exercises of the involved finger without resistance. Warm water baths are of value initially on removal of dressings to give relaxation, ease pain and facilitate movement.

Second week

Continue as above. Add passive extension exercises at the distal joint with the metacarpophalangeal and proximal interphalangeal joints flexed.

Third week

Continue as above. Add active extension exercises without resistance.

Fourth week

As above. Begin flexion and extension exercises against resistance.

The aim is a return to work 8 weeks after operation.

Some adherence of the graft may develop and lanolin massage can be given to help mobilize the tissues. If flexion contractures develop, it may be necessary to fit a splint which can be worn at night to help stretch the contractures. Occupational therapy is started at this stage with specific activities to make use of the range of tendon glide.

Amputations (see also Chapter 17)

Amputation of a finger may affect the mobilization of the other fingers and the patient should be encouraged to use the hand early. In a partial digital amputation, the remaining joints of that finger will readily stiffen unless the patient is taught specifically to mobilize these as well as general mobilization of the hand. Digital amputees should be referred to occupational therapy following removal of stitches. Patients are naturally cautious about pressure on the scar, and it must be stressed that the part will become less sensitive as it is used. It is never too soon to start activity and as soon as the skin is healed a sand bowl can be used to begin the toughening up process. Dusting and gardening are suitable follow up home activities. Tapping the stump end is a method of toughening nerves and desensitizing painful neuromata but must be carried out at least three times a day for a few minutes to be effective. Many patients with digital amputation suffer psychological distress and are concerned that the ugly stump will remain swollen and be of little use to them; many reject it and will not even look at it. The inclusion of the patient in small groups with similar conditions will, with the reassurance from the therapist, help to allay these fears. Suitable activities give practical proof of normal usage.

Division of nerves

Loss of sensation can be even more disabling than loss of power, and even small patches of insensitive skin can interfere with normal function. If the area is functionally important, for example the ulnar side of the thumb or radial side of the index finger, simple repetitive tasks in the occupational therapy department requiring gross and pinch grip should be instituted using vision to compensate for the deficit. A short period of treatment is usually sufficient for the average patient, providing these measures are applied to some definite tasks at home.

Compensation for larger areas of sensory loss, e.g. full median or ulnar distribution, takes longer. Initially the patient is taught to use residual sensory areas to identify and manipulate objects, together with the aid of visual training as a supplementary method to help develop a near-normal pattern of use. The programme is based on the activities used in the initial assessment and progresses from the level of identification.

The therapist must understand the dangers associated with sensory loss and reinforce the warnings already given by medical staff that the skin may be at risk from lack of sensory protection when smoking, striking matches, handling hot dishes, cooking and washing up.

Sensory retraining by the occupational therapist is divided into three sections covering shape, texture and weight but training sessions are not sufficient in themselves and the sensory appreciation must be applied to an overall activity, preferably where both hands are needed.

Continued use of the hand is the most effective way of alleviating hypersensitivity. Tapping initiated under supervision is helpful in this and also in desensitizing scars.

Management of specific nerve injuries (see also Chapter 12)

Radial

A lively extensor splint (Fig. 37.11) is fitted and requires a practical assessment of its effectiveness in allowing the patient to use the hand normally whilst wearing it. If work is heavy, the splint may not be strong enough and the patient should seek temporary alternative employment.

Median

A full sensory training programme enables the patient to make the best use of the hand. An opponens splint prevents web contracture and retains thumb mobility allowing the use of pinch grip (see Fig. 37.2b).

Ulnar

Diminished pinch and grasp can usually be compensated except for fine discriminatory work or when a powerful grasp is required. The sensory deficit is seldom of great importance.

Dupuytren's contracture (see also Chapter 32)

Physiotherapy starts before removal of the stitches, all joints being put through a full passive range of flexion and the patient encouraged to do active movements. Gentle stretching into extension is started and on removing stitches, local massage to the scar. There is often some superficial necrotic and dry skin which will be loosened by the massage and should be removed.

A plaster or metal night splint may be required to help maintain extension and prevent the healing scar from contracting (see Fig. 32.16).

Rheumatoid arthritis (see also Chapter 25)

The role of the therapist is to take part in assessment of function, prevention of deformity and treatment.

Assessment

Function of the hand in daily living and work activities is assessed routinely showing whether normal or adaptive methods are present and the degree to which pain, weakness or joint deformity affect normal usage. Pre-operative assessment which gives an objective picture to supplement clinical findings, is essential where surgery is contemplated.

Prevention of deformity

Advice at an early stage of the disease about aids to daily living and the provision of suitable splints to allay pain and prevent deformity is an important part of the work of the occupational therapist.

Treatment

Any period of inaction will be followed by loss of power and diminution of function and the therapist can make a valuable contribution to a programme aimed at mobilising, increasing power and building up confidence. The emphasis is on a slow and gentle progress otherwise more painful and swollen joints will be the result. A post operative assessment of daily living activities and hand function to compare with the pre-operative assessment is required and may indicate whether further treatment is needed.

The hemiplegic hand (see also Chapter 29)

Facilitation techniques employed in an integrated physiotherapy/occupational therapy programme ensure the diminution of spasm and prevention of flexion contractures at wrist and elbow. Carefully selected activities are given as useful function returns, ensuring that they do not induce spasm and that abnormal patterns of movement are avoided. In some cases, useful gross grip may return with partial sensation.

Resettlement and retraining

The expectation of the vast majority of patients with injuries of the hand coincides with the goal of treatment which is a return to their previous work. Where this proves impossible, alternative employment is the only answer. This may imply retraining; the therapist's report on the patient's abilities are a necessary contribution to the Disablement Resettlement Officer's final decision.

Compensation (see also Chapter 39)

Experience shows that a pending claim for compensation results in poor attendance for treatment and a passive attitude on the patient's part, which has unfortunately sometimes been engendered by legal advice. Since effective recovery is dependent upon the full involvement of the patient, this attitude often leads to a poor return of function which may adversely affect the patient's whole life.

REFERENCE

[1] WYNN PARRY, C. B. *Rehabilitation of the Hand*, 3rd Ed. London, Butterworths, 1973.

CHAPTER 37

Orthoses for the Hand

MARGARET ELLIS

An orthosis is an appliance used to give support and optimal possible function to a weakened part of the body [1]. Thus any external device, excluding prosthesis (p. 543), may be termed orthosis.

Wood, metal and leather were used most commonly in construction of the early splints. With the development of thermoplastic and other materials, orthotic construction can be of greater variety and more acceptable to the patient.

Indications for a specific orthosis should be clearly defined [2], as otherwise the patient may become merely an appendage to his splint [3]. Grasp efficiency, precision and sensation are diminished with interposition of any material between the hand's surface and the object [4].

Classes of orthoses

(1) *Static* i.e. rigid or immobilizing; no moving parts,
(2) *Dynamic* i.e. lively [5] or mobilizing; moving parts; power provided by the patient or external force.

Major indications for an orthosis

Immobilization: to relieve pain, to prevent contractures, to stabilize a fracture, to discourage movement.

Mobilization: to prevent or stretch contractures, to encourage active movement, to provide passive movement.

Presurgical assessment: to simulate result of surgery, e.g. prior to joint arthrodesis or tendon transfer.

Provision of continuous pressure to the hand: to avoid formation of hypertrophic scars, and prevent contracture.

Principal factors in consideration, preparation and use of an orthosis

(1) Co-operation of the patient, (2) assessment of the condition, (3) functional aspects of the device, (4) prescription form, (5) method of provision, (6) reassessment of the preceding factors when the orthosis is ready, (7) instructing the patient, and (8) regular reassessment.

Patient co-operation

This is all important [6]. The necessity for the orthosis must be explained clearly; showing a sample will make the explanation simpler. The patient must know how many appointments will be necessary during construction and be given details about the overall prognosis as well as length of time the device will need to be worn each day. The ability to work temporarily or permanently, wearing the orthosis, may be a major factor in its acceptability. Unless the patient is enthusiastic and co-operative during the preliminary discussions, it is better not to proceed. Heavy, bulky orthoses are more likely to be put into cupboards than used; sometimes an orthosis may be less efficient mechanically but more acceptable cosmetically. The test of the usefulness and good design of a splint is whether the patient wears it voluntarily [3].

Assessment of the condition

Diagnosis of a primary condition may cover a surprising variety of functional deficit. It is too easy to assume that two patients with a median nerve injury will have the same disability. Careful individual assessment is essential. The therapist must make a full chart of range and power of movement and stereognosis, and comment on the salient features of the condition [7]. Sometimes it is contraindicated to carry out full assessment as immediately after a tendon suture. Acceptance of a common terminology in assessment is important and that of the International Federation [8] is used throughout this chapter. The assessment provides a clear picture of the condition and facts, rather than a hazy impression, serve as a base line for comparison during further treatment. It also gives a basis for choice of the type of the orthosis.

Functional aspects of the device

The facts available from the assessment must be considered in conjunction with the anatomy (chap. 1) and physiology (chap. 6) of the hand in order to formulate the detailed prescription for the orthosis. Consideration must be given to the mechanical factors required [9]. The hand is not a flat plate in any of the functioning positions and if the patient is required to use the hand while wearing the orthosis it is useless to provide anything which is flat. Wrist dorsiflexion of 25–30° should be possible if grip and digital function is not to be interfered with, and to prevent contractures, the hand and the wrist must be carefully positioned (p. 2). Bunnell recognized incorrect ways of splinting the hand [10], and it seems incredible that splints which he said wrecked the hand are still being advocated [11]. Some orthoses with extended metacarpophalangeal and flexed interphalangeal joints may prove to be self-defeating and tend to induce rather than prevent contractures [12]. Occasionally compromises have to be made [13], but this should be only in extreme cases such as severe burns.

Prescription forms

For orthoses these are as variable as those dealing with

assessment of joint movement. The National Academy of Sciences in U.S.A. set up a group to clarify orthotic terminology [14]. The detail in the orthotic recommendation section is currently accepted in the United States of America [15] and should become universal. In order to avoid basic pitfalls, it is essential that the prescription form is complete in every detail including the mechanical aspects such as forces required. However, where there is a close contact between the clinician and the orthotist, a simpler prescription form may well be acceptable; the aim and function of the device as well as the details about the part of the limb involved could well be sufficient. Whichever method is preferred, it is essential that the clinician discharges his responsibility for provision of a prescription. Where possible, the advice of the whole rehabilitation team should be available so that expertise can be pooled.

Method of provision

The expertise of local orthotic or therapy workshop may well be the deciding factor. This is discussed below.

In the United Kingdom many conventional orthoses are included in the Standard List of Appliances [16]. These can be ordered and are supplied by approved local surgical appliance contractors. Misunderstandings can take place as requisitions pass from the clinician to a clerk. There is little check on the success of the provided devices [17], and often lengthy waiting periods between prescription and provision. Where there is close liaison between clinician and orthotist the end results may be highly satisfactory. Where this is not possible, arrangements should be made for a trained therapist to be responsible for checking the orthoses. Accurate reports on any changes required could be relayed to the manufacturer and difficulties overcome.

Many surgical appliance companies provide designs for prefabricated orthoses. These are advertised usually through catalogues and obtainable on request. There is a great variation in the detailed information both in the catalogues and in further literature about individual devices. Some give excellent detail on measuring, adjusting, assembly and fitting [18]. Others list only general aspects, e.g. splint for radial nerve injury, right or left hand and vague classification into small, medium and large. There is often little information provided about adaptation of the device to the individual. Far more use could be made of these types of orthoses were better instructions available. Malick reminds us that a splint which fits everyone fits no one [19]. Occasionally universal splints have to be used in emergency but not for maintaining position over a long period [13].

Some centres have devised kit forms of orthoses for local assembly [20, 21]. Variations on the form of the orthosis can be made using only some parts of the kit. Instructions on assembly are also available. Skilled operators can assemble these quickly, but those less skilled may find it is easier and quicker to start from scratch with other materials. With the introduction of thermoplastic materials perhaps the need for metal orthoses has been superceded.

If the necessary training and expertise are available, the most successful way of production is by locally made orthoses supplied by orthotists or therapists. There has been an increase in the number of organized training courses [22, 23] and a wider variety of orthoses is available. Costs and time involved can be reduced as patient and therapist are in the same place [24]. Discussions are easier between clinician and therapist, and alterations to the orthosis carried out quickly. Most of the specific orthoses described in detail later in the chapter can be made locally. It is not intended to give detailed information on making orthoses. However, some aspects of production have to be considered when prescribing the orthosis. The therapist, orthotist or other person making the orthosis have to consider factors which involve expertise in handling materials. The following items should be considered: (1) selection of material(s), (2) method of construction, and (3) special considerations.

Selection of the materials

This will depend on:

(1) *Availability*: an increased range of materials is being used, including plaster of Paris, epoxy resins, fibreglass, silicone, isoprene rubber, polythene, polypropylene and metals.

(2) *Local workshop facilities*, may be limited, e.g. although polypropylene can be moulded by hand it is easier to deal with it when vacuum moulded.

(3) *Expertise of the maker*. However experienced the therapist or orthotist, moulding can be quite difficult on an abnormal hand. Adequate training is necessary.

(4) *Direct or indirect moulding*. Manufacture will be easier where direct moulding is possible. Indirect moulding may be necessary if: (a) a high temperature material is used, (b) if the patient does not live locally and is unavailable for regular fittings, (c) there is a particularly painful or unstable condition.

(5) *Urgency of provision*. Immediate provision is often necessary and valuable and quickly moulded materials are essential. A more robust device can be provided later.

(6) *Appearance*. Lightweight materials easily kept clean are more acceptable to the patient. A strong material does not necessarily have to be heavy. Outriggers and complex strappings may be desirable from a mechanical viewpoint, but are unpopular with patients as they will not easily slip into sleeve or coat pocket.

(7) *Cost*. Some orthotic materials are expensive, but may need less staff time and thus ultimately be cheaper. The overall costs of an orthosis may be small compared with other medical care. If expensive surgery or inpatient care can be avoided, the saving may be enormous.

Method of construction

A well-made pattern is desirable to provide the basic shapes from which the orthosis can be made. There are many sources of information on pattern making [9, 19, 24, 25].

Particular points of construction will depend on the material and the adaptability. Each description of an orthosis later in this chapter includes some details of construction.

Special considerations

These include areas of potential pressure, areas where function may be adversely affected, safety factors, and the training of the patient. Important considerations for each orthosis are given later.

Reassessment of the produced orthosis

Prescription is no guarantee of satisfaction [17]. An orthosis which solves the original problem but introduces three others will not be acceptable. Proper reassessment of the provided device is essential and only then should the patient be allowed to wear the orthosis for any length of time.

Instructing the patient

Clear instructions on the fitting and use of the orthosis prevent many misunderstandings. A simple instruction sheet (Fig. 37.1) should be given to all patients. Many materials used in orthoses are highly inflammable and require instruction for safe use.

Continued reassessment

Few patients have static conditions and consideration must be given to how often they should be reassessed. No patient with an orthosis should be finally discharged. As the original prescription of an orthosis is the clinician's responsibility, so is the follow-up care.

DESCRIPTION OF SOME ORTHOSES FOR THE HAND

Each is described using sections for type, function of device, indications, material, construction and special considerations.

Static thumb orthosis (thumb post) (Fig. 37.2)

Type. Hand orthosis (HO).

Function. To position the thumb for prehension (Fig. 37.2a).

THE LONDON HOSPITAL
Occupational Therapy Department

INSTRUCTIONS FOR SPLINTS

WEARING   you must only wear your splint for:
(1)   minutes per hour in the day.
(2)   hours per day.
(3) during the night.
increasing to:
(1)   minutes per hour in the day.
(2)   hours per day.
(3) during the night.

CARE OF SPLINT

You must *not* alter the splint in any way.
Your appointment is on   at
It is important that you attend for your appointment so that we can report your progress to the Doctor.
If you have any problems, or pain please telephone: 01-247 5454 Ext. 110 and speak to:

FIG. 37.1. Patient instruction sheet.

Indications.

(1) Immobilize painful carpometacarpal joint.

(2) Immobilize carpometacarpel joint following arthrodesis or arthroplasty.

(3) Mobilize interphalangeal joint while immobilizing carpometacarpal joint.

(4) Presurgical assessment prior to arthrodesis of carpometacarpal joint.

Material. Plastic.

Construction. A circle of plastic round the proximal-phalanx controls movement while not interfering with touch between thumb pulp and other fingers.

Special considerations. The thumb web must not be stretched.

Static thumb orthosis (C bar)

Type. Hand orthosis (HO).

Function. To hold the thumb for prehension. To stretch the thumb web space (Fig. 37.2b).

Indications.

(1) To immobilize thumb web providing best functional position following trauma, median nerve injury and surgery for pollicization.

(2) To apply even pressure to thumb web space following contracture.

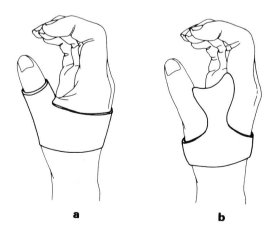

FIG. 37.2. Static thumb orthosis (a) thumb post, (b) C bar.

Material. Plastic.

Construction. A C-shaped bar is moulded into the thumb web space to achieve optimum functional position. Movement at the interphalangeal joint of the thumb is not interrupted.

Special considerations. Thumb web stretching may have to be introduced gradually.

Static distal interphalangeal orthosis (Oakley) [26] (Fig. 37.3a)

Type. Hand orthosis (HO).

Function. To hold the distal interphalangeal joint in extension.

Indications. Following trauma, e.g. mallet finger deformity.

Materials. Plastic or metal.

Construction. Formed to make total contact with the finger. Proximal interphalangeal movement is not interfered with.

Special considerations. The terminal joint should be maintained in extension until the orthosis is discarded. The orthosis should be removed only for washing.

Static proximal interphalangeal orthoses. (1) Ring, Fig. 37.3b, (2) Spiral, Fig. 37.3c

Type. Hand orthosis (HO).

Function. To hold the proximal interphalangeal joint in extension.

Indications.

(1) To immobilize painful proximal interphalangeal joint.

(2) To immobilize proximal interphalangeal joint in Boutonnière deformity [27].

(3) Pre-surgical assessment prior to arthrodesis of proximal interphalangeal joint.

Materials. Plastic or metal.

Construction. Made to have close skin contact but not to interfere with other joints' movement.

Special considerations. The edges of the material should be moulded away from the finger so as not to cause pressure areas.

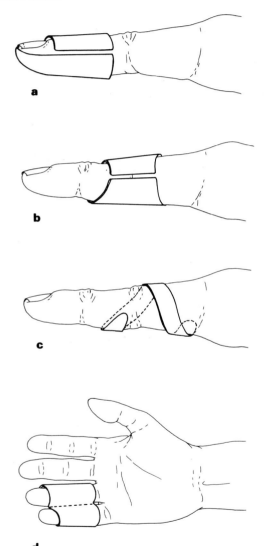

FIG. 37.3. Static distal interphalangeal orthoses (a) Oakley, (b) ring, (c) spiral, (d) dynamic proximal interphalangeal flexion assist orthosis (Siamese or Shotgun).

Dynamic proximal interphalangeal flexion-assisted orthosis (Siamese or shotgun) (Fig. 37.3d)

Type. Hand orthosis (HO).

Function. To assist flexion in proximal interphalangeal joint in one finger by the active function in the adjacent one.

Indications. To mobilize proximal interphalangeal joint flexion following trauma or flexor tendon grafts [3].

Material. Cotton or nylon webbing or fine leather.

Construction. The stitching separates the two fingers. Accurate measurements required from the active finger as well as the injured one. If necessary a small wrist band and linking band can be added to keep orthosis in position during heavy work.

Special considerations. Orthosis should not be used for long periods.

Dynamic proximal interphalangeal flexion-assist orthosis (Odstock) [28, 29] (Fig. 37.4a)

Type. Hand orthosis (HO).

Function. To assist flexion in proximal interphalangeal joint.

Indications.
    (1) To mobilize proximal interphalangeal joint following trauma or surgery.
    (2) To mobilize for specific exercise in proximal interphalangeal joints with extension resisted.

Materials. Spring wire, two plastic pads with lining, plastic tubing.

Construction. Power is provided by a figure of eight spring wire threaded through the pads and tubing. Amount of power depends on grade of wire used.

Special considerations. Wrongly graded wire may provide too little or too much power. The patient must be instructed on extending length of time orthosis is worn. Not usually fitted after fractures.

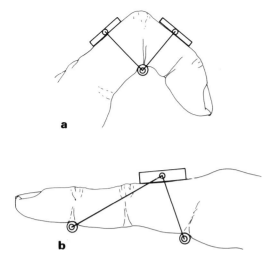

a

b

FIG. 37.4. (a) Dynamic proximal interphalangeal flexion assist orthosis (Odstock). (b) Dynamic proximal interphalangeal extension assist orthosis (Odstock).

Dynamic proximal interphalangeal extension-assist orthosis (Odstock) [28, 29] (Fig. 37.4b)

Type. Hand orthosis (HO).

Function. To assist extension in proximal interphalangeal joint.

Indications.
 (1) To mobilize proximal interphalangeal joint following trauma or surgery.
 (2) To mobilize for specific exercise in proximal interphalangeal joint with flexion resisted.
 (3) To mobilize in correct functional position following Boutonnière deformity.

Materials. Spring wire, one plastic pad with lining, plastic tubing.

Construction. Power is provided by a figure of eight spring wire threaded through the pad and the two tubes. Amount of power depends on the grade of wire used.

Special considerations. Wrongly graded wire may provide too little or too much power. The patient must be instructed on extending length of time orthosis is worn. Not usually used following fractures.

Dynamic flexion-assist metacarpophalangeal joint orthosis [30, 31] (Fig. 37.5a)

Type. Hand orthosis (HO).

Function. To assist flexion in ring and little fingers.

Indications. To mobilize following ulnar nerve injury providing assisted functional position.

Materials. Spring wire, plastic.

Construction. The power is provided by wire threaded through plastic pads and coiled over the axis of the metacarpophalangeal joints. Amount of power depends on grade of wire used.

Special considerations. Care must be taken not to allow the coil to brush the skin. Incorrect choice of wire grade will result in too much or too little power. The orthosis must be made in the corrected position.

Dynamic extension-assist metacarpophalangeal joint orthosis (Fig. 37.5b)

Type. Hand orthosis (HO).

Function. To assist extension in ring or little fingers.

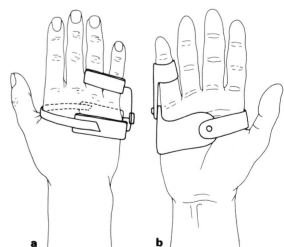

a **b**

FIG. 37.5. (a) Dynamic flexion assist metacarpophalangeal joint orthosis. (b) Dynamic extension assist metacarpophalangeal joint orthosis.

Indications. To mobilize following Dupuytren's contracture providing assisted extension.

Materials. Spring wire, plastic.

Construction. The power is provided by the spring wire threaded through to form a hinge on the plastic bars.

Special considerations. Care must be taken not to allow the hinge to brush the skin in motion. The orthosis must be assembled in the corrected position. Incorrect choice of wire grade will result in too much or too little power.

Dynamic flexion assist metacarpophalangeal joint orthosis (knuckle duster) [29] (Fig. 37.6a)

Type. Hand orthosis (HO).

Function. To assist flexion in the metacarpophalangeal joints.

Indications.
(1) To mobilize metacarpophalangeal joints following trauma or surgery.
(2) To mobilize metacarpophalangeal joints following intrinsic paralysis where the thumb is not involved.
(3) To mobilize for specific exercise in metacarpophalangeal joints with extension resisted.

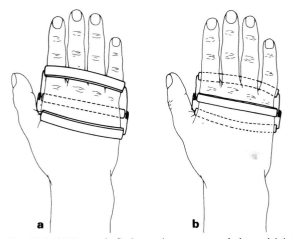

FIG. 37.6. (a) Dynamic flexion assist metacarpophalangeal joint orthosis (knuckle duster). (b) Dynamic extension assist metacarpophalangeal joint orthosis (reverse knuckle duster).

Materials. Spring wire, plastic, plastic strapping.

Construction. Power is provided by the figure of eight spring wire threaded through the dorsal and palmar pads. Amount of power depends on grade of wire used. Dorsal and palmar pads must be moulded to curves of the hand.

Special considerations. The spring wire must not brush the lateral borders of the hand in function. Periods of hand use without the orthosis must be programmed. There should be a gradual increase in the length of time the orthosis is used each waking hour.

Dynamic extension assist metacarpophalangeal joint orthosis (reverse knuckle duster) (Fig. 37.6b)

Type. Hand orthosis (HO).

Function. To assist extension in the metacarpophalangeal joints.

Indications
(1) To mobilize following trauma or surgery.
(2) To mobilize following contractures at the metacarpophalangeal joints.
(3) To mobilize for specific exercise in the metacarpophalangeal joints with flexion resisted.

Materials. Spring wire, plastic, plastic strapping.

Construction. Power is provided by the figure of eight spring wire threaded through the dorsal and palmar bars. Power assistance depends on grade of wire used. If the hand is to function without restriction dorsal and palmar bars must be moulded to allow for palmar curves.

Special considerations. The spring wire must not brush the lateral borders of the hand in function. Incorrect choice of wire grade will result in too much or too little power. Periods of hand use without the orthosis must be programmed. If for specific exercise there should be a gradual increase in the length of time the orthosis is used each waking hour.

Dynamic orthosis to resist ulnar drift [32] (Fig. 37.7a)

Type. Hand orthosis (HO).

Function. To assist adduction of the ring and little fingers in rheumatoid arthritis.

Indications.
(1) To mobilize the ring and little fingers with assisted adduction where ulnar phalangeal drift is present.
(2) To wear during exacerbation of rheumatoid arthritis in order to prevent increase of deformity.

Materials. Plastic, hinged rivet.

Construction. Plastic is moulded to the shape of the little and ring fingers. Assisted adduction is provided by the placing of the riveted hinge. Alignment of the hinge with the joint is important. Flexion and extension at the metacarpophalangeal joints should be free.

Special considerations. The correction of ulnar drift may need to be done gradually; there may be too much pressure built up if the position is corrected straight away. Tolerance of the patient for the orthosis should be programmed to be increased gradually. If worn during a rheumatoid arthritis 'flare up' the development of oedema may cause pressure.

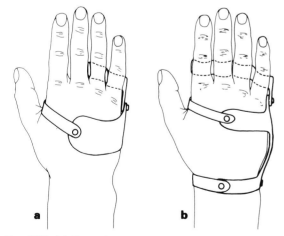

FIG. 37.7. (a) Dynamic adduction orthosis for ring and little fingers. (b) Dynamic orthosis to assist neutral position.

Dynamic orthosis to assist neutral position (Fig. 37.7b)

Type. Wrist hand orthosis (WHO).

Function. To control the wrist and metacarpophalangeal joints while allowing free flexion and extension.

Indications.
Used particularly in rheumatoid arthritis.
(1) To mobilize in an improved functional position in cases where the zig-zag deformity [33] is present.
(2) To mobilize during 'flare ups' of the rheumatoid arthritis to try to avoid increased deformity.

Materials. Plastic or metal, hinged rivets.

Construction. The alignment of the lateral hinges with the joint axes is important. The finger bar is carefully moulded to contour round each one. Flexion and extension should be free at the wrist and metacarpophalangeal joints.

Special considerations. The correction of deformity may have to be done by degrees. Orthotic tolerance will have to be carefully programmed.

Static interphalangeal and metacarpophalangeal joint orthosis [34] (Fig. 37.8a)

Type. Wrist hand orthosis (WHO).

Function and indications. To immobilize and assist extension of the interphalangeal and metacarpophalangeal joints following Dupuytren's contracture [25].

Materials. Plastic, metal wire.

Construction. Careful measurements of the wire finger support are taken. The ends of the metal wire are sandwiched between the plastic layers of the wrist band. The latter is moulded to the wrist.

Special consideration. The patient may be disconcerted by sighting the open palmar wound following surgery.

Dynamic finger wrist orthosis (Fig. 37.8b)

Type. Wrist hand orthosis (WHO).

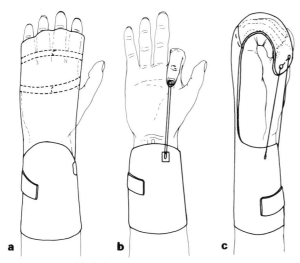

FIG. 37.8. (a) Static interphalangeal and metacarpophalangeal joint orthosis. (b) Dynamic finger wrist orthosis. (c) Dynamic finger flexion orthosis (finger flexion cuff).

Function. To assist flexion and resist extension in a finger.

Indications.
   (1) To mobilize a finger following surgery after, for example, flexor tendon repair [35].
   (2) To mobilize the finger with resisted extension.

Materials. Elastic band or plastic and fibre finger cover.

Construction. The plastic wrist band is moulded on the patient's wrist prior to operation. The traction may be fixed to the nail and the length of the elastic band adjusted in the operating theatre.

Special considerations. Construction in the operating theatre requires sterilization of component parts. The elastic band should not overstretch the finger. The length of wound will determine whether the fibre finger cover can be used. If used it is important not to overstretch the elastic band or the finger cover will apply excessive traction.

Dynamic finger flexion orthosis (finger flexion cuff) [36] (Fig. 37.8c)

Type. Wrist hand orthosis (WHO).

Function. To assist flexion of the fingers at the interphalangeal and metacarpophalangeal joints.

Materials. Plastic, sheepskin, elastic.

Construction. The sheepskin cuff must fit the hand snugly. The plastic wrist band is moulded onto the wrist. The elastic must be carefully measured so as not to overstretch the fingers.

Special considerations. Lateral movement of the fingers needs careful control or they will slip out of the cuff. Wearing of the orthosis must be carefully planned probably to alternate with some form of extension device.

Static proximal and distal interphalangeal flexion assist orthoses (Edinburgh) [21] (Fig. 37.9 a & b)

Type. Wrist hand orthoses (WHO).

Function. To assist flexion at interphalangeal joints by enabling specific flexion exercises, for example, following surgery or trauma. Movement at wrist and metacarpophalangeal joints prevented.

Materials. Plaster of Paris, retaining strap. Epoxy resin if necessary.

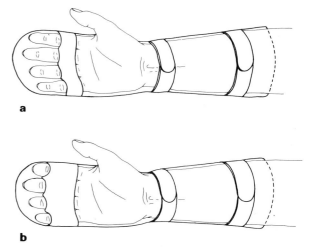

FIG. 37.9. (a) Static proximal interphalangeal joint flexion assist orthosis (Edinburgh). (b) Static distal interphalangeal joint flexion assist orthosis (Edinburgh).

Construction. A dorsal plaster of Paris slab is crossed by a carefully moulded palmar bar. The wrist strap keeps the hand accurately positioned. Epoxy resin coating can be applied to strengthen the plaster of Paris.

Special considerations. The palmar bar must carefully contour the appropriate crease so as not to interfere with joint flexion. Orthotic use must be graded so that patient exercises regularly each waking hour.

Static wrist hand orthosis [13] (Fig. 37.10a)

Type. Wrist hand orthosis (WHO).

Indication. To immobilize the wrist and hand in a 'safe' position following disease, trauma, surgery or burns [13, 37, 38].

Materials. Plastic, strapping.

Construction. The wrist is positioned in about 25° of extension, the metacarpophalangeal joints flexed as fully as possible and the interphalangeal joints fully extended. The thumb is held in abduction and extension. In a painful condition a thin padding layer may be required.

Special considerations. For painful rheumatoid arthritis its use must alternate with periods of activity [25]. Following burns good hygiene is essential; the orthosis must be cleaned at least two/three times daily.

Static wrist extension assist orthoses (Figs. 37.10b and 37.10c)

Type. Wrist hand orthosis (WHO).

Indications. To immobilize the wrist:
   (1) Following trauma, e.g. radial nerve injury.
   (2) For pain, for example in rheumatoid arthritis [30].
   (3) While awaiting surgery, for example carpal tunnel syndrome. If symptoms are relieved surgery can be avoided.
   (4) For presurgical assessment prior to arthrodesis of the wrist.

Materials. Plastic, strapping.

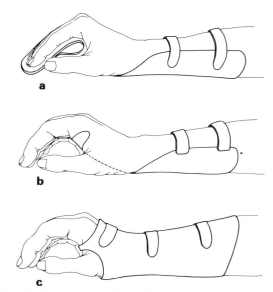

FIG. 37.10. (a) Static wrist hand orthosis. (b & c) Static wrist extension assist orthoses.

Construction. If to be worn during function the wrist should be moulded in 25–30° extension. If to be worn at night only then a neutral position at the wrist is desirable. If for carpal tunnel compression the wrist may be placed in 10–15° flexion to avoid pressure on the flexor retinaculum. The contouring should not interfere with metacarpophalangeal joint flexion and extension.

Special considerations. Wearing of the orthosis should be alternated by periods of exercise. If to be used during function and at night two devices should be provided.

Static wrist thumb extension assist orthosis (as in Fig. 37.10c, but including proximal phalanx of thumb)

Type. Wrist hand orthosis (WHO).

Indication. To immobilize the wrist and thumb during pain [36] and to encourage function.

Material. Plastic, strapping.

Construction. Moulded in 20–30° wrist extension with thumb in opposition and its interphalangeal joint crease left free. The distal palmar crease should be left free so that finger flexion is not interfered with. Spherical grasp should be maintained when moulding the palmar section.

Dynamic wrist extension assist orthosis [39] (Fig. 37.11a)

Type. Wrist hand orthosis (WHO).

Indication. To mobilize following trauma, peripheral nerve injury [40].

Material. Plastic, spring wire, strapping.

Construction. The wrist is held in extension of approximately 25°. The palmar pad should be small and curved

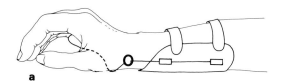

a

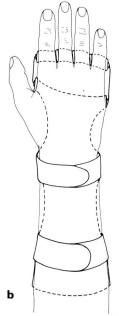

b

FIG. 37.11. (a) Dynamic wrist extension assist orthosis. (b) Static wrist dynamic metacarpophalangeal joint extension assist orthosis.

to allow spherical grasp and not interfere with the distal palmar crease. Power is provided by coiled spring wire of appropriate gauge.

Special considerations. Periods of exercise without the orthosis should alternate with wearing the device.

Static wrist dynamic metacarpophalangeal joint extension assist orthosis [7] (Fig. 37.11b)

Type. Wrist hand orthosis (WHO).

Indications.
   (1) To mobilize the metacarpophalangeal joints following arthroplasty [41], providing specific resisted exercises for short periods, or controlling ulnar drift.
   (2) To immobilize the wrist following surgical repair of extensor tendons allowing mobilization of the metacarpophalangeal joints.

Materials. Plastic, spring wire, strapping.

Construction. The wrist is held in extension of approximately 25°. The palmar bar is curved to allow the fingers to function. Power is provided by the spring wire coil over the axis of the metacarpophalangeal joints. Lateral finger movement can be controlled by individual finger stops. Thumb movement must be free.

Special considerations. Incorrect gauge wire will result in too little or too much resistance. Spring wire coils shold be aligned with joint axis. They should not brush the lateral borders of the skin.
   Ulnar drift at metacarpophalangeal joints can be corrected as required by finger stops and angling of the lateral coils. For specific resisted exercise this orthosis may be alternated with flexion cuff [36].

Dynamic wrist driven flexor hinge orthosis [43] (Fig. 37.12a)

Type. Wrist hand orthosis (WHO).

Indications.
   (1) To mobilize the metacarpophalangeal joints using active wrist power.
   (2) Presurgical assessment prior to tenodesis.

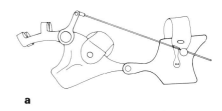

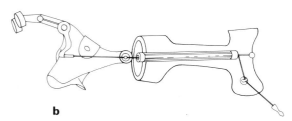

Fig. 37.12. (a) Dynamic wrist driven flexor hinge and orthosis. (b) Dynamic power assisted flexor hinge orthosis.

Materials. Plastic, metal, strapping.

Construction. The axis of the hinges must be aligned with wrist and metacarpophalangeal joints. 20–30° wrist extension is required to facilitate function. The thumb and fingers should be able to flex and extend to obtain skin touch. Manufacture may be easier from a plaster cast with final fitting only taking place on the patient. Prefabricated parts may be used [20, 21].

Special considerations. Non-alignment of hinges will hinder movement. Active wrist extension is needed to power the grip movement.

Dynamic power assisted flexor hinge orthosis [31, 42–45] (Fig. 37.12b)

Type. Wrist hand orthosis (WHO).

Indications. To mobilize the hand and wrist (following trauma) for example, brachial plexus lesion.

Materials. Plastic, metal, strapping.
Power provided by one of the following:
(1) electric motor and battery pack,
(2) artificial muscle with gas cylinder,
(3) cable operated by abduction of opposite scapula.

Construction. The axis of the hinges must be aligned with the patient's metacarpophalangeal joints. The thumb and fingers should be able to flex and extend to obtain pinch. Prefabricated parts may be used not only for the power source but also for the hand components [20, 21]. Selection and siting of power source will depend on availability and suitability for the patient concerned.

Special considerations. Careful patient selection. To avoid early rejection in the early stages usage should be limited to short periods for specific purposes such as feeding. Training of patient in orthotic usage. Local maintenance is essential. Siting of any control switch mechanisms will depend on patient. Orthotist must ensure excellent fitting.

Burns pressure garment [46, 47]

Indications.
(1) To apply continuous pressure following burns.
(2) To prevent contracture formation.
(3) To reduce formation of hypertrophic scars.

Materials. 'Lycra' or 'Dacron spandex bobbinette', zip fasteners and strapping.

Construction. Careful measurements of area concerned can either be:
(1) made into a pattern and the orthosis constructed locally from 'Lycra',
(2) sent off to the manufacturer for fabrication.

Special considerations. Accurate measurement prior to fabrication is essential. Garment must be worn continuously for 6–12 months. Therefore two or three garments necessary at one time to allow washing. Garments should be applied as soon as skin healing takes place.

REFERENCES

[1] British Orthopaedic Association. *Report of Committee on Prosthetic and Orthotic Services in England, Wales and Northern Ireland*, 1974.
[2] Rose, G. K. Definition of Orthosis—Classification and some Mechanical Considerations. A paper presented at BOA Instructional Course, 1974.

[3] WYNN PARRY, C. B. *Rehabilitation of the Hand*, 3rd ed., Chaps. 2, 3, 39 and 90. London, Butterworth, 1973.

[4] PERRY, J. Prescription principles. In *Atlas of Orthotics*. St. Louis, Mosby, 1975.

[5] CAPENER, N. C. Splints and other appliances for the hand. In *Operative Surgery Service Volume*, Part X, pp. 35–48, 1964.

[6] ELLIS, M. A Survey of Splintage of the Hand. A paper presented at ISPO Meeting, Cambridge, 1974.

[7] ELLIS, M. Hand Splinting. A paper presented at British Society for Surgery of the Hand, Instructional Course, London, 1975.

[8] INTERNATIONAL FEDERATION OF SOCIETIES FOR SURGERY OF THE HAND. In *Terminology for Hand Surgery*, ed. H. G. Stack. Edinburgh, Livingstone, 1971.

[9] BARR, N. *The Hand—principles and techniques of simple splint making in rehabilitation*, pp. 71–83. London, Butterworth, 1975.

[10] BUNNELL, S. *Hand Surgery—Conclusions on care of injured hands*, 25. Publication Office of the Surgeon General Medical Department US Army Surgery in World War II, 1955.

[11] MUCKART, R. D. Finger splints. In *The Advance in Orthotics*, ed. G. Murdoch. London, Edward Arnold, 1976.

[12] ENGEN, T. J. Upper extremity orthotics for hand and forearm. In *The Advance in Orthotics*, ed. G. Murdoch. London, Edward Arnold, 1976.

[13] VON PRINCE, K. M. P. AND YEAKEL, M. H. *The Splinting of Burn Patients*, Chaps. 3, 40, 54 and 97. Springfield, Ill., Charles C. Thomas, 1974.

[14] HARRIS, E. E. A new orthotics terminology. *Orthotics and Prosthetics*, 1973, **27**, 6.

[15] McCOLLOUGH, N. C. AND SARRAFIN, S. K. Biochemical analysis system. In *Atlas of Orthotics*. St. Louis, Mosby, 1975.

[16] *Department of Health and Social Security Surgical Appliances Contract Handbook*, 1979.

[17] JAY, P. AND DUNNE, M. A patient's viewpoint—An Action for the Crippled Child Monograph, 1976.

[18] STEEPER, H. *The Roehampton Flail Arm Splint*. Steeper Ltd.

[19] MALICK, M. H. *Manual on Static Hand Splinting*. Hamarville Rehabilitation Centre, 1970.

[20] NICKEL, V. L., PERRY, J. AND SNELSON, R. *Handbook of Hand Splints*. Rancho Los Amigos Hospital.

[21] SAVILL, D. L. Bracing in the surgical management of rheumatoid arthritis. In *Advance in Orthotics*, ed. G. Murdoch. London, Edward Arnold, 1976.

[22] BRITISH ASSOCIATION OF OCCUPATIONAL THERAPISTS. *Basic and Intermediate Orthotic Courses Outline*, 1976.

[23] UNIVERSITY OF STRATHCLYDE. Courses in Prosthetics and Orthotics 1979–80 at the National Centre for Training and Education in Prosthetics and Orthotics, 1979.

[24] MAYERSON, E. F. The occupational therapists role in splinting. In *Splinting Theory and Fabrication*. 1971.

[25] MALICK, M. H. *Manual on Dynamic Hand Splinting with Thermoplastic Materials*, 99. Harmarville Rehabilitation Centre, 1970.

[26] MIKIC, Z. AND HELAL, B. The treatment of the mallet finger by the Oakley splint. *The Hand*, 1974, **6**, 76.

[27] STACK, H. G. Buttonhole deformity. *The Hand*, 1971, **3**, 152.

[28] ELLIS, M., JONES, C. AND RUDDICK, R. The London Hospital version of the Odstock Splint—a film available from the London Hospital Photographic Department, 1973.

[29] GLANVILLE, H. J. A versatile lively splint. *Lancet*, 1962, **i**, 252.

[30] SOUTER, W. A. Splintage of the rheumatoid hand. *The Hand*, 1971, **3**, 146.

[31] ZRUBECKY, G. Orthosis for restoration of prehensile function in tetraplegics. *The Hand*, 1972, **4**, 72.

[32] MANNERFELT, L. AND FREDRIKSSON, K. *The Effect of Commercial Orthosis on Rheumatically Deformed Hands*. STU Report 47—1976. Styrelsen Fur Teknisk Utveckling, 1976.

[33] STACK, H. G. AND VAUGHAN JACKSON, O. J. The zig zag deformity in the rheumatoid hand. *The Hand*, 1971, **3**, 67.

[34] McCASH, C. R. The open palm technique in Dupuytren's contracture. *British Journal of Plastic Surgery*, 1964, **17**, 3.

[35] KLEINERT, H. E., KUTZ, J. E., ATASOY, E. AND STROMAY, A. Primary repair of flexor tendons. *Orthopaedic Clinics of North America*, 1973, **4**, 867.

[36] SWANSON, A. B. Silicone rubber implants for the replacement of arthritic or destroyed joints in the hand. *Surgical Clinics of North America*, 1968, **5**, 1113.

[37] LARSON, D. L. *et al. The Prevention and Correction of Burn Scar Contracture and Hypertrophy*. Shriners Burns Institute, 1973.

[38] WILLIS, B. Custom splinting of the burned patient. In *Symposium on Burns*. St. Louis, Mosby, 1973.

[39] WYNN PARRY, C. B. *et al.* New types of lively splints for peripheral nerve lesions affecting the hand. *The Hand*, 1970, **2**, 31.

[40] BARTON, N. J. Radial nerve lesions. *The Hand*, 1973, **5**, 200.

[41] NICOLLE, F. V. AND PRESSWELL, D. R. A valuable splint for the rheumatoid hand. *The Hand*, 1975, **7**, 67.

[42] KARCHAK, A. AND ALLEN, J. R. Investigation of externally powered orthotic devices. Final Project Report RD, 1461–M–67, 1968.

[43] PARRISH, J. G. Recent developments in functional bracing of the upper extremities. *Annals of Physical Medicine*, 1963, **7**, 87.

[44] GUILFORD, C. G. AND PERRY, J. Orthotic components. In *Atlas of Orthotics*. American Academy of Orthopaedic Surgeons, 1975.

[45] LAMB, D. W. AND LANDRY, R. The hand in quadriplegia. *The Hand*, 1971, **3**, 31.

[46] MALICK, M. H. Management of the severe burned patient. *Occupational Therapy Journal*, 1975, **38**, 76.

[47] WILLIS, B. *Burn Scar Therapy—a treatment method*, Form 129, 7311–15. Jobst Institute Inc., 1973.

CHAPTER 38

Prosthetic Replacement

D. C. SIMPSON and D. W. LAMB

For many years a common philosophy has been to interchange a cosmetic hand with a functional split hook [1]. From time to time, complex hands, attempting to provide both function and appearance, have been designed but have seldom withstood the test of time. In some of these hands attempts have been made to simulate normal movements of the hands in a most ingenious way but, in our opinion, it is a mistake to make the mechanism of the artificial hand too complicated [2, 3].

Other hands seem to have been made, not as a serious attempt to replace the hand itself, but rather as a demonstration of some kind of control system [4, 5]. The great popularity in the 1960s of the hands controlled by electromyographic signals has been very much a case in point [6, 7]. The apparent early success from fitting these hands seems to have been due to the pleasure of the amputee in the appearance and movement of the artificial hand rather than the operation of the device itself.

There seems very little reason why a hand prosthesis should not be as functional as the amputee requires, as well as being light and satisfactory in appearance (Fig. 38.1). This combination of function and cosmesis in one device is accepted in other branches of prosthetics and it is probable that the different view which has been taken on prosthetic replacement of the hand stems from the underlying difficulty of this task, which has forced compromise on the designer [8].

A basic problem is that the artificial hand in order to be functional, must be on continuous display, and because it cannot be hidden, cosmesis plays a very important element in patient acceptance. While the amputee would like to be normal and to have a 'flesh and blood' arm and hand, if this is not possible one would prefer to at least appear normal, or to attract the least attention [9]. Cosmesis in a limb, however, is not just the 'static cosmesis', i.e. the appearance of the prosthesis when at rest or in an illustration, but includes a much more important component, and one which is difficult to simulate, the appearance of the prosthesis when in motion—a feature which has been called the 'dynamic cosmesis'.

This appearance of compliance and movement pattern

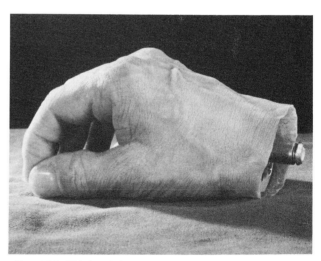

FIG. 38.1. This hand developed in the Bio-Engineering unit at Princess Margaret Rose Orthopaedic Hospital combines attractive cosmesis and useful function.

is difficult to simulate because this is itself not a simple quality—it is made up of both the pattern of movement, which should correspond to the normal pattern, and the spatial configuration or positions taken by the different parts of the hand or arm under the influence of outside forces such as gravity or internally occurring forces such as those arising from inertia. Usually in prosthetic design, very little attention is paid to these factors but it is often the absence of the correct pattern, or the presence of an incorrect pattern, which destroys any illusion based purely on the static cosmesis. In saying this, however, one must not underestimate the difficulty of trying to build any such passive movements or compliance into a prosthesis and it is often hoped that the active movements in a functional hand may be adequate to prevent the impression of lifelessness in the hand.

The alternative approach, common in Britain over many years, of providing an artificial hand covered by a glove which almost advertises its artificial nature, permits the perception of that artificiality very much more quickly with less disturbing initial consequence to the observer but surely this is not desirable for the user even if there is a superficial resemblance to the normal hand inside a glove.

The importance to the patient of cosmesis, in all its aspects, is still not sufficiently appreciated and although cosmetic gloves can be provided to cover non-functional artificial hands and some cosmetic replacements of partial hand loss are available, the artificial nature of the devices is not fully disguised. Although the argument can be, and has been, made that a well designed split hook is a functional and attractive device in its own right, our clinical experience has shown us that what the user wants is a good functional and cosmetically acceptable hand.

In a survey of over 7000 arm amputees, 48 per cent said they would prefer a functional hand in contrast to 7 per cent who preferred a hook, 30 per cent who preferred interchangeable devices and 15 per cent who did not know [10].

A final consideration is that the appearance of the hand will set the appearance of the whole arm. When the arm is covered by normal clothing, an artificial hand, which has good static, kinetic and dynamic cosmesis if it deceives the observer at all, will make him believe the rest of the arm is normal too; you cannot have a natural hand on an artificial arm.

In an attempt at functional replacement we have already stated that we think it is a mistake to attempt to simulate the normal manipulative hand function. While it is possible to incorporate joints which could conceivably allow this type of movement, the control of these joints would be difficult if not impossible and the type of construction requires a mechanism which is somewhat vulnerable to injury. Most designers of functional hands have therefore concentrated on providing a simple prehension pattern basing their approach on the finding that thumb to index and middle finger is the commonest form of grip [11]. No doubt they were also influenced by the fact that this hand shape is particularly adaptable for cosmetic glove cover. In practice however, this type of prehension gives an artificial hand which is not particularly effective in function. This is partly due to the fact that the hand obscures the user's view, and vision is so important when there is no sensation in the artificial hand. In addition, the positioning of the thumb makes it difficult to grip and pick up objects from a flat surface, a difficulty which is further compounded by the rigidity of the gripping surfaces of the average artificial hand with its resultant inefficiency in gripping potential [12].

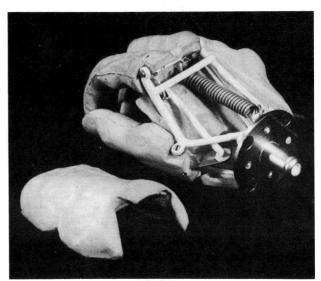

FIG. 38.2. Showing basic mechanical structure of the hand shown in Fig. 38.1. Linked movement at the base of the hand and metacarpophalangeal joints of the index and long fingers brings the thumb pulp into apposition to those of index and middle fingers.

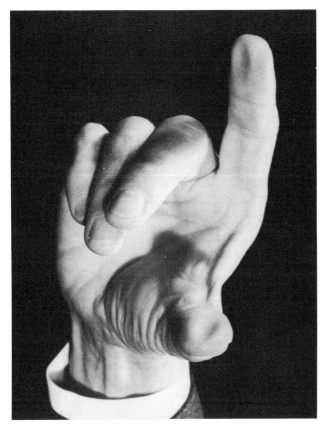

FIG. 38.3. Showing how the normal pulps are indented to facilitate gripping.

If an efficient prehension mechanism for an artificial hand is to be provided, it is necessary to give the user good visibility of the object which is to be picked up or held and to provide a shape and action that can be covered for good cosmesis.

These ideals can be achieved by using a lateral movement of the thumb against the side of the index or index and middle fingers (see Fig. 38.1) [13, 14]. This simulates the function so often seen in the hand which has been impaired by various paralytic conditions and other diseases such as rheumatoid arthritis. In the artificial hand, this provision of a 'key' pinch has several advantages; firstly, the user can see both the object and the thumb action readily; secondly, the thumb moves in a plane much more nearly aligned with the horizontal; thirdly, it provides a good engineering base for a

suitable grip and can allow a long object such as a pen, to be held satisfactorily. Fourthly, this can be achieved by a very simple mechanism.

The basic mechanical structure is illustrated (Fig. 38.2) and can accommodate for a fairly wide variety of objects. The ring and little fingers are flexible but do not actively conform to the shape of the object being held and do not obstruct the action of prehension. In order to provide a desirable degree of resilience in the gripping surfaces, the finger tips have been adapted to simulate the normal indentation of the human pulp to aid gripping and holding (Fig. 38.3). Small sacks of powder incorporated in the finger and thumb tips (Fig. 38.4) [12] allow the finger tip to be shaped by the object and when the grip is under pressure, frictional forces stiffen the flow of the powder. This type of gripping action is extremely firm and for the same forces applied between the digits will provide a more rigid grip than the normal.

Although good cosmetic appearance and functional

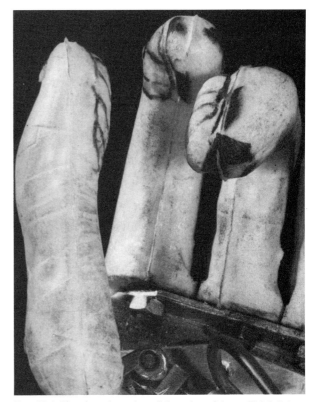

FIG. 38.4. Showing adaptation of the pulps of the artificial digits. The marked areas illustrate the site of the powder sacks.

efficiency for prehension are the properties of the hand which can be seen to be achievable, the one function presenting the greatest difficulty of achievement is the replacement of the tactile and proprioceptive information which normally stems from the hand. In its normal function, the feedback from the hand by its contact with the outside world is responsible for much of its efficiency and the term tactilegnosis accurately portrays the significance of this [15]. Even where motor function is good, the loss of sensation makes the hand so very much less efficient. The lack of sensory appreciation in an artificial hand reduces its efficiency very significantly and the user is entirely dependent upon visual interpretation of the objects which are being handled. The simulation in an artificial hand of a neural network which could give a real sense of touch and not just an indication of pressure must be considered in present day practical terms still to be beyond the bounds of feasibility and even if achieved, it is likely that it would be far in the future before any device could be produced economically for general use.

In this situation therefore, it is essential that the proprioceptive and sensory information arising from the hand itself is replaced by some other parallel source which can give knowledge of the way the hand is functioning. The only method which at present is practical and suitable for application is to employ the one which is to some extent used in the normal biological situation, that is to use vision. From the design point of view therefore, it is important that vision has a chance to operate and that the hand does not itself act in an obstructive way to prevent visual monitoring of the success or failure of the act of prehension.

The production of artificial hands on the principles described should meet many of the needs of the unilateral amputee, but because it will rely on both the material from which the glove is constructed and the movement of the hand to produce an illusion of reality and life, it is hoped that the research which is at present going on into the covering and materials for the hand prosthesis can be extended to help the individual with a partial or mutilated hand. The need for a very simple finger prosthesis to restore appearance in these cases has long been recognized but it is only recently that is has been possible to provide devices which can, in any measure meet this requirement, and in this respect the work of Pillet is outstanding [16]. Further development, particularly of materials, may make it more practical, from an economic point of view, to extent these benefits to a wide population.

The replacement of the hand by a cosmetic and functional hand prosthesis would therefore seem practical and not necessarily expensive provided that the ambition of the design is realistically restrained. It is important to remember that the function of such a hand will be largely limited to holding and carrying and that individual finger movements or manipulative ability would be beyond the bounds of practical feasibility.

REFERENCES

[1] KLOPSTEG, P. AND WILSON, P. D. *Human Limbs and their Substitutes*, New York, McGraw-Hill, 1954.

[2] GILLIS, L. *Amputations*. London, Heinemann Medical, 1954.

[3] COLLINS, D. W. Some new thoughts on hand prostheses. *The Hand*, 1971, **3**, 9.

[4] PEIZER, E. External power in prosthetics, orthotics and orthopaedic aids. *Prosthetics International*, 1971, **4**.

[5] TOMOVIC, R. *Modern Trends in Biomechanics*, Ed. D.C. Simpson, London, Butterworth, 1970.

[6] BATTYE, C. K., NIGHTINGALE, A AND WHILLIS, J. The use of myo-electric currents in the operation of prostheses. *Journal Bone and Joint Surgery*, 1955, **37B**, 506.

[7] MCKENZIE, D. S. The Russian myo-electric arm. *Journal Bone and Joint Surgery*, 1965, **47B**, 418.

[8] FLETCHER, M. J. AND LEONARD, F. Principles of artificial hand design. *Artificial Limbs*, 1955, **2**, 78.

[9] DEMBO, T. AND TANE-BASKIN, E. The noticeability of the cosmetic glove. *Artificial Limbs*, 1955, **2**, 47.

[10] MURDOCH, G. AND SIMPSON, D. C. (Personal communication: unpublished statistics.)

[11] KELLER, A., TAYLOR, C. AND ZAHN, V. Studies to determine functional requirements for hand and arm prostheses. Department of Engineering. U.C.L.A. July 1947. University College of Los Angeles.

[12] SIMPSON, D. C. Gripping surfaces for artificial hands. *The Hand*, 1971, **3**, 12.

[13] KENWORTHY, G. An artificial hand incorporating function and cosmesis. *Biomedical Engineering*, 1974, **9**, 559.

[14] DAVIES, W. A cosmetic functional hand incorporating a silicone rubber cosmetic glove. *Prosthetics and Orthotics International*, 1977, **1**, 89.

[15] MOBERG, E. Objective methods for determining the functional value of sensibility in the hand. *Journal of Bone and Joint Surgery*, 1958, **40B**, 454.

[16] PILLET, J. (Personal communication.)

CHAPTER 39

Medicolegal Assessment

A. H. C. RATLIFF

There are three essential ways of assessment of the results of an injury to the hand.

The surgeon, perhaps naturally, is interested in the anatomical objective result. He desires to know whether his skill has met the challenge and, for example, how far a digit can flex after a tendon graft operation. The result is often classified as good, fair or poor. If the latter, he desires to know why and is usually self critical of his own technique and how it can be improved.

The patient is essentially interested in function and whether he can return to his pre-accident employment, and when.

The judge is interested in a fair assessment of a financial claim for possible damages.

Usually these assessments correlate but the surgeon, the patient and the lawyer examine the problem from a different point of view. For example, the surgeon is seldom interested in the detailed cause of the accident but simply the immediate diagnosis and management of the problem. The law must know exactly how the accident occurred and whether it was the fault of the plaintiff or the insured. Anatomical and functional results have been discussed elsewhere in this book and will not be mentioned in detail. The whole subject of *Medical Evidence in Personal Injury Cases* has been discussed by Dix and Todd [1], but little mention is made of hand injuries.

The aim of this chapter is to discuss the practical preparation of medical reports and to present some comments on how these are assessed by lawyers. It will conclude with various examples which illustrate the damages which have been obtained after certain injuries.

The contents of medical reports

It is principally upon the medical report that the judge will decide how much the case is worth in damages. The surgeon's duty is to produce a practical description of the injury and its consequences. The doctor can measure the impairment of function that results from injury, but the effect of this impairment (i.e. the disability) is purely an administrative and judicial decision. Questions must be directed solely to the elucidation of the *medical* facts of the case. Among the various aspects which are taken into consideration are:

(1) pain and suffering,

(2) permanent residual physical and/or mental disability,

(3) future working ability. This has become of enormous significance in recent years; for example, if a young man will be unable to carry out his pre-accident job by reason of his injuries and so has to take a lower paid job, he may be entitled to a considerable sum under this heading,

(4) disability which may develop in the future, and

(5) diminution of life expectancy; this is seldom, if ever, of importance in hand injuries.

Except under the heading of opinion and prognosis where expert opinion is presented based on probabilities, the remainder of the report should be strictly factual and must not be weighted either for the plaintiff or for the defendant. Even if the report is given for the plaintiff and he is apparently exaggerating the significance of the claim, nevertheless the legal profession always require the exact facts. It should always be remembered that a number of sources of opinion are always available and sooner or later these facts will be revealed, if not by the writer of the report, then by the surgeon preparing such a report for the opposing side.

Damages will seldom, if ever, be settled if a final prognosis cannot be given and in the majority of cases this is relatively easy in the assessment of hand injuries. If the patient has not returned to work or further treatment is necessary, then an intermediate report has to be prepared.

The details necessary in a medical report on hand injuries

Every surgeon appears to have his own particular style of writing a report. Nevertheless it is perhaps fair to note that the legal profession, especially barristers, often have to assimilate the contents very rapidly and therefore clear headings are necessary.

Important contents of any report include:

(1) The age and sex of the patient.

(2) Date of accident.

(3) Date of report.

(4) Pre-accident occupation.

(5) Present occupation.

(6) Side of dominant hand. It should be pointed out that in some highly skilled manual workers this may be of great importance and in others perhaps of less significance.

(7) The mechanism of injury. This is obviously of great importance. An accident may be the plaintiff's own fault or entirely due to negligence of others or perhaps due to a mixture of circumstances which are not easily clarified. Sometimes the plaintiff describes complicated circumstances in which the use of highly skilled machines is mentioned. He is usually naturally anxious that these conditions are accurately described by the surgeon. Fortunately the surgeon may be helped by a detailed statement of the claim sent with the request. This is entirely the province of the law and the surgeon must endeavour to produce a simple description which is correct and satisfies the plaintiff. It is not necessary or desirable to discuss or record circumstances which led up to the causation of the accident but only to record the *mechanism of the actual accident*. It may be introduced with the prefix of 'the patient states', so that this will not be a reason for later debate and possible failure to agree medical reports.

A patient will often be very willing to volunteer statements of the faulty methods of working of his employer, or the bad driving of a motorist, but these should find no place in the medical report; that is for others to investigate.

(8) The diagnosis (a factual list is presented).

(9) The history of treatment.

(a) An indication of pain and suffering which is attributable to the injury itself and consequential medical treatment. This is important and carefully considered by the lawyer. Long periods in hospital as an in-patient, especially with multiple plastic operations, require short and clear description. It is not necessary to enter into details of surgical operations; it will suffice if their purpose and result be indicated. Complicated medical terms should be avoided or if necessary, explained in simple practical words.

(b) The duration of time as an in-patient and the period off work are necessary and sometimes need explanation and comment, especially if unduly long.

(c) Has the plaintiff returned to his original job and if not, why not? Is there a change of ability or speed in operating a machine? This requires careful description. It may be due to circumstances out of his control, for example redundancy, or retirement, or it may be due directly to the disability resulting from the accident.

(10) Previous history of injury. Experience shows that a previous accident to the hand or upper limb has seldom occurred and this section is therefore usually not relevant.

(11) Present complaints.

These are listed as described by the patient.

(a) Effect on occupation.

(b) Other effects, e.g. ability to drive, eat, write, dress and do up buttons, and to perform housework, sewing and knitting. Impairment of day to day function is personal to each patient and his occupation. These disabilities are essentially, loss of pinch, power or hook grip.

(c) The cosmetic appearance. There appears to be a remarkable variability of complaints due to the cosmetic appearance dependant on such factors as the age, sex, temperament and degree of mutilation of the injured hand. In the most severe cases, especially in young women, a deformity may be constantly masked by the wearing of a glove.

(d) Recreations and effect on social life and employment. Common examples are ability to keep a garden, to play all types of sport, including darts and skittles, and to be a handyman in the home.

(12) Objective examination.

At the end of this comprehensive book it would be superfluous to discuss examination of the hand (Chapters 5 and 6). Features which must be included are those of deformity, scars with measurements, contractures, active and passive movements, sensation, tenderness and especially pinch and power grip. It will be recalled that pinch grip essentially requires the thumb, index and middle fingers, whereas power grip requires in addition the use of ring and little fingers.

(13) General function.

The above description does not complete the examination because it gives no indication of practical function as assessed by the observer and what Capener has stressed as 'the orchestration of the hand' [2]. The writer completes a report on hand injuries by the observation of simple tests performed in the consulting room. These include the picking up of paper clips or pins, writing, the observation of dressing and undressing including the tying of a tie and the fastening of buttons; power grip may be simply tested by the lifting of a heavy chair with the injured hand. These objective tests are useful for two reasons: (1) a description may be given in a practical way of what the patient can do, and (2) this examination usually provides an immediate indication of evidence of exaggeration of symptoms and signs. For example, a recent patient with only a mallet deformity of a little finger, deliberately avoided the use of this finger in the gripping of a heavy chair.

The opinion and prognosis

This is undoubtedly the most important section of a medical legal report and is therefore given a separate heading. It is in this part that the writer's professional knowledge and experience and perhaps his knowledge of human nature should show to the greatest advantage. It will be necessary in some instances to explain the course of events or the line of treatment which was adopted always remembering there may be various points of view concerning the value of any given treatment. The treatment should not be criticised adversely because the examiner himself does not favour it, providing that it is

a reasonable and approved method of treatment. Perhaps one of the most fascinating aspects of hand injuries is the different disability which can result from similar injuries to different patients. Every case must therefore be considered on its own merits. Some of this section will be fact and some will be expression of expert opinion. In giving opinions it should always be remembered that lawyers are initially concerned with probabilities and not possibilities, although the latter may have to be mentioned.

Facts which the legal profession need to know under this section are:

(1) The nature of the injury, an indication of its severity, and the contributory condition of the patient to the accident sustained.

(2) Is there a permanent disability and if so, its degree?

(3) Has the patient returned to his previous occupation or not? Will improvement occur or will he have to accept a different occupation for life? The examiner must, therefore, appreciate conditions of the work and for example whether delicate pinch grip is or is not essential. Conditions of work are especially important in connection with jobs which require to be performed at high speed and one in which the patient is one member of a skilled team.

(4) The effect of the injury on his recreation and social life.

(5) Is arthritis likely to develop and if so will further treatment be necessary?

(6) Is any further deterioration likely to occur and if so will treatment be necessary?

(7) Is the patient genuine or is there any evidence of exaggeration of symptoms (see later).

Analysis of these details will enable an assessment to be made of loss of earnings capacity.

Exaggeration of symptoms, malingering and hysteria

These subjects are highly controversial and debatable and will be briefly mentioned.

Exaggeration

This is a very common occurrence amongst witnesses. The patient has often sustained an injury which is not his fault and perhaps, not unnaturally, he is conscious of his disability and seeks maximal financial retribution. The apparent disability may then be exaggerated. This may be revealed in many ways, e.g. the presentation of a list of a multitude of symptoms some of which are quite trivial; another is to deliberately avoid using the injured digit as indicated in the previous section. It is best to be on one's guard when a patient is asked which is his dominant hand and he replies, 'I use both hands'. In these circumstances almost invariably the hand which is not dominant is injured. Fortunately it is the author's impression that exaggeration of symptoms after a hand injury is a relatively small problem compared with its occurrence after other injuries, such as those to the lumbar spine or multiple injuries with superimposed anxiety states.

Hysteria

Pulvertaft described hysteria as 'a functional disturbance in which symptoms are assumed for a personal advantage without the patient being fully conscious of this motive' [3]. In making this diagnosis it is essential to exclude organic disease and this may be difficult when hysteria is superimposed upon an organic disorder. In a limb the presenting feature is usually an anaesthetic area or alternatively paralysis which does not accord with anatomy. In a resistant case there should be no hesitation in seeking psychiatric advice.

Malingering

Pulvertaft stated, 'there are those who deliberately set out to deceive and the border line between true hysteria and malingering is sometimes difficult to determine. I have avoided the term when composing a medical report and have used phrases such as "I am unable to find a satisfactory explanation for this man's complaints". When a remark of this kind follows an examination which clearly has been thoroughly performed, the reader of the report or judge may safely be left to draw his own conclusions' [3]. It should be remembered that judges are always very unwilling to brand a plaintiff as a malingerer unless the accusation is ruled beyond all possible doubt.

It is unwise to state in the opinion and prognosis of the actual report that the patient is hysterical or malingering for these are strong words and the legal profession is then likely to be presented with failure to agree

medical reports and a probable direct confrontation in court. Malingerers are occasionally very clever and frauds may be difficult to detect but they are as a rule persons of poor intelligence and their efforts are crude. The medical witness may be 'morally' certain that a patient is malingering without being capable of proving it. He would be very foolish if he makes that diagnosis in court under these conditions. A diagnosis of malingering should only be offered in cases which can be supported by clear, unarguable evidence.

A covering letter

It will be appreciated that compulsory exchange of expert opinion of medical reports occurs before the trial of an action. A confidential letter presented with a medical report may be very useful since it informs the legal profession of more personal views and yet still allows the sharing of medical reports. Various phrases may be used to indicate exaggeration of symptoms, such as, 'it is likely that some of the patient's symptoms will become less once this claim is settled', or 'the patient is clearly conscious of the legal significance of this claim'. It appears that the legal profession welcome this type of short covering letter and it may be very helpful in the rapid settlement of a claim.

The legal assessment of a claim

From the judge's point of view, whose sole concern is to measure damages fairly, there are three important sections.

Special damages

These are items of loss which should be calculated exactly; for example, loss of earnings and expenses already incurred.

General damages

These are difficult to define but include:

(1) *Permanent disability*. This is probably the most important heading under general damages. In hand injuries it is essentially loss of one or more types of pinch, power, or hook grip and its consequences for permanent loss of function of the hand.

(2) The expected future loss of earnings and the effect on working capacity.

(3) The effect on recreation and social life.

It is stressed that only the law can decide these difficult aspects.

Pain and suffering

This includes both the past and the future, including mental suffering because the capacity for enjoyment of life may have been curtailed by physical handicaps [4]. A description of the degree of pain is helpful, including the nature and quantity of analgesics; the time in hospital and number of operations are other objective indications of suffering. Damages can be recovered for mental or nervous shock even where there is no physical impact providing the shock is not too remote and is really a result of the wrongdoing. It must be more than shock in the popular sense of fright.

The author is not qualified to delve deeper into the many legal problems which may develop after the final medical report has been presented. However, many readers may not know of the *Current Law Year Book* [5] which is published every year and gives an estimation of damages of all types of civil action where cases are held in front of a judge and where there is no debate concerning liability. A legal colleague has drawn my attention to the fact that this book is of special importance since the assessment is that of a judge and not that of a solicitor or barrister, who may be partial to his client. In each *Current Law Year Book* there is a small section concerned with almost every type of injury including hand injuries; three examples will be quoted briefly since they show how the law summarises a claim and what the final damages were. It is of some interest to note the facts included in the summary and the small amount of damages which some patients receive following hand injuries.

Case 1

FINLAYSON v BOWATER SCOTT CORPORATION
(June 26 1975: Kerr J.)
Male, aged 22 at date of accident, 23 at date of trial. Employed as backman (factory hand).
Right middle finger trapped in running machinery.

Half the terminal segment of the digit removed by surgery. Substantial effect on amenities, an amateur rugby league player with some capability and a keen darts player.
Agreed Special Damages: £151.18
General Damages: £800
(The award was reduced by twenty per cent for contributory negligence). (Ex rel: Brian Thompson, Solicitor)

Case 2

SOMAJI v S.K.F. (UK)
(May 5 1975: Judge Norman Richards)
Male, aged 41. Former machine operator. Right hand trapped in machine in accident in December 1972. Index, middle and ring fingers injured, former so severely that it had to be amputated five months later. Grip reduced by 50 per cent. Now worked as storeman. If he lost that job he might have difficulty finding another. Loss of future earnings assessed at £500, potential disability on labour market at £1000 and pain and suffering and loss of amenities at £2000.
Agreed Special Damages: £402
Total General Damages: £3500

Case 3

WAGER v GAUNSON
(June 10 1975: Kenneth Jones J. Leeds)
Female aged 15 at date of accident, now 17.
Dominant right hand trapped in electric appliance that stuck labels on to garments. Serious burning and crushing to ring finger. Attempts at repair failed and whole of finger amputated.
Further skin grafting required leaving unsightly scars on two donor areas (left forearm and inside right thigh).
Cosmetic disability caused embarrassment but there was little functional disability apart from a tendency for coins and other small objects to drop through hand. No loss of earnings capacity. Eight weeks away from work.
No Special Damages.
General Damages: £1500
(Ex rel: Peter Hunt. Barrister)

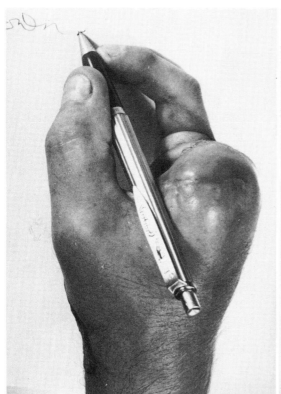
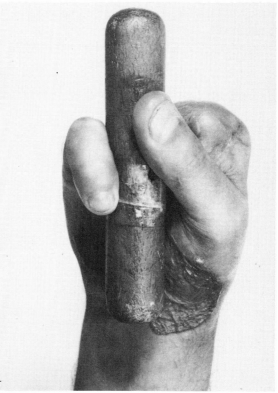
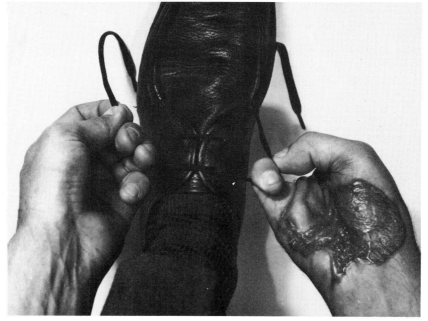

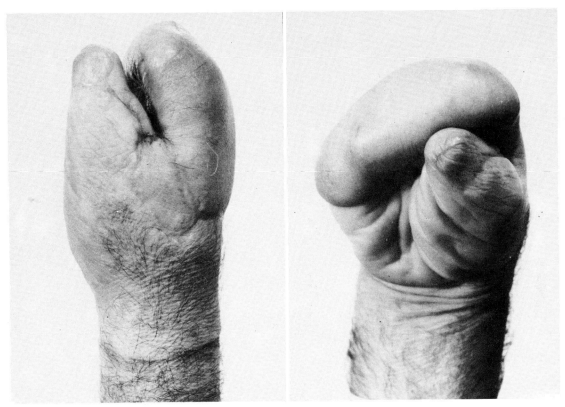

FIG. 39.2. Photograph of the hand of a man aged 55 who had sustained a severe crush injury with degloving of all digits. Several operations were required for a pedicle flap from the opposite shoulder. He was off work for 10 months. Before injury he was an Inspector of plastics and right-handed. He is now virtually 'one handed' working in the same factory but simply oiling machines. Fortunately there is no continuing loss of earnings.

Special Damages: Nil (Paid by Ministry benefits whilst away from work)

General Damages: £7500 (settled 1975).

Opposite

FIG. 39.1. The hand of an assistant mill manager aged 49. He had sustained a severe crush injury to the right hand in a machine with loss of the index, middle and ring fingers and multiple fractures. Dorsal skin from the fingers was used to partially cover the palm of the hand. Primary healing occurred. He was well motivated and he was off work for only 6 weeks.

Special Damages: Nil

General Damages: £3750 (settled 1976).

(If there had been no contributory negligence then the damages would have been about £6000)

It will be appreciated that, with inflation, damages are increasing at a considerable rate and therefore one example is given, taken from the *Current Law Year Book* of December 1978, including a relatively recent settlement:

Case 4
MUKTA PUJARA v JENSON BOOK CO.
(July 27 1978: Park J.)
Female, aged 45. Right-handed. Injured during course of her work on bookbinding and sewing machine. Sustained a compound fracture of the proximal phalanx of the right index finger involving lacerations and crushing of the tissue. Off work for 15 weeks.

Residual stiffness in joints, extending into arm and shoulder. Slightly restricted grip, flexion, etc. Not able to work at her previous speed. Award of £750 for her future risk in the open labour market.
Agreed Special Damages: £162.57.
General Damages: £2000.
(Ex. rel. Messrs. Robin Thompson & Partners, Solicitors)

Finally, it may be of interest to many surgeons to see the illustrations (Figs. 39.1 and 39.2) of two examples of injuries which have been reported on by the author and in which the final assessment of damages is known.

REFERENCES

[1] DIX, A. AND TODD, S. *Medical Evidence in Personal Injury Cases*, 1961.
[2] CAPENER, N. The hand in surgery. *Journal of Bone and Joint Surgery*, 1956, **38B**, 128.
[3] PULVERTAFT, G. Psychological aspects of hand injuries. *The Hand*; 1975, 7, 93.
[4] WINFIELD, F. *Jolowcz on Tort*. London, Sweet and Maxwell, 1975.
[5] CURRENT LAW YEAR BOOK. London, Sweet and Maxwell, 1975.

Index

Italics denote illustrations. T stands for table.